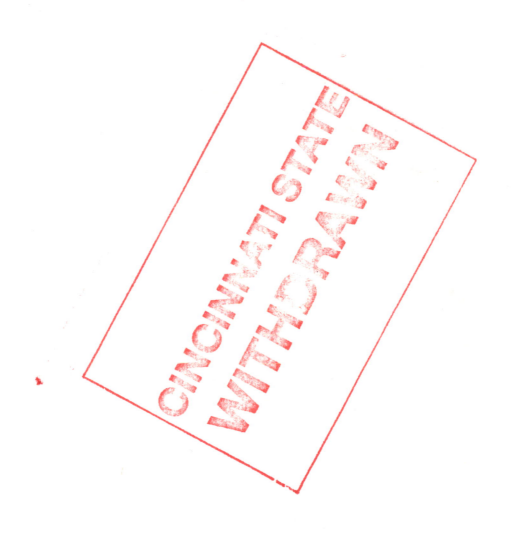

PHYSICAL ACTIVITY EPIDEMIOLOGY

Rod K. Dishman, PhD

The University of Georgia

Richard A. Washburn, PhD

The University of Kansas

Gregory W. Heath, DHSc, MPH

The University of Georgia

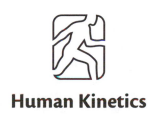

Human Kinetics

Library of Congress Cataloging-in-Publication Data

Dishman, Rod K.
    Physical activity epidemiology / Rod K. Dishman, Richard A. Washburn,
Gregory W. Heath.
        p. ; cm.
Includes bibliographical references and index.
    ISBN 0-88011-605-6 (hard cover)
    1. Exercise--Health aspects.   2. Health behavior.   3. Epidemiology.
    [DNLM: 1. Exercise.   2. Epidemiologic Methods.   3. Health Promotion.
QT 255 D612p 2004]   I. Washburn, Richard A., 1947-   II. Heath, Gregory.
III. Title.
    RA781.D5485 2004
    613.7'1--dc21

                                                            2003008212

ISBN: 0-88011-605-6

The Web addresses cited in this text were current as of June 2003, unless otherwise noted.

Acquisitions Editor: Michael S. Bahrke, PhD; **Developmental Editor:** Jennifer Clark; **Assistant Editors:** Amanda Gunn and Derek Campbell; **Copyeditor:** Karen Bojda; **Proofreader:** Erin Cler; **Indexer:** Robert Swanson; **Permission Manager:** Dalene Reeder; **Graphic Designer:** Fred Starbird; **Graphic Artist:** Denise Lowry; **Photo Manager:** Kareema McLendon; **Cover Designer:** Jack W. Davis; **Photographer (cover):** © Levine-Roberts; **Photographer (interior):** © Human Kinetics, unless otherwise noted; **Art Manager:** Kelly Hendren; **Illustrator:** Accurate Art, Inc.; **Printer:** Sheridan Books

Printed in the United States of America   10   9   8   7   6   5   4   3   2   1

Human Kinetics
Web site: www.HumanKinetics.com

United States: Human Kinetics, P.O. Box 5076, Champaign, IL 61825-5076
800-747-4457
e-mail: humank@hkusa.com

Canada: Human Kinetics, 475 Devonshire Road Unit 100, Windsor, ON N8Y 2L5
800-465-7301 (in Canada only)
e-mail: orders@hkcanada.com

Europe: Human Kinetics, 107 Bradford Road, Stanningley, Leeds LS28 6AT, United Kingdom
+44 (0) 113 255 5665
e-mail: hk@hkeurope.com

Australia: Human Kinetics, 57A Price Avenue, Lower Mitcham, South Australia 5062
08 8277 1555
e-mail: liahka@senet.com.au

New Zealand: Human Kinetics, P.O. Box 105-231, Auckland Central
09-523-3462
e-mail: hkp@ihug.co.nz

To serious students.
To Henry J. Montoye and Ralph S. Paffenbarger Jr., for lighting the fire
and stoking it. To Sharon and our scholar-athletes Jessica, Corinne,
Adrienne, and Philip. To my mother, Virginia, and the memory of my father,
Willard, a hardworking farmer who knew about quality of life
and far outlived his birth cohort.

Knowing is not enough; we must apply.
Willing is not enough; we must do.
—Johann Wolfgang von Goethe

Rod K. Dishman

To Henry J. Montoye and Ronald E. LaPorte, for fostering my interest in the study
of the association between physical activity and health. To my wife, Susan,
and our two children, who have put up with me for all these years.

Richard A. Washburn

To my mother, Lovell, and the memory of my father, Ernest, who as a physician
taught me that good science has hands and a heart. To John Holloszy
and Ken Powell, who did their best to equip me
as an applied physiologist and epidemiologist.

A student is not above his teacher,
but everyone who is fully trained will be like his teacher.
—Saint Luke 6:40

Gregory W. Heath

Contents

Part 1   Introduction to Physical Activity Epidemiology   1

Chapter 1   Origins of Physical Activity Epidemiology   3

Chapter 2   Concepts and Methods in Physical Activity Epidemiology   13

Chapter 3   Measurement and Surveillance of Physical Activity and Fitness   33

Preface

Physical activity has endured as an important part of hygiene in many cultures since antiquity. This book is about how the methods of epidemiology are being used to scientifically confirm that physical inactivity is a burden on public health and what can be done about it. Epidemiology is the study of the distribution of disease and other health events in a population. Behavioral epidemiology is the observation and study of behaviors that lead to disease or premature death and of the distribution of these behaviors. In this way, behavioral epidemiology goes beyond the traditional focus of epidemiology on infectious diseases, the containment of bacterial and viral contagion. Though traditional epidemiology is concerned with preventive measures, the emphasis is on environmental intervention (e.g., sewage disposal, water purification, or inoculation programs for viruses). In behavioral epidemiology, the focus shifts to understanding behaviors that increase or decrease the risk of people developing diseases (e.g., hand washing, medical screening for tumors, or sharing hypodermic needles by drug abusers). The importance of behavioral epidemiology is especially important for understanding and preventing chronic diseases, which develop over periods of years largely as a result of people's habits, such as physical inactivity.

Physical activity epidemiology is a specific branch of behavioral epidemiology. Thus, physical activity epidemiology is composed of two main features. The first is the study of relationships between physical activity, and conversely physical inactivity, and disease using the traditional methods of epidemiology. The second feature is the study of the distribution and putative determinants of physical activity in a population. Once it is established by convincing epidemiologic evidence that physical activity appears causally linked with disease, injury, or early death, the next goal of physical activity epidemiology is to determine how physical activity can be altered in order to reduce the frequency of disease, injury, or early death.

Physical activity epidemiology is a new field, about 30 years old, but it has evolved from old ideas dating to the use of structured exercise for health promotion in China around 2500 B.C., the ancient Indian Ayurveda system of medicine of the ninth century B.C., and the use of vigorous exercise (gymnastics) by ancient Greek physicians Herodicus, Hippocrates, Asclepiades, and Galen. Even during the Middle Ages in Europe, when the influence of Greek writings was obscured until the Renaissance, the Greek medical tradition of using exercise was preserved by the Arabs and later translated from Arabic into Latin medical manuals, the *Tacuinum Sanitatis*. The work, *Sirr al-asrar*, reportedly written by Aristotle, is believed to be the basis of the famous poem of medicine, *Regimen Sanitatis Salernitanum*, which was published at the medical school at Salerno, Italy, in the 12th century and mentioned the healthful benefits of physical activity. Rabbi Moses ben Maimum, the Jewish philosopher of the 12th century and physician to Saladin, the sultan of Egypt, advocated healthful exercise in the *Mishnah Torah*. During the Renaissance, scholars in Italy renewed interest in classical Greek gymnastics and recommended it as a fundamental part of education. The 14th-century Italian poet laureate, Francesco Petrarca, encouraged exercise as a natural remedy to replace medicines that "poison the body" in his 1354 work, *Invective Contra Medicum* (Protest Against the Doctor). In 1772 Benjamin Rush, Philadelphia physician and father of American psychiatry, delivered a "Sermon on Exercise" in which he recommended sports and exercises for people of all ages. His plan of a Federal University included exercise, laying the foundation for exercise and fitness in preventive medicine, which was perpetuated during the mid-to-late 19th century by early American physician educators at Harvard and Yale universities.

The modern history of physical activity epidemiology is short, however. Though many researchers have contributed, modern physical activity epidemiology has its roots in the studies by Dr. Jeremy Morris, professor emeritus of public health at the London School of Hygiene and Tropical Medicine of the University of London, who found in the early 1950s that the highly active conductors on London's double-decker buses were at lower risk of coronary heart disease than the drivers, who sat through their shifts at the steering wheel. That work was followed shortly in the 1960s and 1970s by the first of many studies by Dr. Ralph Paffenbarger, professor emeritus of medicine at Stanford University, who found that the risk of heart disease was inversely related to the amount of work done by San Francisco longshoremen and the amount of leisure-time physical activity among Harvard alumni. During that time, Henry Montoye began his pioneering development of measures of physical activity and fitness for use in epidemiologic studies. The impact of their work was especially noteworthy at the time because physical activity was not yet considered by epidemiologists to be an important influence on public health worthy of study.

Despite traditional epidemiologists' lack of acceptance that physical activity has a proven benefit to health, in 1980 the U.S. Public Health Service identified physical fitness and exercise as one of 15 areas of focus of the national objectives for improving people's health. Recognizing, however, that the scientific basis of physical activity as a national health objective was not yet solid, the Centers for Disease Control (CDC) created the Behavioral Epidemiology and Evaluation Branch (BEEB) within the Center for Health Promotion and Education of the Division of Health Education. Under the direction of Dr. Kenneth Powell, its main purpose was monitoring progress of the nation's 1990 goals for physical activity and fitness. To help with this purpose, the Behavioral Risk Factor Surveillance System (BRFSS) was begun to monitor activity in most of the United States, and the Workshop on Epidemiologic and Public Health Aspects of Physical Activity and Exercise was held in Atlanta on September 24 and 25, 1984, which culminated in the publication of summaries of current knowledge and directions for future research in physical activity epidemiology.

Another historical focal point in the modern history of physical activity epidemiology was the first International Conference on Exercise, Fitness, and Health organized by Professor Claude Bouchard under the auspices of the Canadian Association of Sport Sciences and the Ontario Ministry of Tourism and Recreation. Held in Toronto in the spring of 1988, the conference resulted in scientific consensus statements summarizing the world's knowledge about exercise, fitness, and health. The widespread impact of that conference and the resulting book, as well as a rapidly growing knowledge base, led to the Second International Consensus Symposium on Physical Activity, Fitness, and Health, held again in Toronto in May 1992, that updated the knowledge summarized in the first conference.

Key documents published in the United States include a position statement by the American Heart Association in 1992 recognizing physical inactivity as an independent risk factor for coronary heart disease and recommendations on physical activity and public health prepared jointly by the Centers for Disease Control and Prevention and the American College of Sports Medicine and published in the *Journal of the American Medical Association* in 1995. In the historical benchmark *Physical Activity and Health: A Report of the Surgeon General* published in 1996, nearly 100 experts, led by Steven Blair, then director of epidemiology and clinical applications at the Cooper Institute for Aerobics Research in Dallas, outlined the consensus in the scientific community about the beneficial effects of physical activity. That capstone publication signaled the maturation of the field of physical activity epidemiology by providing a scientific footing for the development of public health guidelines and policy about physical activity and by outlining a host of questions for future study.

The purpose of this book is to summarize that knowledge, the methods used to obtain it, its implications for public health, and the important questions that remain. A unique feature of the book is application of the cardinal principles used by epidemiologists to infer cause-and-effect relationships about physical activity and health risk. Other novel features of the book are chapters that specifically address the measurement and surveillance of physical activity and fitness in a population and the problem of motivating large numbers of youth and adults to become more physically active in their leisure time.

The social significance of exercise and other forms of physical activity in developed and developing nations has never been greater. In the United States, physical inactivity is a burden to the public's health, accounting for an estimated 200,000 deaths annually from coronary heart disease, type 2 diabetes mellitus, and colon cancer. The combined effect of physical inactivity and excess caloric intake accounts for an estimated 300,000 deaths each year and is a key contributor to the 50% increase in the prevalence of obesity, and a similar increase in the risk of type 2 diabetes, among U.S. adults and youth during the past decade. For the first time, obesity is a bigger world health problem than malnutrition. Growing evidence also supports that physical inactivity is a risk factor for poor mental health, especially depression, which the World Health Organization has projected will be second only to cardiovascular disease as the world's leading cause of death and disability by the year 2020.

The promotion of leisure-time physical activity has emerged as an important initiative for public health and quality of living in many economically developed nations. *Healthy People 2010,* the national health goals of the U.S. Department of Health and Human Services, includes several objectives that collectively call for increasing physical activity in all segments of the U.S. population. Similar policy statements about the health importance of physical activity have been issued during the decade in Australia, Canada, and Europe. It is especially noteworthy that the theme for World Health Day in 2002 was "Move for Health."

Nonetheless, leisure-time physical activity levels have remained below recommendations in nations that keep population statistics about physical activity. In the U.S., insufficient levels of leisure-time physical activity have not changed appreciably during the past decade. Despite widespread attempts to increase physical activity in the general population, 30% to 40% of U.S. adults aged 18 years or older do not participate in leisure-time physical activity. Only about 25% participate at a recommended level for health. Less than two thirds of American youth participate in vigorous physical activity three or more days a week. A recent study found that by ages 16 or 17 nearly a third of white American girls and more than half of African-American girls said they did not participate in any regular, leisure physical activity.

This book is dedicated to understanding how leisure-time physical activity can be effectively promoted to enhance people's quality of life. The book is intended to be used as the first textbook for upper-level undergraduates and master's degree students who are being introduced to physical activity epidemiology for the first time or as a companion text for broader-based courses in public health or health promotion and education that include physical activity among other health-related behaviors.

A textbook's worth is judged by how well it serves teaching. A good introductory textbook should raise a lot of questions but answer most of them. It should also instruct beginning students that knowledge is an ever-growing and changing thing. We think that key ingredients to effective teaching are common to an effective text: namely, up-to-date, logically sequenced content illustrated by clear examples. Keeping those ingredients in mind, we have strived to avoid merely presenting superficial summaries of trendy topics and reviews of research literatures rendered uninformative after being watered down to be easily read by a lay audience. We have selected classical and contemporary topics that we feel have a sufficiently large body of knowledge to justify inclusion in a textbook and that we felt capable of presenting with at least a modest degree of competence. Certainly, other topics have public health importance and would be of interest to many people. Examples include osteoarthritis, lung cancer, chronic obstructive lung disease, chronic fatigue, chronic pain, and quality of life and independent living among older adults. Each is an emerging area of study that we didn't feel ready to address in this edition of the book. Perhaps we'll have the good fortune to include those and other emerging topics in a subsequent edition of the book. Our undergirding purpose has been to provide a text that has fidelity with the science but translates that science in ways that will engage, inform, and challenge serious students. We hope to dispel the myth that researchers don't write textbooks and can't teach.

Acknowledgments

We will accept the blame when the book falls short of its goals. When it succeeds, we must share the credit with the many people who offered material for the book, ideas about what that material should be or how it would be best presented, and an environment that permitted the book to become a reality. Those people include the pioneers of physical activity epidemiology who served as mentors and exemplars; students who imparted to us questions and tactics for attacking them; colleagues who motivate us to constantly raise the standard of excellence; and our families, who nurture us and sustain our pursuit of that excellence.

We also gratefully acknowledge the helpful advice given by peer reviewers, including I-Min Lee and Donald L. Evans, and the people of Human Kinetics Publishers: Michael Bahrke, acquisitions editor; Jenn Clark, developmental editor; Dalene Reeder, permissions manager; as well as Karen Bojda, the copyeditor who superbly forced us to be clear and accurate.

Introduction

When meditating over a disease, I never think of finding a remedy for it, but instead, a means of preventing it.

—Louis Pasteur

I propose that the theme for World Health Day 2002 be "Move for Health." This will give particular visibility to ways in which individuals and communities can influence their own health and well being.

—Gro Harlem Brundtland, Director-General, World Health Organization

The essence of epidemiology is captured by the opening words of the French chemist Louis Pasteur. This book is about the role played by physical activity in public health, namely, preventing chronic diseases and premature death. It is about population medicine more than clinical medicine, which focuses on the care of individuals, usually people who are already sick. The main goals of clinical medicine are diagnosis and treatment of disease. Treatment can take the form of secondary prevention, which is reducing the odds that a disease will recur, or tertiary prevention, which is minimizing the negative impact of a disease on a person's quality of daily life. Epidemiology is more aligned with population medicine, which focuses on a community of individuals and includes those who are not sick. The main goals of population medicine are the control and primary prevention of disease within a large group of people. People who are at risk for developing a disease are identified, and measures are then taken to reduce those odds by identifying and altering factors that cause disease.

> ●●● *This book is about why physical inactivity is a burden on public health and what can be done about it.*

The role of physical activity in promoting the longevity and health of the public has become increasingly important for most developed, and many developing, nations around the world (McGinnis 1992), as evidenced by the theme of World Health Day 2002, "Move for Health," sponsored by the World Health Organization in São Paulo, Brazil, on April 7, 2002. In addition to the cost of human suffering resulting from poor health, figure 0.1 illustrates that the financial burden of

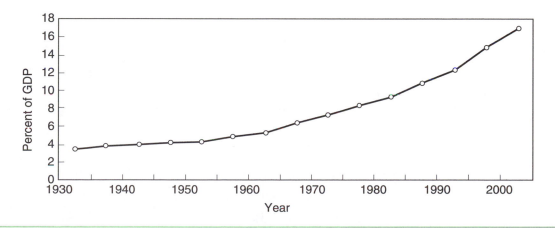

Figure 0.1 U.S. health costs expressed as a percent of gross domestic product (GDP).

poor health has increased steadily during the past 50 years, from about 4% of the gross domestic product in the 1940s to about 17% in 2003. This means that 17 cents of every dollar spent in the United States is spent on some aspect of health care. Containment of health care costs in the United States is a national priority. The burden of cardiovascular disease illustrates this clearly. Not only are cardiovascular diseases the most common (affecting about 38 million Americans each year) and the most deadly (accounting for nearly 925,000 deaths each year, or 43% of all deaths), they are the most expensive, costing nearly $300 billion each year.

Other diseases that are common, deadly, and costly in the United States and that can be helped by physical activity are listed in table 0.1. The statistics provided in this table illustrate the three main ways by which the health impact of diseases, and the health-promoting potential of physical activity, are traditionally judged in the field of epidemiology. In other words, coronary heart disease (CHD) is a prime concern for public health not only because of its frequency of occurrence (ranking near the top) but also because it ranks first in annual mortality and nearly first in economic cost among all diseases. In contrast, cancer and diabetes are about as costly as CHD, but they are less common or account for many fewer deaths. Osteoporosis and depression each has comparably high prevalence rates, but they are less costly and do not have directly attributable death rates as high as those of CHD and diabetes. Hence, the number of people affected, odds of death, and overall financial burden make a strong case that the highest priority for public health is determining whether and to what extent physical activity protects against coronary heart disease.

Certainly, other criteria can be used to render such judgments (such as lost function and lowered quality of life), but this example provides one way to reach decisions about allocating resources for research and policy regarding physical activity in public health. It also partly explains, as will become quickly apparent in subsequent chapters dealing with specific chronic diseases, why more is currently known about the association between physical activity and risk for coronary heart disease than for other chronic diseases. Heart disease has received more research attention. For these reasons, the evidence that physical activity and physical fitness reduce the risk of coronary heart disease mortality is presented in chapter 4 as the model of how behavioral epidemiologists study the association between physical activity and disease and make decisions about whether the scientific evidence permits cause-and-effect conclusions. We will see that indeed the association between physical activity and health is sufficiently strong to justify the inclusion of physical activity and fitness as key indicators of health promotion in the United States.

Disease is medically defined as reduced, abnormal, or lost structure or function of cells, organs, or systems of the body. The main adverse effects of disease include impairment of bodily functions, disfigurement, and death. Diseases usually have distinctive signs (i.e., objective measures), symptoms (i.e., what people feel and can report), causes, and courses of treatment, though the cause may not be known and the treatment may be only partly effective.

However, many chronic diseases, such as coronary heart disease or acquired immunodeficiency syndrome (AIDS), that lead to dysfunction of

TABLE 0.1 DISEASE STATISTICS, UNITED STATES, 2001			
Disease	Annual prevalence	Annual deaths	Cost (U.S. dollars)
Heart disease	12 million	700,000	100 billion
Cancer	3.5 million	550,000	170 billion
Diabetes	17 million (plus 6 million undiagnosed)	71,000	98 billion
Osteoporosis	10 million (plus 18 million with low bone mass)	60,000 (after hip fractures alone)	30 billion (from hip, vertebral, and wrist fractures)
Depression	10 million	29,000 (suicide)	45 billion
Overweight/obesity	70 million (25+ yr)	300,000	118 billion

Adapted from National Center for Health Statistics; CDC

organs or systems are progressions from cellular diseases that initially have no outward signs or symptoms. Hence, a person can appear healthy yet have diseased coronary vessels without heart dysfunction or be infected with the human immunodeficiency virus (HIV) that causes AIDS without impairment of the immune system sufficient to result in the overt signs and symptoms that characterize AIDS. In either case, the person has a disease but is not yet overtly ill or infirm.

> ••• *The main goals of population medicine are the control and primary prevention of disease within a large group of people.*

Conversely, health is not simply defined as the opposite of disease. In 1946, the World Health Organization defined **health** as a "state of complete physical, mental, and social well-being and not merely the absence of disease or infirmity" (World Health Organization 1946). Hence, health is relative rather than absolute in nature. Lost function results from illness, but it can also occur in the absence of disease. For example, lost strength and mobility can result from wasting of muscle and reduced joint flexibility after insufficient use regardless of whether someone is free from disease.

Much of this book is about aging, because the odds that a person will develop a chronic disease increase directly as a person ages. Though people of the same age can certainly differ in risk for disease, exposure—the primary risk factor for disease and death—naturally increases with age. Expressed cynically, the longer you live, the closer you are to dying.

Though longevity has been a longstanding benchmark in the field of epidemiology, the World Health Organization recently adopted the concept of healthy life expectancy as a better index of health around the world (figure 0.2). This concept is based on disability-adjusted life expectancy, which subtracts years according to the prevalence and severity of diseases that impair human functioning and quality of living (Murray and Lopez 1997a, 1997b; Mathers et al. 2001). This is not a new idea, though. Plutarch, the Greek essayist of the first century A.D., wrote in *Consolation to Apollonius,* "The measure of a man's life is the well spending of it, and not the length." Based on a recent study by the United Nations Global Program on Evidence for Health Policy, the United States ranked 24th, with a per

capita healthy life expectancy of 70 years, compared with the highest-ranked countries Japan, Australia, France, Sweden, Spain, and Italy, that had healthy life expectancies ranging from 74.5 years to around 73 years. The focus of the chapters that follow is on the evidence that physical activity can help reduce the risks of major chronic diseases that impact negatively on healthy life expectancy. Most of those diseases increase in prevalence as people age, so the importance of physical activity to public health will surely continue to increase as the population ages during the coming years. The World Health Organization and the United Nations have predicted that the portion of U.S. adults older than 60 years will nearly double from its current 16% to 27% by the year 2050.

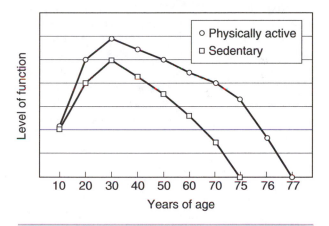

Figure 0.2   Healthy life expectancy.

> ••• *The World Health Organization has defined healthy life expectancy as disability-adjusted life expectancy; the United States ranks 24th worldwide, with a per capita healthy life expectancy of 70 years.*

Loss of function, which contributes to disability, increases with increasing age but usually geometrically; the loss is proportionally greatest in the later years rather than in the middle years of life. The ultimate goals of community medicine and epidemiology (figure 0.2) are to find and implement ways to lessen the slope of the decline of the aging curve, to square off the rapidly accelerating loss in the later years of life, and add a few healthy years as well. Put simply, the goals are to get sick later, lose function slower, live longer, and then die quickly when it's time. Thus, this book is about the quality of years lived, as well as the number of years lived. As the American philosopher Samuel Johnson was quoted in 1769, "It matters not how a man dies, but how he lives. The act of dying is not of importance, it lasts so short a time" (Boswell 1769).

This book presents the theory and the evidence that a habit of physical activity contributes in a meaningful way to both quantity and quality of life. It also teaches you how to think like an epidemiologist and critically evaluate cause and effect from research studies conducted in the field of epidemiology.

The book is organized into six parts: part I, "Introduction to Physical Activity Epidemiology"; part II, "Physical Activity and Disease Mortality"; part III, "Physical Activity and Risk Factors"; part IV, "Physical Activity and Chronic Diseases"; part V, "Physical Activity, Cancer, and Immunity"; and part VI, "Physical Activity and Special Concerns." The first chapter in part I, "Origins of Physical Activity Epidemiology," provides an abridged history of physical activity and health, which provides the background for appreciating the modern field of physical activity epidemiology. Chapter 2, "Concepts and Methods in Physical Activity Epidemiology," and chapter 3, "Measurement and Surveillance of Physical Activity and Fitness," introduce the traditions and techniques used by behavioral epidemiologists to study the distribution and causes of chronic diseases, including the measurement and surveillance of physical activity and physical fitness in segments of a population. Part II deals with all-cause and coronary heart disease mortality (chapter 4) and mortality from cerebrovascular disease and stroke (chapter 5). Chapters 6, 7, and 8 in part III address the impact of physical activity on reducing hypertension, hyperlipidemia, and obesity, respectively. Each of these conditions is a disease in its own right but also is a major risk factor for the development of cardiovascular diseases. Parts IV and V are composed of chapters that describe the effects and etiology of major chronic diseases and the evidence that physical activity offers protection against these diseases: chapter 9 (diabetes), chap-

ter 10 (osteoporosis), chapter 11 (cancers of the colon, breast, and prostate), and chapter 12 (the immune system). Part VI covers special concerns, including mental health (chapter 13), disabilities (chapter 14), hazards that people face when they are physically active (chapter 15), and the challenge of promoting an active lifestyle (chapter 16). A glossary of terms is also provided.

A special feature of all the chapters is discussion of the cardinal principles used by epidemiologists to judge the strength of evidence that physical activity or physical fitness reduces the risk of chronic disease in a direct, causal way that can be explained biologically. Finally, a unique feature of the book is the discussion in chapter 16 of the features of people, environments, and even physical activity itself that are associated with physical inactivity during leisure time. The chapter addresses the crucial problem of motivating the large numbers of people who are sedentary to begin and sustain a regular habit of physical activity in their leisure time. Though a good argument can be made that moderate physical activity is one of the most important behaviors for improving the health of people who live in developed nations, it is possibly the least commonly practiced of all health behaviors. In sum, this book is designed to show why physical inactivity is a burden on public health and what can be done about it.

Bibliography

Boswell, J. 1769. *Boswell's Life of Johnson*. London: Oxford University Press, 1946.

Mathers, C.D., R. Sadana, J.A. Salomon, C.J. Murray, and A.D. Lopez. 2001. Healthy life expectancy in 191 countries, 1999. *Lancet* 357: 1685–1691.

McGinnis, J.M. 1992. The public health burden of a sedentary lifestyle. *Medicine and Science in Sports and Exercise* 24 (6 Suppl.): S196–200.

Murray, C.J., and A.D. Lopez. 1997a. Alternative projections of mortality and disability by cause 1990–2020: Global Burden of Disease Study. *Lancet* 349: 1498–1504.

———. 1997b. Global mortality, disability, and the contribution of risk factors: Global Burden of Disease Study. *Lancet* 349: 1436–1442.

World Health Organization. 1946. Constitution of the World Health Organization. Geneva, Switzerland.

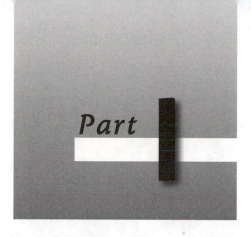

INTRODUCTION TO PHYSICAL ACTIVITY EPIDEMIOLOGY

This book is dedicated to understanding how leisure-time physical activity can enhance people's quantity and quality of life. The promotion of leisure-time physical activity has emerged as an important initiative to improve public health and quality of living in many economically developed nations. The U.S. Surgeon General's report on physical activity and health, published in 1996, provided the scientific consensus on the benefits of physical activity for chronic diseases and mental well-being, and the subsequent Surgeon General's report on mental health, published in 1999, acknowledged a role for physical activity as part of mental hygiene. *Healthy People 2010,* the national health goals of the U.S. Department of Health and Human Services, includes several objectives that collectively call for increasing physical activity in all segments of the U.S. population. Similar policy statements about the importance of physical activity to health were issued during the 1990s in Australia, Canada, and Europe. It was especially significant that World Health Day 2002, sponsored by the World Health Organization, was dedicated to physical activity and fitness. The chapters in this section provide historical and contemporary views of the field of physical activity epidemiology and how it is applied to determine whether physical activity is causally linked with health and longevity.

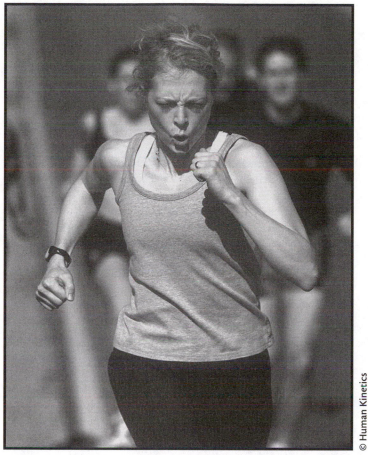

© Human Kinetics

Origins of Physical Activity Epidemiology

Health is the vital principle of bliss,
And exercise, of health.

—James Thomson, The Castle of Indolence, 1748

Physical activity epidemiology has emerged as a new field of study and intervention during the past 20 years as its scientific undergirding has grown. However, the ideas that underlie the field are not new but are based in antiquity, dating to the use of structured exercise for health promotion in China around 2500 B.C. (Lyons and Petrucelli 1978). The main purpose of this chapter is to recount key events in the ancient and modern history of physical activity and health so as to provide perspective on the present and future of physical activity

epidemiology through an understanding of its past.

Ancient History of Physical Activity and Health

Allen J. Ryan, MD, founding editor of the primary care journal *The Physician and Sportsmedicine* and a pioneer in the field of sports medicine at the University of Wisconsin during the 1960s and 1970s, wrote one of the first modern accounts of the history of physical activity and health. In it he concluded that "the concept of health is older than knowledge about the causes of disease" (Ryan 1984).

In his book *De Sanitate Tuenda* (On Hygiene), the second-century Greco Roman physician Claudius Galen, a.k.a. Galen (1951), extolled the virtues of exercise:

> *The uses of exercise, I think, are twofold, one for the evacuation of the excrements, the other for the production of good condition of the firm parts of the body. For since vigorous motion is exercise, it must needs be that only these three things result from it in the exercising body, hardness of the organs from mutual attrition, increase of the intrinsic warmth, and accelerated movement of respiration.*

Exercise As Medicine

The written history about the use of physical activity and exercise for the protection and rehabilitation of health can be traced back to the ancient Indian system of medicine of the ninth century B.C., the **Ayurveda** (Sanskrit for "the knowledge of living"), which recommended exercise and massage for the treatment of rheumatism (Guthrie 1945). Around 480 B.C., the Greek physician Herodicus specialized in therapeutic **gymnastics** (one of three classes of medical practice at that time). He based his therapies mainly on vigorous exercise. Though Hippocrates (460–377 B.C.), the "father of medicine," criticized Herodicus for his reliance on exercise, Hippocrates was influenced by him and later acknowledged the values of exercise, prescribing it for mental as well as physical illness. In his writings *Regimen in Health,* Hippocrates wrote:

> *Eating alone will not keep a man well; he must also take exercise. For food and exercise, while possessing opposite qualities, yet work together to produce health. . . . And it is necessary . . . to discern the power of various exercises, both natural exercises and artificial, to know which of them tends to increase flesh and which to lessen it; and not only this, but also to proportion exercise to bulk of food, to the constitution of the patient, to the age of the individual. . . . Exercise should be many and of all kinds, running on the double track increased*

> *gradually, . . . sharp walks after exercises, short walks in the sun after dinner, many walks in the early morning, quiet to begin with, increasing till they are violent and then gently finishing.*

Herophilus and Eristratus of Alexandria, Egypt, in the fourth century B.C. recommended moderate exercise, and Asclepiades of Bithynia, a Greek reformer of Hippocratic therapy in the first century B.C., recommended walking and running for his patients (Vallance 1995). Later, Aristotle, the Greek philosopher and tutor of Alexander the Great in the court of Macedonia, extended those views, stating, "The following are examples of the results of action: bodily health is the result of a fondness for gymnastics; a man falls into ill health as a result of not caring for exercise" (Aristotle 1908).

Even during the Middle Ages in Europe, when the influence of Greek writings was obscured until the Renaissance, the Greek medical tradition of using exercise was preserved by the Arabs and later translated from Arabic into Latin medical manuals, the *Tacuinum Sanitatis* (Arano 1976). The work, *Sirr al-asrar,* reportedly written by Aristotle, is believed to be the basis of the famous poem of medicine, *Regimen Sanitatis Salernitanum,* which was published at the medical school at Salerno, Italy in the 12th century and mentioned the healthful benefits of walking after a meal and the use of exercise as a purgative (Cummins 1976). Rabbi Moses ben Maimum (also known as Maimonides), the Jewish philosopher–physician of the 12th century who was chief rabbi in Cairo and physician to Saladin, the sultan of Egypt, wrote in the Mishnah Torah: "Anyone who lives a sedentary life and does not exercise . . . even if he eats good foods and takes care of himself according to proper medical principles—all his days will be painful ones and his strength shall wane . . . The most beneficial of all types of exercise is physical gymnastics to the point that the soul rejoices" (Maimonides 1990).

Exercise and Health Education

During the Renaissance, scholars in Italy renewed interest in classical Greek gymnastics and recommended it as a fundamental part of education. The 14th-century Italian poet laureate, Francesco Petrarca, encouraged exercise as a natural remedy to replace medicines that "poison the body" in his 1354 work, *Invective Contra Medicum* (Protest Against the Doctor) (Struever 1993).

In the mid-1400s Leon Battista Alberti recommended physical exercise beginning in early infancy for strengthening the muscles, stimulating the circulation, and adapting the nervous system. He also stated that exercise for those purposes became even more important with increasing age. Maffeus Vegius, in his 15th-century *Education of Children and Their Good Habits,* made a distinction between light recreational exercises from heavy exercise designed to strengthen the body and advised moderation in all physical activity.

Although the great educators of the 15th century recommended exercise as a lifelong habit, contemporary physicians did not embrace exercise. This was changed during the Renaissance by the Italian physician Hieronymus Mercurialis, who urged all people who led sedentary lives to exercise. His *Six Books on the Art of Gymnastics,* printed in 1569, laid the foundation for modern rehabilitative medicine by recommending that convalescents and weakened older people should do special exercises, based on specific diagnoses, that should not worsen their infirmities.

For the purpose of health, Mercurialis replaced passive exercises, which had been recommended by early Renaissance experts, with vigorous exercise involving heavy breathing and physical effort, including mountain climbing among three types of walking. He considered running, jumping, rope climbing, and wrestling to be healthy forms of exercise and suggested ball games to strengthen the upper body.

One of the first physicians since the classical Greeks to attempt an explanation of the benefits of exercise was the French-born Swiss pharmacologist Joseph Duchesne, who in 1648 wrote in *Ars Medica Hermetica,* "The essential purpose of gymnastics for the body is its deliverance from superfluous humors, the regulation of digestion, the strengthening of the heart and joints, the opening of the pores of the skin, and the stronger circulation of blood in the lungs by strenuous breathing."

In 1772 Benjamin Rush, Philadelphia physician and father of American psychiatry, delivered a "Sermon on Exercise," in which he recommended sports and exercises for young and old alike. His "Plan of a Federal University" included exercises to improve the body's strength and health (Runes 1947). Soon after, in 1802, the British physician William Heberden reported a case history of heart disease in which he concluded,

"I know one who set himself a task of sawing wood half an hour every day, and was nearly cured" (Heberden 1802). But it was not until the years between the U.S. Civil War and World War I that physicians became the main proponents of exercise to promote good health. Their influence was the basis for our present-day acceptance of the relationship between exercise and a more rewarding and healthier life and for our contemporary knowledge about the developing science of exercise as a form of preventive medicine.

After Edward Hitchcock Jr. (1828–1911) graduated from Harvard Medical School in 1853, he and his father published a description of the relationship between exercise and health for boys and girls, which argued that gymnastics was as important to schools and colleges as were academic libraries (Hitchcock and Hitchcock 1860). Hitchcock was appointed director of the Department of Physical Education and Hygiene at Amherst College in 1861 and kept the position for 50 years, lecturing on anatomy, physiology,

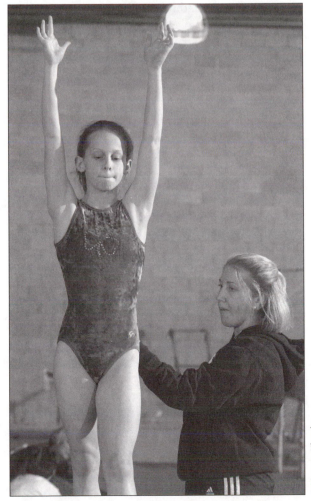

physical culture, and **hygiene.** In 1885 he was elected as the first president of the Association for the Advancement of Physical Education.

The role of physical fitness in preventive medicine was advocated further by Dudley Sargent, an 1878 graduate of Yale Medical School who was the first director of the Hemenway Gymnasium at Harvard in 1880. One of the first men he tested for fitness at Harvard was Theodore Roosevelt. Sargent also established a private gymnasium in Cambridge, Massachusetts, known as the Sanatory Gymnasium, where he directed an exercise program for the female Harvard students who studied in the Harvard Annex, which later became Radcliffe College. Sargent published *Health, Strength, and Power* in 1904 in which he argued for the importance of regular vigorous exercise for health and presented exercises for children and men of all ages designed to increase fitness.

R. Tait McKenzie (1867–1938), a Canadian who completed his undergraduate and medical degrees at McGill University, sustained Hitchcock's impetus. After graduation and a short medical practice, McKenzie returned to McGill as a lecturer in anatomy and became medical director of physical education. He moved to the University of Pennsylvania in 1904, where he was professor and director of physical education. McKenzie published *Exercise in Education and Medicine* in 1909, which discussed the physiology of exercise and systems used for physical conditioning. He also described physical education for people with disabilities. The second half of the book discussed the use of exercise to treat diseases, providing the foundation of modern physical medicine and rehabilitation.

The impetus provided by those early physician-educators continued in the United States and Europe during the first half of the 20th century and culminated in the founding of the American College of Sports Medicine in 1954. Though many contributors to the application of physiological methods and principles to the study of physical activity and fitness are noteworthy and have been chronicled elsewhere (e.g., Buskirk 1992; Costill 1994; Tipton 1998), much of their work focused on performance or secondary prevention of disease and rehabilitation. The pioneering efforts of Thomas K. Cureton are especially noteworthy as they relate to the role of fitness in the primary prevention of chronic diseases and the maintenance of physical function with aging. After his appointment as Director of the Physical

Fitness Research Laboratory at the University of Illinois in 1944, Dr. Cureton's seminal studies on the physiology of fitness laid the cornerstone for today's recognition that multiple components of fitness are each related to the public's health. He led by example, too, holding 14 World and National Masters Swimming Records, beginning at age 72 winning 5 gold medals at the first National Masters Swimming Championships in Chicago in 1973 (Berryman 1996). Moreover, the subsequent contributions of his many doctoral students, including Henry Montoye (recipient in 1949 of the first PhD awarded in Physical Education in the United States) and five presidents of the American College of Sports Medicine (Montoye, Charles Tipton, James Skinner, Michael L. Pollock, and William Haskell), to the study of physical activity, fitness, and health provided, and continue to provide, much of the experimental evidence that supports the modern epidemiological study of physical activity. The legacy of exercise physiologists to understanding of mechanisms whereby physical activity contributes to health has grown exponentially since the impetus provided by Dr. Cureton, extending to the molecular biology of exercise and disease (Booth et al. 2002).

Modern History of Physical Activity and Health

The modern history of physical activity epidemiology is short; its beginnings can be traced to the late 1940s and a growth spurt in the mid-1980s that has continued exponentially up to the present time (Paffenbarger, Blair, and Lee 2001). Though many researchers have contributed, modern physical activity epidemiology has its roots in the work of Dr. Jeremy Morris, professor emeritus of public health at the London School of Hygiene and Tropical Medicine of the University of London, and Dr. Ralph Paffenbarger, professor emeritus of medicine at Stanford University and adjunct professor emeritus at Harvard University. Their impact was heightened because they were respected epidemiologists at a time when physical activity was not considered by their peers to be an important influence on public health worthy of study.

Dr. Morris served for many years as professor of social medicine and director of the Medical Research Council's Social Medicine Unit at the London Hospital Medical College, where he authored *Uses of Epidemiology* (1957), the first text to apply classical epidemiology to emerging health problems of chronic, noncommunicable disease. Dr. Morris and his co-workers helped establish the epidemiologic method for the collection, analysis, and interpretation of data on the causes of chronic diseases.

Dr. Paffenbarger also made important scientific contributions to epidemiology prior to his studies of physical activity. Early in his career, Dr. Paffenbarger worked with Dr. David Bodian at Johns Hopkins University on the mechanisms of transmission and the pathogenesis of poliomyelitis, one of the most disabling and fatal childhood diseases of the first half of the 20th century. Dr. Paffenbarger also did some of the earliest research on postpartum depression and other mental illnesses more than 30 years ago. His work on potential causes of reproductive cancers included some of the first studies of leisure physical activity and cancer risk. Dr. Paffenbarger has also led by example. A distinguished masters athlete, he has run more than 150 races of marathon distance (42.2 km) or farther, including completion of the Western States 100-mile (161-km) run 5 times and the Boston Marathon more than 20 times.

Landmark Research

The association of physical activity and physical fitness with reduced risk of chronic diseases was not understood scientifically until Dr. Morris and his colleagues began to study **coronary heart disease (CHD)** in the late 1940s. In the early 1950s Morris formulated the hypothesis that "men in physically active jobs suffer less coronary—ischaemic—heart disease than comparable men in sedentary jobs, such disease as the active do develop is less severe and strikes at later ages" (Morris et al. 1953).

The hypothesis evolved when Morris observed what appeared to be a protective effect of occupational physical activity against CHD, observations that were viewed skeptically by the scientific community at the time.

The first study by Morris and colleagues (1953) found that the highly active conductors on London's double-decker buses were at lower risk of CHD than the drivers, who sat through their shifts at the steering wheel. If conductors developed the disease, it was less severe and occurred at later ages. The London bus study sparked the modern era of physical activity epidemiology. Morris later reported a similar observation, that postmen delivering the mail on foot had lower

rates of CHD than sedentary office clerks and telephone operators.

Several important studies of occupational and leisure-time physical activity and disease began around the world after the findings by Dr. Morris, including studies of Finnish lumberjacks (Karvonen 1962), U.S. railroad workers (Taylor et al. 1969), and CHD in men in the Seven Countries Study (Keys 1967). Studies of entire communities—such as the Framingham (Massachusetts) Heart Study, begun in 1948 (Dawber, Meadors, and Moore 1951; Kannel 1967), and the Tecumseh (Michigan) Community Health Study, begun in 1957 (Montoye 1975)—soon added measures of fitness and physical activity.

Framingham Heart Study

This ongoing community study began in 1948, when a random sample of 5,209 men and women aged 30 to 62 years who lived in Framingham, Massachusetts, located 20 miles west of Boston, agreed to participate in a long-term study funded by the National Heart Institute (now the National Heart, Lung, and Blood Institute) of the National Institutes of Health. The original participants underwent physical examinations every two years, including a resting electrocardiogram, chest X ray, and urine and blood tests. In 1971 the Offspring Study of 5,135 adult children of the original participants and their spouses began, and in 1995, 500 of Framingham's minority residents were added to begin the Omni Study. Thus, although 75% of the original participants have died, mainly from cardiovascular disease, these new recruits will ensure that the Framingham Study will continue to provide important information about health risks. Notably, data from the Framingham study linked physical activity with reduced risk of heart disease (Kannel 1967), soon after it had been discovered in 1960 and 1961 that cigarette smoking, cholesterol, and high blood pressure were risk factors for heart disease.

Tecumseh Community Health Study

In the 1940s Dr. Thomas Francis Jr., an epidemiologist at the University of Michigan, had the idea that a study of an entire community, including the biological, physical, and social environment, might reveal how some people maintain good health while others are more susceptible to disease (Francis 1961; cf. Montoye 1975). With funding from the state of Michigan and later from the National Institutes of Health, such a community study was started in 1957 in Tecumseh, Michigan, a mixed rural–urban community with a population of about 9,500 located 55 miles southwest of Detroit. There were three cycles of health examinations. From 1959 to 1960, over 8,600 people (88% of those eligible for the study) aged 20 years or older underwent physical examinations, including resting electrocardiograms, lung function tests, chest X rays, anthropometric tests, and blood and urine tests. A second cycle of testing from 1961 to 1965 reexamined most of the original participants and added 2,500 new residents. In addition to adding hand and cervical X rays to the examination, the physical activity of men aged 16 to 69 also was assessed by a questionnaire and interview, and a simple submaximal step test was used to estimate fitness from heart rate response and recovery after exercise. A treadmill exercise test was later added for some participants during a third testing cycle, conducted from 1967 to 1969. Montoye (1975) published a comprehensive summary of the relationships among physical activity, fitness, and health risk factors discovered in this study.

Longshoremen and College Alumni Studies

The most sustained and compelling studies of physical activity and health were conducted in the United States by Dr. Paffenbarger, who is most recognized for his seminal reports from the San Francisco Longshoremen Study and the ongoing College Health Study (at Harvard College and the University of Pennsylvania) begun in the 1960s and 1970s (Paffenbarger et al. 1966, 1970, 1978). Those large studies helped fuel scientific and public interest in physical activity as an important component of health promotion and focused the broader fields of preventive medicine and public health on physical inactivity as a significant public health problem.

Contemporary Physical Activity Epidemiology

Despite the growing evidence that physical activity is linked with lowered risk for heart disease, in 1975 Milton Terris, former president of the American Public Health Association, concluded in a keynote address at the Sixth Annual Meeting of the Society for Epidemiologic Research that "physical fitness and physical education have

no respected place in the American public health movement." He stated:

> *On the subject of physical fitness I speak with no authority. Having spent a large portion of my life seated at a desk, I have no personal acquaintance with the concept. On a more intellectual level, I have been far too bound by the philosophical rigidities of the American public health movement to become knowledgeable in the literature of this field, and am therefore in no position to judge the relation of physical exercise and physical fitness to performance of activities of daily living and to "physical, mental and social well-being," that is, to "positive health," vitality, and joy of life. These are issues which are eminently worth studying.*
> —Terris 1975, 1039

Despite traditional epidemiologists' lack of acceptance that physical activity was a proven benefit to health, in 1980 the U.S. Public Health Service identified physical fitness and exercise as one of 15 areas of focus of the national objectives for improving people's health (U.S. Department of Health and Human Services 1980). Recognizing, however, that the scientific basis of physical activity as a national health objective was not yet solid, the Centers for Disease Control (CDC) created the Behavioral Epidemiology and Evaluation Branch (BEEB) within the Center for Health Promotion and Education of the Division of Health Education. Under the direction of Dr. Kenneth Powell, its main purpose was monitoring progress of the nation's 1990 goals for physical activity and fitness. To help with this purpose, the Behavioral Risk Factor Surveillance System (BRFSS) was begun to monitor activity in most of the United States. This system is still operating today. The BEEB staff organized and conducted the Workshop on Epidemiologic and Public Health Aspects of Physical Activity and Exercise in Atlanta on September 24 and 25, 1984, which culminated in the publication of summaries of current knowledge and directions for future research in 10 areas (Powell and Paffenbarger 1985).

International Consensus

Another historical focal point in the modern history of physical activity epidemiology was the first International Conference on Exercise, Fitness, and Health organized by Professor Claude Bouchard under the auspices of the Canadian Association of Sport Sciences and the Ontario Ministry of Tourism and Recreation and held in Toronto in the spring of 1988. Sixty-two papers from that conference, together with scientific consensus statements summarizing the world's knowledge about exercise, fitness, and health, were published (Bouchard et al. 1990). The widespread impact of that conference and the resulting book, as well as a rapidly growing knowledge base, led to the Second International Consensus Symposium on Physical Activity, Fitness, and Health, held again in Toronto in May 1992 as part of Canada's celebration of 125 years of confederation. A sequel book, titled *Physical Activity, Fitness, and Health: International Proceedings and Consensus Statement*, contained 70 chapters that updated the knowledge summarized in the first conference and book (Bouchard, Shephard, and Stephens 1994), and it was an important prelude to *Physical Activity and Health: A Report of the Surgeon General* (U.S. Department of Health and Human Services 1996).

U.S. Government Reports

Key documents published in the United States include a position statement by the American Heart Association in 1992 recognizing physical inactivity as an independent risk factor for coronary heart disease (Fletcher et al. 1992) and recommendations on physical activity and public health prepared jointly by the Centers for Disease Control and Prevention and the American College of Sports Medicine (Pate et al. 1995).

In the historical benchmark, *Physical Activity and Health: A Report of the Surgeon General* (U.S. Department of Health and Human Services 1996), nearly 100 experts, led by Steven Blair, director of epidemiology and clinical applications at the Cooper Institute for Aerobics Research in Dallas, outlined the consensus in the scientific community about the beneficial effects of physical activity on overall mortality, cardiovascular diseases, cancer, type 2 diabetes, osteoarthritis, osteoporosis, obesity, mental health, health-related quality of life, risk of musculoskeletal injury, and risk of sudden death.

Another clear testament to the modern acceptance of physical activity epidemiology occurred in 1996, when Drs. Morris and Paffenbarger jointly received the first Olympic Prize in Sports Science awarded by the Medical Commission of the International Olympic Committee. The Olympic Prize is the "Nobel Prize" of sport and exercise science.

Health Goals for the Nation

Behavioral epidemiologists are helping shape public health policy for the purpose of promoting participation in physical activity by the public. In each decade since 1980, the U.S. Department of Health and Human Services has published a set of health objectives for the nation, policy goals for improving the nation's health. Objectives for increasing physical activity and physical fitness have figured prominently among these objectives. The main objectives for physical activity pertaining to health status and risk reduction for the year 2000 are listed in table 1.1. For realistic national objectives to be set, surveillance systems are necessary for monitoring progress. Such systems have only been available since the mid-1980s.

The status of the 13 objectives for physical activity established in 1990 for the year 2000 was recently evaluated by the Centers for Disease Control and Prevention (2000). While progress was made in five areas (e.g., deaths from coronary heart disease were reduced by about 20%, from 135 to 108 per 100,000 people; the death rate from stroke declined by 12%; the number of work-site fitness programs increased; more people are resistance-training; and there were modest gains in moderate and vigorous physical activity), no change was seen in two areas (e.g., the proportion of sedentary adults remained at 24% of the population), and there was movement away from the target objectives in four areas (e.g., overweight adults increased from 26% to about 35% of the population, and physical activity during school physical education appears to have decreased). Other areas could not be evaluated because a surveillance system was not in place. The proportion of objectives for physical activity that were met (38%) was lower than all other priority areas except diabetes and disabling conditions (22%), immunization and infectious diseases (37%), and clinical preventive services (25%), and substantially lower than the average success rate across all the priority areas (57%).

Based on that evaluation, physical activity objectives were recently established for the year 2010 and are provided for comparison in table 1.2.

TABLE 1.1 PHYSICAL ACTIVITY OBJECTIVES FOR THE NATION 2000

Core objective	2000 Target	Baseline
HEALTH STATUS		
Deaths from coronary heart disease	≤100 per 100,000	135 per 100,000
Overweight	≤20% of adults	26% ages 20–74
RISK REDUCTION		
Regular physical activity	≥30% ages 6+	22% ages 18+
Vigorous physical activity	≥20% ages 18+	12% ages 18+
Sedentary lifestyle	≤15% ages 6+	24% ages 18+
People age 65 or over	22%	43%
People with disabilities	20%	35%
Strength/flexibility activity	≥40% ages 6+	Unknown
Overweight reduction	≥50% ages 12+	<30% ages 18+
SERVICES AND PROTECTION		
Daily school physical education	≥50% grades 1–12	36% grades 1–12
Physical education time exercising	≥50% class time	27% class time
Work-site fitness programs	≥50% work sites of 250–759 employees	32% work sites
Outdoor fitness trails	≥1 per 10,000 people	1 per 71,000 people
Routine counseling on exercise	≥50% primary-care providers	30% providers

Adapted from *Healthy People 2000* (U.S. Department of Health and Human Services 1991).

Summary

Acknowledgment of the potential health benefits of physical activity is as old as recorded history. Since the inclusion of physical activity in the practice of ancient medicine in China, India, and Greece, its recognition in the Bible and the Mishnah Torah, its preservation in medical practice by the Arabs, and its reintroduction to Western medicine of the 16th through 18th centuries by physicians such as the Italian physician-educator Mercurialis, the French pharmacologist Duchesne, the British cardiologist Heberden, and the American physician Rush, physical activity has endured as an important part of hygiene in many cultures. However, physical activity epidemiology as a formal field of research has a short history of about 25 years. British epidemiologist Jeremy Morris is credited with the seminal research that spawned modern physical activity epidemiology in the late 1940s, and his work was expanded by Ralph Paffenbarger and other investigators in the United States and Europe during the late 1960s and 1970s. Systematic inquiry into physical activity epidemiology did not gather full steam until landmark scientific consensus meetings in Atlanta in 1984, organized by Ken Powell of the Centers for Disease Control, and in Toronto in 1988, organized by Claude Bouchard and the Canadian government. The capstone publication of the report of the U.S. Surgeon General, *Physical Activity and Health,* spearheaded by Steven Blair, signaled the maturation of the field by summarizing current knowledge pertinent to public health guidelines and policy and by outlining a host of questions for future study. The purpose of the chapters that follow in this book is to summarize that knowledge, the methods used to obtain it, its implications for public health, and the important questions that remain.

TABLE 1.2	HEALTHY PEOPLE 2010 OBJECTIVES

PHYSICAL ACTIVITY BY ADULTS (18 years and older)

Objective 1: Reduce the proportion of adults who engage in no leisure-time physical activity.
1997 baseline: 40% **2010 target: 20%**

Objective 2: Increase the proportion of adults who engage regularly, preferably daily, in moderate physical activity for at least 30 minutes per day.*
1997 baseline: 15% **2010 target: 30%**

Objective 3: Increase the proportion of adults who engage in vigorous physical activity that promotes cardiorespiratory fitness for 20 or more minutes three or more days a week.
1997 baseline: 23% **2010 target: 30%**

Objective 4: Increase the proportion of adults who perform physical activities that enhance and maintain muscular strength and endurance.
1998 baseline: 18% **2010 target: 30%**

Objective 5: Increase the proportion of adults who perform physical activities that enhance and maintain flexibility.
1998 baseline: 30% **2010 target: 43%**

PHYSICAL ACTIVITY BY CHILDREN AND ADOLESCENTS

Objective 6: Increase the proportion of adolescents who engage in moderate physical activity for at least 30 minutes on five or more of the previous seven days.
1999 baseline: 27% **2010 target: 35%**

Objective 7: Increase the proportion of adolescents who engage in vigorous physical activity that promotes cardiorespiratory fitness three or more days per week for 20 or more minutes per occasion.
1999 baseline: 65% **2010 target: 85%**

Objective 8: Increase the proportion of the nation's public and private schools that require daily physical education for all students.
1994 baseline: 17% (grades 6–8) **2010 target: 25% (grades 6–8)**
2% (grades 9–12) **5% (grades 9–12)**

Objective 9: Increase the proportion of adolescents who participate in daily school physical education.
1999 baseline: 29% (grades 9–12) **2010 target: 50%**

Objective 10: Increase the proportion of adolescents who spend at least 50% of school physical education class time being physically active.
1999 baseline: 38% (grades 9–12) **2010 target: 50%**

U.S. Department of Health and Human Services (2000).

*This objective has been redefined by CDC/NCHS to recommend either moderate or vigorous physical activity. For tracking purposes, the baseline rate of the new recommended activity is 32% and the target for 2010 is 50%. http://wonder.cdc.gov/data2010/focus.htm

Bibliography

Aristotle. 1908. *The works of Aristotle.* Translated by W.D. Ross. Oxford: Clarendon Press, 1908–1952.

Arano, L.C. 1976. *Tacuinum sanitatis.* Milan: Electa Edifice.

Berryman, J.W. 1996. Thomas K. Cureton, Jr.: Pioneer researcher, proselytizer, and proponent for physical fitness. *Research Quarterly for Exercise and Sport* 67: 1–12.

Booth, F.W., M.V. Chakravarthy, S.E. Gordon, and E.E. Spangenburg. 2002. Waging war on physical inactivity: Using modern molecular ammunition against an ancient enemy. *Journal of Applied Physiology* 93: 3–30.

Bouchard, C., R.J. Shephard, and T. Stephens, eds. 1994. *Physical activity, fitness, and health: International proceedings and consensus statement.* Champaign, IL: Human Kinetics.

Bouchard, C., R.J. Shephard, T. Stephens, J.R. Sutton, and B.D. McPherson, eds. 1990. *Exercise, fitness, and health: A consensus of current knowledge.* Champaign, IL: Human Kinetics.

Burton, R. 1632. *The anatomy of melancholy.* Printed by Ion Lichfield for Henry Cripps.

Buskirk, E.R. 1992. From Harvard to Minnesota: Keys to our history. *Exercise and Sport Sciences Reviews* 20: 1–26.

Centers for Disease Control and Prevention, National Center for Health Statistics. 2000. *Healthy people 2000 review, 1998–99.* Washington, DC: U.S. Government Printing Office.

Costill, D.L. 1994. Applied exercise physiology. In *40th Anniversary Lectures,* 69–80. Indianapolis: American College of Sports Medicine.

Cummins, P.W. 1976. *A critical edition of* le regime tresutile et tresproufitable pour conserver et garder la santé du corps humain. Chapel Hill, NC: North Carolina Studies in the Romance Languages and Literatures.

Dawber, T.R., G.F. Meadors, and F.E.J. Moore. 1951. Epidemiological approaches to heart disease: The Framingham Study. *American Journal of Public Health* 41: 279–286.

Fletcher, G.F., S.N. Blair, J. Blumenthal, C. Caspersen, B. Chaitman, S. Epstein, H. Falls, E.S. Froelicher, V.F. Froelicher, and I.L. Pina. 1992. Statement on exercise: Benefits and recommendations for physical activity programs for all Americans. A statement for health professionals by the Committee on Exercise and Cardiac Rehabilitation of the Council on Clinical Cardiology, American Heart Association. *Circulation* 86: 340–344.

Francis, T. Jr. 1961. Aspects of the Tecumseh Study. *Public Health Reports* 76: 963–966.

Galen, C. 1951. *De sanitate tuenda.* Translated by R.M. Green. Springfield, IL: Charles C Thomas.

Guthrie, D. 1945. *A history of medicine.* London: Thomas Nelson.

Heberden, W. 1802. *Commentaries on the history and cure of diseases.* London: T. Payne, News-gate.

Hitchcock, E., and E. Hitchcock Jr. 1860. *Elementary anatomy and physiology for colleges, academies, and other schools.* New York: Ivison, Phinney & Co.

Joseph, L.H. 1949. Gymnastics from the middle ages to the 18th century. *Ciba Symposia* 10 (March–April): 5.

Kannel, W.B. 1967. Habitual level of physical activity and risk of coronary heart disease: The Framingham Study. *Canadian Medical Association Journal* 96: 811–812.

Karvonen, M.J. 1962. Arteriosclerosis: Clinical surveys in Finland. *Proceedings, Royal Society of Medicine* 55: 271–274.

Keys, A. 1967. Epidemiological studies related to coronary heart disease: Characteristics of men aged 40–59 in seven countries. *Acta Medica Scandinavica* 460 (Suppl.): 1–392.

Lyons, A.S., and R.J. Petrucelli. 1978. *Medicine: An illustrated history.* New York: Harry N. Abrams, p. 130.

Maimonides, M. [1199] 1990. *Three treatises on health.* Translated by F. Rosner with bibliographies by J.I. Dienstege. Haifa, Israel: Maimonides Research Institute.

McGinnis, J.M. 1992. The public health burden of a sedentary lifestyle. *Medicine and Science in Sports and Exercise* 24 (Suppl. 6): S196–S200.

McKenzie, R. 1909. *Exercise in education and medicine.* Philadelphia: W.B. Saunders.

Montoye, H.J. 1975. *Physical activity and health: An epidemiologic study of an entire community.* Englewood Cliffs, NJ: Prentice Hall.

Morris, J.N. 1957. *Uses of epidemiology.* London: Churchill Livingstone.

Morris, J.N., J.A. Heady, R.A.B. Raffle, C.G. Roberts, and S.W. Parks. 1953. Coronary heart disease and physical activity of work. *Lancet* ii: 111–120, 1053–1057.

Paffenbarger, R.S. Jr., S.N. Blair, and I.M. Lee. 2001. A history of physical activity, cardiovascular health and longevity: The scientific contributions of Jeremy N Morris, DSc, DPH, FRCP. *International Journal of Epidemiology* 30: 1184–1192.

Paffenbarger, R.S. Jr., M.E. Lauglin, A.S. Gima, and R.A. Black. 1970. Work activity of longshoremen as related to death from coronary heart disease and stroke. *New England Journal of Medicine* 282: 1109–1114.

Paffenbarger, R.S. Jr., A.L. Wing, and R.T. Hyde. 1978. Chronic disease in former college students: XVI. Physical activity as an index of heart attack risk in college alumni. *American Journal of Epidemiology* 108: 161–175.

Paffenbarger, R.S. Jr., P.A. Wolf, J. Notkin, and M.C. Thorne. 1966. Chronic disease in former college students: I. Early

precursors of fatal coronary heart disease. *American Journal of Epidemiology* 83: 314–328.

Pate, R.R., M. Pratt, S.N. Blair, W.L. Haskell, C.A. Macera, C. Bouchard, D. Buchner, W. Ettinger, G.W. Heath, A.C. King, et al. 1995. Physical activity and public health: A recommendation from the Centers for Disease Control and Prevention and the American College of Sports Medicine. *Journal of the American Medical Association* 273: 402–407.

Powell, K.E., and R.S. Paffenbarger Jr. 1985. Workshop on epidemiologic and public health aspects of physical activity and exercise: A summary. *Public Health Reports* 100: 118–126.

Runes, D. 1947. *Selected writings of Benjamin Rush.* New York: Philosophical Library.

Ryan, A.J. 1984. Exercise and health: Lessons from the past. In *Exercise and health: The academy papers,* edited by H.M. Eckert and H.J. Montoye. Vol. 17, pp. 3–13. American Academy of Physical Education. Champaign, IL: Human Kinetics.

Sargent, D.A. 1904. *Health, strength, and power.* New York: Dodge.

Struever, N. 1993. Petrarch's invective contra medicum: An early confrontation of rhetoric and medicine. *Modern Language Notes* 108: 659–679.

Taylor, H.L., H. Blackburn, V. Puchner, R.W. Parlin, and A. Keys. 1969. Coronary heart disease in selected occupations of American railroads in relation to physical activity. *Circulation* 40 (Suppl. 3): 202.

Terris, M. 1975. Approaches to an epidemiology of health. *American Journal of Public Health* 65: 1037–1045.

Tipton, C.M. 1998. Contemporary exercise physiology: Fifty years after the closure of Harvard Fatigue Laboratory. *Exercise and Sport Sciences Reviews* 26: 315–339.

U.S. Department of Health and Human Services. 2000. *Healthy people 2010: Understanding and improving health.* 2nd edition. With *Understanding and improving health* and *Objectives for improving health.* 2 vols. Washington, DC: U.S. Government Printing Office.

U.S. Department of Health and Human Services. 1996. *Physical activity and health: A report of the Surgeon General.* Atlanta: U.S. Department of Health and Human Services, Centers for Disease Control and Prevention, National Center for Chronic Disease Prevention and Health Promotion.

U.S. Department of Health and Human Services. 1991. *Healthy people 2000: National health promotion and disease prevention objectives.* DHHS Publication No. [PHS] 91-50212. Washington, DC: U.S. Government Printing Office.

U.S. Department of Health and Human Services. 1980. *Promoting health/preventing disease: Objectives for the nation.* Washington, DC: U.S. Government Printing Office.

Vallance, J.T. 1995. *The lost theory of Asclepiades of Bithynia.* Oxford: Clarendon Press.

Web Sites

www.cdc.gov/nccdphp/sgr/sgr.htm. This web page of the National Center for Chronic Disease Prevention and Health Promotion of the Centers for Disease Control and Prevention provides access to *Physical Activity and Health: A Report of the Surgeon General.*

www.healthypeople.gov/Publications/. This site provides a description of and access to *Healthy People 2010* and other *Healthy People* publications.

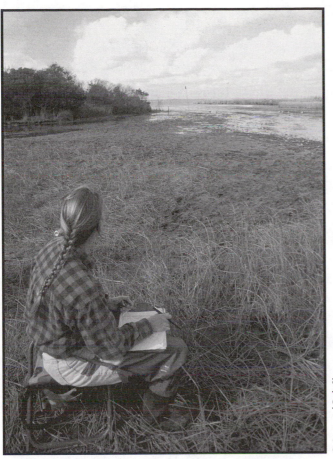

© Ann and Rob Simpson

Chapter 2

Concepts and Methods in Physical Activity Epidemiology

Nothing has such power to broaden the mind as the ability to investigate systematically and truly all that come under thy observation in life.

—*Marcus Aurelius (*A.D.* 121–180), Meditations*

The term **epidemiology** is derived from the Latin roots *epi* (upon) and *demo* (the community). In simple terms, epidemiology is the study of the distribution of disease in a population. More specifically, the term is defined as the application of the scientific method to the study of the distribution and dynamics of disease in a population for the purposes of identifying factors that affect this distribution and then modifying these risk factors in order to reduce the frequency of **morbidity** and mortality from the disease. A **risk factor** is a characteristic that,

if present, increases the probability of disease in a group of individuals who have that characteristic compared with a group of individuals who do not have that characteristic. Epidemiology has three distinct goals: (1) to describe the distribution of disease, for example, who gets the disease and when and where the disease occurs; (2) to analyze this descriptive information in order to identify risk factors that are associated with an increased probability of disease occurrence; and (3) to prevent disease occurrence by modifying the identified risk factors.

Physical activity epidemiology studies factors associated with participation in a specific behavior—that is, physical activity—and how this behavior relates to the probability of disease or injury. Examples of this study include description of the level of physical activity in a population, comparison of levels of physical activity among populations, determination of factors that are associated with participation in physical activity, and the investigation of the association between physical activity and the risk for chronic diseases such as coronary heart disease (CHD), stroke, diabetes, osteoporosis, and cancer.

> ••• *Epidemiology is the use of the scientific method to study the distribution of disease in a population, to identify risk factors that likely cause the disease, and then to change the risk factors in order to reduce sickness and death from the disease.*

Epidemiologic Measures

A fundamental measurement in epidemiology is the frequency with which an event under study occurs, usually an injury, disease, or cause of death in a population. **Incident cases** are the new occurrences of these events in the study population during the time period of interest. In other words, incident cases are those cases in which health status changes—that is, from alive to dead, from not injured to injured, or from not sick to sick—during the period of observation. In contrast, **prevalent cases** represent the number of persons in the population who have a particular disease or condition at some specific point in time. Prevalence of a disease is a function of both incidence and duration. The prevalence of a disease can increase as a result of an increase in either the number of new cases (incidence) or the length of time that individuals have the disease before they die or recover.

If the incidence or prevalence of a condition is known, the incidence rates and prevalence rates can be calculated. The rate is simply the frequency or number of events that occur over some defined time period divided by the average size of the population at risk. The usual estimate of the average number of people at risk is the population at the midpoint of the time interval under study. The general formula for calculating a rate is

$$Rate = \frac{Number\ of\ cases}{Average\ population\ size}$$

Because incidence and prevalence rates are usually less than 1, they are generally expressed per some power of 10 (e.g., per 100 [percent], per 1,000, or per 10,000) for ease of discussion. Therefore, if the death rate in the United States was calculated to be 0.009 deaths per year, 0.009 could be multiplied by 1,000 and expressed as 9 deaths per 1,000 individuals in the population per year.

Incidence rates are the number of incident cases over a defined time period divided by the population at risk over that time period. Incidence rates provide a measure of the rate at which people without disease develop disease over a specified time interval. Likewise, prevalence rates are calculated as the number of prevalent cases divided by the size of the population at a particular time. Prevalence rates indicate only how many people have a particular disease or engage in a behavior, such as physical activity or smoking, at a certain time. Prevalence rates are useful for planning purposes. For example, a survey of a city might find that the prevalence of people with CHD is particularly high. Therefore it may be economically feasible for a local hospital to consider opening a cardiac rehabilitation program. However, prevalence data are not useful when trying to determine factors that may be related to an increased probability of disease because high prevalence does not necessarily indicate high risk; it could reflect increased survival. For example, the high prevalence of CHD in a city survey might not necessarily indicate that people in that city are at increased risk of getting coronary heart disease but could reflect high-quality emergency services and medical care that increase the rate of survival. In contrast, low prevalence might simply reflect rapid death or rapid cure, not low incidence. The problem of using prevalence data alone is that you don't know which of the possible interpretations is true.

It is particularly important to be sure that the information you use to make comparisons among groups is based on actual rates. This may seem obvious, but this fact was overlooked in a number of real-world examples. For example, a sports medicine physician reports that he has seen 100 cases of ruptured patellar tendons in runners over the past year. Does this indicate that running is the cause of this problem and that indeed it is a large problem that needs to be dealt with? The answer is that, with information only on the number of cases (numerator) and no information regarding the number of people at risk (denominator), it is impossible to tell. To make these assessments, you need to know how many runners visited the clinic over the course of the year. If 100 runners were seen and 100 cases of ruptured patellar tendons were diagnosed, then the incidence would be 100%, a potentially serious problem! On the other hand, if 1,000 runners were seen, the rate would be only 10%, a completely different interpretation. The use of numerator data, the number of cases, without considering the size of the population at risk should be avoided. However numerator data of this nature can often be found in the sports medicine literature.

Crude, Specific, and Standardized Rates

There are three general categories of rates that are commonly used in epidemiology: crude, specific, and standardized. Rates that are based on a total population without consideration of any of the population characteristics, such as the distribution of age, sex, ethnicity, and so on, are referred to as *crude rates*. When rates are calculated separately for population subgroups (typically age, sex, and ethnicity), they are called *specific rates* (e.g., age-specific rates, sex-specific rates). Standardized rates are crude rates that have been standardized (adjusted) for some population characteristic, such as age or sex, to allow valid comparisons of rates among populations where the distribution of the given characteristic may be quite different.

Crude rates, because they depend on the characteristics of the population from which they are calculated, can often be misleading. For example, the crude prevalence of participation in vigorous physical activity in Boulder, Colorado, would be expected to be higher than that in a community such as Sun City, Arizona, simply because of the difference in the age distribution of residents in those communities. Likewise a comparison of breast cancer rates in two populations where the sex distribution varies greatly could be misleading. There are two solutions to this problem. First, valid comparisons among populations can be made if specific rates are used. In the preceding examples, it would be reasonable to compare the rates of participation in vigorous physical activity between Boulder and Sun City by five-year age groups, or the rates of breast cancer for men and women separately. Although the use of specific rates provides a valid comparison, the procedure can become cumbersome, particularly when numerous categories, such as five-year age groups over a large age range, need to be compared. Therefore, to make comparisons of rates between two populations with unequal distributions of risk factors, standardized rates should be used.

Standardized rates, which are also referred to as adjusted rates, are simply crude rates that have been adjusted to control for the effect of some population characteristic, such as age or sex. The most common method for the adjustment is called direct standardization. In practice, the standardization process is performed by readily available computer software packages. The following example is an illustration of how the direct standardization process actually works. The data in table 2.1 represent the death rates from two different populations. The crude death rate in population A is 4.51% and in population B is 3.08%. This is curious, and misleading, when you consider that the age-specific death rates in population B are twice that of population A. An inspection of the age distributions in these populations suggests the problem. Population A has a higher proportion of individuals in the older age group, where the age-specific death rate is highest, than population B does. To make a valid comparison of the death rates in these two populations, death rates need to be adjusted to account for the difference in age distribution. The direct standardization method involves applying the age-specific rates of the populations to be compared to a single standardized population. The standard population can be any reasonable or realistic population. In this example, the standard population is simply the combination of populations A and B. In practice, the population of a particular state or the entire United States is often used. Because the age distribution in the standard population is the same for all the age-specific death rates that are applied to it, the effect of the different age distribution in the two actual populations being compared is eliminated. This procedure allows the overall death rates in the two populations to be compared without the **bias** introduced by differences in the age distribution.

As illustrated in table 2.1, after adjustment for age, the overall death rate in population B

TABLE 2.1   ILLUSTRATION OF THE PRINCIPLE OF DIRECT STANDARDIZATION OF CRUDE RATES FROM TWO HYPOTHETICAL POPULATIONS

Age group	Number	Population A age-specific death rate	Expected	Number	Population B age-specific death rate	Expected
CALCULATION OF CRUDE RATE						
20–49	2,000	0.001	2	8,000	0.002	16
50–79	10,000	0.01	100	10,000	0.02	200
80 and over	8,000	0.1	800	2,000	0.2	400
Total	20,000		902	20,000		616
Crude death rate	902/20,000 = 4.51%			616/20,000 = 3.08%		
CALCULATION OF STANDARDIZED RATES USING THE COMBINED POPULATION TO FORM THE STANDARD POPULATION						
20–49	10,000	0.001	10	10,000	0.002	20
50–79	20,000	0.01	200	20,000	0.02	400
80 and over	10,000	0.1	1,000	10,000	0.2	2,000
Total	40,000		1,210	40,000		2,420
Standardized death rate	1,210/40,000 = 3.03%			2,420/40,000 = 6.05%		

(2,420/40,000 = 6.05%) is twice that of population A (1,210/40,000 = 3.03%), accurately reflecting the fact that the age-specific death rates in population B are twice as high as those in population A. The same principles of direct standardization can also be used to compare incidence rates of disease or injury in populations that differ in their distributions of sex, health status, **cholesterol** or blood pressure level, or any other characteristic that might bias the rate comparison. Though standardized rates are useful for making valid comparisons across populations, it must be remembered that they are fictional rates. The adjusted rates can vary, depending on the standard population that is used in the adjustment process. Therefore, the adjusted rate can be misleading and should be used only for comparison purposes.

Research Design in Epidemiologic Studies

A **research design** is the way that participants are grouped and compared according to behavior or attributes (e.g., physical activity or fitness), the health-related events being studied, time, and factors other than physical activity or fitness that could explain the occurrence of health-related events. The goal of a design in physical activity epidemiologic research is to make sure that comparisons of groups based on differences in physical activity or fitness are not biased by other factors. Said another way, the research design used determines whether it is reasonable to infer that physical inactivity was a direct, or the only, explanation for the occurrence of an injury, disease, or death.

In a true research design, passage of time is needed between the change in the **independent variable** (i.e., the manipulated or fluctuating variable, such as physical activity, thought to be associated with the outcome) and the subsequent change in the **dependent variable** (i.e., the outcome variable, such as heart disease). When the change occurs as the result of **natural history** (i.e., it is self-initiated by the people being studied), the design is observational. When change in the independent variable is manipulated by the investigator, the design is experimental. When the independent and dependent variables are observed or manipulated across a period of time, the design is longitudinal or prospective. When the study looks back in time after the occurrence of injury, disease, or death in an attempt to reconstruct an influencing factor, such as physical activity habits, the design is retrospective.

> ••• *The research design used is an important consideration in evaluating the likelihood of a cause-and-effect association between physical activity and the occurrence of death or disease.*

There are several types of research designs commonly used in epidemiologic research: cross-sectional surveys, case–control studies, cohort studies, and randomized controlled trials (table 2.2). The actual design employed in

any particular study depends on the questions to be answered, the time and financial resources available, and the availability of data. The major advantages and disadvantages of the commonly used epidemiologic study designs are summarized in table 2.3.

Definitions of Study Designs

• **Cross-sectional study.** Both risk factors and the presence or absence of disease are measured at the same point in time.

• **Case–control study.** Participants are selected based on the presence (i.e., cases) or

TABLE 2.2   STUDY DESIGNS

Type of study	Past	Present	Future
		TIME	
Cross-sectional		Assess risk factors and disease outcome	
Case–control	Inquire about exposure to risk factors	Assess outcome, i.e., case or control	
Prospective cohort		Assemble cohort Assess risk factors	Assess outcomes
Randomized trial		Randomly assign to experimental groups	Assess outcomes

TABLE 2.3   STUDY DESIGNS IN EPIDEMIOLOGIC RESEARCH: ADVANTAGES AND DISADVANTAGES

Design	Advantages	Disadvantages
Cross-sectional surveys	Quick and easy to conduct. Appropriate for hypothesis generation.	No temporal relationship between risk factors and disease. Not appropriate for hypothesis testing.
Case–control studies	Appropriate for the study of rare events. Can study multiple risk factors. Inexpensive and quick to perform.	Cannot determine absolute risk. Subject to recall bias. Can study only one disease at a time. Temporal relationships may be uncertain.
Cohort studies	Provide an absolute measure of risk. Allow the study of multiple disease outcomes.	Expensive and time-consuming to conduct. Not appropriate for studying rare outcomes. Results can be affected by loss to follow-up. Can assess the effect only of risk factors obtained at baseline.
Randomized controlled trials	Investigator has control over the research process. Is the gold standard for evaluation of interventions.	Expensive and time-consuming to conduct. Generalizability is often limited. Lack of compliance and dropouts can cause problems.

absence (i.e., **controls**) of a disease of interest. Cases and controls are matched on several possible causes of disease, then a comparison of the frequency of past exposure to other potential risk factors for the disease is made between the two groups.

- **Prospective cohort study.** A group of individuals is selected at random from a defined population. After the **cohort** is selected, baseline information on potential risk factors is collected, and individuals are followed over time to track the incidence of disease between those people subsequently exposed or not exposed to the risk factors of interest.

- **Randomized controlled trial.** Participants are selected and randomly assigned to receive an experimental manipulation or a control condition. Baseline and outcome measurements are obtained to determine the size of changes after the experimental manipulation compared with the control condition.

Cross-Sectional Surveys

Cross-sectional surveys, sometimes called prevalence studies, measure both risk factors and the presence or absence of disease at the same point in time. Although this approach is expedient and relatively inexpensive, it cannot determine the temporal relationship of a potential cause-and-effect relationship. For example, in a cross-sectional survey of 556 female participants in the Health and Religion Project, Eaton et al. (1995) reported significant negative correlations between physical activity and body mass index, systolic and diastolic blood pressure, and total cholesterol. While those results indicate that the women with lower levels of physical activity had higher levels of important cardiovascular disease risk factors, it is not possible to deter-mine whether low activity or high risk factors came first. The use of a cross-sectional study design precludes our knowing whether the women were less active because they had high body mass, blood pressure, or cholesterol, or whether they had high levels of these risk factors because they were less active. Cross-sectional surveys can be useful for generating hypotheses regarding potential associations between risk factors and diseases and also for assessment of the prevalence of risk factors or behaviors in a defined population. For example, the U.S. Centers for Disease Control and Prevention, in cooperation with state health departments, conducts a

Behavioral Risk Factor Surveillance Survey each year to determine the prevalence of several disease risk factors, including smoking and sedentary behavior. An **ecological study** is a specific type of cross-sectional survey in which the frequency of some risk factor of interest, for instance sedentary behavior, is compared with an outcome measure, such as obesity, in a particular geographic region, for example a city, county, or state. For example, surveys conducted in a particular state might find high rates of sedentary behavior as well as high rates of obesity. Though this type of information may suggest the hypothesis that sedentary behavior results in obesity, drawing this conclusion is unjustified. Data from this type of survey should never be used to make any conclusion regarding cause and effect because these data are not associated with individual persons. There is no way to know whether the individuals who are sedentary are the same individuals who are obese. This problem is referred to as the **ecological fallacy,** that is, erroneously concluding that an association between variables exists based on an ecological study.

Case–Control Studies

In a case–control study, subjects are selected based on the presence of a disease of interest and matched with controls without the disease. After cases and controls are selected, the frequency of past exposure to potential risk factors for the disease and the odds of having the risk factors between the case and control groups are compared. Risk-factor information is typically obtained by personal interview or a review of medical records. A number of case–control studies are available in the physical activity epidemiology literature, particularly in the area of physical activity and cancer. The case–control methodology is ideal for the study of diseases like cancer that occur rather infrequently and have a long latent period between exposure to a risk factor and actual manifestation of the disease. Prospective study designs are not practical if the period between the exposure to a risk factor and the development of a disease is long, as the investigator would have to wait up to 20 years in many cases before having any cases of disease to study.

For example, a group of investigators in the Netherlands reported on a case–control study of physical activity as a risk for breast cancer in women ages 20 to 54 years. A sample of 918 women who had been diagnosed with invasive breast cancer between 1986 and 1989 were selected from a cancer registry. Each patient was matched by age and region of residence with a control subject. Both cases and controls were interviewed in their homes to collect information about lifetime physical activity and other risk factors, including reproductive and contraceptive history, family history of breast cancer, smoking, alcohol use, and premenstrual and menstrual complaints. To ensure recall of past behavior over the same time interval in cases and controls, control subjects were assigned a date of pseudodiagnosis, that is, a date that corresponded with the date on which the controls were the same age as their matched case subject at actual diagnosis. The analysis was restricted to risk events that occurred prior to actual diagnosis or pseudodiagnosis to ensure the correct temporal association between the risk factor and disease. Results indicated that women who were more active than their peers at ages 10 to 12 years were at significantly reduced risk of breast cancer. Also, women who had ever engaged in recreational physical activity at any point prior to diagnosis were also at significantly reduced risk for breast cancer. These data support the hypothesis that recreational physical activity decreases the risk of breast cancer in women, but the results must be interpreted in the light of potential problems associated with the case–control study design, including recall bias and nonrepresentativeness of the control group.

There are several disadvantages to the case–control study design. As discussed later in this chapter in the section on evaluating associations, the case–control design does not allow a direct determination of the **absolute risk** of the disease because the incidence rates are not available; a group of individuals is not followed over time. However, an estimate of the risk of disease in those exposed to the risk factor compared with those not exposed can be calculated. An additional disadvantage of the case–control design is difficulty in obtaining a truly representative control group. To obtain a representative group of controls that are generally matched with cases by age, sex, and race, controls are often obtained from the same setting as the cases (i.e., the hospital where the cases were diagnosed or the same neighborhood where the cases reside). Investigators often use multiple control groups to increase the probability of obtaining a representative comparison group. Another limitation of case–control studies is recall bias, which may result in a spurious association between a risk factor and disease. Recall bias is the phenomenon that individuals who have experienced an adverse event (e.g., cancer, heart attack) may think more about why they had this problem than healthy individuals and thus might be more likely to recall exposure to potential risk factors. Case–control studies of mortality are also vulnerable to recall bias because information must be obtained from a witness to past behavior, such as a spouse. The spouse or other close relatives of the deceased might be more likely to recall previous risk behaviors than individuals who have not lost a loved one. Another disadvantage of case–control studies is the inability to study more than one disease outcome at a time.

Case–control studies offer several advantages over other epidemiologic study designs. They are relatively quick and inexpensive to conduct, are useful for studying rare disease outcomes, require a relatively small number of subjects, and allow the study of multiple risk factors. These advantages make this design particularly useful for the initial development and testing of hypotheses to determine whether conducting a more time-consuming and expensive cohort study or randomized trial is warranted.

Prospective Cohort Studies

The term *cohort* comes from the Latin word for a division of a Roman army consisting of 300 to 600 soldiers. In epidemiology, a cohort is a clearly identified group to be studied. Prospective cohort studies, sometimes referred to as *incidence* or *longitudinal follow-up studies,* involve the selection of a group of individuals at random from some defined population or the selection of groups exposed or not exposed to a risk factor of interest. After the cohort is selected, baseline information on potential risk factors is collected, and individuals are followed over time to track the incidence of disease. A number of prospective cohort studies—for example, the Nurses' Health Study, the Framingham Heart Study, the Harvard Alumni Study, the Honolulu Heart Study, the Physicians' Health Study, and the Aerobics Center Longitudinal Study—have generated valuable information regarding the association of physical activity, physical fitness, and health outcomes. For example, the Aerobics Center Longitudinal Study to date has measured physical fitness, defined as endurance time on a treadmill test, in over 10,000 men and 3,000 women when they visited the Cooper Clinic in Dallas, Texas, for preventive medical examination. In one analysis, total mortality in the cohort was assessed for about eight years of follow-up. During the period of observation, 240 deaths among men and 43 deaths among women occurred after about 110,000 **person-years** of exposure (one person followed for one year equals one person-year). Age-adjusted death rates (per 10,000 person-years of exposure) from all causes were lower with each successive level of fitness, from the least fit (64 deaths among men and 40 deaths among women) to the most fit (19 deaths among men and 9 deaths among women). The effects of higher fitness were independent of age, smoking, cholesterol level, systolic blood pressure, blood sugar, and parental history of CHD. Much of the decrease in the total mortality rate in the fitter subjects was explainable by reduced rates of cardiovascular disease and cancer.

The prospective approach is more costly and time-consuming than either a cross-sectional survey or a case–control study, it cannot be used to study diseases that occur infrequently, and it can assess the effects only of risk factors that were measured at baseline (i.e., the beginning of the study). The major advantage of the prospective study is that the risk profile is established before the outcome is assessed. Therefore, any information obtained at baseline cannot be biased by the knowledge of results. Prospective studies also allow the investigator to control the data collection as the study proceeds, to assess changes in risk factors over time, to classify the disease end points (e.g., CHD, diabetes, osteoporosis) correctly, and to study multiple disease outcomes, some of which may not have been planned at the outset of the study. Perhaps most important, a prospective design allows the estimation of the true absolute risk of developing a disease. Definition and measurement of risk are discussed later in this chapter.

Randomized Controlled Trial

The randomized controlled trial is the gold standard of research designs for testing a research hypothesis. This design gives the researcher more control than any of the other epidemiologic research designs. In a randomized controlled trial, participants are selected for study and randomly assigned to receive an experimental manipulation or a control condition. Measurements are made before and after the intervention period in both groups to assess the difference in the outcomes of interest between the intervention and control conditions. The key to this approach is randomization, which ensures that the experimental and control groups are comparable with respect to all factors, known or unknown, except for the factor being studied by the experimental intervention.

Although the randomized controlled trial is the optimal research design, actually conducting these trials poses a number of challenging problems. For example, potential participants in a randomized trial must agree to participate without knowing whether they will be assigned to the intervention or control group. This can be particularly problematic in an exercise intervention trial in which the motivation to participate is to receive the intervention, not to be assigned to a control condition. If possible, it is best to conduct a randomized trial in a double-blind manner; that is, neither the participants nor the observers who collect the data are aware of group assignments. The double-blind approach is obviously not possible in exercise intervention research, for which only single-blind trials (in which only data-collection personnel are unaware of group assignments) are feasible. Biases can be introduced by poor compliance with the intervention (i.e., some experimental participants fail to take or to participate in the intervention) and by dropouts in either the intervention or control group (i.e., groups are no longer equivalent by the end of the study). Because of the difficulty in recruiting participants for large randomized trials, these trials are often conducted using highly select samples. This reduces external validity, the ability to generalize the study results to other populations. For example, the Physicians' Health Study, which was conducted to determine the **effectiveness** of aspirin on cardiovascular disease and of beta carotene on cancer and which included a measurement of physical activity, had as subjects mostly white, healthy, middle-aged, male physicians. The generalizability of these results to other groups, such as young men, women, minorities, or non-physicians, is questionable.

Although the randomized controlled trial is the research design of choice for hypothesis testing, many important questions in physical activity epidemiology cannot be answered with this approach. For example, researchers may be interested in knowing what type, frequency, intensity, and duration of exercise are most beneficial for reducing the incidence of CHD. In theory, an experiment could be conducted in which individuals are randomly assigned to a specific exercise regimen or a control condition and followed for incidence of heart disease. This approach is not practical for several reasons. First, the risk of a first **myocardial infarction** in healthy middle-aged men is about 7 per 1,000 per year. Hence, the study would need to involve about 20,000 men, randomly assigned to an exercise intervention group and a control group and followed over a one-year period, to obtain 140 potential cases of myocardial infarction for study! All 20,000 men would need to undergo extensive evaluation prior to randomization to ensure that they were free from heart disease. Steps would have to be taken to ensure that the exercise group adhered to the exercise frequency, intensity, and duration stipulated in the program and that the control group did not start an exercise program during the intervention year. Given the large numbers of subjects needed, a study of this type would have to be conducted at multiple sites across the country, adding additional complexity to maintaining quality control over both the intervention program and other measures of interest (e.g., risk factors). It is obvious that such a study would be exceedingly expensive and a logistical nightmare. Needless to say, a trial of this type has never been and most likely will never be undertaken. The randomized trial has a place in physical activity studies, where smaller, more manageable trials can be conducted on the effects of different levels of physical activity or exercise training on muscle performance, balance, gait, CHD risk factors (such as lipid levels, obesity, blood pressure, insulin levels), and so on.

Summary

The ultimate goal of a research design is to assess the degree to which change in an independent variable (e.g., physical activity or fitness) is causally associated with change in a dependent variable (e.g., injury, disease, or death). It is important to remember the inherent strengths and weaknesses of the various study design options as we discuss the evidence for physical activity in reducing the risk of chronic disease.

Evaluating Associations in Epidemiologic Studies

Conceptually, epidemiologic research is simply a comparison of groups formed based on the presence or absence of a risk factor under study, the independent variable (e.g., physical activity, smoking, obesity), and the presence or absence of a disease or condition of interest, the dependent variable (e.g., CHD, diabetes, osteoporosis). The goal is generally to identify the risk factors for a particular disease and to determine how much of an impact those factors have on the probability of disease. In practice, the situation can easily become much more complex in that it is often desirable to study several independent variables at the same time and to determine how those variables interact to affect disease risk. For example, epidemiologists are interested in studying the association of physical activity and the incidence of type 2 diabetes while considering the influence of age, sex, body fat, family history of diabetes, diet, smoking, and so on. They may also be interested in assessing the effect of different levels of exercise (i.e., low-, moderate-, or high-intensity) and durations of exposure to a risk factor on disease outcome.

Regardless of how complex the issues under study become, most epidemiologic research can be conceptually framed in a standard 2 × 2 table (see table 2.4). There are slight differences in the interpretation of the 2 × 2 table, depending

TABLE 2.4   THE 2 × 2 TABLE FOR ASSESSING THE ASSOCIATION BETWEEN RISK FACTORS AND DISEASE

		DISEASE STATUS		
		Present	Absent	Total
Risk factor	Present	a	b	$a + b$
Status	Absent	c	d	$c + d$
	Total	$a + c$	$b + d$	$a + b + c + d$

a = Subjects with both risk factor and disease
b = Subjects with risk factor but no disease
c = Subjects with no risk factor and disease
d = Subjects with no risk factor and no disease
$a + b$ = All subjects with risk factor

$c + d$ = All subjects with no risk factor
$a + c$ = All subjects with disease
$b + d$ = All subjects with no disease
$a + b + c + d$ = All subjects

on whether data were obtained from a prospective cohort or a case–control study. Both study designs are discussed in further detail in the following sections.

Prospective Cohort Study

The interpretation of the 2 × 2 table for a prospective cohort study is presented in table 2.5. Recall that in a prospective cohort study, a population is selected, baseline measurements are obtained, and the population is followed over time to document the development of disease. Table 2.6 provides data from a hypothetical prospective cohort study on the association between physical activity at baseline and the incidence of CHD to illustrate the process of assessing the strength of the association between a risk factor and disease.

In the example, 500 men in the total sample of 10,000 developed CHD. The overall incidence rate is then 500 cases per 10,000 population, or 0.05 (5%). The question of interest is, What impact does risk-factor status (i.e., level of physical activity) have on the incidence of disease? To answer this question, we need to calculate the incidence of disease in both the active and sedentary groups. The incidence rate, or risk, for CHD in the sedentary group is $a/(a + b) = 400/(400 + 5,600) = 400/6,000 = 0.067$, or 6.7%. The incidence rate, or risk, of disease in the active group is $c/(c + d) = 100/(100 + 3,900) = 100/4,000 = 0.025$, or 2.5%. With this information, the effect of sedentary behavior

on CHD risk can be evaluated. The **risk difference** is simply the risk of disease in the group exposed to the risk factor minus the risk of disease in the unexposed group. In the example, the risk in the exposed (sedentary) group is 6.7%, and the risk in the unexposed (active) group is 2.5%, so the risk difference is 6.7% – 2.5% = 4.2%. Obviously, if the levels of risk in the exposed and unexposed groups are the same, the risk difference is zero. If exposure to the risk factor is harmful, as is the case for sedentary behavior in the example, then the risk difference is greater than zero. If exposure is protective (e.g., exposure to a drug that lowers cholesterol level), then the risk difference is less than zero. The risk difference is also called the **attributable risk;** it is an estimate of the amount of risk attributed to the risk factor. In the example, 4.2% of the risk of CHD in this population is attributed to exposure to the risk factor of sedentary behavior. The **relative risk (RR),** or **risk ratio,** is the ratio of the risk in the exposed group to the risk in the unexposed group. In the example, the relative risk of CHD between the exposed (sedentary) group and the unexposed (active) group is

$$RR = [a/(a + b)]/[c/(c + d)]$$
$$= [400/(400 + 5,600)]/[100/(100 + 3,900)]$$
$$= 0.067/0.025 = 2.68$$

If the risk of disease in both the exposed and unexposed groups is the same, the relative risk is 1.0. If the risks in the two groups are not the

TABLE 2.5 THE 2 × 2 TABLE FOR A PROSPECTIVE COHORT STUDY					
		FOLLOW-UP			
		Develop disease	**Do not develop disease**	**Total**	**Incidence rate of disease**
Risk factor	Present	a	b	$a + b$	$a/(a + b)$
Status	Absent	c	d	$c + d$	$c/(c + d)$

TABLE 2.6 HYPOTHETICAL COHORT STUDY ON PHYSICAL ACTIVITY AND CORONARY HEART DISEASE				
		FOLLOW-UP		
		Develop disease	**Do not develop disease**	**Incidence rate of disease**
Risk factor	Present (sedentary)	$a = 400$	$b = 5,600$	6.7%
Status	Absent (active)	$c = 100$	$d = 3,900$	2.5%
	Total	500	9,500	

same, calculation of the relative risk provides an easily interpretable method of demonstrating, in relative terms, how much greater or smaller the risks are. In the example, the risk of CHD in the sedentary group is 2.68 times higher than in the active group. When considering risk assessments, it is important to remember the difference between absolute and relative risk. In the example, the absolute risk for developing CHD—that is, the true risk in the exposed (sedentary) group—is 6.7%, but that level of risk is 2.68 times higher than the absolute risk in the active group (2.5%). In some cases the relative risk can be extremely high even while the absolute risk in both groups is rather low. For example, the relative risk of a myocardial infarction after heavy physical exertion in a group of men and women who do not exercise regularly has been shown to be approximately 100 times the risk of myocardial infarction in men and women who are regular exercisers. This is an extremely high relative risk; however, the absolute risk of myocardial infarction following heavy exertion, even for sedentary individuals, is actually quite low. Considering that the absolute risk of a myocardial infarction during any given hour in a healthy, middle-aged adult man is approximately one per million, even with a hundredfold increase, the absolute risk is still quite small (0.000001 × 100 = 0.0001, or an absolute risk of 1 per 10,000).

The **odds ratio (OR)** can also be calculated for a prospective study, but as will become evident from the subsequent discussion, this measure is typically associated with the case–control design. The odds ratio is calculated by dividing the odds of exposure to the risk factor in the diseased group by the odds of exposure to the risk factor in the nondiseased group:

$$OR = (a/c)/(b/d)$$
$$= ad/bc$$

Odds and risk are conceptually different. In the standard 2 × 2 table (see table 2.4), the risk of disease in the exposed group, as discussed previously, is $a/(a + b)$, whereas the odds of disease in the exposed group (i.e., the chance of having versus not having the disease) in the exposed group is simply a/b. Based strictly on the mathematics, if a is small compared with b, which it often is, then the odds and the risk are quite similar. This is illustrated by calculating the odds ratio for the hypothetical data in table 2.6. Here the odds ratio is $(400 × 3,900)/(100 × 5,600) = 1,560,000/560,000 = 2.79$, which is quite similar to the relative risk of 2.68. Therefore, when using a case–control design, in which a measure of disease incidence cannot be obtained, the odds ratio provides a reasonable estimate of relative risk.

Case–Control Study

Recall that in a case–control study, participants are selected based on disease status (i.e., whether the disease is present or absent). A 2 × 2 table illustrating the organization of data from a case–control study is shown in table 2.7. The analysis in a case–control study is a comparison of the proportion of cases exposed to a suspected risk factor, $a/(a + c)$, with the proportion of controls exposed to the same risk factor, $b/(b + d)$. If exposure to the risk factor is positively related to the disease, then the proportion of cases exposed to the risk factor should be greater than the proportion of controls exposed to the risk factor. In a case–control study, the only measure of the strength of the association between the risk factor and disease is the odds ratio (ad/bc). Conceptually, the odds ratio is an estimate of the risk of disease given the presence of a particular risk factor compared with the risk of disease if the risk factor is not present. In most instances, the odds ratios from well-conducted case–control studies are good estimates of the relative risk that would have been derived from a prospective cohort study, provided that the overall risk of disease in the population is low (i.e., less than 5%).

TABLE 2.7 THE 2 × 2 TABLE FOR A CASE–CONTROL STUDY		Cases (disease)	Controls (no disease)
Risk factor status	Present	a	b
	Absent	c	d
Proportion exposed		$a/(a + c)$	$b/(b + d)$

Interpreting Relative Risks and Odds Ratios

If the risk of disease is the same in the groups exposed and not exposed to the risk factor, the relative risk and odds ratio will be 1.0. Typically, when calculating relative risk, the incidence of disease in the exposed group is placed in the numerator and the incidence of disease in the unexposed group in the denominator, as was done with the data from the hypothetical prospective cohort study in table 2.6, where the calculated relative risk was 2.68. This makes sense because as the impact of the risk factor increases (in this case the impact of sedentary behavior on CHD incidence), the relative risk increases. However, it is also acceptable to reverse the fraction and place the incidence of disease in the exposed group in the denominator. Then the relative risk would be 0.025/0.067 = 0.37, indicating that the risk in the active group is about one third that of the sedentary group.

Although the formula for calculating the odds ratio is different from that for calculating relative risk, the interpretation of magnitude of the actual value is virtually the same. Usually the odds ratio is expressed with the group exposed to the risk factor in the numerator. However, the interpretation of the strength of the observed odds ratio is not changed if the exposed group is placed in the denominator. The 95% **confidence interval** is a measure of the degree of confidence that the observed relative risk or odds ratio is meaningful. The 95% confidence interval gives an estimate of the lowest and highest values that might be expected 95 times if the study were to be repeated 100 times using other samples of the same number of people. The confidence interval can be used to determine whether the observed relative risk or odds ratio differs statistically from 1.0. A relative risk or odds ratio of 1.0 indicates that there is no difference in the risk of disease between those exposed and not exposed to the risk factor. If the relative risk of CHD in sedentary individuals (2.68 in our hypothetical study) has a 95% confidence interval ranging from 0.72 to 3.15, the relative risk would not be statistically significant because the confidence interval includes a value of 1.0. However, if the same relative risk had a 95% confidence interval ranging from 1.5 to 3.5, the relative risk would be significantly different from 1.0 because 1.0 does not fall within the calculated confidence interval.

Attributable Risk

An important function of epidemiologic research is to estimate the amount of disease burden in a population that results from a potentially modifiable risk factor. For example, researchers might ask: In the U.S. population, how much CHD mortality is the result of sedentary behavior, high blood pressure, obesity, and other modifiable risk factors? This type of information is extremely important for making decisions about which risk factors intervention efforts should target to maximize the benefits to public health. Also, the public may be more interested and likely to comply with intervention efforts if the importance of such efforts to their individual health can be demonstrated.

Several epidemiologic measures are used to assess the impact of exposure on disease risk factors. These include the attributable risk percentage in the exposed group, **population attributable risk,** and population attributable risk percentage. The following paragraphs describe these measures using the hypothetical data in table 2.6 as an illustration.

Attributable risk (AR) percentage in the exposed. The AR percentage estimates the total risk of disease that results from a risk factor among those who are exposed to that risk factor. Either of two formulas can be used to calculate the AR percentage:

(1) AR% = $(\text{Risk}_{\text{exposed}} - \text{Risk}_{\text{unexposed}})/\text{Risk}_{\text{exposed}}$

(2) AR% = $(RR - 1)/RR$

Using the data from table 2.6 with formula (1) to calculate the AR percentage of CHD among the sedentary,

$$\begin{aligned} AR\% &= (0.067 - 0.025)/0.067 \\ &= 0.042/0.067 \\ &= 0.6268 \\ &= 62.7\% \end{aligned}$$

Using formula (2),

$$\begin{aligned} AR\% &= (2.68 - 1)/2.68 \\ &= 1.68/2.68 \\ &= 0.6268 \\ &= 62.7\% \end{aligned}$$

Therefore, among those who are sedentary, 62.7% of the risk for CHD is attributable to sedentary behavior. The AR percentage in the exposed can also be calculated for a case–control study by substituting the odds ratio for the relative risk in formula (2).

Population attributable risk (PAR). Population attributable risk is the risk of disease in the total population minus the risk in the unexposed group. In the CHD example of table 2.6, the calculation of the PAR allows a determination of how much of the total risk of CHD is attributable to sedentary behavior. In this example, the risk of CHD in the total population is 500/10,000 = 0.05, or 5 per 100 per year. The risk of disease in the active group is 100/4,000 = 0.025, 2.5 per 100 per year. Therefore, PAR = 5 – 2.5 = 2.5; in other words, 2.5 cases per 100 population per year are attributable to sedentary behavior.

Population attributable risk (PAR) percentage. PAR percentage is the percentage of the risk of a disease that is attributable to a particular risk factor. It is PAR expressed as a percentage rather than an absolute value.

$$PAR\% = (Risk_{total} - Risk_{unexposed})/Risk_{total}$$

Using the data from table 2.6,

$$PAR\% = (5 - 2.5)/5$$
$$= 0.5$$
$$= 50\%$$

Therefore, 50% of the total risk for CHD in this population is attributable to sedentary behavior.

From a public health perspective, this formula is a more useful approach to the calculation of PAR percentage:

$$PAR\% = (P_{exposed})(RR - 1)/[1 + (P_{exposed})(RR - 1)]$$

Where $P_{exposed}$ is the proportion of the population exposed to the risk factor and RR is the relative risk of disease associated with the risk factor. This formula allows a comparison of the impact of different risk factors on disease risk in a population. For example, the proportion of CHD risk due to sedentary behavior could be compared with that due to cigarette smoking. Let us assume that the relative risk for coronary heart disease associated with sedentary behavior is 2.0 and that 50% of the U.S. population is sedentary ($P_{exposed}$). Let us also assume that the relative risk of CHD associated with cigarette smoking is 5.0 and that 20% of the U.S. population smokes. With this information, the PAR percentage for both sedentary behavior and cigarette smoking can be calculated as follows:

$$PAR\% \text{ (sedentary behavior)} = 0.5(2.0 - 1)/$$
$$[1 + (0.5)(2.0 - 1)]$$
$$= 0.5/1.5$$
$$= 0.333$$
$$= 33.3\%$$

$$PAR\% \text{ (smoking)} = 0.2(5.0 - 1)/[1 + (0.2)(5.0 - 1)]$$
$$= 0.2(4)/[1 + (0.2)(4)]$$
$$= 0.8/(1 + 0.8)$$
$$= 0.444$$
$$= 44.4\%$$

Thus, in this example, approximately 33% of the CHD in the population is attributable to sedentary behavior and 44% to cigarette smoking. In theory, if all sedentary individuals become active, there would be 33% fewer cases of CHD in the population. Similarly, if all the cigarette smokers quit, there would be 44% fewer CHD cases. PAR percentage thus allows the comparison of the impact of risk factors that vary in relative risk and prevalence in the population. A risk factor might have a very high relative risk but a low prevalence in the population; modification of that risk factor thus would have limited impact on public health. The PAR percentage of sedentary behavior as it relates to several disease outcomes, including CHD and cancer, is evaluated in subsequent chapters.

Models in Physical Activity Epidemiology

To understand the role of physical activity and fitness in health, it is necessary to view these factors in the context of the models used by epidemiologists to understand the independent and interactive causes of disease, injury, or death. The three most commonly used models for this purpose are presented in figure 2.1. The first and most common model is the epidemiologic triangle, consisting of the host (i.e., the person), the environment (e.g., physical, social) and the agent (e.g., physical activity or fitness). This model evolved from the early days of infectious disease epidemiology and has been superseded by more recent models that are more applicable to chronic disease epidemiology, in which the cause of disease is generally multifactorial. The web of causation holds that a disease has no single, isolated cause. Hence, a study of physical activity and fitness as risk factors for a disease must consider how they interact with other potential causes of the disease. The strength of the web—namely, its acknowledgment that the causes of disease interact with each other—is also its weakness, because its complexity makes it hard to understand the etiology of disease and to predict health outcomes. The wheel is probably the most valid model of epidemiologic inquiry because it views the development of the host as intertwined with the environment, and it recognizes that the host develops from a genetic core that is modifiable to varying degrees by the biological, physical, and social environments to which the host is exposed.

Exercise scientists Claude Bouchard and Roy Shephard have integrated the traditional epidemiologic models to illustrate how the independent and interactive effects on health of heredity, habits other than physical activity, the physical environment, the social environment, and personal attributes might be conceptualized (Bouchard and Shephard 1994). Their model is presented in figure 2.2 and simplified in figure 2.3.

As shown in figures 2.2 and 2.3, heredity, or genetic factors, is directly associated with all

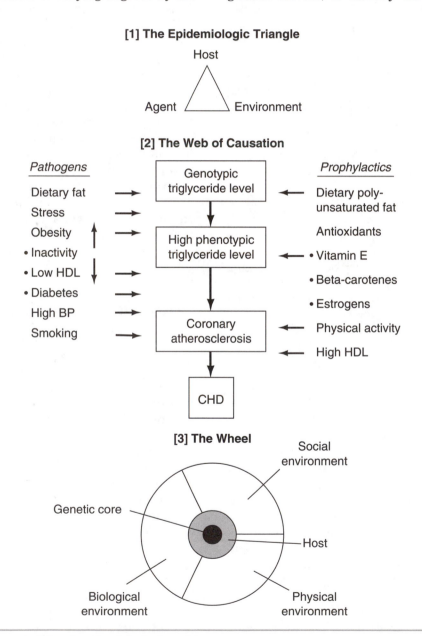

[1] The Epidemiologic Triangle

[2] The Web of Causation

[3] The Wheel

Figure 2.1   The three traditional epidemiological models.

Adapted from Mausner and Kramer 1985.

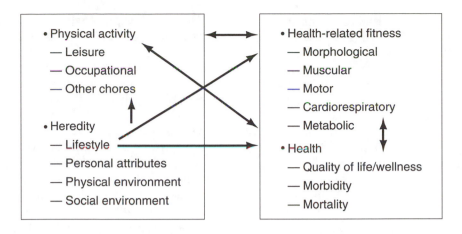

Figure 2.2 Plausible causal paths for physical activity, fitness, and health.

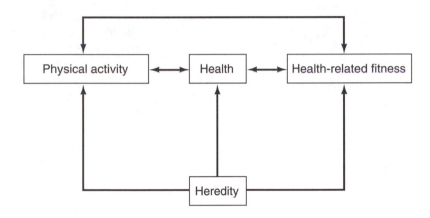

Figure 2.3 An integration of the traditional epidemiological models illustrates how the independent and interactive effects on health of heredity, habits other than physical activity, the physical environment, the social environment, and personal attributes might be conceptualized.

other parts of the model. Although we cannot alter genetic factors, at least at this point in time, it is important to be aware of the role that genetic factors might play in the association of physical activity and health. Humans differ widely in genetic makeup. For example, there appears to be as much variation in DNA sequence within each race as there is among the races. Given these circumstances, an equal state of health and of physical and mental well-being is unlikely to be achieved for all. Individuals of a particular genetic makeup are less susceptible to disease and disability than others. Genetic predisposition explains, at least in part, why we are not equally prone to hypertension, atherosclerosis, diabetes, osteoporosis, cancer, or heart attacks. Genetic factors also may play a significant role in determining an individual's level of physical activity and physical fitness (muscular strength,

aerobic capacity, etc.) and explain a major part of the difference in people's physiological response (e.g., body fat, cholesterol, blood pressure, aerobic capacity) to identical diets or exercise training programs.

There is equally wide variation in the physical and social environments to which people are exposed among and within societies. Those differences can be in climate, population density, natural resources, economy, educational level, and cultural values. All these factors can singly and collectively affect exposure to disease risk factors (including behaviors) and disease vulnerability. These influences are evidenced by the fact that only about 20% of the variation in people's physical activity and about 40% of the variation in their cardiorespiratory fitness is explainable by variation in **genotypes** (i.e., genetic inheritance). Moreover, even among monozygotic (i.e., identical) twins, biological adaptations to vigorous physical activity, including fitness changes, can vary by as much as 50% (Bouchard et al. 1994). Hence, even gene expression in response to physical activity is apparently influenced by the environment during the life span. On the other hand, although age, sex, and ethnicity are not strong influences on adaptations to physical activity, people's initial phenotypes (i.e., their observable **traits**) are major predictors of responses to exercise training for some variables (e.g., submaximal heart rate and blood pressure) but not others (e.g., maximal oxygen uptake and high-density lipoprotein cholesterol; Bouchard and Rankinen 2001).

Determining Cause in Epidemiologic Studies

The epidemiologic models previously described provide a framework for considering the association among variables in an attempt to determine cause and effect. In the context of epidemiology, causal association can be defined as an association between categories of events or characteristics in which an alteration in the frequency or quality of one category is followed by a change in the other category. To determine whether an observed association between a risk factor and disease is likely causal, it is first necessary to demonstrate that there is a statistical association between the risk factor and disease outcome. Even when a strong and statistically significant association between a risk factor and disease is demonstrated, there is always the possibility that the observed association is noncausal. Two issues, confounding and effect modification, can result in noncausal associations.

Confounding

Confounding is the confusion of the effect of the presumably causal variable under study with the effects of other extraneous variables so that all or part of the supposed causal effect of the "causal" variable on the dependent variable is actually explainable by the extraneous variables. For example, in men, baldness is associated with the risk of myocardial infarction; however, this is most likely not a causal association. Age increases both the likelihood of baldness and the risk of myocardial infarction; thus, age confounds the association between baldness and myocardial infarction. Con-

founding takes place when two or more potential risk factors co-occur in a group so that it is not possible to determine the independent effect of either risk factor. Said another way, if a physically active group of people were observed to have a lower rate of disease than a sedentary group but they also were younger and smoked less tobacco, it would not be possible to conclude that physical activity protected against disease independently of age and smoking. Rather, the higher rate of disease in the sedentary group might be explainable by older age and smoking, not by the group's low physical activity.

The possibility of confounding is higher in observational studies, which are common in physical activity epidemiology, than in randomized controlled trials because the random assignment of participants to groups in randomized trials reduces the likelihood that the comparison groups (e.g., exposed versus not exposed) differ with regards to a potential confounding variable.

For example, many observational studies have shown greater physical activity at baseline to be associated with lower risk of all-cause mortality. Does increased physical activity cause the lower mortality risk, or are more-active people generally in better health and therefore at lower risk of dying? Does overall health status confound the observed association between more physical activity and decreased mortality? Most well-conducted observational studies use statistical techniques to adjust, or attempt to adjust, for indicators of health status such as blood pressure, lipid levels, obesity, and cigarette smoking to determine whether the association of physical activity with morbidity or mortality risk has **independence** of confounders. However, the possibility that some confounding still plays a role in the observed association is open to question. It is possible that the measurement of **confounders** was imprecise or that potential confounders were not considered.

Nevertheless, many studies report that the association of physical activity and all-cause mortality still persists after adjustment for the measured confounders. However, this association may still be the result of confounding, as most studies do not measure all potential confounders. For example, other diseases that may affect both physical activity and mortality, such as diabetes or depression, are often not taken into consideration. This points to the difficulty for any single observational study to account for all potential confounders and therefore to provide definitive evidence that the apparent effect of physical activity in reducing risk is wholly independent of other possible explanations for the reduced risk. The accumulation of results of numerous investigations using different samples and measuring different confounding variables adds weight to a causal association between physical activity and chronic disease risk.

Effect Modification

In addition to confounding, effect modification, also called *interaction,* needs to be considered when evaluating the possibility of causal associations. Effect modification in epidemiology describes a situation where two or more risk factors modify one another's effects on an outcome. For dichotomous variables (variables with only two levels or categories, e.g., yes or no, sedentary or active), effect modification means that the effect of the exposure on the outcome depends on the presence of another variable. For example, the effect of the physical activity categories sedentary or active on the presence or absence of CHD might differ depending on some third factor, such as sex; physical activity might reduce the risk of disease among men but not in women. In such a case, sex would be termed an **effect modifier.** The effect modification of continuous variables can be evaluated by determining the extent to which the effect of exposure on outcome depends on the level of some other variable. For example, the effect of physical activity assessed by questionnaire on the risk for CHD may depend on the body mass index (BMI, body weight in kilograms divided by the square of height in meters). The risk of disease among the least active people might be greatest among those having the highest BMI. If so, BMI would be considered an effect modifier in the association between activity and CHD.

Determining the degree to which certain factors act as effect modifiers can provide important information for the development of preventive strategies. For example, if it were demonstrated that individuals with high BMIs are at higher risk of CHD only if they also are relatively inactive compared with those with normal or low BMIs, the evidence for effect modification might be sufficient to prompt interventions designed specifically to increase physical activity among individuals with high BMIs.

The potential for confounding and effect modification increases the difficulty of inter-

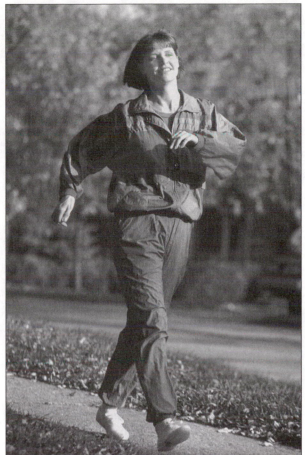

© Jim and Mary Whitmer

preting epidemiologic studies of the direct effects of physical activity on health. Age can be a confounder because of a direct association between age and increased risk for death and most chronic diseases. Therefore, to examine the association between physical activity and health outcomes, the effect of age needs to be removed. Age can also change the magnitude of risk associated with other variables. Thus, age is also considered an effect modifier. For example, the risk of CHD increases with age, increased blood pressure, and decreased levels of physical activity. But age is also associated with decreased physical activity and increased blood pressure. Therefore, to determine whether there is an association between physical activity and CHD risk, the effect of both age and blood pressure must be controlled. In epidemiologic studies, this type of control is typically done by statistical analysis. When you read and interpret information about the association of physical activity and health outcomes, it is important to be aware of the potential consequences of confounding (i.e., the confusion of two supposedly causal variables) and effect modification (i.e., the influence of a third variable on the strength or direction of the association between two other variables) and to determine whether these issues have been satisfactorily addressed.

Criteria for Causation

When a statistical association between a risk factor and a disease outcome can be demonstrated and the results of confounding and effect modification have been accounted for, there are several criteria that, if satisfied, increase the probability that the association is causal. These criteria can be traced to the work of John Stuart Mill, *A System of Logic: Ratiocination and Induction,* published in 1843, in which he discussed five Canons of Induction used to judge causal relationships: method of agreement, method of difference, joint method of agreement and difference, method residues, and the method of concomitant variation (Stebbing 1875). Applied to contemporary epidemiology, the following criteria are referred to as **Mill's canons.** If met, an observed association is more likely to be causal: (1) temporal sequence, (2) strength of association, (3) consistency, (4) dose response, and (5) biological plausibility.

Mill's Canons

1. **Temporal sequence:** Exposure to the risk factor must precede development of the disease with sufficient time to account for disease progression.

2. **Strength of association:** There is a large and clinically meaningful difference in disease risk between those exposed and those not exposed to the risk factor.

3. **Consistency:** The observed association is always observed if the risk factor is present (e.g., regardless of sex, race, age, or methods of measurement).

4. **Dose response:** The risk of disease associated with the risk factor is greater with stronger exposure to the risk factor.

5. **Biological plausibility:** The observed association is explainable by existing knowledge about possible biological mechanisms of the disease, which may be alterable (e.g., by physical activity).

The determination of a causal relationship in the absence of direct experimental evidence, as is often the case for the association of physical activity and health outcomes, is not easy, nor is it entirely objective. Individuals often have different interpretations of the available evidence. In this text we summarize and present, to the best of our ability, the evidence that physical activity and fitness have a causal association with major chronic diseases and injury.

Summary

This chapter on methods and concepts presented the rudimentary principles and skills of logical inquiry that epidemiologists use to study physical activity. Odds ratios, relative risks, and attributable risks help determine whether physical activity can reduce the rate of disease or death among people at risk. The research design used in an epidemiologic study—whether a cross-sectional, case–control, or cohort observational design or an experimental, randomized controlled trial—determines the strength of the inference that lower risk is explainable solely by physical activity or fitness and not by other confounding or effect-modifying factors. Ultimately, the strength of the evidence for concluding that there is a cause and an effect is judged by Mill's canons: temporal sequence, strength of association, consistency, dose–response relationship, and biological plausibility. This chapter provided the foundation for understanding how epidemiologists determine whether people's attributes or behavior influences their risk of disease and death. The next chapter on behavioral epidemiology discusses the definition and measurement of physical fitness and physical activity, the attributes and behavior central to physical activity epidemiology.

Bibliography

Bouchard, C., and T. Rankinen. 2001. Individual differences in response to regular physical activity. *Medicine and Science in Sports and Exercise* 33 (Suppl. 6): S446–S451.

Bouchard, C., and R.J. Shephard. 1994. *Physical activity, fitness, and health: International proceedings and consensus statement.* Champaign, IL: Human Kinetics.

Bouchard, C., A. Tremblay, J.P. Despres, G. Theriault, A. Nadeau, P.J. Lupien, S. Moorjani, D. Prudhomme, and G. Fournier. 1994. The response to exercise with constant energy intake in identical twins. *Obesity Research* 2: 400–410.

Caspersen, C.J. 1989. Physical activity epidemiology: Concepts, methods, and applications to exercise science. *Exercise and Sport Sciences Reviews* 17: 423–474.

Dean, A.G. 1999. Epi Info and Epi Map: Current status and plans for Epi Info 2000. *Journal of Public Health Management and Practice* 5 (4): 54–57.

Dean, A.G., J.A. Dean, D. Coulombier, K.A. Brendel, D.C. Smith, A.H. Burton, R.C. Dicker, K. Sullivan, R.F. Fagan, and T.B. Arner. 1996. *Epi Info, version 6.04a, a word processing, database, and statistics program for public health on IBM-compatible microcomputers.* Atlanta: Centers for Disease Control and Prevention.

Eaton, C.B., K.L. Lapane, C.E. Graber, A.R. Assaf, T.M. Lasater, and R.A. Carleton. 1995. Physical activity, physical fitness, and coronary heart disease risk factors. *Medicine and Science in Sports and Exercise* 27: 340–346.

Jekel, J.F., J.G. Elmore, and D.L. Katz. 1996. *Epidemiology, biostatistics and preventive medicine.* Philadelphia: Saunders.

MacMahon, B., and D. Trichopoulos. 1996. *Epidemiology: Principles and methods.* 2nd edition. Boston: Little, Brown.

Mausner, J., and S. Kramer. 1985. *Mausner and Bahn epidemiology: An introductory text.* 2nd edition. Philadelphia: Saunders.

Mittleman, M.A., M. Maclure, G.H. Tofler, J.B. Sherwood, R.J. Goldberg, and J.E. Mullen. 1993. Triggering of acute myocardial infarction by heavy exertion: Protection against triggering by regular exertion. *New England Journal of Medicine* 329: 1677–1683.

Paffenbarger, R.S. Jr. 1988. Contributions of epidemiology to exercise science and cardiovascular health. *Medicine and Science in Sports and Exercise* 20: 426–438.

Stebbing, W. 1875. *Analysis of Mr. Mill's system of logic.* New edition. London: Longmans, Green, and Co.

Szklo, M., F.J. Nieto, and F. Javier. 2000. *Epidemiology: Beyond the basics.* Gaithersburg, MD: Aspen.

Web Site

www.cdc.gov/epiinfo/. This site describes Epi Info, a series of programs for Microsoft® Windows® developed by the Centers for Disease Control and Prevention for use by public health professionals in conducting outbreak investigations and managing databases and statistics for public health surveillance (Dean 1999; Dean et al. 1996). Click Download to see further instructions for downloading Epi Info to a personal computer, or browse the Epi Info pages to learn more about the programs.

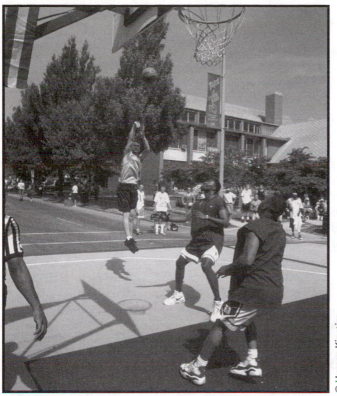
© Human Kinetics

Chapter 3

Measurement and Surveillance of Physical Activity and Fitness

The office of the scholar is to . . . guide men by showing them facts amidst appearances. He plies the slow, unhonored, and unpaid task of observation. . . . He is the world's eye.

—Ralph Waldo Emerson, 1837

Behavioral epidemiology is the observation and study of behaviors, including physical inactivity or sedentariness, that lead to disease or premature death and of the distribution of these behaviors. Thus, behavioral epidemiology encompasses two main features. The first is the study of relationships between behavior and disease, the traditional approach introduced in chapters 1 and 2. The second feature is the study of the behavior, its distribution in a population, and its determinants (Mason and Powell 1985). Once it is established, using epidemiologic methods, that a behavior appears causally linked with disease, injury, or early death, the next critical step is to determine how the behavior can be altered. In this way, behavioral epidemiology goes beyond traditional infectious disease epidemiology, which mainly is concerned with the containment of bacterial and viral contagion. Though traditional epidemiology is concerned with preventive measures, the emphasis is on environmental intervention (e.g., sewage disposal, inoculation programs for school children, etc). In behavioral epidemiology, the focus shifts to understanding behaviors that increase or decrease the risk of people developing the disease (e.g., hand washing or sharing hypodermic needles by drug abusers, which can spread diseases). Behavioral epidemiology is especially important for understanding and preventing chronic diseases that develop over periods of years largely as a result of people's habits. The discussion of behavioral epidemiology in this book focuses on who is physically active or inactive and why and on how health professionals and public policy makers can help the physically inactive to become active in ways that reduce chronic diseases and premature death and promote health. This chapter introduces a fundamental step in the application of behavioral epidemiology to physical activity, namely the measurement and **surveillance** of physical activity and fitness. Chapter 16 concludes this book by describing environmental and personal factors that are associated with physical activity and interventions designed to increase it.

> *••• Behavioral epidemiology is the study of behaviors, including physical inactivity or sedentariness, that lead to disease or premature death and of the distribution of these behaviors.*

Why Is Behavioral Epidemiology Important?

Until the middle of the 20th century, the major threat from disease was infectious contagion. For example, the great flu **epidemic** of 1918 killed 40,000,000 people worldwide, including 675,000 Americans, in just 11 months. Fears over such **pandemic** (i.e., an epidemic that spreads widely across a region or the world) catastrophes spurred growth in the field of epidemiology. Indeed, in 1927, the physician Wade Hampton Frost defined epidemiology as the science of the mass phenomena of infectious diseases. Similar concerns exist today about AIDS and deadly hemorrhagic diseases caused by viruses, such as the Ebola virus, which kills 80% of those infected. Infectious diseases remain a serious threat to public health, ranking as the third leading cause of death worldwide. Failure to maintain public sanitation and vaccination could lead to an exponential growth of death from infectious disease in a short period of time.

Despite the importance to public health of sustaining efforts to observe and control infectious and contagious diseases, the early definition of epidemiology no longer suffices. Noninfectious diseases are now the top causes of illness, disability, and death. Though early epidemiologists were concerned mainly about infectious contagions resulting directly from physical and chemical **pathogens** (e.g., bacteria and viruses that cause diseases that can spread to humans) arising from environmental conditions or contaminants, most infectious diseases are now controllable. Modern-day epidemiologists are equally concerned about chronic diseases. Chronic diseases may be partly caused by pathogens such as bacteria or viruses, but they are diseases that usually require many years to fully develop; their signs and symptoms manifest themselves usually in middle age or later. Their gradual adult, rather than congenital or adolescent, onset suggests that environmental factors other than direct exposure to pathogens are very important in determining the age of their onset and their severity. For example, non-insulin-dependent diabetes (i.e., type 2 diabetes) has traditionally been also called adult-onset diabetes. However, the increasing rate of type 2 diabetes among youth is reaching epidemic status in the United States and other developed nations probably because of increasing obesity linked to overeating and physical inactivity. Indeed, it is now known that about half the mortality from the top 10 leading causes of death in the United States can be traced directly or indirectly to behavior. Hence, it is now understood that certain behaviors, such as insufficient physical activity, can be pathogenic. Today, epidemiologists are as concerned with the prevention of behaviors that cause disease as with containing diseases once they occur. This is evidenced by the 1992 name change by the federal Centers for Disease Control, established in 1946, to the Centers for Disease Control and Prevention.

What Is Physical Activity?

Physical activity is defined as "any bodily movement produced by skeletal muscle that results in energy expenditure" (Caspersen, Powell, and Christenson 1985); it includes occupational work, chores, leisure activity, playing sports, and **exercise** that is planned for fitness or health purposes. Physical activity is the most variable component of an individual's total daily energy expenditure, which consists of basal metabolic rate (i.e., the energy needed to maintain the body at rest) and the thermic effect of food (i.e., the energy required to digest food) in addition to physical activity. The high degree of both intra- and interindividual variability in daily physical activity makes the assessment of this behavior in free-living populations a very difficult task. Without a valid and reliable measure of daily physical activity, epidemiologists would be unable to evaluate the association between physical activity and the risk for chronic disease. In addition, measures of physical activity are needed for the **descriptive epidemiology** of physical activity (i.e., the assessment of variation in physical activity by age, sex, ethnicity, health status, and geographic location), for surveillance systems that track population trends in physical activity over time, and for assessing mediators of physical activity and the effectiveness of interventions designed to increase the level of physical activity.

Measures of Physical Activity

Several potential methods are available for physical activity assessment, including occupational classification, behavioral observation, physiological markers (heart rate, doubly labeled water), dietary intake, motion sensors, and self-report questionnaires. Prior to 1970, 20 of the 24 epidemiologic studies of the association between physical activity and coronary heart disease used occupational classification as the measure of physical activity. Although these studies provided interesting information on the potential association between physical activity and heart disease, they ignored the influence of leisure-time physical activity. It was not until the mid-1960s that Dr. Henry J. Montoye quantified both the occupational and leisure-time physical activity habits recalled by participants using a questionnaire interview in the Tecumseh (Michigan) Community Health Study (Montoye 1975). Since that time, about 50 physical activity questionnaires have been developed.

Before discussing the specifics of physical activity questionnaires, it is important to consider the problem of establishing the validity of these instruments. Using physical activity questionnaires, epidemiologists can obtain data on the physical activity habits of a large number of people in a very cost- and time-efficient manner. However, how do we know that the questionnaire provides a valid assessment of physical activity? The problem in answering this question is that there is no acceptable criterion measure or gold standard with which to compare questionnaire results. Though direct observation of behavior might provide such a criterion, it is impractical, and socially unacceptable, to implement objective round-the-clock surveillance of people. Therefore, epidemiologists must be satisfied with assessing questionnaire validity using imperfect measures of physical activity, such as dietary intake, physiological variables, such as doubly labeled water and heart rate monitoring, motion sensors, direct or indirect **calorimetry,** or using other variables influenced by physical activity, such as body fat, blood pressure, blood lipids, muscular strength and endurance, or aerobic power.

The goal of most physical activity questionnaires is to estimate the energy expenditure attributable to participation in specific types of physical activity, such as household, occupational, or leisure activity. Energy expenditure in kilocalories or kilojoules (1 kcal is the amount of heat required to increase the temperature of 1 kg of water 1 °C; 1 kcal = 4.2 kJ) can be accurately measured using direct or indirect calorimetry. An average daily energy expenditure of about 4.3 kcal/min or greater is frequently used to classify individuals as physically active in epidemiologic studies. Direct calorimetry involves the measurement of heat production of an individual in a sealed, insulated chamber. This technique is highly accurate (<1% error); however, the engineering problems associated with developing and maintaining a direct calorimeter are substantial, and the size of the chamber limits the potential for physical activity. Therefore, this technique is infrequently used in the development or validation of physical activity questionnaires. **Indirect calorimetry** involves estimating energy expenditure from oxygen consumption and carbon dioxide production by applying the caloric equivalent of oxygen: 5 kcal per liter of oxygen consumed. Laboratory systems to measure energy expenditure by indirect calorimetry have been in use for decades; however, in the recent past, light, portable systems, such as the Cosmed K4b[2], capable of measuring oxygen during unrestricted physical activity outside the laboratory have become available. These devices are particularly useful for assessing the energy costs of specific activities that can be used in developing scoring algorithms for physical activity questionnaires and for assessing the validity of a variety of motion-sensing devices as measures of physical activity.

TABLE 3.1 CHARACTERISTICS OF PHYSICAL ACTIVITY ASSESSMENT PROCEDURES

| Activity assessment procedure | GROUP | | STUDY COSTS[1] | | SUBJECT COSTS[1] | | | Probability of interfering[1] | ACCEPTABILITY | | Activity specifics |
	Size	Age	Money	Time	Time	Effort		Personal	Social	
Calorimetry:											
Direct	Single	Infant–elderly	VH	VH	VH	H–VH	H–VH	No	No	Yes
Indirect	Single–small	Young adult–elderly	H–VH	VH	VH	M–VH	H–VH	No	No	Yes
Job classification	Large	Employed only	L–M	L–M	L	L	L	Yes	Yes	?
Surveys:											
Indirect calorimetry diary	Single–small	Young adult–elderly	M–H	M–H	M–H	M–H	VH	No	No	Yes
Task-specific diary	Small–large	Adolescent–elderly	L–M	L–M	H–VH	VH	VH	?	Yes	Yes
Recall questionnaire	Small–large	Adolescent–elderly	L–M	L–M	M–H	M–H	L	Yes	Yes	Yes
Quantitative history	Small–large	Adolescent–elderly	L–M	L–M	L–M	L–M	L	Yes	Yes	Yes
Physiological markers:											
Cardiorespiratory fitness	Small–large	Child–elderly	M–VH	M–H	M–H	M–VH	L	?	?	No
Doubly labeled water	Single–small	Infant–elderly	H–VH	M–VH	M	M	L–H	Yes	Yes	No
Behavioral observation	Single–small	Infant–elderly	H–VH	H–VH	H–VH	L–H	L–VH	?	?	Yes
Mechanical and electronic monitors:											
Heart rate	Single–small	Infant–elderly	H–VH	M–VH	M–H	M–H	L–M	Yes	Yes	No
Stabilometer	Single–small	Infant	M–H	M	H–VH	L	L	Yes	Yes	No
Horizontal time monitor	Single–small	Child–elderly	M–H	M	H–VH	L–M	L–M	?	Yes	No
Pedometer	Single–large	Child–elderly	L–M	L	L	L	L–M	Yes	Yes	No
Gait assessment	Single–small	Child–elderly	H–VH	M–VH	L–M	M–H	L–M	?	Yes	No
Electronic motion sensor	Single–large	Child–elderly	M–H	L	L	L	L–M	Yes	Yes	No
Accelerometer	Single–large	Infant–elderly	L–M	L–M	L	L	L–M	Yes	Yes	No
Dietary measures	Large	Adolescent–elderly	M–H	M	M–H	M–H	L	Yes	Yes	No

[1] L = low, M = moderate, H = high, VH = very high, ? = unclear whether the approach has personal or social acceptability

From LaPorte et al, 1985.

Currently, three methods of physical activity assessment—doubly labeled water, heart rate monitoring, and motion sensors—are commonly used both as measures of physical activity in small-scale studies and as criterion measures for validation of physical activity questionnaires. Heart rate monitors and motion sensors are the most popular because they are accurate and feasible to use. Doubly labeled water is expensive and not very feasible for most applications, but it is the most accurate and unobtrusive measure of energy expenditure that can be used in natural settings. The following sections provide a detailed description of these methods. Table 3.1 rates methods by cost, interference with normal activity, acceptability, and whether they measure specific features of physical activity, including type, **intensity,** duration, frequency, and timing.

> ••• *A good measure of physical activity provides reliable and valid information on specific features of physical activity, including type, intensity, duration, frequency, and timing.*

Doubly Labeled Water

At the present time, the **doubly labeled water (DLW)** technique is the best overall measure of total daily energy expenditure (Schoeller 1999). This technique was developed by Lifson and colleagues at the University of Minnesota based on their observation that the oxygen atoms exhaled in carbon dioxide and those in body water were in isotopic equilibrium (Lifson, Gordon, and McClintock 1955). Thus, it was assumed that the kinetics of water elimination and respiration were linked. To use this method, the participant drinks a measured amount of water that has been labeled with stable isotopes of hydrogen and oxygen ($^2H^1H^{18}O$). These isotopes are tracers that transform the body's water into a virtual metabolic recorder that integrates H_2O output and CO_2 production. Urine samples are obtained over a 7- to 14-day period, and the overall energy expenditure over the evaluation period can be estimated from CO_2 production without having to collect respiratory gases. When the labeled water is drunk, the two isotopes are rapidly distributed in body water and start to be eliminated from the body. The ^2H is eliminated as ^2HHO and is a measure of water flux. The ^{18}O is eliminated from the body as both $H_2^{18}O$ and $C^{18}O_2$ and is

thus a measure of water and carbon dioxide flux. The difference between these elimination rates is, thus, an estimate of carbon dioxide flux, as shown in figure 3.1. Using the equations of indirect calorimetry and assuming a value for the respiratory quotient (RQ), energy expenditure can be estimated by the known oxidative cost, and hence caloric expenditure, of burning fat, carbohydrate, and protein. This is explained later in this chapter in the section on lipid metabolism as a component of physical fitness. In addition, assumptions regarding the amount of total body water and the amount of body water lost in the evaporation of sweat and through the respiratory tract must be made.

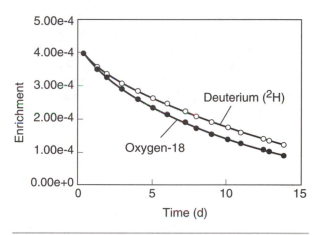

Figure 3.1   Doubly labeled water. The Δ between slopes of ^2H and ^{18}O = CO_2 production, an indirect measure of metabolic rate, which can be converted to calories of Joules based on the chemical composition of food being oxidized (which affects the energy equivalence of each liter of CO_2 produced).

Adapted, by permission, from A.M. Prentice, 1990, *International atomic energy agency NAHRES-4, IAEA, Vienna (1990)* (Lausanne, Switzerland: I/D/E/C/G International Dietary Energy Consultancy).

The DLW method was validated first under laboratory conditions in mice (McClintock and Lifson 1957) and was later shown to be feasible for use with humans (Lifson et al. 1975; Schoeller and van Santen 1982). Theoretically, the coefficient of variation of the DLW method is between 4% and 8%; however, the error is exaggerated when normal metabolism is disrupted, which can easily occur in individuals in uncontrolled field settings.

The DLW technique has the advantage of using nonradioactive isotopes, and it allows the assessment of energy expenditure over a relatively long time period (one to two weeks) in an unobtrusive manner. The major disadvantages are cost (about $750 per person), the need for expensive equipment (ratio mass spectrometer) for analysis of urine samples, and the lack of direct information on energy expenditure from physical activity, its specific components, or the pattern of energy expenditure over time. Although the DLW technique is often considered the most accurate measure of daily energy expenditure in free-living humans, a number of sources of error with this technique must be considered (Prentice 1990). For example, a change in body water, which can be estimated from changes in body weight, increases the error in estimated total energy expenditure. Approximately 4% of the ^2H molecules and 1% of the ^{18}O molecules are incorporated into nonaqueous tissue, which results in an overestimation of their dilution space in body water. Deuterium isotopes are lost as vapor at a slower rate than ^1H molecules, which can result in approximately a 2.5% error in estimated energy expenditure. Approximately 2% of the isotopes are lost in feces rather than in urine. Each variation in RQ of 0.01 from an assumed value of 0.85 results in a 1% error in estimates. This can be especially problematic in individuals who consume large amounts of alcohol, because hydrogen used in the metabolism of ethanol reduces the difference in the elimination rates of ^2H and ^{18}O, which results in an underestimation of energy expenditure.

Since the mid-1980s, use of the DLW technique has become more common in studies of human energy expenditure (Westerterp et al. 1984, 1988; Westerterp 1998); however, its primary value is as a validation measure against which to compare other physical activity assessment methods. It provides the best measure of total energy expenditure that can be obtained while people live naturally outside a laboratory. However, the high cost of the ^{18}O tracer isotope and the need for a ratio mass spectrometer to determine its rate of elimination in the urine make the DLW method infeasible in epidemiologic studies with large numbers of participants.

Heart Rate Monitors

A variety of heart rate monitors are currently available commercially. The most useful heart rate monitors measure the electrical activity of the heart, typically by attaching a transmitter with chest electrodes to a chest strap that transmits the electrocardiographic signal to a digital wrist-watch receiver. A computer chip in the wristwatch uses the R-R interval (the period of the heart beat measured as the time difference in milliseconds between successive R-waves of the electrocardiogram) to calculate the minute-by-minute heart rate and stores this information in a memory cell, which can be downloaded to a personal computer for analysis. Studies have indicated that this type of heart rate monitor provides a highly accurate measure of heart rate when compared with the heart rate determined from the conventional hard-wired electrocardiogram.

However, the conversion of heart rate to a measure of energy expenditure, which is based on a linear association between heart rate and oxygen consumption, is problematic. Typically, a linear regression is calculated between heart rate and oxygen consumption measured during exercise on a treadmill or cycle ergometer, sometimes along with heart rate and oxygen consumption measured during sitting, standing, or other typical daily physical activities. The mean heart rate during daily activities is then used with the laboratory-developed regression equation to estimate oxygen consumption and thus energy expenditure. Considerable error in energy expenditure estimates can occur because the average daily heart rate is typically at the low end of the heart rate–oxygen consumption calibration, where the association between those variables is not linear. The need to develop calibrations for each participant makes the use of heart rate to estimate energy expenditure both time-consuming and expensive and thus impractical for large-scale studies. In addition, the heart rate–oxygen consumption relationship varies with posture, environmental temperature, emotional state, type of muscular contraction (static or dynamic, small or large muscle mass), level of cardiovascular fitness, and fatigue, all of which are potential sources of error. It has been suggested that the difference between an individual's resting heart rate and mean daily heart rate may provide a useful index of physical activity. The utility of heart rate monitors may be in assessing the pattern of physical activity over the course of a day to assess the intensity of physical activity.

Motion Sensors

The pedometer, a device for counting steps, was first conceived by Leonardo da Vinci over 500 years ago. Research using older, gear-driven, mechanical pedometers indicated that these devices show poor validity and **reliability** as a step counter, even under highly controlled laboratory conditions (Gayle, Montoye, and Philpot 1977; Washburn, Chin, and Montoye 1980). However, research on the reliability and validity of newer electronic pedometers, such as the Digi-Walker (manufactured by Yamax, Inc., Tokyo), is more encouraging. For example Bassett et al. (1996) reported that the Digi-Walker recorded the number of both left and right steps during outdoor walking in 20 adults with only a trivial 1% overestimate of actual steps taken. Similarly, Welk et al. (2000) showed that the mean step counts from the Digi-Walker during both walking and running on a treadmill and a track by 31 adult volunteers were within 3% to 5% of the actual values. However, in the same sample, Welk et al. (2000) reported a rather low correlation ($r = 0.34$) between the average daily step count over a one-week period and average daily energy expenditure assessed by the Stanford Seven-Day Physical Activity Recall Questionnaire. When participants removed the Digi-Walker during all structured vigorous and moderate physical activity, the correlation between the step counts and energy expenditure estimated by the recall questionnaire was near zero ($r = -0.07$). In general, there are some concerns about the interunit reliability of these devices. Also, currently available pedometers do not have a time stamp or data storage capacity; thus, participants must record numbers from the devices at the beginning and end of the day. It has been suggested that pedometers may serve as a useful criterion measure for validating self-report estimates of walking and as motivational devices for interventions designed to increase walking.

The development of portable **accelerometers** as physical activity assessment devices was prompted by laboratory studies conducted in the late 1950s that suggested an association between the integral of vertical acceleration with respect to time and energy expenditure (Brouha and Smith 1958; Montoye, Servais, and Webster 1986). Montoye and colleagues at the University of Wisconsin–Madison were the first to use this principle to develop the prototype for a portable accelerometer later marketed under the name Caltrac. The Caltrac, like most portable accelerometers, uses a transducer, made of two layers of piezoceramic material with a brass center layer. When the body accelerates, the transducer, mounted on a cantilever beam, bends, producing an electric charge proportional to the force exerted. An internal computer chip integrates the

area under the acceleration–deceleration curve over a defined time interval, stores that value in computer memory, and resets the integrator.

Though pedometers are simply event counters, portable accelerometers, designed to be worn on a belt at the waist, provide a measure of both frequency and intensity of movement. Currently available portable accelerometers have the advantage of collecting and storing data sequentially over time so that the pattern of physical activity over a day or a number of days can be assessed. The disadvantages of these devices include their cost (approximately $300 to $500 per unit), their unsuitability for aquatic activities, and their unresponsiveness to static activity or activities that involve minimal movement of the body's center of gravity, such as rowing or cycling. Despite these limitations, portable accelerometers are a useful addition to the methodology of physical activity assessment.

The Caltrac, unlike the newer generation of portable accelerometers, does not store data in a time sequence but provides only an estimate of total physical activity in a given time period. A number of studies, in both laboratory and field settings, have shown Caltrac readings to be significantly associated with energy expenditure measured by indirect calorimetry during walking and running on level surfaces ($r = 0.68$ to 0.94) and with energy expenditure during daily activities measured by doubly labeled water over a seven-day period. The lack of data storage capability, the rather large size, and poor quality control in manufacturing have led researchers away from using the Caltrac to using more sophisticated portable accelerometers, such as the one made by Computer Science and Applications, Inc. (CSA, in Shalimar, Florida), the Biotrainer, and the Tritrac.

The CSA Model 7164 portable accelerometer (now marketed as the Actigraph by Manufacturer's Technology, Inc., in Fort Walton Beach, Florida) is a small ($5.1 \times 3.8 \times 1.5$ cm, 43 g), single-plane portable accelerometer that uses a piezoelectric transducer. Data can be downloaded via an optical interface to the serial port of a personal computer for analysis. The investigator can set the start time and data collection interval. The Actigraph accelerometer can store minute-by-minute data for up to 22 days.

Studies have indicated moderate associations between the Actigraph accelerometer's counts per minute and energy expenditure measured by indirect calorimetry during both treadmill and overground walking and running at increasing speeds (r = 0.66 to 0.82; Hendelman et al. 2000; Melanson and Freedson 1995). Like all portable accelerometers, however, the Actigraph accelerometer's counts per minute do not reflect increases in energy cost due to increased grade. The association between Actigraph accelerometer readings and energy expenditure during other types of physical activity, such as housecleaning, golf, and yard work, are lower (r = 0.59; Hendelman et al. 2000; Welk et al. 2000).

The Biotrainer (manufactured by IM Systems, Baltimore, Maryland) is a single-plane accelerometer similar in size to the Actigraph accelerometer, while the Tritrac (made by Reining International, Madison, Wisconsin) is a three-plane accelerometer that is considerably larger than the others (170 g). Welk et al. (2000) compared Actigraph accelerometer, Biotrainer, and Tritrac output with energy expenditure measured by indirect calorimetry from 52 adults who completed two 30-min activity scenarios, including treadmill walking or jogging and simulated lifestyle activities. The correlation between accelerometer readings and energy expenditure was higher for treadmill activity (mean r = 0.86) than for lifestyle activities (mean r = 0.55). Correlations among the Actigraph accelerometer, Biotrainer, and Tritrac were high for both treadmill (r = 0.86) and lifestyle activity (r = 0.70), suggesting that similar information is obtained from all three accelerometers. In theory, a multiplane accelerometer should provide a better estimate of body movement and thus energy expenditure; however, recent studies (e.g., Welk et al. 2000; Hendelman et al. 2000) have shown little advantage to using the larger and more complex three-plane Tritrac accelerometer over smaller and less complex single-plane accelerometers (such as the Actigraph and the Biotrainer).

In the future, the use of motion sensors in epidemiologic research will most likely increase. As the price of this technology declines, the feasibility of monitoring a large number of individuals over several days will increase. In the meantime, portable accelerometers will continue to be a useful criterion measure for the validation of self-reported physical activity instruments.

To provide a better understanding of the dose–response relationship between physical activity intensity and chronic disease risk, better self-report measures of physical activity intensity must be developed. Heart rate monitoring and portable accelerometers have been suggested as criterion measures for assessing the intensity of daily physical activity. Several investigators have attempted to define cut points for Actigraph accelerometer counts per minute that correspond to various levels of activity measured in metabolic equivalents, or **METs;** however, the results of these studies have not been encouraging. For example, activity intensity of 3 METs or greater varied from 191 to 1,952 Actigraph accelerometer counts per minute, a 10-fold difference between reports! Further work is needed to more clearly define these cut points for activity intensity and to clearly delineate the physical activity characteristics for which the cut points are valid. Technologies such as global positioning systems and body-mounted cameras are also beginning to be used for physical activity assessment. New technologies will provide researchers additional options for future work on the validation of self-report instruments to assess physical activity.

Physical Activity Questionnaires

The most practical and often-used method of assessing physical activity in epidemiologic studies is self-report physical activity questionnaires or interviews. This method allows researchers to obtain physical activity information from a large number of individuals in a time- and cost-efficient manner. Since the early 1970s, over 30 survey instruments have been developed for physical activity assessment, including a new International Physical Activity Questionnaire (IPAQ) developed to permit standardized measurement of physical activity across nations (Booth 2000). Pereira et al. (1997), Montoye et al. (1996), and Washburn and Montoye (1986) published descriptions of survey instruments and information on their reliability and validity. These questionnaires differ on several important factors, such as the time period over which activity is assessed (from the past week to the respondent's lifetime), type of activity assessed (leisure, household, transportation, occupation), length of the questionnaire, administration mode (interview or self-administered), and outcome measurement (e.g., kilocalories, MET-hours, unitless score). Three questionnaires are commonly used in epidemiology research: the Minnesota Leisure Time Physical Activity Questionnaire (MLTPAQ), the Harvard Alumni/Paffenbarger Physical Activity Survey, and the Stanford Seven-Day Physical Activity Recall Interview.

Minnesota Leisure Time Physical Activity Questionnaire

The MLTPAQ is an interview-administered instrument that asks respondents to recall their participation in a list of leisure-time physical activities over the past year. Respondents are asked to provide the number of months, average number of times per month, and the average amount of time spent on each occasion of each activity reported. The outcome is scored as an activity metabolic index per week based on MET values associated with each reported activity. A number of studies have indicated reasonable validity and reliability for this instrument. Physical activity assessed by the MLTPAQ has been associated with reduced risk of coronary heart disease in two reports from the Multiple Risk Factor Intervention Trial (Leon et al. 1987; Leon and Connett 1991).

Harvard Alumni/Paffenbarger Physical Activity Survey

This instrument was designed for a study of the association of physical activity habits and chronic disease risk in a population of Harvard University alumni (Paffenbarger, Wing, and Hyde 1978). The time frame can range from the past week to several past years. The survey is brief and contains the following items: "How many city blocks do you normally walk each day? How many flights of stairs do you climb up each day? List any sports or recreation you have actively participated in during the past year." Values in kilocalories are assigned to walking, stair climbing, and recreational activity and summed to obtain a score in kilocalories per week. Physical activity assessed with this survey has been associated with reduced risk for chronic disease in the Harvard alumni population (Paffenbarger, Hyde, et al. 1993; Lee, Hsieh, and Paffenbarger 1995; Lee and Paffenbarger 2000; Lee, Sesso, and Paffenbarger 2000; Sesso, Paffenbarger, and Lee 2000).

Stanford Seven-Day Physical Activity Recall Interview

This instrument was designed for use in the Stanford Five-City Project (Sallis et al. 1985; Blair et al. 1985). It is an interviewer-administered survey that requests information on sleep and physical activity, such as aerobic exercise, work-related activity, gardening, walking, and leisure-time physical activity of moderate intensity or greater, over the past seven days. Respondents are shown a list of possible activities in each category. The amount of time remaining each day after accounting for activities of moderate intensity or greater is assumed to have been spent performing light-intensity activity. The outcome is expressed in kilocalories per kilogram (or simply kilocalories if the respondent's body weight is known) per week or per day.

An important issue to consider when evaluating the epidemiologic literature on the association between physical activity and health outcomes is the physical activity assessment method that was used. Did the investigators use an instrument with established validity and reliability for the type of sample under study? If not, do the authors provide any evidence for the validity and reliability of the instrument that was used? Many large epidemiologic studies that provide physical activity and health information were designed to evaluate other health risk factors; physical activity was only of secondary interest in many such studies, and thus the physical activity assessment methods were often less than optimal and sometimes of poorly established validity and reliability. For example, the Physicians' Health Study was a randomized, double-blind, placebo-controlled trial designed to determine whether aspirin in low doses decreases the risk of coronary heart disease and whether beta-carotene decreases the risk of both coronary heart disease and cancer. Physical activity in this study was assessed by the question, "How often do you exercise vigorously enough to work up a sweat?" Response categories were "daily," "5 to 6 times/week," "2 to 4 times/week," "once/week," "1 to 3 times/month," or "rarely/never." There is some evidence for the validity of this item as an indicator of physical activity level (Siconolfi et al. 1985; Washburn et al. 1990), and activity assessed with "sweat" questions has been associated with health outcomes (Manson et al. 1992). However, this item assesses a very specific type of physical activity in which only a small and highly select segment of the population may engage. The Nurses' Health Study is a prospective study begun in 1976 of health and lifestyle factors in 121,700 female registered nurses. In addition to other types of leisure-time physical activity, respondents are asked to report the average amount of time spent in walking or hiking outdoors per week during the past year and to estimate their usual walking pace as easy or casual, average, brisk, or very brisk. The validity and reliability of self-reports of walking distance and speed have not been established.

> ••• *Self-reports of physical activity are the most feasible method for measuring physical activity in national surveys and surveillance systems. Objective measures, such as motion sensors, heart rate monitors, and doubly labeled water, can estimate different components of physical activity and are commonly used to validate self-report measures.*

There are currently a number of well-established **physical activity surveys** for individuals of all ages, from adolescents to adults over 65 years old. However, physical activity surveys specifically for women and ethnic minorities or to assess specific aspects of physical activity that may be related to health outcomes, such as high-load weight-bearing activities or activities that increase muscular strength, have yet to be validated.

It is generally thought that individuals tend to overestimate participation in vigorous activities and underestimate participation in light- to moderate-intensity activities (Sallis and Saelens 2000). Further work needs to be done to enhance recall of physical activity intensity on self-report measures so that the amount and intensity of physical activity required to reduce chronic disease risk can be determined.

What Is Physical Fitness?

Physical fitness is an attribute that has a genetic basis but is also sensitive to changes in type and amount of physical activity, especially as people age. It is important to measure fitness both as an outcome of physical activity and as a **moderator** or mediator of physical activity's effect on disease morbidity and mortality and injury. The measurement of fitness should become an important part of surveillance systems that track physical activity and risks for disease or injury. Defining physical fitness is a harder task than one might first think. The World Health Organization has defined fitness as "the ability to perform muscular work satisfactorily." That definition does not specify the ways that physical, social, and psychological circumstances can vary to determine what is satisfactory, nor does it acknowledge that several abilities exist, rather than a single overall ability. Physical fitness is better understood by defining the specific components that can be measured and the circumstances in which those components relate

to bodily function and health or reduced disease. According to scientific consensus from the Second International Conference on Physical Activity, Fitness, and Health (Bouchard, Shephard, and Stephens 1994), the components of **health-related physical fitness,** listed in table 3.2, can be categorized as morphological, muscular, motor, cardiorespiratory, and metabolic.

Fitness can be classified as performance related when the ability to perform (e.g., competitive sports, military maneuvers, or occupational work) is considered. Tests of **performance-related fitness** are designed to measure psychomotor skills, maximal and submaximal cardiorespiratory power, muscular strength, power and endurance in the limbs and trunk for propulsion, body size, and body composition. High scores on

---

TABLE 3.2   THE COMPONENTS OF HEALTH-RELATED FITNESS

Morphological component
Body mass for height
Body composition
Subcutaneous fat distribution
Abdominal visceral fat
Bone density
Flexibility
Muscular component
Power
Strength
Endurance
Motor component
Agility
Balance
Coordination
Speed of movement
Cardiorespiratory component
Submaximal exercise capacity
Maximal aerobic power
Heart functions
Lung functions
Blood pressure
Metabolic component
Glucose tolerance
Insulin sensitivity
Lipid and lipoprotein metabolism
Substrate oxidation characteristics

Reprinted, by permission, from C. Bouchard, R.J. Shephard, and T. Stephens, 1994, *Physical activity, fitness, and health: International proceedings and consensus statement* (Champaign, IL: Human Kinetics), 81.

these tests depend on genetic endowment as well as good nutrition and high motivation to train and perform maximally during the testing. Measures of performance-related fitness show only a limited relationship to health, with the exceptions of cardiorespiratory capacity and body composition.

Health-related fitness components are more easily improved by regular physical activity and more directly relate to health. In addition to maximal cardiorespiratory power and body composition, which are important for both performance and health, health-related fitness components include body mass for height, subcutaneous fat distribution, abdominal visceral fat, bone density, strength and endurance of the muscles in the abdomen and low back, heart and lung functions, blood pressure, glucose and insulin metabolism, blood lipoproteins, and the ratio of lipid to carbohydrate oxidation.

Morphological Component

Many population-based studies have found associations between disease or death rates and measures of body size, shape, and composition. Understanding these associations is important for evaluating the biological plausibility that increased physical activity or physical fitness decreases rates of disease and death.

Fatness

The human body is governed by the first law of thermodynamics, that is, the principle of conservation of energy. Hence, changes in a person's body fat mass are determined by the balance between energy intake from food and energy expenditure, which results from basal or resting cell metabolism, the thermic effect of digestion, and physical activity. The amount of energy released by the body can be expressed in absolute terms (in kilojoules or kilocalories) or as a ratio relative to body mass and the estimated surface area of the body (e.g., per kilogram of body mass or fat-free mass). The relationship of body mass with fatness is most commonly expressed as Quetelet's body mass index (BMI; body mass in kilograms divided by height in meters squared). A high BMI is a risk factor for all-cause mortality and increases risk for high blood pressure, high **triglycerides,** high cholesterol, impaired glucose tolerance, and high insulin levels. A BMI from 20 to 25 is considered normal or desirable for young to middle-aged adults. A very low BMI increases risk for all-cause death, but it is not clear that the risk is independent from smoking or wasting effects associated with disease. Most

population studies have defined overweight as a BMI exceeding 27 for males and 28 for females, because those levels are associated with a doubling of risk for all-cause death. New standards define overweight and obesity as a BMI exceeding 25 and 30, respectively, for both men and women. For children, overweight is defined as a BMI above the 95th percentile for age; the 85th percentile marks at-risk for overweight.

It is important to distinguish *overweight,* indicating high total mass, from *overfat,* indicating that a high percentage of total mass is fat. Proportions of constituents that comprise fat-free body mass are about 73% water, 7% mineral, 19% to 20% protein, and less than 1% carbohydrate. These proportions vary little among people. In contrast, the rest of body mass is fat, which varies widely and commonly comprises 30 to 60% of total body mass in people who are obese. The association between increased risk for disease and death and BMI is assumed to be because BMI estimates percent body fat accurately to within about ±5% in 7 of every 10 people in the population. Nonetheless, the use of BMI as an index of fatness is not appropriate among athletes or otherwise well-conditioned people who have a large fat-free body mass, or among frail elderly or pregnant women.

Population-based studies that measure percent body fat and its association with disease or death have not been conducted, but clinical studies with small groups have shown that percent body fat and total fat mass are significantly correlated with high blood pressure and high blood levels of triglycerides, cholesterol, and insulin.

The distribution of fat mass throughout the body is another risk factor for cardiovascular disease

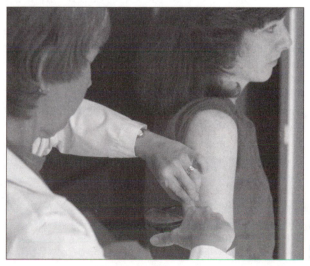

© Tom Pantages

and death and for type 2 or non-insulin-dependent diabetes mellitus (NIDDM). A concentration of regional fat predominantly on the trunk is more common among men and is referred to as an android pattern, or apple shape. A concentration of regional fat predominantly on the hips is more common among women and is referred to as a gynoid pattern, or pear shape. Based on girth measurements, waist-to-hip ratios of 0.85 or lower for women and 0.95 or lower for men are regarded as normal in terms of health risk. In both men and women, waist-to-hip ratios exceeding those values are associated with high blood pressure, insulin resistance, elevated blood insulin levels, high blood triglycerides, and high cholesterol.

The elevated risk for premature death posed by upper-body fat can be partly explained by fat cells in the abdomen that drain into the portal circulation to the liver, thus affecting insulin levels and the metabolism of glucose, triglycerides, and cholesterol.

Bone Mass

Bone mass is typically measured by the density of mineral per area of bone (in grams per centimeter squared) using **dual X-ray absorptiometry (DXA)**, a special X-ray scan. The potential maximal bone mineral density seems to be determined by young adulthood and peaks in women from ages 30 to 40 years and in men from ages 40 to 50. After those ages, new bone is formed at a slower rate than old bone is absorbed by the body, leading to bone involution, which is a risk factor for developing clinical osteoporosis. Aside from body deformities, the main health problem resulting from osteoporosis is increased risk of fractures associated with falls among the elderly. Risk factors for osteoporosis include inherited susceptibility (80% of the cases are older women, especially white women), decreased estrogen levels (usually after menopause or in young women who have amenorrhea), low dietary intake of calcium, and a low level of physical activity. Bone mineral content is higher in people with a high fat-free body mass and is increased by weight-bearing and resistance exercises, most specifically in the body areas most used during those exercises. The effects of physical activity on bone mass are discussed in chapter 10.

Flexibility

Flexibility is generally defined as the range of motion at a specific joint or linked joints during both passive and dynamic movements. Flexibility is determined by the structure of bone and its surface, including cartilage, and the soft tissues around the articulating surfaces of the joint. As a measure of physical fitness, flexibility is usually distinguished from the laxity of a joint, which is a measure of joint instability governed largely by the tightness of ligaments. Flexibility for fitness is improved mainly by stretching muscles, their surrounding connective tissues, and tendons. The loss or gain of flexibility is very specific to each joint and its customary range of motion.

Muscular Component

Muscular strength, power, and **endurance** are the three main features of muscular fitness that are most related to physical performance and health. In sedentary men and women, a marked loss of fat-free body mass accompanies aging. This wasting is largely the result of lack of use of muscles and contributes to loss of mobility. In the frail elderly, important activities of daily living—such as lifting objects from the floor or over the head, carrying groceries, or rising out of a chair or bed—become impossible. Even a moderate amount of muscular fitness permits a person to engage in daily chores or leisure-time recreational activities with greater endurance, less subjective fatigue, and better circulation to exercising muscles. Maintaining muscular fitness in the trunk may also reduce the risk for low back pain, which is very common among adults in developed industrialized nations that have come to depend on technology for lifting and transporting objects, apparently causing a decline in normal trunk strength and endurance.

> ••• *By maintaining strength as they age, people can do daily chores and leisure physical activity with more endurance and less fatigue. Trunk strength can also reduce risk of low back pain, which is a prevalent health complaint in middle-aged and older adults.*

Motor Component

Speed of movement, agility, balance, and coordination are the principal components of motor fitness, which is more accurately termed *psychomotor fitness* because those components are influenced by the senses. Motor fitness is especially important for children because it enhances exploring and challenging the physical environment during growth and maturation.

Motor fitness is a limiting factor in the process of acquiring basic psychomotor skills. Children's performance on tests of other components of fitness is limited by their degree of motor fitness. Low motor fitness in childhood may have a long-lasting impact, contributing indirectly to sedentary living among adults who did not develop the psychomotor skills needed for many leisure physical activities. Though motor fitness does not appear to explain differences in health among young adults, poor coordination and balance increase the risks of falls and fractures and the subsequent loss of independence or years of life among frail elderly men and women.

Cardiorespiratory Component

From the late 1950s to the early 1990s, most physicians and exercise scientists came to regard **cardiorespiratory fitness** as the most important component of fitness for health. This occurred mainly because it was most logically related to heart disease, the most prevalent killer of adults; because it could be defined and measured with greater precision than other components of fitness; and because, among single components of fitness, it provided the best explanation of why some people can sustain more work than others. For those reasons, and because it is the only component of fitness to be measured and associated with reduced death rates from all causes and from CHD specifically in population-based epidemiologic studies, cardiorespiratory fitness still holds the premier position among health-related components of fitness. However, epidemiologists now place more emphasis on measuring other components of fitness in studies of disease, injury, and death in order to obtain a more complete view of how physical fitness is related to health.

Maximal Aerobic Capacity

Population-based studies have defined cardiorespiratory fitness mainly as **maximal aerobic power,** or maximal oxygen uptake (i.e., $\dot{V}O_2$), during an exercise test consisting of gradual increments of intensity until a peak or plateau of oxygen uptake by skeletal muscles or until voluntary fatigue that appeared to the testers to be maximal. Today, a broader view of cardiorespiratory fitness and how it may relate to health is emerging.

Submaximal Exercise Capacity

Aerobic endurance performance is defined as the ability to sustain an intensity of power output ranging from moderate to high, but below maximal, for a prolonged period of time.

Cardiac Function

Heart function is usually assessed by measuring cardiac muscle functions, including the heart rate for a given power output (adjusted for body mass), cardiac ejection fraction, myocardial shortening rate, stroke volume, and cardiac output, using exercise electrocardiography and imaging techniques.

Pulmonary Function

Lung function is clinically assessed by measuring static and dynamic lung volumes. These include tidal volume (amount of air inspired or expired during a normal breath), minute ventilation (volume of air expired in 1 min), vital capacity (the maximal volume of air that can be expired after a maximal inspiration), forced expiratory volume (FEV_1; volume of air expired during the first second of vital capacity), and peak flow (highest rate of expired air volume during vital capacity). Though maximal oxygen uptake depends in part on maximal minute ventilation, cardiorespiratory fitness in most healthy adults is limited by heart function, not by differences among people in lung function. Exceptions are cases of severe chronic obstructive lung diseases (COPD; diseases characterized by persistent slowing of airflow during forced expiration) such as cystic fibrosis, emphysema, and asthma.

Blood Pressure

Regular exercise lowers blood pressure at rest and during exercise at submaximal intensities. This is an important part of physical fitness for two reasons: (1) High resting blood pressure is associated with an increased risk of heart attack, stroke, ruptured arteries, kidney failure, death from CHD, and sudden cardiac death not necessarily resulting from coronary disease. (2) Lowered systolic blood pressure at a given heart rate during exercise provides a rough index that the oxygen consumption of the heart is lower, thus lowering the risk of arrhythmia and ischemia during exercise.

Metabolic Component

Metabolic fitness is the newest component of fitness recognized by exercise physiologists and epidemiologists who study health. It appears especially useful for understanding the potential health benefits of physical activity for preventing diabetes and atherosclerosis, the disease process leading to CHD and stroke.

Glucose Tolerance

People with impaired glucose tolerance are at risk for developing type 2 diabetes, a leading cause of cardiovascular disease and death and of circulatory diseases of the eye, kidneys, and extremities. Regular physical activity affects glucose metabolism in ways that appear to protect against glucose intolerance. These include normalizing hormonal secretion of insulin and glucagon from the pancreas, increasing the sensitivity of muscle cells to insulin, and an insulin-like action of muscle contraction that enhances glucose uptake from the blood.

Blood Lipid and Cholesterol Profiles

High blood levels of triglycerides, total cholesterol, and low-density lipoprotein cholesterol (LDL-C) and low blood levels of high-density lipoprotein cholesterol (HDL-C) are risk factors for CHD and stroke. Because regular physical activity affects lipid metabolism in ways that apparently lead to lowered triglycerides and elevated HDL-C, the concept of metabolic fitness can help explain how physical activity helps protect against atherosclerotic diseases that lead to CHD and stroke.

> ••• *Metabolic fitness is the newest component of fitness recognized by exercise physiologists and epidemiologists who study health. It is especially useful for understanding the potential health benefits of physical activity for preventing diabetes and cardiovascular disease.*

Lipid Oxidation

The ratio of carbon dioxide exhaled to oxygen consumed each minute is known as the respiratory exchange ratio (RER), which provides an index of the relative oxidation of lipids to carbohydrate in the cell, the respiratory quotient (RQ). At rest, RER is approximately 0.83 for a person whose diet has the usual mixture of calories from protein, carbohydrate, and fat. An RER of 0.70 would indicate that only fat was oxidized, while an RER of 1.0 would indicate that only carbohydrate was oxidized. A relatively low RER at rest or during prolonged submaximal exercise indicates that a person is burning more lipids than carbohydrates as fuel. A high rate of lipid oxidation also appears to alter cholesterol metabolism and reduce body fat so as to reduce risk of cardiovascular disease and premature death.

Sustained muscular effort for prolonged periods of time depends on high initial levels of glucose stored in the liver and muscle as glycogen and on normal levels of glucose maintained in the blood during exercise. However, using fat as a fuel in cell respiration is also important for endurance performance by helping spare glucose.

Exercise Training

Exercise is a specific type of physical activity performed regularly usually for the purpose of improving or maintaining physical fitness, physical skills, or health. Enough is known about the ways in which some biological systems (e.g., cardiorespiratory and neuromuscular) respond to differing amounts of exercise that professional guidelines have been adopted for optimal exercise prescription by exercise and health professionals. The most established exercise training guidelines, which outline the recommended frequency, intensity, time, and type or mode of exercise for fitness (cleverly referred to as the F.I.T.T. principles), were pronounced by the American College of Sports Medicine (ACSM) in 1978 and revised in 1990 and 1998 (table 3.3; Pollock et al. 1998). Those guidelines generally encompass recommendations for moderate physical activity endorsed by the ACSM and the CDC and adopted in the Surgeon General's report on physical activity and health (U.S. Department of Health and Human Services 1996). The key difference between the guidelines of the ACSM and those of the Surgeon General is the emphasis on gradual progression to vigorous-intensity exercise for fitness in the ACSM guidelines and the emphasis on moderate-intensity physical activity for total energy expenditure in the Surgeon General's guidelines.

> ••• *Exercise training guidelines for fitness endorsed by the ACSM focus on the F.I.T.T. principles: recommended frequency, intensity, time, and type or mode of exercise for fitness.*

Frequency

The recommended frequency of exercise depends on a person's goals. A range of three to five days per week is recommended for increasing cardiorespiratory fitness or decreasing body fat, although a sedentary person can improve by exercising two days per week during the first few

ACSM Guidelines for Fitness 1998	Surgeon General's Report 1996
Broadened types	30 min or more
20 to 60 min	Most days of the week (≥5)
Continuous	45–85% capacity
3–5 days/wk	>1,000 kcal/wk
40/50–85% capacity	Emphasis on moderate activity
Progression to vigorous activity	

TABLE 3.3   ACSM 1998 AND U.S. SURGEON GENERAL'S REPORT 1996 GUIDELINES

weeks of training. Gains are proportional to frequency within the range of three to five days. A frequency beyond five days each week increases risk for injury, even among people who are well conditioned.

Muscular strength and endurance, fat-free body mass, and flexibility can be increased and maintained by participating in resistance exercise (e.g., weightlifting) at least two to three days per week.

Intensity

Because people differ in their initial level of fitness, the recommended intensity of exercise is always relative to a person's maximal capacity. For cardiorespiratory fitness, the recommended intensity of training ranges from 50% to 85% of maximal oxygen uptake reserve, which is calculated by adding 50% to 85% of the difference between resting and maximal $\dot{V}O_2$ measured during exercise testing to a person's resting $\dot{V}O_2$. For very sedentary, older, or obese people, 40% may be a more appropriate and effective beginning intensity. Because heart rate (HR) reserve (a percentage, usually 50% to 85%, of the difference between maximal exercise HR and resting HR, added to resting HR) is linearly related to $\dot{V}O_2$ reserve in the 50% to 85% range and is much more practical to use, an intensity of 50% to 85% of HR reserve can be used as a surrogate for percent $\dot{V}O_2$ reserve. A range of 65% to 90% of maximal heart rate is equivalent to 50% to 85% of HR reserve.

For increasing or maintaining muscular strength and endurance and fat-free body mass, the intensity of resistance exercise has traditionally been expressed relative to a person's one-repetition maximum (1RM). Some experts recommend that the resistance used fall within a range of percentages of 1RM, such as the range of 50% to 85% proposed for cardiorespiratory fitness. Another common approach is to use the highest resistance that can be repeated a certain number of times before fatigue (commonly 8RM–15RM). A lower RM value (i.e., a higher resistance) promotes strength more so than endurance, while a higher RM (i.e., a lower resistance) promotes more endurance. The ACSM recommendations do not specify intensity; rather, they suggest a minimum of 8 to 10 different resistance exercises using the major muscle groups. People under 50 years of age are advised to complete 8 to 12 repetitions of each exercise, and people over 50 are advised to complete 10 to 15 repetitions.

For flexibility training, the ACSM recommends that the joints involved with the major muscle groups be stretched, using both static and dynamic methods, but no mention is made of intensity. In common practice, intensity is judged by the person based on the sensation of stretch without pain.

Time or Duration

The recommended daily time or duration for exercise for increasing or maintaining cardiorespiratory fitness or reducing body fat ranges from 20 to 60 min. While fitness improvements are proportional to exercise time within those ranges, the risk of injury, especially musculoskeletal injuries and heat injury in hot or humid environments, also increases with longer durations. The ACSM has not offered specific recommendations for the duration of resistance and stretching exercises, probably because the benefits of training for strength and flexibility depend more on the number of repetitions than on the rate at which the repetitions are completed, unlike exercise training for cardiorespiratory fitness, in which improved fitness is proportional to the rate of energy expenditure. However, some recent research suggests that several intermittent bouts of aerobic exercise (e.g., three separate sessions of 10 min each) can increase cardiorespiratory fitness.

Type or Mode

The type or mode of exercise refers to the form of the activity, its rate or pace, and its continuity. Activities that involve large muscle groups (e.g., walking or hiking, running or jogging, cycling, cross-country skiing, aerobic dance or aerobic group exercise, rope skipping, rowing, stair climbing, swimming, skating, and endurance games), are performed rhythmically, and can be sustained continuously for 20 to 60 min at a time are recommended when the goals of exercise are cardiorespiratory fitness or fat loss. When the frequency, intensity, and time spent are similar, gains in cardiorespiratory fitness and fat loss are similar, regardless of the type of physical activity. Resistance exercises (e.g., weightlifting) are used for muscular strength and endurance, and stretching exercises are used for flexibility training. Because body systems respond in very specific ways to the challenges imposed by different modes of exercise, a well-balanced exercise training program includes several modes.

> ••• *The percent gains in fitness after exercise training are very similar for males and females of all ages. The effects of frequency, intensity, and duration on fitness are interrelated. For example, similar increases in fitness can occur at relatively lower intensities if the frequency and duration of the activity are increased. Similarly, by increasing the intensity of the exercise, the frequency and duration can be reduced. This algebraic relationship among intensity, duration, and frequency permits the exercise training program to be individualized based on initial fitness or readiness for exercise, age, and personal fitness goals.*

Certain types of physical activity that affect specific components of physical fitness might be especially effective in reducing the risk of specific diseases (table 3.4).

Dose Response of Physical Activity and Health

Observe moderation.
> —Hesiod, eighth century B.C.

Keep the Golden Mean.
> —Cleobu'los, king of Rhodes (630–559 B.C.)

Not too strong, not too fast, not too often, not too long.
> —T.L. De Lorme, 1945

Establishing dose response is one of Mill's canons for determining the causality of a health risk factor and also has practical importance for public policy recommendations about the types and amounts of physical activity that are healthful. Subsequent chapters discuss the dose–response evidence for each aspect of health covered in this book. Here we provide an overview of the current evidence.

Since the Second International Consensus Symposium on Physical Activity, Fitness, and Health in Toronto in 1992 (Bouchard, Shephard, and Stephens 1994), worldwide attention has been paid to the question of whether, and in what forms, dose–response relationships exist between the frequency, intensity, and duration of

TABLE 3.4 DIMENSIONS OF PHYSICAL ACTIVITY WITH PROPOSED MECHANISM OF EFFECT, DISEASES OR CONDITIONS AFFECTED, AND POTENTIAL SURVEILLANCE DEFINITIONS

Physical activity dimension	Possible mechanisms	Diseases or conditions affected	Potential operational definitions for surveillance purposes
Caloric expenditure	Energy use	CHD, type 2 diabetes, obesity, cancer	Kilocalorie score; total time spent in or pattern of regular, sustained activities
Aerobic intensity	Enhanced cardiac function	CHD, type 2 diabetes, cancer	Kilocalorie score; total time spent in or pattern of intense activities
Weight bearing	Gravitational force	Osteoporosis	Total time spent in or pattern of weight-bearing activities
Flexibility	Range of motion	Disability	Total time spent in or pattern of activities that promote or require flexibility
Muscular strength	Muscle force generation	Disability	Total time spent in or pattern of activities that promote or require muscular strength

Reprinted, by permission, from C.J. Caspersen, R.K. Merritt, and T. Stephens, 1994, International physical activity patterns: A methodological perspective. In *Advances in Exercise Adherence*, edited by R.K. Dishman (Champaign, IL: Human Kinetics), 90.

different types of physical activity and reduced risks of disease, injury, and premature death. Hypothetical dose–response relationships between the amount of physical activity and several risk factors for CHD (Haskell 1994) and between intensity of physical activity and general health benefits and hazards (Dehn and Mullins 1977) are depicted in figures 3.2 and 3.3, respectively. As illustrated next, whether the apparent health-protective effects of physical activity are best described by a linear, dose-dependent relationship was controversial in the past decade and remains undecided today.

••• *Establishing dose response is one of Mill's canons for determining the causality of a health risk factor, but it is also important for public policy recommendations about the types and amounts of physical activity that are healthful.*

National Runners' Health Study

Circumstantial evidence supportive of a linear dose–response relationship between activity and health outcomes was provided by the

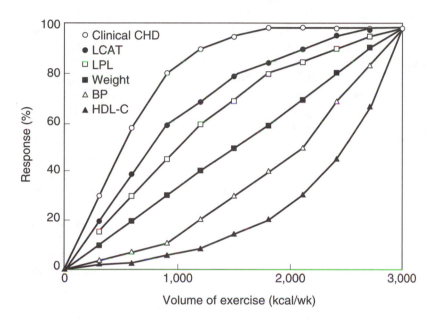

Figure 3.2 Hypothetical dose–response relationships between the amount of physical activity and several risk factors for coronary heart disease and general health benefits and hazards of moderate to heavy physical activity are depicted.

Reprinted, by permission, from W.L. Haskell, 2001, Dose-response issues from a biological perspective. In *Physical activity, fitness, and health: International proceedings and consensus statement,* edited by C. Bouchard, R.J. Shephard, and T. Stephens (Champaign, IL: Human Kinetics), 1037.

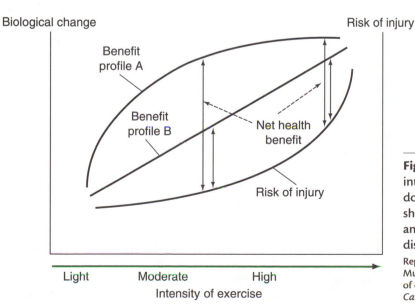

Figure 3.3 The relationship of exercise intensity to biological change (for two dose–response profiles) and risk injury is shown. Net health benefit for moderate- and high-intensity exercise is also displayed.

Reprinted, by permission, from M. Dehn and C. Mullins, 1977, "Physiologic effects and importance of exercise in patients with coronary heart disease," *Cardiovascular Medicine* 2: 365.

National Runners' Health Study conducted at the University of California at Berkeley. This cross-sectional study included about 2,600 female (Williams 1996) and over 8,200 male runners (Williams 1997). After runners with history of heart attack or medication that might affect CHD, smokers, and vegetarians were excluded, 1,837 women and 7,059 men remained in the study for data analysis. Participants completed a two-page questionnaire, which was distributed at races and sent to subscribers of *Runner's World* magazine. The questionnaire obtained information on demographic characteristics (age, race, and education); running history (age when the participant began running at least 12 miles per week, average weekly distance run and number of marathons run in the preceding five years, best marathon and 10-km times); weight history (highest and current weight; weight when the participant started running; lowest weight as a runner); circumferences of the chest, waist, and hips; diet (whether vegetarian; weekly intake of alcohol, red meat, fish, fruit, vitamin C, vitamin E, and aspirin); current and past cigarette use; history of heart attack and cancer; and medications taken to treat high blood pressure, thyroid conditions, high cholesterol levels, or diabetes. In addition to the questions asked of the men, women were asked about menstrual history (whether currently having periods and age at menarche) and hormone use (birth control pills, postmenopausal estrogen replacement, or progesterone). The questionnaire also requested permission to obtain the participants' height, weight, plasma cholesterol and triglyceride concentrations, blood pressure, and heart rate at rest from their physicians. Risk for CHD was estimated using the Framingham Heart Study equation for predicting CHD risk by combining runners' scores on blood levels of cholesterol, triglycerides, uric acid, and glucose.

Among men, results indicated a linear reduction in estimated overall risk for CHD with each successive 16-km (about 10-mile) increment in weekly running distance, from less than 16 km up to 80 km (about 50 miles) per week. Risk was 30% lower in male runners who averaged 64 km or more each week than in those running less than 15 km each week. Nonetheless, male runners covering 80 km or more per week had the same CHD risk as those running 64 to 79 km per week.

The results for women also suggested a dose–response relationship between reduction in CHD risk and physical activity as distance run each week increased. There was a 30% reduction

in the overall risk of CHD and a 45% reduction in risk of CHD death among the women who ran the most. Those risk reductions were statistically independent of BMI, age, education, menstrual status, alcohol consumption, diet, estrogen, progesterone, and the use of birth control pills. The clearest findings were for increased HDL-C: The women who ran the most (more than 64 km each week) had HDL-C levels that were nearly 10 mg/dl (0.25 mmol/L) higher than the women who ran the least (16 km or less each week).

Whether there was a dose–response relationship for running intensity and health outcome was also examined, based on runners' reports of pace (in kilometers per hour) during their best recent 10-km race; this was used as a surrogate measure of their exercise intensity during training (Williams 1998b). After adjustments for weekly running distance, age, consumption of alcohol, and diet, both men and women who ran faster (i.e., at greater intensity) had lower blood pressures; triglyceride levels; ratios of total cholesterol to HDL-C; BMIs; and waist, hip, and chest girths. Relative to the effect of running distance, running velocity was associated with a 13.3 times greater effect on systolic blood pressure, a 2.8 times greater effect on diastolic blood pressure, and a 4.7 times greater calculated effect on waist circumference. Among women, running velocity was associated with a 5.7 times greater effect on systolic blood pressure. In contrast, running distance had a more than sixfold greater calculated effect on HDL-C levels in both sexes than did running velocity.

Other findings from the National Runners' Health Study suggest that associations between running distance and reduced risk factors extended to older runners (Williams 1998a). Among 935 men in their 60s and 175 men in their 70s, the associations of weekly running distance with higher levels of plasma HDL-C and lower plasma triglycerides, lower ratio of total cholesterol to HDL-C, lower systolic and diastolic blood pressure, and lower BMI were similar to those seen in runners younger than age 60. In contrast, the inverse relationship between running distance and LDL-C was smaller than observed among younger men.

An important question is whether these results are generalizable to the U.S. population at large. Because all subjects were runners, even the least-active subjects in the study were more active than the least-active subjects in other studies of physical activity and CHD risk that included sedentary subjects. Hence, the National Runners' Health Study suggested a dose–response reduction in CHD that is linear for most runners, but it did not permit a test of whether there is a proportionately greater reduction in risk when comparing low-mileage runners with sedentary peers. Also, the study predicted risk based on 10 years of running experience at the time of the survey (the average subject had been running about eight and a half years), but the study did not actually observe the runners for 10 years nor were actual CHD events measured; the likelihood of CHD events was computed using a prediction formula derived from men in the Framingham Heart Study. Moreover, the National Runners' Health Study showed a benefit plateau at about 50 miles run per week. That finding is pertinent for evaluating the public health benefits versus costs of exercise; we later consider the risk of injuries among runners, which appears to increase with increased running distance.

The results of the National Runners' Health Study and many other studies suggest that regular physical activity has great potential for reducing health risk factors that are associated with all-cause and coronary heart and vascular disease (CVD) mortality in a dose–response manner. However, it was a cross-sectional study, not a prospective cohort or controlled trial, and was limited to relatively high-distance runners who expended many more calories than the typical person, who might benefit from less physical activity.

Current Scientific Consensus

A consensus symposium on the dose–response relationship between physical activity and health was held in October 2000 at Hockley Valley Resort near Toronto (Bouchard 2001). Twenty-four invited experts from six countries reviewed the available research literature and evaluated the cumulative evidence in several areas of health according to four scientific categories that considered the quality of the research designs and the quantity and agreement of findings in each area. Consensus was reached that an inverse and generally linear relationship exists between physical activity and rates of all-cause mortality and mortality attributable to CVD and CHD incidence and mortality, and the incidence of type 2 diabetes.

Consensus was not reached about dose response for the other health outcomes evaluated, mainly because (1) in some areas not enough studies examined the dose–response question, (2) measures of physical activity were imprecise, (3) some responses to physical activity were too small to examine the dose influence, and (4) confounding influences such as genetic variability and body fatness were inadequately controlled. Moreover, given the wide variability in people's adaptations to similar physical activity stimuli, it is not too surprising that as yet it has been difficult to define precisely a dose–response pattern for physical activity and many health outcomes. For example, as figures 3.4 and 3.5 show, changes

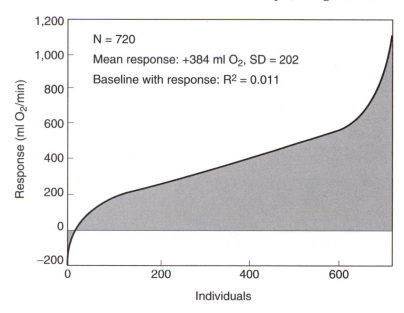

Figure 3.4 Heterogeneity of $\dot{V}O_2$max training response in the HERITAGE Family Study. Individual differences in response to regular physical activity.

Reprinted, by permission, from C. Bouchard and T. Rankinen, 2001, "Individual differences in response to regular physical activity," *Medicine and Science in Sports and Exercise* 33 (Suppl. 6): S446-S451.

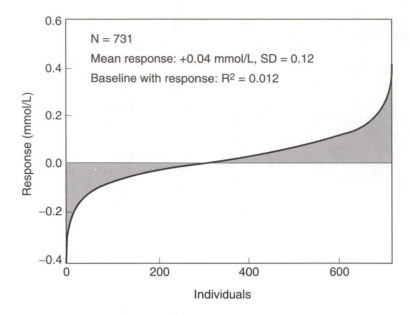

Figure 3.5 Heterogeneity of the training responses of HDL cholesterol in the HERITAGE Family Study. Individual differences in response to regular physical activity.

Reprinted, by permission, from C. Bouchard and T. Rankinen, 2001, "Individual differences in response to regular physical activity," *Medicine and Science in Sports and Exercise* 33 (Suppl. 6): S446-S451.

in maximal oxygen uptake and HDL-C in response to exercise training in the HERITAGE Family Study of several hundred sedentary adults varied widely, despite subjects' exposure to the same exercise stimulus (i.e., 20 weeks of cycling exercise three days per week at an intensity of 65% of maximal oxygen uptake; Bouchard and Rankinen 2001).

Similarly, wide variations have been found for other outcomes of exercise training. The HERITAGE Family Study found that responses to training are relatively the same for adults regardless of age, sex, and race. However, people's initial levels are a strong predictor of training response for some attributes, including submaximal exercise heart rate and blood pressure, but weakly influence changes in maximal oxygen uptake and HDL-C. Moreover, family inheritance (i.e., shared environment and genetics) is a significant influence on variation in people's response to regular physical activity (Bouchard and Rankinen 2001).

Current conclusions about people's average responses in specific health outcomes to various amounts of physical activity are categorized in table 3.5 according to the strength of the evidence: strong, agreement among numerous randomized controlled trials; substantial, agreement or mixed evidence among limited number of randomized controlled trials or among nonrepresentative samples; moderate, agreement among uncontrolled trials or observational studies (Kesaniemi et al. 2001).

Surveys and Surveillance of Physical Activity

Before physical activity can be increased in a population, the prevalence rates of physical activity and its trends across time among geographic regions and subgroups within the population must be established. Surveys are used to determine the prevalence of physical activity by asking a sample of the population about their physical activity habits. Trends in physical activity prevalence are determined by surveillance systems, which repeatedly and regularly conduct the same survey in a population every year or every several years. Surveillance is necessary to measure **secular trends** (i.e., naturally occurring change in the population) and response to public health interventions. Surveys and surveillance systems that measure and track changes in physical activity prevalence are necessary to determine population segments that need intervention and to judge the effectiveness of population-based intervention.

In the following section, some surveys and surveillance systems in developed nations worldwide are discussed, followed by their estimates of physical activity prevalence. Next, key national surveys and surveillance systems in the United States, and their results, are presented. Though

TABLE 3.5   SUMMARY OF EVIDENCE FOR DOSE–RESPONSE EFFECTS OF PHYSICAL ACTIVITY ON HEALTH

Health outcome	Strength of the evidence	Consensus conclusion
All-cause mortality	Moderate	Inverse and roughly linear reduction, with a threshold around 1,000 kcal/wk
Coronary heart and vascular disease	Moderate	Inverse and linear reduction in incidence and mortality
Blood pressure (normotensive and hypertensive participants)	Substantial to strong	Window of benefit: about 50%–70% of capacity; no apparent dose gradient
Blood lipids (+HDL-C; –LDL-C; –triglycerides)	Substantial	Window of benefit: about 50%–80% of capacity; no apparent dose gradient
Hemostatic factors (–platelet adhesion; –fibrinogen; +tPA)	Moderate to substantial	No evidence for dose response
Overweight and obesity	Strong	Linear reduction in weight in studies lasting 4 months or less with controlled diet; no dose response in studies lasting 6 months or more
Type 2 diabetes	Moderate	Inverse linear reduction
Osteoporosis	Substantial Strong	No evidence for peak bone mass No evidence for slowing bone loss after menopause
Cancer	Moderate	Inverse linear reduction for colon cancer
Depression	Moderate to substantial	No evidence for dose response

it is tempting to compare nations, varying definitions and methods used by many of the different surveys make it, as yet, nearly impossible to make direct comparisons that are precise. The International Consensus Group for Physical Activity Measurement met in Geneva, Switzerland, in 1998 to launch the development of a set of valid instruments that can be used internationally to obtain comparable estimates of physical activity worldwide (Booth 2000). Subsequently, an International Physical Activity Prevalence Study is under way. Until data are available from that study, comparisons of low, moderate, and high physical activity levels among several industrialized nations can be made cautiously, based on the frequency of participation in activities of differing intensities. Finally, differences in the prevalence of physical activity in the United States according to region of the country and demographic groups are presented.

National Surveys in Developed Nations

The World Health Organization (WHO) MONICA Optional Study of Physical Activity (MOSPA) was developed and is managed by the CDC for the purpose of comparing estimates of physical activity among nations that participate in the WHO MONICA surveillance system, which monitors cardiovascular disease trends worldwide. Thirteen of the 40 WHO MONICA survey sites in Europe and Asia participated from 1988 to 1994.

In addition, for the past decade seven countries, including the United States, have included questions about leisure-time physical activity in national surveys about health and behavior. Those surveys provide a basis for comparing prevalence of physical activity among population subgroups and changes in prevalence over time. Table 3.6 describes the features of the surveys in each nation. Figure 3.6 illustrates participation rates estimated by each country.

Pan–European Union Survey

In 1997, the 15 nations that constituted the inaugural European Union (Austria, Belgium, Denmark, Finland, France, Germany, Greece, Ireland, Italy, Luxembourg, the Netherlands, Portugal, Spain, Sweden, and the United Kingdom) aggregated physical activity information from about 1,200 household interviews of people ages 15 years or older. People were categorized into four groups by how much time in an average week they reported spending in 18 different activities (none, <1.5 h,

TABLE 3.6	FEATURES OF POPULATION SURVEYS OF PHYSICAL ACTIVITY IN SEVEN NATIONS				
Country, survey name (reference), year(s) of survey	**Mode of administration**	**Sample size**	**Age of sample**	**Recall period**	
Australia National Physical Activity Survey (Armstrong et al. 2000), 1997, 1999	Telephone interview	3,841	18–75	Past week Average week in past 6 months	
Canada National Population Health Survey (Health Canada 1999), 1994–1995, 1996–1997	Household interview	69,524	>12	Past 3 months	
England National Health Survey for England (Prior 1999), 1994–1995, 1998–1999	Computer-assisted household interview	1,908	≥16	Past 4 weeks	
Finland National Health Behaviour Monitoring System (Helakorpi et al. 1999), 1978–1999	Postal survey	3,371	15–64	Past 4 weeks Past year Usual work day	
Ireland Happy Heart National Survey (Irish Heart Foundation 1994), 1992	Household interview	1,798	30–69	Usual work day NR Usual work day NR NR	
New Zealand Life in New Zealand Survey (Hopkins et al. 1991; Russell and Wilson 1991), 1989–1990	Phase I: Postal survey Phase II: Interviewer-administered survey at health examination	11,295	≥15	Past 4 weeks	
United States National Health Interview Survey (U.S. Dept. of Health and Human Services 1996), 1985, 1990, 1991	Household interview	36,399–43,732	≥18	Past 2 weeks	

Adapted from tables 10 and 11 (pp. 24–29) of H. Vainio and F. Bianchini, eds. 2002. *Weight control and physical activity.* Vol. 6 of *IARC handbooks of cancer prevention.* Lyon, France: IARC Press.

1.5–3.5 h, or >3.5 h each week). Figure 3.7 provides an international comparison of how many people did not participate in leisure physical activity (European Commission 1999; Kearney et al. 1999).

The United States

The first surveillance system for estimating and monitoring leisure-time physical activity in the United States was the Behavioral Risk Factor Surveillance System (BRFSS), which was developed by the Behavioral Epidemiology and Evaluation Branch of the Division of Health Education of the CDC's Center for Health Promotion and Educa-

tion (Bradstock et al. 1984) and is administered and supported by the Division of Adult and Community Health of the National Center for Chronic Disease Prevention and Health Promotion.

Behavioral Risk Factor Surveillance System

The BRFSS uses a population-based telephone survey and has provided estimates of national and state trends in physical activity, as well as obesity and fruit and vegetable consumption, since 1984. Its creation was prompted mainly by the 1990 health objectives for the nation established in 1980 (U.S. Department of Health and Human Services 1980), which emphasized physical

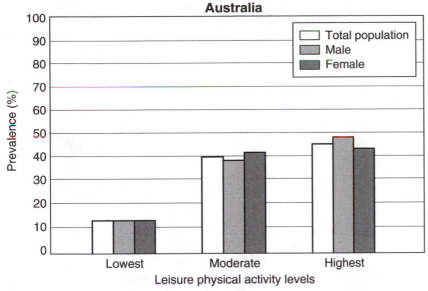

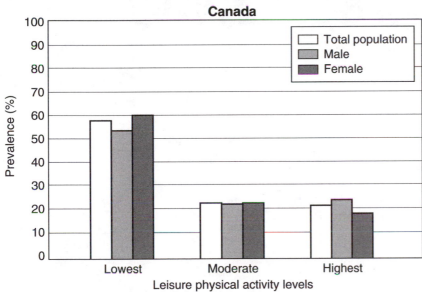

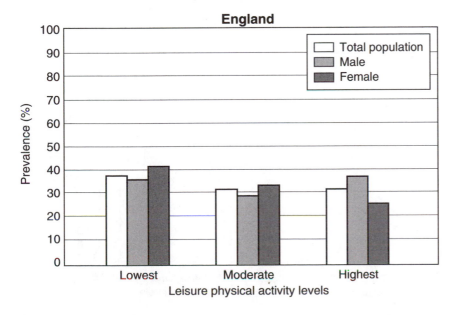

(continued)

Figure 3.6 Prevalence of low, moderate, and high levels of leisure-time physical activity in seven nations.

Data from table 12 (pp. 32–33). Vainio, H. & Bianchini, F. (Eds.) Weight control and physical activity. *IARC Handbooks of Cancer Prevention.* Vol 6. World Health Organization. International Agency for Research on Cancer. Lyon, France: IARC Press, 2002.

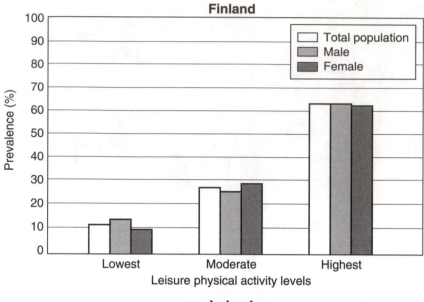

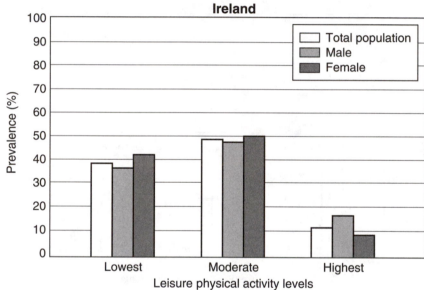

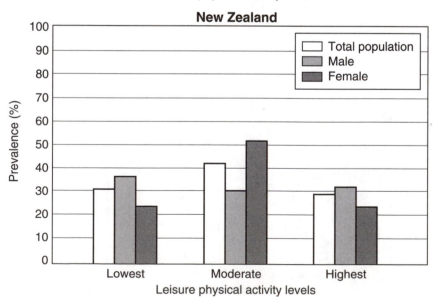

(continued)

Figure 3.6 *(continued)*

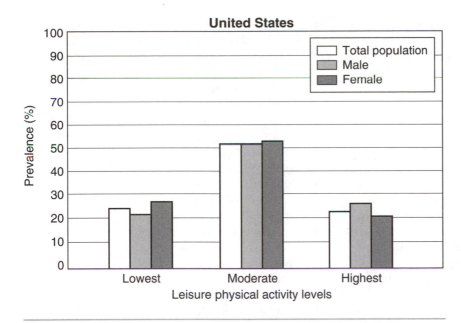

Figure 3.6 *(continued)*

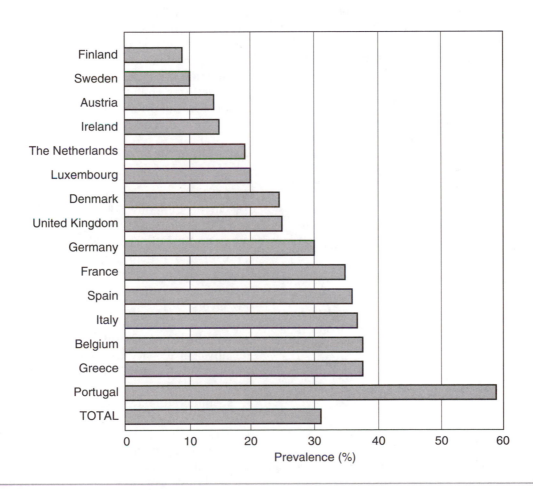

Figure 3.7 Prevalence of sedentary leisure time in the inaugural European Union.

Adapted, by permission, from H. Vainio and R. Bianchini, 2002, *IARC Handbooks of Cancer Prevention Vol 6* (Lyon, France: IARC Press), 34.

activity and fitness for the first time. Those objectives highlighted the need to estimate current and future prevalence rates of physical activity in order to judge whether the participation objectives were appropriate and could be met. National estimates of physical activity and other health risk behaviors among adults had been provided by surveys regularly conducted by the National Center for Health Statistics (NCHS), but those surveys had not emphasized physical activity and health behaviors and were not designed to provide estimates for individual states, which might differ from the national average. Initially, from 1981 to 1983, BRFSS conducted point-prevalence surveys in 28 states and the District of Columbia. By 1994, all states, the District of Columbia, and three territories were participating in the BRFSS.

National Health Interview Survey

The National Health Interview Survey (NHIS) is a household survey conducted since 1957 by the NCHS that uses family interviews to provide national health statistics. It provided the baseline estimates of physical activity prevalence in the *Healthy People 2010* objectives of the U.S. Department of Health and Human Services (2000).

Youth Risk Behavior Surveillance System

The Youth Risk Behavior Surveillance System (YRBSS) is a national school-based survey conducted biannually by state, local, and U.S. territorial schools. It was begun in 1990 to monitor physical activity, nutrition, and other health risk behaviors among youths in grades 9 to 12.

Nationwide Personal Transportation Survey

The U.S. Department of Transportation conducts the Nationwide Personal Transportation Survey (NPTS) to provide estimates of the amount and nature of daily travel by household members in the United States (e.g., how children get to and from school, how workers get to and from their jobs). Trends in walking and bicycling have been provided since 1969 and are currently being used by the Active Community Environments Initiative to promote physical activity through environmental change.

Physical Activity in the United States

Physical activity levels in the United States seem generally similar to those in other economically developed nations that have a surveillance system for estimating the prevalence of leisure physical activity. Estimates from the 1994 BRFSS survey of over 105,000 U.S. adults from the District of Columbia and all states except Rhode Island indicated that about 60% of adults fail to participate in the level of leisure-time physical activity recommended by the CDC (20 min of moderate physical activity on each of three or more days per week). Nationwide, 30% of adults do not participate in any leisure-time physical activity. Just 15% of adults engage in at least 30 min of moderate physical activity three or more days a week. A third of adolescents participate less than 20 min of vigorous physical activity three days a week. Recent estimates from other surveys are even less encouraging. The latest NCHS survey of 68,556 U.S. adults aged 18 years and older estimated that in 1997 to 1998, 70% of U.S. adults failed to participate in either half an hour of light to moderate physical activity at least five times a week or in 20 min of vigorous exercise three times a week. Nearly 40% reported no leisure-time physical activity at all (Schoenborn and Barnes 2002). About 24% said they engaged in vigorous physical activity three or more times each week; other estimates indicate that only 10% of American adults are active at that level (Caspersen, Merritt, and Stephens 1994). Figure 3.8 illustrates that these participation rates are well below the public health goals for the United States for the year 2010.

Geographic Variation

Figure 3.9 illustrates a wide variation in sedentary living across the United States, ranging from 18% in the state of Washington to 49% in Washington, DC, in the most recently compiled estimates from the 1998 BRFSS survey (Centers for Disease Control and Prevention 1999). The distinction of being least active belongs to the District of Columbia, an irony that will not be lost on most taxpayers.

Figure 3.10 illustrates a similarly wide variation across the United States in participation in regular physical activity, defined as either 20 or more minutes of vigorous physical activity (e.g., 6 METs or more) on three or more days each week or sustained physical activity of any intensity for about 30 min on five or more days each week. Generally, the Rocky Mountain and northwestern states are most active, and the southeastern states least active. The average participation rate for both men and women is 27%, ranging from a high of 36% in Oregon to a low, once again in the District of Columbia, of 16%.

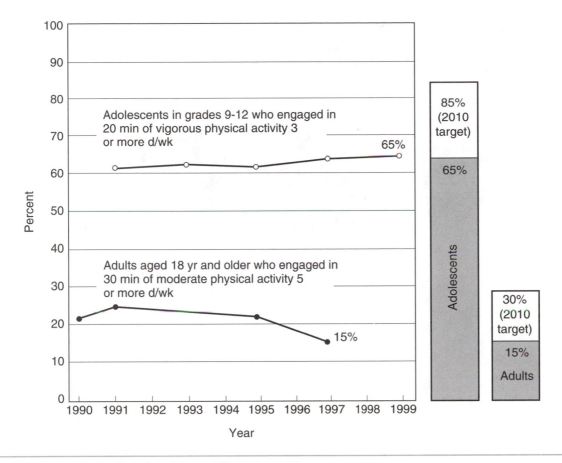

Figure 3.8 Percentage of physical activity at differing intensities.

Sources: Center for Disease Control and Prevention. Youth Risk Behavior Surveillance System. 1991–1997. Centers for Disease Control and Prevention, National Center for Health Statistics. National Health Interview Survey. 1990–1999. U.S. Department of Health and Human Services (2000). *Healthy People 2010: Understanding and improving health.* 2nd Edition.

Population Subgroups

Within the United States, physical activity differs by race or ethnic group, sex, age, and education level, as illustrated by the 1997 baseline participation rates for the *Healthy People 2010* objectives of decreasing sedentariness and increasing vigorous physical activity among adults (figures 3.11 through 3.14). Generally, whites are more active than American minority groups, and men appear to be more active than women. Also, physical activity decreases with age but increases with education level.

Demographic characteristics such as race or ethnicity, sex, and age can be misleading, though, if they are influenced by differences in education, income, social influences, and geographic region. Likewise, some of the geographic variation in physical activity could be explained by differences in the geographic distributions of racial or ethnic groups, ages, and education levels across the nation. American adults with the least formal education tend to be sedentary regardless of their age, and adolescents who are sedentary tend to have sedentary parents.

After entering adolescence, girls in the United States and several European countries show a bigger reduction in both school-based and leisure physical activity than do boys. Whether this is explainable by social factors is not yet known, but there seems to be nothing biologically inherent about being female that would cause girls and women to be less active than males. Though girls become fatter than boys after puberty, cultural factors seem more likely than biology to explain most of the reduced activity.

••• *Secular changes in culture can strongly influence the prevalence of physical activity. Examples are increased television viewing and computer use among youths and a decrease in daily physical education during the past decade.*

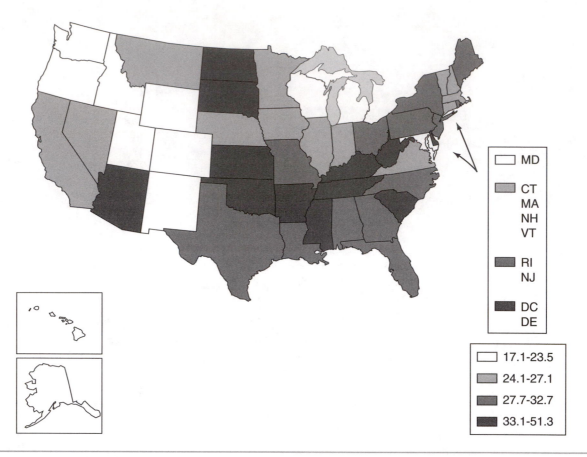

Figure 3.9 Percentage of adults who reported no leisure-time physical activity in 1998.

Source: Chronic diseases and their risk factors: The nations leading causes of death. U.S. Department of Health and Human Services. Centers for Disease Control and Prevention. 1999.

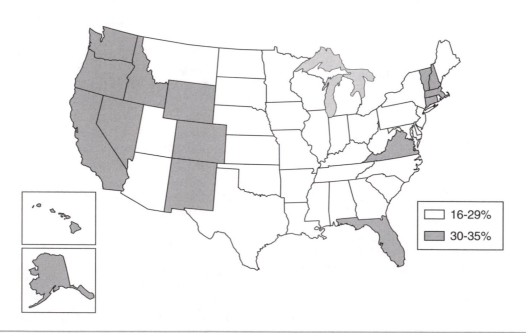

Figure 3.10 Who's physically active? Activity meeting either the recommendation for regular vigorous physical activity (≥20 min per day on ≥3 days per week) or regular sustained moderate activity (an average of ≥30 min per day ≥5 days per week).

Source: Data from the Centers for Disease Control and Prevention, 1996, *MMWR*, 45 (31): 674.

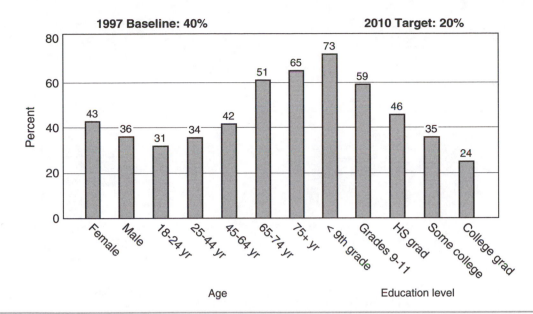

Figure 3.11 Percentage of adult population by age and education level who engage in no leisure-time physical activity. Based on the *Healthy People 2010* Objective 1: Reduce the proportion of adults who engage in no leisure-time physical activity.

Data from U.S. Department of Health and Human Services (2000). *Healthy People 2010 Objectives*. U.S. Government Printing Office.

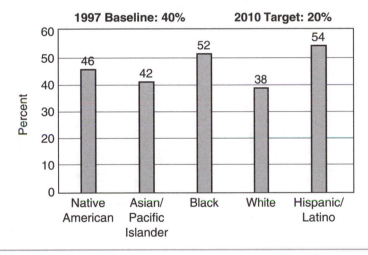

Figure 3.12 Percentage of adult population by ethnicity who engage in no leisure-time physical activity. Based on the *Healthy People 2010* Objective 1: Reduce the proportion of adults who engage in no leisure-time physical activity.

Data from U.S. Department of Health and Human Services (2000). *Healthy People 2010 Objectives*. U.S. Government Printing Office.

Mixed positive and negative trends in physical activity among youths during the 1990s seem to support the hypothesis that long-term trends in the culture are strong influences on youth. The results from the YRBSS shown in figure 3.15 show increases in the proportion of youth who participated in strength or resistance exercise between 1991 and 1999 but a smaller percentage who attended daily physical education classes. Both of these trends are plausibly explained by social factors.

Physical Activity and Aging

Though it seems reasonable that people will become less active as they age, perhaps as a result of lost mobility, it is probably incorrect to assume that age is an independent and unavoidable cause of reduced activity. Figure 3.16 illustrates this by comparing changes from 1962 to 1977 in the percentage of Harvard alumni who were judged to be active according to age cohort or birth cohort. Population studies that extend

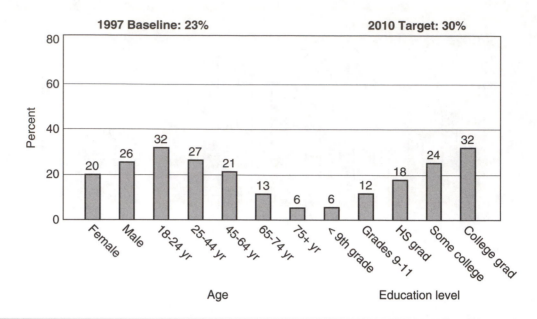

Figure 3.13 Percentage of adult population by age and education level who engage in vigorous physical activity that promotes cardiorespiratory fitness for 20 or more minutes 3 or more days a week. Based on the *Healthy People 2010* Objective 3: Increase the proportion of adults who engage in vigorous physical activity that promotes cardiorespiratory fitness for 20 or more minutes 3 or more days a week.

Data from U.S. Department of Health and Human Services (2000). *Healthy People 2010 Objectives*. U.S. Government Printing Office.

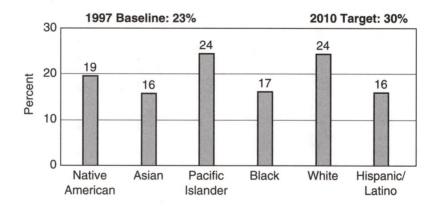

Figure 3.14 Percentage of adult population by ethnicity who engage in vigorous physical activity that promotes cardiorespiratory fitness for 20 or more minutes 3 or more days a week. Based on the *Healthy People 2010* Objective 3: Increase the proportion of adults who engage in vigorous physical activity that promotes cardiorespiratory fitness for 20 or more minutes 3 or more days a week.

Data from U.S. Department of Health and Human Services (2000). *Healthy People 2010 Objectives*. U.S. Government Printing Office.

over many years often begin keeping records in different years on different waves of people. People are frequently placed into the same age cohort for analyses, even though they were born in different years. A birth cohort contains only people born in the same year. Figure 3.16 shows the common observation that the percentage of each age group that is physically active steadily declines from the youngest age group (34–39 years) to the oldest age group (65–69 years). In

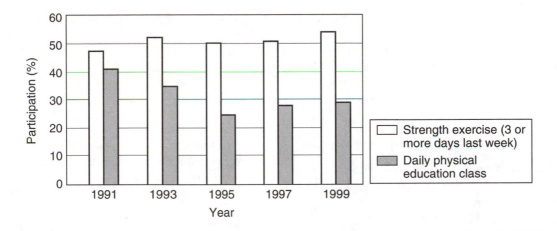

Figure 3.15 The Youth Risk Behavior Survey indicates that there were increases in the proportion of youth that participated in strength or resistance exercise between 1991 and 1999, but less youth attended daily physical education classes.

Source: Data from Youth Risk Behavior Survey, Centers for Disease Control and Prevention, 2002.

	Percentage of subjects by age						
Activity and survey year	35-39	40-44	45-49	50-54	55-59	60-64	65-69
Climbed 50 or more steps per day:							
1962	67	68	57				
1966	68	70	64	67	65	65	58
1977		66	69	62	60	60	57
Walked 5 or more blocks per day:							
1962	78	76	78				
1966	77	74	75	77	79	79	76
1977		72	75	75	72	77	73
Participated in any sport activity:							
1962	50	52	38				
1966	54	52	55	54	47	38	34
1977		91	93	88	85	82	81
Participated in vigorous sport activity:							
1962	38	38	27				
1966	46	42	40	38	26	18	14
1977		83	82	70	71	62	55

Figure 3.16 Birth- versus age-cohort effect on physical activity with aging. Changes over time in specific physical activities among Harvard alumni by cross-sectional age group and by cohort, 1962–1977.

Reprinted, by permission, from K.E. Powell and R.S. Paffenbarger, 1985, "Workshop on epidemiologic and public health aspects of physical activity and exercise: A summary," *Public Health Reports* 100(2): 118-126.

contrast, however, the lines connecting birth cohorts as they aged shows that in most instances men born in the same year maintained their level of stair climbing and walking as they aged and that in many instances they increased the time they spent playing sports as they aged.

> ••• *Though surveys typically show that physical activity declines when groups of older people are compared with younger people, this can be an artifact of using absolute intensity rather than relative intensity, which adjusts for decreasing fitness with age. Harvard alumni who were tracked individually actually increased physical activity during the transition from middle age to old age.*

Studies have overestimated the decline in physical activity at older ages because they have used the same absolute standards of the rate of energy expenditure for young and old people alike, despite the fact that a person's maximal rate of energy expenditure declines linearly with increasing age. Dr. Carl Caspersen, a physical activity epidemiologist with the CDC, elegantly showed the impact of inappropriately using such absolute standards for gauging trends in physical activity patterns among older people (Caspersen et al. 1994). In his analysis of data on U.S. men from the 1985 National Health Interview Study (NHIS), the trend of declining physical activity with age that appears when the commonly used recommendation of 3 kcal per kilogram per day of energy expenditure is used as the standard did not appear with another common recommendation based on frequency, duration, and rate of energy expenditure relative to capacity. Based on the relative standard, the decline in the proportion of men participating in physical activity was less steep than for the decline in the absolute standard, and men actually became more active after age 75.

Likewise, the trend for declining participation by older men in physical activities requiring 6 METs or more was reversed among men aged 75 years or older when a relative standard of activities requiring 60% or more of maximum METs was used. The concept of METs was introduced in 1936 by exercise physiologist David Bruce Dill to express exercise intensity relative to metabolic rate and independently of body mass. Basal or resting metabolic rate represents 1 MET, which is the equivalent, on average, of 3.5 ml of O_2 consumed per kilogram of body mass per minute or $1 \text{ kcal} \cdot \text{kg}^{-1} \cdot \text{h}^{-1}$. Exercise intensity is expressed as a multiple of a MET. For example, a woman with a maximal aerobic capacity of $35 \text{ ml } O_2 \cdot \text{kg}^{-1} \cdot \text{min}^{-1}$ would, on average, raise her metabolism 10 times above its resting level while exercising at her peak capacity.

Participation rates among older men in the aforementioned NHIS study were underestimated because they were based on standard activities that simply are too intense for the older men, who apparently were choosing activities that, though lower in absolute intensity, were appropriately intense relative to the men's declining fitness levels. Though the analysis was limited to men, the general idea should apply equally to older women.

Summary

This chapter introduced the commonly accepted definitions and measures of physical activity and physical fitness. The descriptive epidemiology of differences in physical activity by geographic region, race or ethnic group, sex, age, and education level was introduced. Surveillance of physical activity prevalence and trends among groups and regions is necessary to monitor progress toward public health objectives for increasing physical activity.

Because physical activity occurs in many forms, intensities, and amounts, it is possible that its relationship with the development of disease and with premature death might differ according to those features. Determining whether that is so is fundamentally necessary in order to satisfy Mill's canon of dose response. It is also practically important for public policy about recommended types and amounts of physical activity and to determine which components of physical fitness are related to the risk of mortality or to the development of specific diseases. Determining whether physical fitness has specific effects on disease risk is also important for forming public policy and for satisfying Mill's canon of biological plausibility. That is, it is expected that many physiological adaptations to physical activity that favorably influence the pathophysiology of diseases would also be reflected in changes in some component of physical fitness. The following chapters address these issues, starting in chapter 4, "All-Cause and Coronary Heart Disease Mortality."

Bibliography

Armstrong, T., A. Bauman, and J. Davies. 2000. *Physical activity patterns of Australian adults: Results of the 1999 National Physical Activity Survey.* Canberra, Australia: Australia Institute of Health and Welfare.

Bassett, D.R., B.E. Ainsworth, S.R. Leggett, C.A. Mathien, J.A. Main, D.C. Hunter, and G.E. Duncan. 1996. Accuracy of five electronic pedometers for measuring distance walked. *Medicine and Science in Sports and Exercise* 28 (8): 1071–1077.

Bassett, D.R. Jr., B.E. Ainsworth, A.M. Swartz, S.J. Strath, W.L. O'Brien, and G.A. King. 2000. Validity of four motion sensors in measuring moderate intensity physical activity. *Medicine and Science in Sports and Exercise* 32 (Suppl. 9): S471–S480.

Blair, S.N., W.L. Haskell, P. Ho, R.A. Paffenbarger Jr., K.M. Vranizan, J.W. Farquhar, and P.D. Wood. 1985. Assessment of habitual physical activity by seven-day recall in a community survey and controlled experiments. *American Journal of Epidemiology* 122 (5): 794–804.

Booth, M.L. 2000. Assessment of physical activity: An international perspective. *Research Quarterly for Exercise and Sport* 71: 114–120.

Bouchard, C. 2001. Physical activity and health: Introduction to the dose–response symposium. *Medicine and Science in Sports and Exercise* 33 (Suppl. 6): S347–S350.

Bouchard, C., and T. Rankinen. 2001. Individual differences in response to regular physical activity. *Medicine and Science in Sports and Exercise* 33 (Suppl. 6): S446–S451.

Bouchard, C., and R.J. Shephard. 1994. Physical activity, fitness, and health: The model and key concepts. In *Physical activity, fitness, and health: International proceedings and consensus statement,* edited by C. Bouchard, R.J. Shephard, and T. Stephens, pp. 77–88. Champaign, IL: Human Kinetics.

Bouchard, C., R.J. Shephard, and T. Stephens, eds. 1994. *Physical activity, fitness, and health: International proceedings and consensus statement.* Champaign, IL: Human Kinetics.

Bradstock, M.K., J.S. Marks, M. Forman, E.M. Gentry, G.C. Hogelin, and F.L. Trowbridge. 1984. Behavioral risk factor surveillance, 1981–1983: CDC surveillance summaries. *Morbidity and Mortality Weekly Report* 33 (1): 1SS–4SS.

Brouha, L., and P.E. Smith Jr. 1958. Energy expenditure of motions (abstract). *Federation Proceedings of the American Society for Experimental Biology* 17: 20.

Caspersen, C.J. 1989. Physical activity epidemiology: Concepts, methods, and applications to exercise science. *Exercise and Sport Sciences Reviews* 17: 423–475.

Caspersen, C.J., R.K. Merritt, and T. Stephens. 1994. International physical activity patterns: A methodological perspective. In *Advances in exercise adherence,* edited by R.K. Dishman. Champaign, IL: Human Kinetics.

Caspersen, C.J., K.E. Powell, and G.M. Christenson. 1985. Physical activity, exercise, and physical fitness: Definitions and distinctions for health-related research. *Public Health Reports* 100 (2): 126–130.

Centers for Disease Control and Prevention. 1996. State-specific prevalence of participation in physical activity—Behavioral Risk Factor Surveillance System, 1994. *Morbidity and Mortality Weekly Report* 45 (31): 673–675.

Dehn, M., and C. Mullins. 1977. Physiologic effects and importance of exercise in patients with coronary heart disease. *Cardiovascular Medicine* 2: 365.

De Lorme, T.L. 1945. Restoration of muscle power by heavy resistance exercise. *Journal of Bone and Joint Surgery* 27: 645–647.

Dishman, R.K., R.A. Washburn, and D.A. Schoeller. 2001. Measurement of physical activity. *Quest: American Academy of Kinesiology and Physical Education Papers* 53: 295–309.

European Commission. 1999. *A pan-EU survey on consumer attitudes to physical activity, body weight and health.* Luxembourg: Office for Official Publications of the European Communities.

Freedson, P.S., and K. Miller. 2000. Objective monitoring of physical activity using motion sensors and heart rate. *Research Quarterly for Exercise and Sport* 71: 21–29.

Gayle, R., H.J. Montoye, and J. Philpot. 1977. Accuracy of pedometers for measuring distance walked. *Research Quarterly* 48 (3): 632–636.

Haskell, W. 1994. Dose–response issues from a biological perspective. In *Physical activity, fitness, and health: International proceedings and consensus statement,* edited by C. Bouchard, R.J. Shephard, and T. Stephens, pp. 1030–1039. Champaign, IL: Human Kinetics.

Health Canada. 1999. *Physical activity of Canadians. 2.1 Description of the survey and reports.* National Population Health Survey Highlights, no. 2. Ottawa, ON: Health Canada.

Helakorpi, S., A. Uutela, R. Prättälä, and P. Puska. 1999. *Health behaviour and health among Finnish adult population, spring 1999.* Helsinki: National Public Health Institute.

Hendelman, D., K. Miller, C. Baggett, E. Debold, and P. Freedson. 2000. Validity of accelerometry for the assessment of moderate intensity physical activity in the field. *Medicine and Science in Sports and Exercise* 32 (Suppl.): S442–S449.

Hopkins, W.G., N.C. Wilson, D.G. Russell, and G.P. Herbison. 1991. *Life in New Zealand commission report. Vol. 3, Physical activity.* Dunedin, New Zealand: University of Otago.

Irish Heart Foundation. 1994. *Happy Heart National Survey: A report on health behaviour in Ireland.* Dublin: Irish Heart Foundation.

Jacobs, D.R., B.E. Ainsworth, T.J. Hartman, and A.S. Leon. 1993. A simultaneous evaluation of 10 commonly used physical activity questionnaires. *Medicine and Science in Sports and Exercise* 25: 81–91.

Kearney, J.M., M.J. Kearney, S. McElhone, and M.J. Gibney. 1999. Methods used to conduct the pan–European Union survey on consumer attitudes to physical activity, body weight and health. *Public Health Nutrition* 2: 79–86.

Kesaniemi, Y.A., E. Danforth Jr., M.D. Jensen, P.G. Kopelman, P. Lefebvre, and B.A. Reeder. 2001. Dose–response issues concerning physical activity and health: An evidence-based symposium. *Medicine and Science in Sports and Exercise* 33 (Suppl. 6): S351–S358.

Kriska, A.M., and C.J. Caspersen. 1997. Introduction to a collection of physical activity questionnaires. *Medicine and Science in Sports and Exercise* 29 (Suppl. 6): S5–S9.

LaPorte, R.E., H.J. Montoye, and C.J. Caspersen. 1985. Assessment of physical activity in epidemiologic research: Problems and prospects. *Public Health Reports* 100: 131–146.

Lee, I.M., C.C. Hsieh, and R.S. Paffenbarger Jr. 1995. Exercise intensity and longevity in men: The Harvard Alumni Health Study. *Journal of the American Medical Association* 273 (15): 1179–1184.

Lee, I.M., and R.S. Paffenbarger Jr. 2000. Associations of light, moderate, and vigorous intensity physical activity with longevity: The Harvard Alumni Health Study. *American Journal of Epidemiology* 151 (3): 293–299.

Lee, I.M., H.D. Sesso, and R.S. Paffenbarger Jr. 2000. Physical activity and coronary heart disease risk in men: Does the duration of exercise episodes predict risk? *Circulation* 102: 981–986.

Leon, A.S., and J. Connett. 1991. Physical activity and 10.5 year mortality in the Multiple Risk Factor Intervention Trial. *International Journal of Epidemiology* 20: 690–697.

Leon, A.S., J. Connett, D.R. Jacobs Jr., and R. Rauramaa. 1987. Leisure-time physical activity levels and risk of coronary heart disease and death: The Multiple Risk Factor Intervention Trial. *Journal of the American Medical Association* 258 (17): 2388–2395.

Lifson, N., G.B. Gordon, and R. McClintock. 1955. Measurement of total carbon dioxide production by means of $D_2{}^{18}O$. *Journal of Applied Physiology* 7: 704–710.

Lifson, N., W.S. Little, D.G. Levitt, and R.M. Henderson. 1975. $D_2{}^{18}O$ method for CO_2 output in small animals and economic feasibility in man. *Journal of Applied Physiology* 39: 657–663.

Manson, J.E., D.M. Nathan, A.S. Sroleswski, M.J. Stampfer, W.C. Willett, and C.H. Hennekens. 1992. A prospective study of exercise and incidence of diabetes in U.S. male physicians. *Journal of the American Medical Association* 268: 63–67.

Mason, J.O., and K.E. Powell. 1985. Physical activity, behavioral epidemiology, and public health. *Public Health Reports* 100: 113–115.

McClintock, R., and N. Lifson. 1957. Applicability of the $D_2{}^{18}O$ method to the measurement of the total carbon dioxide output of obese mice. *Journal of Biological Chemistry* 226: 153–156.

Melanson, E.L. Jr., and P.S. Freedson. 1995. Validity of the Computer Science and Applications, Inc. (CSA) activity monitor. *Medicine and Science in Sports and Exercise* 27 (6): 934–940.

Montoye, H.J. 1975. *Physical activity and health: An epidemiologic study of an entire community.* Englewood Cliffs, NJ: Prentice Hall.

Montoye, H.J., H.C.G. Kemper, W.H.M. Saris, and R.A. Washburn. 1996. *Measuring physical activity and energy expenditure.* Champaign, IL: Human Kinetics.

Montoye, H.J., S.B. Servais, and J.G. Webster. 1986. Estimation of energy expenditure from a force platform and an accelerometer. In *Sport science,* edited by J. Watkins, T. Reilly, and L. Burwitz, pp. 375–380. London: Spon.

Paffenbarger, R.S. Jr., S.N. Blair, I.M. Lee, and R.T. Hyde. 1993. Measurement of physical activity to assess health effects in free-living populations. *Medicine and Science in Sports and Exercise* 25: 60–70.

Paffenbarger, R.S. Jr., R.T. Hyde, A.W. Wing, I.M. Lee, D.L. Jung, and J.B. Kampert. 1993. The association of changes in physical activity level and other lifestyle characteristics with mortality among men. *New England Journal of Medicine* 328 (February 23): 538–545.

Paffenbarger, R.S. Jr., A.L. Wing, and R.T. Hyde. 1978. Physical activity as an index of heart attack risk in college alumni. *American Journal of Epidemiology* 108: 165–175.

Pereira, M.A., S.J. Fitzgerald, E.W. Gregg, M.L. Joswiak, W.J. Ryan, R.R. Suminski, A.C. Utter, and J.M. Zmuda. 1997. A collection of physical questionnaires for health-related research. *Medicine and Science in Sports and Exercise* 29 (6): S3–S205.

Perusse, L., A. Tremblay, C. LeBlanc, and C. Bouchard. 1989. Genetic and familial environmental influences on level of habitual physical activity. *American Journal of Epidemiology* 129: 1012–1022.

Pollock, M.L., G.A. Gaesser, J.D. Butcher, J.P. Despres, R.K. Dishman, B.A. Franklin, and C.E. Garber. 1998. Recommended quantity and quality of exercise for developing and maintaining cardiorespiratory and muscular fitness, and flexibility in healthy adults. *Medicine and Science in Sports and Exercise* 30: 975–991.

Powell, K.E. 1988. Habitual exercise and public health: An epidemiological view. In *Exercise adherence: Its impact on public health,* edited by R.K. Dishman, pp. 15–40. Champaign, IL: Human Kinetics.

Powell, K.E., and R.S. Paffenbarger. 1985. Workshop on epidemiologic and public health aspects of physical activity and exercise: A summary. *Public Health Reports* 100(2): 118–126.

Prentice, A.M., ed. 1990. *The doubly-labeled water method for measuring energy expenditure: A consensus report by the IDECG working group. Technical recommendations for use in humans.* International Atomic Energy Agency NAHRES-4. Vienna: International Dietary Energy Consultancy Group.

Prior, G. 1999. Physical activity. In *Health survey for England: Cardiovascular disease '98,* edited by B. Erens and P. Primatesta, pp. 181–219. London: Stationery Office.

Russell, D.G., and N.C. Wilson. 1991. *Life in New Zealand commission report.* Vol. 1, *Executive overview.* Dunedin, New Zealand: University of Otago.

Sallis, J.F., W.L. Haskell, P.D. Wood, S.P. Fortmann, T. Rogers, S.N. Blair, and R.S. Paffenbarger Jr. 1985. Physical activity assessment methodology in the five-city project. *American Journal of Epidemiology* 212 (1): 91–106.

Sallis, J.F., and B.E. Saelens. 2000. Assessment of physical activity by self-report: Status, limitations, and future directions. *Research Quarterly for Exercise and Sport* 71: 1–14.

Schoeller, D.A. 1999. Recent advances from application of doubly labeled water to measurement of human energy expenditure. *Journal of Nutrition* 129 (10): 1765–1768.

Schoeller, D.A., and E. van Santen. 1982. Measurement of energy expenditure in humans by doubly-labelled water method. *Journal of Applied Physiology* 53: 955–959.

Schoenborn, C.A., and M.A. Barnes. 2002. Leisure-time physical activity among adults: United States, 1997–98. *Advance Data* 325 (April 7): 1–24.

Servais, S.B., J.G. Webster, and H.J. Montoye. 1984. Estimating human energy expenditure using an accelerometer device. *Journal of Clinical Engineering* 9: 159–171.

Sesso, H.D., R.S. Paffenbarger Jr., and I.M. Lee. 2000. Physical activity and coronary heart disease in men: The Harvard Alumni Health Study. *Circulation* 102: 975–980.

Siconolfi, S.F., T.M. Lasater, R.C.K. Snow, and R.A. Carleton. 1985. Self-reported physical activity compared with maximal oxygen uptake. *American Journal of Epidemiology* 122: 101–105.

Sirard, J.R., and R.R. Pate. 2001. Physical activity assessment in children and adolescents. *Sports Medicine* 31: 439–454.

Strath, S.J., A.M. Swartz, D.R. Bassett Jr., W.L. O'Brien, G.A. King, and B.E. Ainsworth. 2000. Evaluation of heart rate as a method for assessing moderate intensity physical activity. *Medicine and Science in Sports and Exercise* 32 (Suppl. 9): S465–S470.

U.S. Department of Health and Human Services. 1980. *Promoting health/preventing disease: Objectives for the nation.* Washington, DC: U.S. Government Printing Office.

———. 1996. *Physical activity and health: A report of the Surgeon General.* Atlanta: Centers for Disease Control and Prevention, National Center for Chronic Disease Prevention and Health Promotion.

———. 2000. *Healthy people 2010: Understanding and improving health.* 2nd edition. Washington, DC: Government Printing Office.

Vainio, H., and F. Bianchini, eds. 2002. *Weight control and physical activity. Vol. 6 of IARC handbooks of cancer prevention.* Lyon, France: IARC Press.

Washburn, R., M.K. Chin, and H.J. Montoye. 1980. Accuracy of pedometers in walking and running. *Research Quarterly for Exercise and Sport* 51 (4): 695–702.

Washburn, R.A., S.R.W. Goldfield, K. Smith, and J.B. McKinlay. 1990. The validity of exercise induced sweating as a measure of physical activity. *American Journal of Epidemiology* 132: 107–113.

Washburn, R.A., and H.J. Montoye. 1986. The assessment of physical activity by questionnaire. *American Journal of Epidemiology* 123 (4): 563–576.

Welk, G.J., J.A. Differding, R.W. Thompson, S.N. Blair, J. Dziura, and T. Hart. 2000. The utility of the Digi-Walker step counter to assess daily physical activity patterns. *Medicine and Science in Sports and Exercise* 32 (Suppl.): S481–S488.

Westerterp, K.R. 1998. Alterations in energy balance with exercise. *American Journal of Clinical Nutrition* 68 (4): 970S–974S.

———. 1999. Physical activity assessment with accelerometers. *International Journal of Obesity and Related Metabolic Disorders* 23 (Suppl. 3): S45–S49.

Westerterp, K.R., F. Brouns, W.H.M. Saris, and F. Ten Hoor. 1988. Comparison of doubly labelled water with respirometry at low- and high-activity levels. *Journal of Applied Physiology* 65: 53–56.

Westerterp, K.R., J.O. de Boer, W.H.M. Saris, P.F.M. Schoffelen, and F. Ten Hoor. 1984. Measurement of energy expenditure using doubly-labelled water. *International Journal of Sports Medicine* 5 (Suppl.): 74–75.

Williams, P.T. 1996. High-density lipoprotein cholesterol and other risk factors for coronary heart disease in female runners. *New England Journal of Medicine* 334 (20): 1298–1303.

———. 1997. Relationship of distance run per week to coronary heart disease risk factors in 8283 male runners: The National Runners' Health Study. *Archives of Internal Medicine* 157: 191–198.

———. 1998a. Coronary heart disease risk factors of vigorously active sexagenarians and septuagenarians. *Journal of the American Geriatric Society* 46 (2): 134–142.

———. 1998b. Relationships of heart disease risk factors to exercise quantity and intensity. *Archives of Internal Medicine* 158 (3): 237–245.

Web Sites

www.cdc.gov. The home page of the federal Centers for Disease Control and Prevention in Atlanta, Georgia, provides quick access to many health databases pertinent to physical activity epidemiology and to the *Morbidity and Mortality Weekly Report.*

www.cdc.gov/mmwr/. *Morbidity and Mortality Weekly Report,* which compiles national health data and reports from state health departments.

www.cdc.gov/brfss/. The site for the Behavioral Risk Factor Surveillance System (BRFSS), the world's largest telephone survey, which tracks health risks, including physical inactivity, in the United States.

www.cdc.gov/nccdphp/dnpa/surveill.htm. The site of the National Center for Chronic Disease Prevention and Health Promotion of the CDC provides access to information about the major survey and surveillance systems for measuring and tracking physical activity in the United States.

www.cdc.gov/nchs/nhis.htm. The site for the National Health Interview Survey, which tracks health behaviors in the United States.

www.cdc.gov/nccdphp/dash/yrbs/. The site of the Youth Risk Behavior Survey, which tracks health risks, including physical inactivity, among youth in the United States.

www.fedstats.gov/programs/health.html. This site provides links to statistics from several U.S. federal health agencies, including the National Center for Health Statistics.

www.ipaq.ki.se. This site describes the development and validation of the International Physical Activity Questionnaire.

www.who.int. This site of the World Health Organization in Geneva, Switzerland, provides information on world diseases and lifestyles.

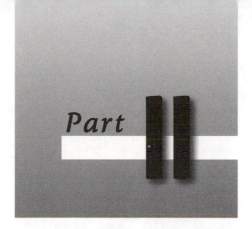

PHYSICAL ACTIVITY AND DISEASE MORTALITY

Today, the average life span of a U.S. citizen, about 74 years for men and 79 years for women, ranks near the lowest among industrialized nations. Because it is accepted that people's behavior influences their health and risk of premature mortality, understanding the role of physical activity in reducing mortality risk has great public health importance in the U.S., as it does in other developed and developing nations. Sedentariness is a burden to the public health in the United States, accounting for an estimated 200,000 deaths each year from all causes, especially from coronary heart disease, type 2 diabetes mellitus, and colon cancer. The chapters in this section focus on the evidence that physical activity protects against premature death from all causes and, more specifically, deaths from coronary heart disease and stroke, which account for about 20% of all deaths worldwide and 50% of deaths in developed nations.

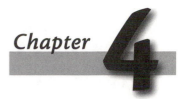

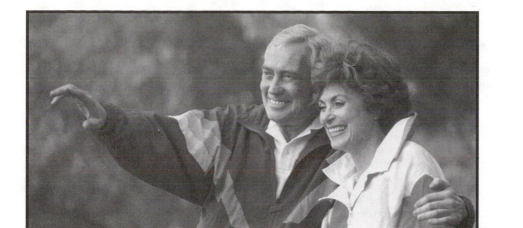

Chapter 4

© Jim and Mary Whitmer

All-Cause and Coronary Heart Disease Mortality

It is not the rich nor the great, not those who depend on medicine, who became old, but such as use much exercise.

—James Easton, 1799

The conclusion by the early English epidemiologist James Easton was drawn in his 1799 book, *Human Longevity,* in which he chronicled the lives of 1,712 people who lived to 100 years of age or older between the years A.D. 66 to 1799 (Easton 1799). This chapter examines whether Easton's view was correct, based on modern epidemiologic evidence. We focus especially on the reduced risk of coronary heart disease (CHD) mortality among people who are physically active. Subsequent chapters of the book present evidence for the association of physical inactivity and the risk of developing other specific major contributors to mortality, specifically hypertension, **hyperlipidemia,** obesity, stroke, type 2 diabetes, osteoporosis, cancer, and depression. In this chapter, we review the evidence to support the hypothesis that physical inactivity increases the risk for both all-cause and CHD mortality. It is not our goal to provide an exhaustive review of these topics but to present a sample of classic and contemporary studies on these topics and to summarize current issues, including dose response and optimal activity intensity to reduce mortality risk. For comprehensive reviews on the topic of physical activity and all-cause and CHD mortality, see Berlin and Colditz (1990), Blair and Wei (2000), Kohl (2001), Lee and Paffenbarger (1996), Lee and Skerrett (2001), and Powell et al. (1987).

All-Cause Mortality

Today, the average life span of a U.S. citizen is among the lowest of industrialized nations. As indicated in table 4.1, in 2001 the highest average life expectancy at birth was in Japan (77.9 years for men, 84.7 years for women), while the United States was 22nd for men (74.3 years) and 19th for women (79.5 years).

Death rates are lower among women than men at all ages in all developed, and in most undeveloped, nations (figure 4.1). Possible, though unproven, explanations include sex hormones: Testosterone has been linked with hazardous behavior and undesirable cholesterol levels, while estrogen is an **antioxidant** (which might protect against cell damage) and appears to regulate enzymes that favorably affect cholesterol metabolism. Evolutionary biologists argue that long life in women is linked with a genetic advantage for childbirth and care of the young (Perls and Fretts 1998). However, many other social and environmental influences might interact to explain the longer life expectancy of women. Paradoxically, females are less active than males. Nonetheless, living longer does not necessarily ensure more years of good health. When data are available, we will discuss how physical activity and fitness affect disease risk and health outcomes similarly and differently in women and men.

TABLE 4.1   LIFE EXPECTANCY BY COUNTRY, 2001

FEMALE		MALE	
Country	**Years of life expectancy**	**Country**	**Years of life expectancy**
Japan	84.7	Japan	77.9
France	82.9	Sweden	77.7
Switzerland	82.8	Australia	77.4
Australia	82.6	Switzerland	77.3
Spain	82.6	Canada	76.6
Sweden	82.3	Singapore	76.5
Italy	82.2	Italy	76.2
Canada	81.9	Israel	76.1
Austria	81.8	New Zealand	76.1
Norway	81.4	Norway	76.1
Belgium	81.2	Austria	75.9
Finland	81.2	The Netherlands	75.8
Germany	81.1	France	75.6

FEMALE			MALE		
Country	**Years of life expectancy**		**Country**	**Years of life expectancy**	
Singapore	81.1		Greece	75.5	
Israel	80.9		Spain	75.3	
Greece	80.8		Germany	75.1	
The Netherlands	80.7		United Kingdom	75.1	
United Kingdom	79.9		Belgium	74.8	
United States	79.5		Denmark	74.8	
			Cuba	74.7	
			Finland	74.5	
			United States	74.3	

World Health Organization. 2003. *The World Health Report 2002.* Geneva, Switzerland.

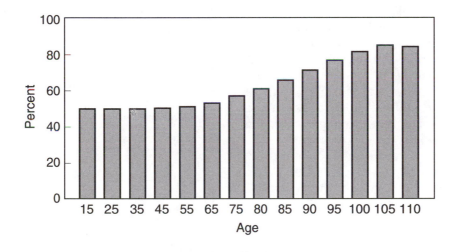

Figure 4.1 Percentage of U.S. population that is female.

Reprinted, by permission, from T.T. Perls and R.C. Fretts, 1998, "Why women live longer than men," *Scientific American,* June. By permission of the author.

Cardiovascular Disease Mortality

Coronary heart disease and **cerebrovascular disease** constitute most of cardiovascular disease (CVD), which is responsible for 20% of all deaths worldwide (about 14 million deaths per year) according to the World Health Organization. CVD accounts for 50% of deaths in developed nations, making it the main cause of mortality. It is the third leading killer in developing nations, accounting for 16% of all deaths. Excluding accidents, which are the third leading cause of death among men in the United States, the three leading causes of death for both men and women are heart disease (mainly coronary heart disease), cancer, and cerebrovascular disease (mainly stroke). Despite steady progress in reducing CVD mortality during the past 40 years, CVD has been the top U.S. killer every year since 1900 except in 1918, the year of the great flu epidemic. In 2001, an estimated 922,000 deaths were attributed to CVD (Centers for Disease Control and Prevention 2003). The economic burden of CVD, including health care costs and lost productivity from sickness and death, was projected to be $298.2 billion in 2001, with CHD costing $100.8 billion and stroke costing $45.4 billion (American Heart Association 2000).

> ••• *Cardiovascular disease is the main cause of death in developed nations and the third leading killer in developing nations, accounting for 20% of all deaths each year worldwide.*

Though CVD prevalence has declined, the rate of decline has not been uniform among all segments of the population. People with lower economic status have higher risk than those who are more affluent. There are race differences in mortality rates in the United States that vary by age and disease. In a nine-year follow-up to the National Longitudinal Mortality Study of adults 25 years of age and older, all-cause and cardiovascular mortality were highest among black persons younger than 65 years, especially between ages 25 to 44 years, independent of socioeconomic status (Ng-Mak et al. 1999). Cause of death also varies by age with heart disease leading the list in individuals age 65 and over (table 4.2).

Over the past 20 years, evidence has accumulated that implicates physical inactivity as a risk factor for a number of the leading causes of death in the United States and thus as a reason for our reduced life spans. The National Center for Health Statistics has estimated that the combination of physical inactivity and poor dietary habits accounted for 300,000 deaths in the United States in 1990, second only to tobacco smoking, which accounts for an estimated 440,000 deaths annually (McGinnis and Foege 1993). An estimated 200,000 deaths linked to physical inactivity

TABLE 4.2　U.S. MORTALITY RATES BY CAUSE AND AGE, 2001

LEADING CAUSES OF DEATH BY AGE GROUP

Younger than 1 year	Number of deaths
Birth defects	5,608
Disorders related to premature birth	4,496
Sudden infant death syndrome	1,972
1–4 years	
Unintentional injuries	1,701
Birth defects	552
Cancer	413
5–14 years	
Unintentional injuries	2,802
Cancer	1,002
Birth defects	366
15–24 years	
Unintentional injuries	13,871
Homicide	5,126
Suicide	3,854
25–44 years	
Unintentional injuries	26,138
Cancer	20,493
Heart disease	15,942
45–64 years	
Cancer	139,908
Heart disease	98,048
Unintentional injuries	19,965
65 years and older	
Heart disease	583,773
Cancer	389,657
Stroke	144,626

Centers for Disease Control and Prevention. National Center for Health Statistics. 2003. *National Vital Statistics Reports* 51(5).

resulted from three diseases: coronary heart disease, colon cancer, and type 2 diabetes (Powell and Blair 1994).

> ••• *Physical inactivity accounts for about 300,000 deaths each year from coronary heart disease, colon cancer, and type 2 diabetes, second only to the 440,000 deaths now attributed to tobacco use.*

Physical Activity and All-Cause Mortality

In a recent review of the cumulative evidence (Lee and Skerrett 2001), 34 of 44 observational studies published between 1966 and July 2000 that included at least three levels of physical activity (38 studies) or fitness (7 studies) suggested a linear reduction in mortality risk with increased level of physical activity. All but 2 of the 17 studies that conducted a statistical test of linear trend found one that was similar in men and women regardless of age. On average, a threshold of about 1,000 kcal per week was accompanied by a 20% to 30% reduction in mortality risk. Further risk reduction was observed with activity expending greater than 1,000 kcal/wk, but there wasn't enough evidence to draw conclusions about the impact of the intensity, duration, and frequency of activity (Lee and Skerrett 2001).

Most of the studies used a prospective cohort design, classifying participants according to activity level at baseline, and compared all-cause mortality rates after follow-up among physical activity categories or compared mortality rates in participants who changed or did not change their physical activity levels over time. The following sections consider studies that compared all-cause mortality in active participants with their sedentary peers.

> ••• *Observational studies have shown an average 20% to 30% reduction in mortality risk when people expend at least 1,000 kcal a week in physical activity.*

U.S. Railroad Workers

In an early study on physical activity, 1,978 white men who had worked in the U.S. railroad industry for at least 10 years by 1951 were classified by level of occupational activity as sedentary (clerks) or active (switchmen or section men, the most active). All-cause mortality from 1955 to 1956 in men ages 40 to 64 years was included in the analysis. The age-adjusted death rates (per 1,000) were 11.8 for clerks, 10.3 for switchmen, and 7.6 for section men. Although the mortality rate was significantly lower for the most-active men, the results should be interpreted cautiously because data on potential confounding factors, such as BMI, blood pressure, smoking, and cholesterol, were not available, and thus the analysis did not adjust for them.

Men and Women in Eastern Finland

Salonen, Puska, and Tuomilehto (1982) observed about 4,000 men ages 30 to 59 years and 3,700 women ages 35 to 59 years from two counties in eastern Finland for seven years. Relative risk of all-cause mortality adjusted for age, BMI, cigarette smoking, diastolic blood pressure, and serum cholesterol in men was 1.9 (95% confidence interval [CI]: 1.5–2.5) for those with low occupational physical activity and 1.5 (95% CI: 1.2–2.0) for those with low leisure-time physical activity. Corresponding relative risks for women were 2.2 (95% CI: 1.5–3.3) and 1.6 (1.0–2.3).

Harvard Alumni Health Study

The Harvard Alumni Health Study, one of the most influential studies of physical activity and chronic disease, is an ongoing cohort study of predictors of chronic disease in men who were undergraduates at Harvard University between 1916 and 1950. The original cohort is composed of 21,582 alumni who returned a mail questionnaire on medical history and health habits in 1962 or 1966. To be eligible for the physical activity and mortality analysis, respondents needed to report no physician-diagnosed cardiovascular disease, cancer, or chronic obstructive pulmonary disease. In addition, respondents had to provide information on physical activity, body weight, height, cigarette smoking, physician-diagnosed high blood pressure and diabetes, vital status of both parents, and the age of parents' death if applicable. Approximately 17,000 alumni satisfied the eligibility criteria. Most were either retired or engaged in sedentary occupations.

Paffenbarger et al. (1986) followed these men for 16 years after they completed a mail survey on their exercise habits, the Harvard Alumni

Physical Activity Survey, which requested information on their usual walking, stair climbing, and sports participation. The exercise self-reports were converted to estimates of caloric expenditure and reported as kilocalories per week. There was a steady decline in all-cause death rates across weekly caloric expenditure categories, from 94 per 10,000 person-years of follow-up for men who expended less than 500 kcal/wk exercising to 43 per 10,000 person-years for men in the 3,000 to 3,499 kcal/wk category. Men 35 to 79 years old who expended less than 2,000 kcal/wk in exercise at the beginning of the study were compared with men who expended 2,000 kcal/wk or more. The active men gained 1.25 years of life up to age 80, compared with the sedentary men. For each hour spent exercising each week, Harvard alumni gained 2 h of life.

> ••• *Among Harvard alumni, men 35 to 79 years old who expended 2,000 kcal/wk or more in exercise at the beginning of the study gained 1.25 years of life up to age 80, compared with men categorized as sedentary.*

Finnish Cohort of Seven Countries Study

Of the 16 cohorts in the Seven Countries Study on cardiovascular diseases, 12 population samples in six countries reached the 20-year follow-up deadline by the mid-1980s. Data on mortality in 8,300 men ages 40 to 59 at entry into the study included two cohorts in Finland (figure 4.2; Menotti et al. 1989). Men classified as highly active at the beginning of the study had about half the mortality rate of low-activity men at each of the first 5-year periods throughout the 20-year follow-up, demonstrating persistent protection against premature death.

The Seventh Day Adventist Mortality Study

The association of self-reported physical activity with all-cause and disease-specific mortality was examined in a study of nearly 9,500 men ages 30 years or older in 1958 who were followed from 1960 through 1985 (Lindsted et al. 1991). All-cause death at age 50 was reduced by participation in either moderate (RR = 0.61, 95% CI: 0.50–0.74) or vigorous (RR = 0.66, 95% CI: 0.50–0.87) physical activity. Moderate physical activity remained associated with reduced mortality rates at age 80; neither moderate nor vigorous activity was protective at age 90.

Cardiovascular Health Study

The Cardiovascular Health Study was a prospective cohort study designed to determine the extent to which subclinical disease, functional health, and personal characteristics jointly predict mortality among adults ages 65 years or older (Fried et al. 1998). A main cohort of 5,201 men and women that was 95% white and a supplemental cohort of 685 African American men and women ages 65 years or older were recruited from four U.S. communities in Sacramento, California; Maryland; North Carolina; and Pittsburgh, Pennsylvania. After five years of follow-up, there were 646 deaths (12%) in the main cohort. Twenty

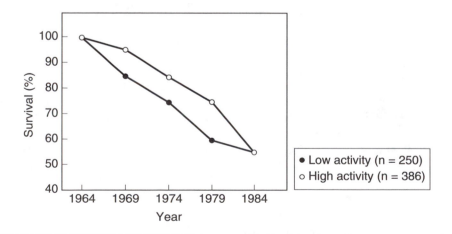

Figure 4.2 Finnish cohort.

Adapted, by permission, from A. Menotti et al., 1989, "Seven countries study. First 20-year mortality data in 12 cohorts of six countries," *Annals of Medicine* 21(3): 175-179.

characteristics of the participants were independently associated with mortality, including increasing age, male sex, income less than $50,000 per year, low weight, smoking for more than 50 pack-years, high brachial systolic blood pressure (>169 mmHg), elevated fasting glucose level (>7.2 mmol/L, or >130 mg/dl), abnormal left ventricular ejection fraction, major electrocardiographic abnormality, and lack of moderate or vigorous exercise. Neither HDL-C nor LDL-C was associated with mortality in this cohort. After adjustment for other factors, the association between age and mortality diminished, but the reduction in mortality for female sex persisted. A prediction equation for mortality computed from the main cohort also accurately predicted mortality during 4.5 years of follow-up in the African American cohort.

Men and women who said they expended more than 4,100 kJ/wk (980 kcal/wk) during moderate to vigorous leisure-time physical activity had two thirds the risk of mortality (RR = 0.72, 95% CI: 0.55–0.93), and those expending more than 7,900 kJ/wk (1,890 kcal/wk) had one half the risk of mortality (RR = 0.56, 95% CI: 0.43–0.75) of those expending less than 280 kJ/wk (67 kcal/wk). The reduced mortality was linearly related to increased physical activity and was adjusted for age, smoking, BMI, alcohol use, blood pressure, serum cholesterol, and chronic diseases.

The Finnish Twin Study

The Finnish Twin Study was begun in 1975 to determine whether genetic factors or family health habits during childhood explain part of the protective effects of physical activity against premature death (Kujala et al. 1998). A cohort of 7,925 healthy men and 7,977 healthy women ages 25 to 64 years responded to a questionnaire asking about physical activity habits and other known risk factors of mortality. Those who reported exercising at least six times per month with an intensity equivalent to at least vigorous walking for an average duration of 30 min were classified as conditioning exercisers. Those who reported no leisure physical activity were classified as sedentary, and other subjects were classified as occasional exercisers. There were 1,253 deaths in the whole cohort and 434 discordant deaths among same-sex twins (i.e., one twin died and the other was still alive) in the period 1977 through 1994.

After controlling for age, sex, smoking, occupation, and alcohol use, the relative risk for death was 0.80 (95% CI: 0.69–0.91) among occasional exercisers in the whole cohort and 0.76 (0.59–0.98)

among conditioning exercisers, compared with sedentary subjects. Also, there was a linear reduction in risk with increasing amounts of physical activity. Among same-sex twin pairs, the discordant death rate was about 65% among occasional exercisers and 45% among conditioning exercisers compared with those who were sedentary. Again, the reduction in risk with increasing physical activity was linear, but it was no longer statistically significant after controlling for smoking and alcohol use. It was not possible to determine whether genetic or familial factors were more influential on the protective effect of physical activity. In only a single instance among the 120 monozygotic twins who were death-discordant was one twin sedentary and the other a conditioning exerciser. The correlation between the estimated daily energy expenditure of twins was about 0.40 for both male and female monozygotic twins, about twice as large as for dizygotic twins. In this study, physical activity was associated with reduced mortality, even after genetic and other familial factors were taken into account.

Physical Fitness and All-Cause Mortality

The imprecise methods available to assess regular physical activity and the use of occupational classification as a surrogate for physical activity probably underestimate the true relationship between physical activity and mortality by misclassifying some inactive people as active and some active people as inactive. Another way to address the exercise–mortality question is to assess physical fitness as a marker of exercise habits. Though physical fitness is partly determined by genetic factors, Canadian research on the inheritance of fitness in monozygotic twins has estimated that the genetically transmissible portion is only about 40% of cardiorespiratory fitness (i.e., maximal oxygen uptake) (Bouchard et al. 1986). Thus, fitness is a good marker of physical activity habits among adults. The following section describes the few reports that have assessed physical fitness and all-cause mortality.

U.S. Railroad Workers

Physical fitness was assessed by the heart rate response to submaximal treadmill exercise in 2,431 men ages 22 to 79 years who were employed in the U.S. railroad industry and were free from cardiovascular disease at the baseline exam (Slattery and Jacobs 1988). The men were followed for mortality from the baseline exam, done from 1957 to 1960, until 1977, during which time there were 631 deaths. Results indicated that the risk for all-cause mortality in the least-fit group was 1.23 times (95% CI: 1.17–1.30) that of the fittest group after adjustment for age, blood pressure, cigarette smoking, and serum cholesterol.

Aerobics Center Longitudinal Study

The Aerobics Center Longitudinal Study is an observational cohort study of over 25,000 men and 7,000 women who received preventive medical examinations at the Cooper Institute in Dallas, Texas. Blair et al. (1989) reported the relationship between maximal treadmill time (an estimate of cardiorespiratory fitness that predicts maximal oxygen uptake with about 80% accuracy) and mortality rates in 10,224 men and 3,120 women from this cohort who were followed for an average of about eight years. The age-adjusted

all-cause mortality rate for the least-fit (first quintile, i.e. the lowest 20% of the cohort) men was three times greater (95% CI: 2.05–5.77) than for the most fit (fifth quintile), and the mortality rate for the least-fit women was 4.65 times greater (95% CI: 2.22–9.75) than for the fittest women (figure 4.3). Mortality rates per 10,000 person-years were 64.0 for men of low fitness (first quintile), 26.3 for moderate fitness (second and third quintiles), and 20.3 for high fitness (fourth and fifth quintiles). For women in the same fitness categories, mortality rates per 10,000 person-years were 39.5, 16.4, and 7.4, respectively.

Analyses of mortality rates in the Aerobics Center Longitudinal Study were extended up to 1994 among 749 women and 1,758 men who were 60 to 89 years old at the time of their first clinic visit and fitness test. During an average of 10 years of follow-up surveillance, 44 women and 270 men died. Though the small number of deaths renders the analysis tentative, particularly for the

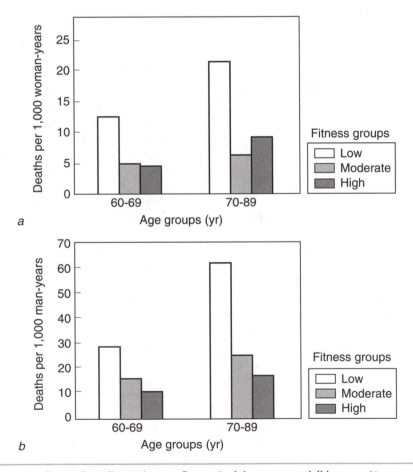

Figure 4.3 All-cause mortality and cardiorespiratory fitness in (a) women and (b) men >60 years of age.

Adapted, by permission, from S. Blair et al., 1989, "Physical fitness and all-cause mortality: A prospective study of healthy men and women," *Journal of the American Medical Association* 262: 2395-2401.

women, the least-fit 20% of both men and women had elevated crude death rates per 1,000 person-years of exposure compared with the fittest 40% (figure 4.4). An apparent linear dose–response gradient in risk reduction by level of fitness was observed for men, whereas an apparent threshold of benefit appeared for the moderately fit women, with no further risk reduction among the fittest women. The reduction in death rate among the highly fit remained after adjustment for age, examination year, BMI, total cholesterol, smoking, high blood pressure, diabetes, and personal and parental history of cardiovascular disease. Should these analyses be confirmed by subsequent studies, the important finding would be that the protective effect of fitness in reducing mortality is not merely a reduction in the rate of premature death among middle-aged people.

> ••• *The lower death rates among highly fit men and women appear to be independent of age, BMI, total cholesterol, smoking, high blood pressure, diabetes, and personal and parental history of cardiovascular disease.*

Another report on 25,341 men and 7,080 women ages 20 to 88 years in the Aerobics Center Longitudinal Study cohort analyzed 690 deaths during an eight-year follow-up and found that the highest 20% of performers on a maximal treadmill test had a relative risk of 0.49 (95% CI: 0.37–0.64) for men and 0.37 (0.19–0.72) for women compared with the lowest 20% of performers and adjusted for age,

year of examination, smoking, chronic diseases, and ECG abnormalities (Kampert et al. 1996).

Norwegian Men

In a prospective study that started in 1972, the physical fitness of 1,960 healthy Norwegian men aged 40 to 59 years was measured as the total work performed during a symptom-limited cycling exercise test (Sandvik et al. 1993). About 16 years later 271 men had died. After adjustment for age, smoking status, serum lipids, blood pressure, resting heart rate, vital capacity, BMI, level of physical activity, and glucose tolerance, the relative risk for all-cause mortality among men in the highest quartile (i.e., the highest 25% of the men) of fitness was less than half (RR = 0.41, 95% CI: 0.20–0.84) the rate observed among men in the lowest quartile, but all-cause mortality was similar among the men in the lowest three fitness quartiles. Physical activity did not influence mortality risk beyond the influence of fitness.

Changes in Physical Activity and Fitness and All-Cause Mortality

Few studies have assessed the impact of changing physical activity habits or physical fitness on the subsequent risk for all-cause mortality. Though not as convincing as evidence from a randomized controlled trial (in which physical activity or fitness are manipulated independently by investigators), demonstrating that a naturally occurring change in an independent variable, such as physical activity or fitness, results in a

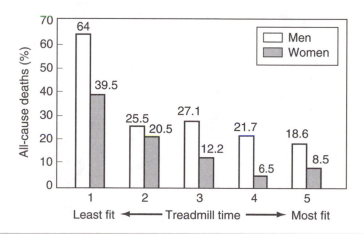

Figure 4.4 The least-fit 20% of both men and women had elevated crude death rates per 1,000 person-years of exposure compared to the 40% who were judged most fit.

Adapted, by permission, from S.N. Blair and M. Wei, 2000, "Sedentary habits, health, and function in older women and men," *American Journal of Health Promotion* 15: 1-8.

change in the dependent variable, such as all-cause mortality, provides strong evidence for the cause-and-effect association of those variables.

> ••• *Few studies have assessed the impact of changing physical activity habits or physical fitness on the subsequent risk for all-cause mortality.*

Harvard Alumni Health Study

A report on 10,269 healthy Harvard alumni ages 45 to 84 years examined the change in mortality risk associated with a change in physical activity assessed with the Harvard Alumni Physical Activity Survey between 1962 and 1966 and again in 1977 (Paffenbarger et al. 1993). During the follow-up period, 1977 to 1985, a total of 476 deaths were recorded (figure 4.5). Results indicated that men who changed from being inactive (<2,000 kcal/wk) to active (≥2,000 kcal/wk) had approximately the same mortality rate as men who were active at both times. Men who did not participate in any moderate physical activity (≥4.5 METs) at baseline but did so in 1977 showed a significant 23% lower all-cause mortality rate (RR = 0.77, 95% CI: 0.58–0.96) compared with those who never reported moderate activity, after adjustment for age, cigarette smoking, hypertension, and BMI.

Men who reported moderate activity at both time points also had a significant 29% reduction in mortality rate.

> ••• *During nearly 10 years of follow-up, all-cause mortality was reduced by nearly a quarter among male Harvard alumni who changed from being inactive to participating in moderate physical activity. Though not as convincing as results from a randomized controlled trial, showing a change in mortality associated with a naturally occurring change in physical activity or fitness strongly suggests causation.*

Nurses' Health Study

The Nurses' Health Study began in 1976, when 121,700 female registered nurses 30 to 55 years of age residing in 11 large U.S. states completed a mail questionnaire regarding their medical history and lifestyle, including physical activity. This group has been followed every two years to update risk factor information and health status.

One report from this cohort (Manson et al. 1999) compared physical activity in 1980 with that in 1986. Among women who were sedentary (exercised less than once per week) in 1980, those who remained sedentary in 1986 had sub-

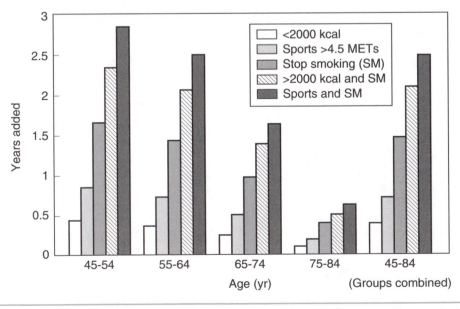

Figure 4.5 This study examines the change in mortality risk associated with a change in physical activity assessed with the Harvard Alumni Physical Activity Survey in 1962–1966 and again in 1977.

Data from R.S. Paffenbarger et al. 1993.

stantially higher rates of CHD events than women who became active. Compared with the risk for women who remained sedentary, the multivariate adjusted risk of coronary deaths from 1986 to 1994 for women in increasing quintiles of total physical activity were, respectively, 0.85 (95% CI: 0.69–1.06), 0.70 (0.62–0.99), 0.67 (0.54–0.88) and 0.60 (0.46–0.77).

> ••• *Among women ages 30 to 55 years, those who remained sedentary over a six-year period had approximately 40% to 66% higher mortality rates than women who increased their physical activity.*

Aerobics Center Longitudinal Study

The Aerobics Center Longitudinal Study included a follow-up of 9,177 men (6,219 healthy and 2,958 unhealthy) ages 20 to 82 years who received two preventive medical exams between 1970 and 1987 (Blair et al. 1995). The mean interval between examinations was 4.9 years. Physical fitness was assessed by time on a treadmill in a maximal exercise protocol; subjects were classified by quintile (Q1, unfit; Q2–Q5, fit). Mortality was assessed during a 5.1-year follow-up starting after the second exam and continuing through 1989. Results indicated that the lowest age-adjusted mortality rates were in men who were fit at both exams, while the highest mortality rates were in those unfit at both exams. Men who changed fitness category, either from unfit to fit or from fit to unfit, showed intermediate mortality rates that were similar for both change groups. For each minute of increased treadmill time (about 1 MET), mortality risk was reduced by 7.9%.

Norwegian Men

A cohort study of 1,428 healthy men ages 50 to 70 years were followed for 13 years after an initial cycling fitness test administered from 1972 to 1975 (Erikssen et al. 1998). During the 13-year follow-up, there were 238 deaths. At a second test administered from 1980 to 1982, a linear reduction in mortality risk was seen when the three highest quartiles of fitness were compared with the lowest. The relative risks were 0.72 (95% CI: 0.52–0.99), 0.48 (0.33–0.71), and 0.45 (0.29–0.69), respectively. Those men who improved their cycling fitness on the second evaluation (over a range of 5 to 10 years) had lower mortality rates, independent of their initial fitness level.

Stanford Men

A recent prospective study of a cohort of 6,213 men referred by a physician for clinical treadmill exercise testing found that exercise capacity was a more powerful predictor of mortality among men than other established risk factors for cardiovascular disease, such as blood pressure (Myers et al. 2002). Of these men, 3,679 had an abnormal exercise test result, a history of cardiovascular disease, or both, and 2,534 had a normal exercise test result and no history of cardiovascular disease. There were 1,256 deaths and an average annual mortality of 2.6%. After adjustment for age, the peak exercise capacity measured in METs was the strongest predictor of the risk of death among both normal subjects and those with cardiovascular disease. Mortality was reduced by 12% for each MET of exercise completed during the test.

Coronary Heart Disease Mortality

Although a high percentage of all-cause mortality is due to CHD, studies evaluating the association of physical activity and all-cause mortality also include deaths from cancer and accidents and deaths secondary to diabetes and other health conditions. In this section we describe the magnitude of the problem of CHD, its risk factors, and its **etiology**.

History and Magnitude of the Problem

The recorded history of coronary heart disease dates to around A.D. 150, when Galen wrote about dyscrasias of the heart (an abnormal condition of the body attributed to materials affecting blood cells). In 1628 the British physician William Harvey explained that blood was pumped by the heart in a circuit. He was the first to describe a myocardial infarction (heart attack). A century later, in 1768, William Heberden coined the term **angina pectoris** to describe the chest pain resulting from inadequate circulation of blood to the heart. Soon after, the English surgeon John Hunter discovered coronary artery disease while conducting an autopsy of a patient who had apparently died in an angry rage. Ironically, Hunter died about 20 years later of a heart attack, reportedly enraged after an acrimonious meeting. In 1912 an American physician, James Harrick, speculated that coronary heart disease resulted from a hardening of the arteries that supplied blood to the heart. Today CHD represents a major public health problem.

According to the National Heart, Lung, and Blood Institute (1998), heart disease (i.e., coronary heart disease, hypertensive heart disease, and rheumatic heart disease) has been the number one cause of death in the United States since the early 1920s. However, mortality from heart disease in the United States has dropped by nearly 65% from a peak of 307 per 100,000 in the 1960s to 108 per 100,000 in 2000. Worldwide, the annual rates of heart attack and coronary death in middle to early old age (35 to 64 years) have dropped in both men (a 2.7% decline) and women (a 2.1% decline) since the 1980s (Tunstall-Pedoe et al. 1999). These U.S. and worldwide trends probably occurred because of reduced cigarette smoking by adults, better medication of hypertension, greater public awareness about the importance of lowering fat and cholesterol in the diet, and better medical treatment for heart attacks.

••• *Mortality from heart disease in the United States has dropped by almost 65%, from a peak of 307 per 100,000 in the 1960s to about 108 per 100,000 in 2000. Nonetheless, CHD remains the number one cause of death in the United States, accounting for about 40% of all deaths annually and costing an estimated $100 billion, more than one third of the costs of all cardiovascular diseases.*

CHD has an annual prevalence in the United States of about 12.5 million people. The annual incidence of acute myocardial infarction (MI) is about 1.1 million, and the annual number of cardiac deaths is about 500,000. Of those, half are sudden cardiac death. CHD accounts for over 50% of cardiovascular deaths and nearly 40% of all deaths each year in the United States. Half of American men and a third of American women will develop CHD (American Heart Association 2001). The average risk among men of having an MI before age 60 is about one in five. Compared with men, women are protected from CHD until menopause. By age 65, the rates of CHD are similar for men and women. Recent findings from the Framingham Heart Study recently indicate that one of three men and one of four women will develop CHD after age 70 (American Heart Association 2001).

Though deaths from CHD have been declining during the past decade, CHD remains the number one cause of mortality in the United States, with an estimated 700,000 deaths in 2001. The economic burden of CHD in the United States also has been high during the past several years, accounting for an estimated $100 billion, or more than one third of the annual cost of all cardiovascular diseases. CHD is a major contributor to disability and lost productivity.

••• *The annual incidence of acute myocardial infarction is about 1.1 million, and the average annual number of cardiac deaths is about 500,000. Of those, half are sudden cardiac death.*

Coronary Heart Disease Risk Factors

The major risk factors for CHD include genetic susceptibility, female sex (postmenopause), age, elevated serum cholesterol, low levels of HDL cholesterol, cigarette smoking, uncontrolled hypertension, obesity, diabetes mellitus, and physical inactivity. Major risk factors that are modifiable by physical activity (e.g., hypertension, hyperlipidemia, obesity, and diabetes) are described in more detail in chapters 6 through 9 of this book.

Major Modifiable Risk Factors for Coronary Heart Disease

- Tobacco smoke
- High blood cholesterol
- High blood pressure
- Physical inactivity
- Diabetes mellitus
- Obesity
- Stress
- High triglycerides
- Alcohol abuse (moderate use, one to two drinks a day, reduces risk)

American Heart Association 2001.

In addition, elevated homocysteine (which is associated with vascular injury), abnormalities in regulatory proteins of the hemostatic system (which control blood clotting mechanisms), and inflammation appear to directly contribute to the pathogenesis of CHD. They are discussed in the following section, which describes the etiology of CHD.

Coronary Heart Disease Etiology

The process that leads to CHD and ischemic stroke is **atherosclerosis,** which is a form of **arteriosclerosis** (i.e., hardening of an artery) characterized by fatty deposits called **atheromas** (from the Greek words *athere,* meaning "gruel," and *oma,* meaning "tumor"), which contribute to narrowing and obstruction of medium and large arteries.

Plaques (large, more solid atheromas) vary in size and shape. They may protrude into the lumen (interior diameter) of a coronary artery but often extend into the artery wall, making them difficult to detect by common clinical tests such as **angiography.** Though vessel occlusion (blockage) by large plaques is the main cause of angina pectoris, smaller plaques covered by scar tissue are more apt to rupture and release cholesterol into the blood, triggering **thrombosis** (clot formation) and increasing the risks of **ischemia,** heart attack, and injury to or death of myocardial cells downstream from the occluded region of the vessel.

The atherosclerotic process in coronary arteries begins in childhood. Its severity is related to the level of blood cholesterol and its **lipoprotein** constituents. Low-density lipoprotein (LDL) accelerates atherosclerosis, while high-density lipoprotein (HDL) retards it. Cigarette smoking, high blood pressure, and dietary intake of **saturated fat** and cholesterol also contribute to atherosclerosis.

Atherogenesis

The process of atherogenesis begins with a lesion of the **intima** (the innermost lining) of a coronary artery. The lesion results from tissue injury to cells of the **endothelium,** which can be physical damage from lipoprotein levels, or chemical damage from tobacco smoke or high homocysteine levels. The initial response to the injury involves a six-step cascade of interactions between circulating blood platelets and arterial endothelial cells: (1) Platelets adhere to **collagen** at the site of injury, which (2) **activates** fibrinogen. (3) Fibrinogen increases platelet aggregation and (4) releases platelet-derived growth factor, which is **chemotactic** for smooth muscle and **fibroblasts.** (5) Smooth muscle and fibroblasts

proliferate into the arterial intima and lead to (6) **fibrosis** by production of collagen, **elastin,** and muco-sugars (figure 4.6).

Renegade LDL

Contributing to the atheromas in response to endothelial injury are abnormal molecules of low-density lipoprotein that have become free radicals after **oxidation** (i.e., LDL + O_2). A **free radical** is an atom or group of atoms that transiently exists in an unstable state by carrying an unpaired electron until an electron can be stolen from another atom. When oxygen loses an electron from one of its four pairs during normal metabolism, it becomes a free radical. Hence, oxidation occurs when another element becomes a free radical by losing an electron as it combines with oxygen. Oxidation of LDL in the atheromas can lead to disintegration of a cell after damaging the cell membrane.

Oxidized LDL stimulates secretion of monocyte chemoattractant protein-1 (MCP-1), which results in a fatal attraction for immune cells known as **macrophages,** already drawn to the arterial lesion to ingest the debris of injured endothelial cells. In this way, the renegade LDL leads to foam-filled macrophages on the endothelium, which contribute to the growing atheroma, which in turn can eventually block arteries or contribute to a coronary thrombosis. Oxidized LDL is also **cytotoxic** to endothelial cells and thus adds to cell injury. Smoking increases renegade LDL, but beta-carotene (vitamin A) and vitamin E are antioxidants. Antioxidants can give up electrons to free radicals without becoming free radicals themselves. Monounsaturated fats, such as olive oil, also prevent LDL from becoming a free radical.

Homocysteine

The American Heart Association considers high levels of **homocysteine** a possible risk factor for CHD (Malinow, Bostom, and Krauss 1999). Homocysteine, a natural intermediate amino acid, is formed during the metabolism of an essential amino acid, methionine. The homocysteine hypothesis of CHD is credited to physician Kilmer McCully (1969), who observed that children with the genetic condition **homocystinuria** (which leads to abnormally high levels of homocysteine because of deficiencies in metabolic enzymes) usually died from arteriosclerosis at an early age. A high blood level of homocysteine is associated with buildups of collagen and calcium, degeneration of elastin, and endothelial cell damage in the

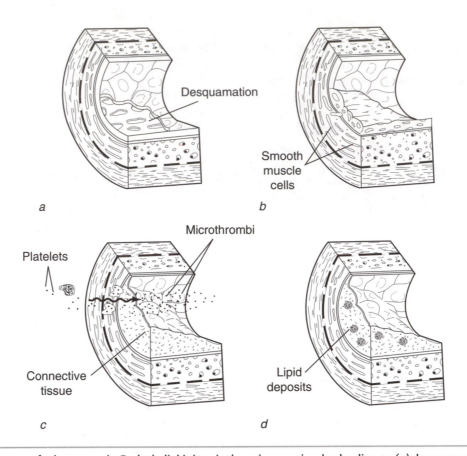

Figure 4.6 Process of atherogenesis. Endothelial injury is the primary stimulus leading to *(a)* desquamation and *(b)* smooth muscle cell migration and proliferation. *(c)* Platelets adhere to the injured endothelium, releasing vasoconstrictive and thrombogenic substances. *(d)* Lipid deposits, primarily LDL cholesterol, accumulate in the lesions.

Adapted, by permission, from R. Ross and J.A. Glomset, 1976, "The pathogenesis of arteriosclerosis," *New England Journal of Medicine* 295: 369, 420.

lumen of coronary arteries, each of which contributes to the formation of atherosclerotic plaques.

The leading hypothesis is that homocysteine damages endothelial cells by producing hydrogen peroxide, which then results in the atherosclerotic cascade of platelet aggregation and blood clotting, leading to arterial occlusion. A recent study of over 1,000 randomly recruited Australian men and women reported that homocysteine level was an independent risk factor for thickening of the wall of the carotid artery and of plaque buildup (McQuillan et al. 1999).

> ••• *High levels of homocysteine, an intermediate of amino acid metabolism, increase risk of coronary heart disease by about 25% to 75%, probably by damaging endothelial cells of arteries. Dietary antioxidants and physical activity can lower homocysteine levels.*

Cumulative results from 15 cross-sectional studies indicate that people with abnormally high levels of homocysteine have a 70% increase in the risk of developing CHD (Homocysteine Lowering Trialists' Collaboration 1998). However, the relative risk averaged from results of prospective studies was smaller, about a 25% increase in risk (Malinow, Bostom, and Krauss 1999). As yet no randomized **clinical trials** have been published that have demonstrated that lowering homocysteine lowers the incidence of CHD.

Nonetheless, the American Heart Association recommends a daily diet containing folic acid and vitamins B_6 and B_{12}, which curb elevations of homocysteine. An enzyme called F1, which remethylates homocysteine to methionine, depends on folic acid and B_{12}. Vitamin B_6 catalyzes other enzymes that metabolize homocysteine to cysteine for excretion in the urine. Folic acid supplements of about 0.5 g per day lower homocysteine levels by 25%. Adding vitamin B_{12} reduces levels by another 7%. Normal levels of homocysteine range from 5 to 15 μmol/L. The American Heart Association recommends a daily dose of 400 μg of folic acid, 2 mg of vitamin B_6, and 6 μg of vitamin B_{12} for people who are at high risk for CHD and do not respond to a change in diet.

Reducing dietary intake of protein and increasing intake of B vitamins are the frontline preventive treatments for moderate elevations in homocysteine. Other factors believed to increase the risk of high homocysteine levels include age, male sex, environmental toxins, high blood cholesterol, and lack of physical activity.

Hemostasis

Studies have shown that hemostatic factors (i.e., factors that regulate blood clotting) are risk factors for CVD. Principal factors that affect **hemostasis** include blood **viscosity**, coagulation factors, platelet aggregability or stickiness, fibrinogenesis, and fibrinolysis. Coagulation or clotting of blood involves platelet aggregation and fibrinogenesis. Platelet stickiness is increased in the morning and by hormones such as adrenaline and noradrenaline and is reduced by aspirin, ethanol, and flavonoids (chemicals such as resveratrol found in the skins of red grapes).

Platelet aggregation is catalyzed by **fibrinogenesis,** which involves the conversion of the blood protein fibrinogen to **fibrin** in the presence of calcium by the hydrolytic **protease** enzyme **thrombin.** Normally, that process is opposed by **fibrinolysis,** which is the hydrolysis of fibrin by the enzyme **plasmin.** Plasmin is formed in the blood from **plasminogen** by **tissue-type plasminogen activator (tPA),** which is released from endothelial cells in blood vessels or by drugs such as streptokinase and **trypsin.** A major contributor to impaired fibrinolysis is a high level in the blood of plasminogen activator inhibitor-1 (PAI-1), which also is released by blood vessel endothelial cells and inhibits tPA.

Results from the Framingham Heart Study have shown that blood **hematocrit,** the percentage of blood volume occupied by cells, is a risk factor for CVD. High hematocrit is associated with increased blood thickness and **coagulability;** these characteristics increase the contact between platelets and endothelial cells, which can promote aggregation.

The concentration of fibrinogen in the blood also is a risk factor for ischemic heart attack and stroke. The cumulative results from 13 prospective, 5 cross-sectional, and 4 case–control population-based studies done in several nations

between 1984 and 1998 indicated that a high level of fibrinogen in blood plasma doubles the risk of developing CVD (when the upper tertile was compared with the lowest) and increases recurrent MI and ischemic stroke by 8%, independently of overall CVD risk status, smoking, and age (Maresca et al. 1999).

Low fibrinogen offers some protection against MI or sudden cardiac death in people who report angina even if they have high serum cholesterol. In contrast, studies have found that high PAI-1 was a risk factor for first heart attack or stroke, a recurrent heart attack among heart attack survivors, and cardiac death among people reporting angina.

> ••• *Blood clotting factors such as fibrinogen and plasminogen activator inhibitor-1 are associated with increased risk of ischemic heart attack and stroke. People who are physically active tend to have lower levels of such clotting factors.*

The association of coagulation factors and fibrinolytic variables with the incidence of MI was examined in the PRIME Study, a prospective cohort study of more than 10,500 men ages 50 to 59 years recruited from three MONICA field centers in France (Lille, Strasbourg, and Toulouse) and Belfast, Northern Ireland. Plasma fibrinogen, clotting factor VII (a risk factor for arterial thrombosis), and PAI-1 activity were measured at the outset of the study. Fibrinogen level increased with age, smoking, waist-to-hip ratio, and LDL cholesterol, and it decreased with educational level, alcohol intake, HDL cholesterol, and leisure-time physical activity. Factor VII activity increased with BMI, waist-to-hip ratio, triglycerides, and HDL and LDL cholesterol, but it did not independently increase the odds of a heart attack. PAI-1 activity increased with BMI, waist-to-hip ratio, triglycerides, alcohol intake, and smoking; it was higher among diabetics; and it decreased with leisure-time physical activity. The odds for MI increased by about 30% to 40% with an elevation of at least one standard deviation in fibrinogen or PAI-1 and remained high after adjusting for the other CVD risk factors (Scarabin et al. 1998).

Inflammation

An emerging body of evidence from laboratory, case–control, and prospective clinical studies during the past decade has shown that atherosclerotic disease involves inflammatory processes (Libby, Ridker, and Maseri 2002) as well as macrophages, as discussed earlier in this chapter. Major risk factors for CVD, including hyperlipidemia, hypertension, diabetes, and obesity, all have pro-inflammatory features, as do bacterial and viral infection. Inflammation also appears to play a role in acute coronary events, such as cardiac sudden death resulting from thrombosis (Rifai and Ridker 2002). Prospective epidemiologic studies have reported that increased risk of vascular disease is associated with elevated levels of cytokines involved with regulation of the acute-phase response to infection and acute-phase markers such as fibrinogen and **C-reactive protein** produced by the liver. Most evidence thus far has focused on C-reactive protein because it is easily measured, has a long half-life (making it stable in the blood over time), and influences several inflammatory responses that plausibly affect the progression of atherosclerosis, including uptake of LDL by macrophages, attraction of **monocytes** to the endothelium of arteries, and production of MCP-1 (Libby, Ridker, and Maseri 2002). A dozen or so prospective population-based studies reported since 1996 have shown that men and women who have high levels of C-reactive protein, a marker of low-grade inflammation, have approximately 2.5 to 4.5 times the risk of developing vascular disease than people with low or normal levels (Albert et al. 2002; Libby, Ridker, and Maseri 2002). Other markers of inflammation, including white blood cell counts and fibrinogen, have also been associated with the development of CHD (Folsom et al. 2002). Finally, several treatments currently used to prevent CHD, including diet, smoking cessation, aspirin, cholesterol-lowering statin drugs, and physical activity, also have anti-inflammatory effects that may explain part of their benefits. The basic immunology of infection and inflammation and the acute inflammatory response to exercise are discussed in chapter 12.

Physical Activity and Coronary Heart Disease: The Evidence

In 1802, Scottish physician William Heberden reported that a patient of his was nearly cured of his angina pectoris after having "sawed wood for half an hour every day" (Willius and Keys 1961). Physical inactivity is recognized by the American Heart Association (Fletcher et al. 1996), the International Society and Federation of Cardiology, and the World Health Organization (Bijnen, Caspersen, and Mosterd 1994) as a major independent risk factor for CHD, with a mean RR of about 2.0 from about 40 population-based studies. The following sections describe early studies on the association between occupational activity and CHD risk and both prospective and retrospective studies on the association of leisure-time physical activity and CHD risk.

> ••• *On average, studies show that leisure-time physical activity during middle age cuts the risk of CHD in half for both men and women.*

In a recent review of the cumulative evidence (Kohl 2001), 20 of 31 reports from 23 observational studies published between 1958 and August 2000 that included at least three levels of physical activity provided at least some evidence for a linear reduction in CHD risk (9 studies examined only fatalities) with increased level of physical activity. Three reports had mixed findings, and eight reports indicated no association. All but three of the studies used a prospective cohort design with observational periods ranging from 3 to 26 years. Only four reports were on women, and just one study examined changes in physical activity.

Occupational Activity and Coronary Heart Disease Risk

British epidemiologist Jeremy Morris began the modern study of exercise and heart disease with his hallmark hypothesis that physical activity protects against CHD and his pioneering research on London transport workers and other occupational groups in the 1950s (Morris et al. 1953).

> ••• *British physician and epidemiologist Jeremy Morris first hypothesized that physical activity was protective against coronary heart disease in the early 1950s.*

London Bus Conductors

The first study by Morris found that the highly active conductors on London's double-decker buses were at lower risk of CHD than the drivers, who sat through their shifts at a steering wheel. If conductors did develop CHD, it was less severe and occurred at later ages. Morris later reported a similar observation that postmen delivering mail on foot had lower rates of CHD than sedentary office clerks and telephone operators. Subsequent studies were conducted to control for other explanations for those initial observations and to determine possible biological mechanisms that might account for the protective effect of physical activity. Blood pressure levels were lower in the conductors, but among men with the same blood pressure, the conductors had fewer heart problems than the drivers. Though bus drivers were more obese, their rate of sudden coronary death was higher regardless of body mass.

San Francisco Dock Workers

In the United States, Ralph Paffenbarger Jr. and W.E. Hale (1975; Paffenbarger et al. 1977) tracked over 6,300 San Francisco longshoremen ages 35 to 74 years for 22 years or until death or age 75. Mortality was determined by official death certificates. Physical activity was classified according to job, and job switches were checked annually. Cargo handlers who loaded and unloaded ships were classified as more physically active than foremen and clerks. Union rules required all workers to serve at least their first 5 years as cargo handlers (the average was 13 years), which helped control for self-selection of unfit men into the easy jobs.

The death rate from CHD expressed per 10,000 person-years of work among men who expended at least 8,500 kcal each week was about half that

of less-active men. Their rate of sudden cardiac death was nearly two thirds lower. After adjustments for cigarette smoking, systolic blood pressure, relative body weight, and glucose tolerance, those relative rates were smaller but remained different (figure 4.7).

Other Studies of Occupational Activity

Incidence and prevalence rates of CHD have been compared among men performing jobs that require different levels of physical activity, including postal workers, railroad workers, farmers, employees of utility companies, civil servants, police officers, and firefighters. Most of these studies reported that physically active workers had one third to three fourths fewer total or fatal CHD events compared with the least-active workers. However, studies of occupational physical activity based on job classifications are difficult to interpret. For example, the actual energy expenditure of people having the same job title can differ widely, and it is hard to keep track of people who switch jobs after the study begins.

Railroad switchmen had a lower rate of CHD than clerks and executives in one study (H.L. Taylor et al. 1962), but the apparently protective effect of physical activity might have been explained by job transfers by sicker workers from more active to inactive jobs. Studies of civil service employees in Los Angeles (Chapman and Massey 1964) and employees of several public utility companies (Hinkle et al. 1968; Mortensen, Stevensen, and Whitney 1959; Paul et al. 1963) observed no association between CHD events and physical activity on the job. That was

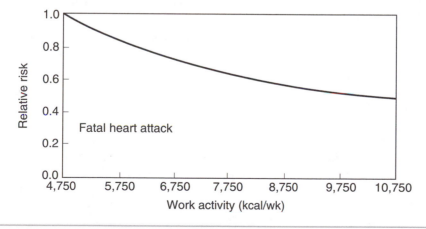

Figure 4.7 The San Francisco Longshoremen study shows the death rate from CHD expressed per 10,000 man-years of work among men who expended at least 8,500 kcal each week was about half that of less-active men.

Reprinted, by permission, from G.S. Thomas et al., 1981, *Exercise and health: The evidence and the implications* (Cambridge, MA: Oelgeschlager, Gunn, and Hain).

probably because most of the jobs at the utility company required a similar, low level of energy expenditure. Leisure-time physical activity was not measured. Also, people who have sedentary jobs might be very active in their leisure, just as laborers might choose to be sedentary during leisure time.

Many of the early studies on occupational activity and CHD risk did not adjust for differences in other CHD risk factors, such as smoking, dietary habits, blood pressure, obesity, or serum cholesterol. For example, in Finland, vigorously active lumberjacks had a higher rate of mortality from CHD and greater frequency of abnormal electrocardiograms than did less-active farmers from the same region (Punsar and Karvonen 1976). However, the lumberjacks smoked more, consumed more saturated fat, and had lower socioeconomic status than the farmers. The high prevalence of the other risk factors may also have offset the potential protective effect of the high daily energy expenditure of lumberjack work. In a study of 62,000 deaths between 1964 and 1978 among Iowa men 20 to 64 years of age, farmers had 10% less CHD and total mortality than nonfarmers (Pomrehn, Wallace, and Burmeister 1982). However, although the Iowa farmers were twice as physically active and more physically fit, they also used less tobacco and alcohol. Those positive habits might have accounted for their better health more than their physical activity did. Farmers in studies in Georgia (Cassell et al. 1971) and North Dakota (Zukel et al. 1959) also smoked less than nonfarmers, which prevents a definitive conclusion that their higher physical activity was an independent explanation for their lower rate of disease.

A retrospective study of Israeli workers in kibbutzim (communal settlements) did a better job of controlling for other risk factors that may have confounded the physical activity–heart disease association (Brunner et al. 1974). Individuals in this study were of similar ethnic origin, lived in the same environment, consumed a common diet, and had the same access to medical care. Nearly 5,300 men and over 5,200 women ages 40 to 64 years were classified as either sedentary or active based on the portion of the workday they spent in manual labor or sitting. The active and sedentary groups had the similar body weights and serum cholesterol and triglyceride levels. The relative risk of nonfatal and fatal heart attacks over a 15-year period was 2.5 times higher among sedentary men and 3 times higher

in sedentary women. These findings were not explained by differences in body weight, serum cholesterol, or triglyceride levels between active and sedentary individuals.

Leisure-Time Physical Activity and Coronary Heart Disease Risk

Nearly all the studies published before 1978 measured only occupational physical activity based on job descriptions. Occupational physical activity decreased precipitously in Western developed nations during the late 1950s to early 1960s as industry moved from manual to mechanized labor. As a result, more attention was directed at understanding whether physical activity in leisure time protects against CHD. In general, the findings of protective effects of leisure-time physical activity against CHD have been more consistent than those reported in studies of occupational physical activity. On average, studies show that leisure-time physical activity during middle age cuts the risk for CHD in half for both men and women. In the following sections, we first describe representative retrospective and case–control studies and then the more methodologically sound prospective cohort studies that have evaluated the association between CHD risk and leisure-time physical activity.

Retrospective and Case–Control Studies

Early studies of physical activity and heart disease risk used retrospective and case–control designs. Though scientifically weaker than prospective designs, positive results from those early studies provided justification for the more costly prospective studies that followed. Case–control studies remain useful today for providing preliminary evidence about new hypotheses that can later be better examined by prospective studies.

Health Insurance Plan of New York. One of the first population studies to assess both leisure-time and occupational physical activity was a retrospective study of 55,000 men ages 25 to 64 years enrolled in the Health Insurance Plan of New York (Shapiro et al. 1969). On-the-job and leisure-time physical activities were assessed by a questionnaire and interviews with the insured or his widow. Subjects' activity levels were classified as light, moderate, or heavy. Considerations were made for time spent walking and sitting at work, transportation to and from work, total working hours, and time spent lifting and carrying objects. The incidence of myocardial infarction in both the heavy- and moderate-activity groups was about half that of the light-activity group; furthermore, the least-active men had a 4.5 times greater mortality rate following MI than the most-active men. The reductions in risk for MI and death after MI were independent of body mass and smoking.

Florida. In a retrospective study similar to the Health Insurance Plan of New York study, physical activity was estimated from interviews with the wives of 568 men from two Florida counties who died from CHD between the ages of 30 and 70 (Hennekens et al. 1977). Matched controls were selected from men living in the same neighborhoods. After controlling for cigarette smoking and hypertension, leisure-time physical activity but not occupational physical activity was associated with decreased risk of death from CHD.

The Netherlands. Nearly 500 heart attack victims in Holland, or their immediate relatives, and 800 controls from the same communities were interviewed about their past physical activity habits (Magnus, Matroos, and Stracklee 1979). A significant inverse association was found between heart attack and habitual (defined as more than eight months per year) walking, cycling, and gardening, but not if those activities were performed only sporadically or seasonally (four to eight months per year). Vigorous exercise did not appear to offer any more protection from CHD than did moderate activities.

King County, Washington. Leisure-time physical activity during the past year was estimated

by interviews with the spouses of 163 people who had suffered primary cardiac arrest and with matched controls ages 25 to 75 who lived in Seattle and suburban King County, Washington (Siscovick et al. 1982). The risk of cardiac arrest was 55% to 65% lower for men and women in the two upper quartiles of high-intensity physical activity than for those who had not engaged in any high-intensity physical activity (figure 4.8).

Prospective Studies

In the past 30 years, a number of prospective cohort studies conducted in Europe and the United States have evaluated the association between leisure-time physical activity and CHD risk. These studies were generally designed to follow representative samples of initially healthy people living in different geographic regions or samples from selected groups, such as Harvard alumni or British civil servants, for extended periods to determine what factors, including physical activity, were associated with the risk of developing CHD. The results of most, but not all, of these studies show that leisure-time physical activity is inversely associated with CHD morbidity or mortality.

Western Collaborative Group Study. The Western Collaborative Group Study was a prospective study of employed California men ages 39 to 59. The main emphasis in this study was the association of behavior patterns and CHD. Leisure-time exercise habits were determined by personal interview. At the four and one half year follow-up, the incidence of CHD and fatal MI was significantly lower in the men with regular exercise habits

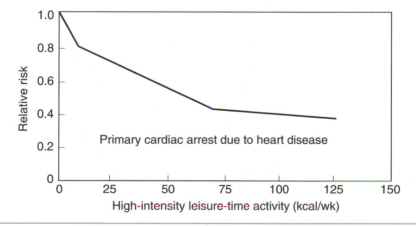

Figure 4.8 The King County, Washington residents study shows the relative risk of primary cardiac arrest due to heart disease versus high intensity leisure-time activity.

Reprinted, by permission, from K.E. Powell, 1988, Habitual exercise and public health: An epidemiological view. In *Exercise adherence: Its impact on public health,* edited by R.K. Dishman (Champaign, IL: Human Kinetics), 30.

(Rosenman et al. 1970). However, after eight to nine years, no significant relation was apparent between physical activity level and CHD for the cohort (Rosenman et al. 1975). However, subgroup analysis indicated that men over 50 years of age who reported exercising daily (including walking) had significantly lower CHD rates than those reporting only occasional exercise.

British Civil Servants. Jeremy Morris and colleagues studied about 18,000 middle-aged executive-level British civil servants who were apparently without CHD and had sedentary desk jobs (Morris et al. 1973, 1980). The men were asked to complete a detailed record of their physical activity during a Friday and Saturday. The activity records were used to classify the men as vigorous exercisers or nonvigorous exercisers. Vigorous exercise was defined as exercise at an intensity of at least 7.5 kcal/min (a level common in heavy industrial work) and included sports, swimming, jogging, rapid walking, hiking, hill climbing, or heavy work around the home. About 20% of the men in the study were classified as vigorous exercisers. Vigorous exercisers reported participating in at least 5 min per day of sports or recreational activities at or above that intensity or at least 30 min of heavy chores, such as digging in the garden. The men were then observed for an average of 8.5 years, providing 150,000 person-years of exposure. During that period, 475 men died from CHD. The rate of CHD death was more than twice as high in the nonvigorous group (2.9%) as in the vigorous group (1.1%), a relative risk of about 2.6. Aerobic exercise (e.g., swimming, brisk walking, and cycling) was associated with lower incidence of CHD, but no apparent protective effect was conferred by time spent in leisure gardening and household chores. Adjustments between the active and less-active men for differences on a wide range of risk factors did not eliminate the main finding that participation in vigorous exercise protected against CHD. Contrary to expectation, the prevalence of heart attack was not lower among people with higher overall leisure-time activity. However, Morris reported a smaller increase with age in both fatal and nonfatal first attacks in the men who reported more exercise, and the protective effect was persistent across the period of observation, eliminating the possibility that the low physical activity resulted from illness.

Morris et al. (1980) also demonstrated that the incidence rates of CHD were low only among men who were active in recent or current times. High rates of CHD were found among those who had stopped previously moderate leisure activity from 5 to over 40 years before the study was conducted. Also, men who played vigorous sports at the time they were questioned had the same low incidence of CHD during follow-up whether or not they had been physically active during the years preceding the study.

Morris and colleagues (1990) reported a study of over 9,000 male British civil servants ages 45 to 64 years, who recalled their physical activity during the preceding month. After 87,500 person-years of observation over a nine-year period, there were 272 deaths from CHD. Another 202 men had nonfatal heart attacks. The rate of CHD events was significantly lower among men who had been classified as vigorous aerobic exercisers. Other physical activities did not appear to protect against either heart attack or CHD death. Lower-intensity aerobic activities were protective for the older men (55 to 64 years at the start of the study), suggesting that dose response varies with age.

Harvard Alumni Health Study. As previously described, this was a prospective cohort study of about 17,000 male alumni of Harvard University who were mainly employed in sedentary occupations or retired (Paffenbarger, Wing, and Hyde 1978). The age-adjusted incidence rate of CHD was inversely related to energy expended by walking, stair climbing, and playing sports and to the composite energy expenditure in kilocalories per week as reported by the men in response to mailed questionnaires. Men expending fewer than 2,000 kcal per week were at a 64% higher risk than their former classmates who were less active (figure 4.9). No additional reduction in CHD rate was found for men who expended more than 2,000 kcal per week. CHD risk decreased about 10% more when the energy expenditure occurred in vigorous sports rather than by walking or climbing stairs. The association between risk of CHD and level of physical activity remained strong when adjustments were made for other risk factors, including cigarette smoking, hypertension, diabetes mellitus, obesity, and parental history of heart attack. Another important finding from the study was that alumni who had been athletes during college and did not continue exercising were at greater risk for CHD than physically active alumni who had not been college athletes. That is, only contemporary physical activity, not prior athletic history in college, was associated with reduced CHD events. Hence, the protective effects of exercise appear to be independent of constitutional factors that would favor success in youth athletics

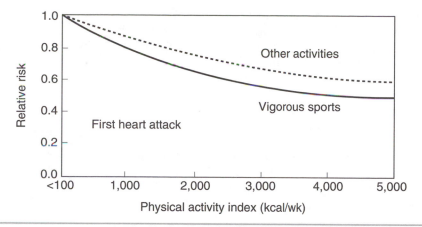

Figure 4.9 The Harvard alumni study shows the relative risk of first heart attack versus physical activity index.

Reprinted, by permission, from K.E. Powell, 1988, Habitual exercise and public health: An epidemiological view. In *Exercise adherence: Its impact on public health,* edited by R.K. Dishman (Champaign, IL: Human Kinetics), 30.

and that might be expected to retard disease in later years.

> ••• *Male Harvard alumni who had been athletes during college and did not continue exercising were at greater risk for CHD than physically active alumni who had not been college athletes. Only contemporary physical activity, not prior athletic history in college, was associated with reduced CHD events.*

The Harvard cohort has provided some of the most well-controlled and long-term data for examining the association between leisure physical activity and all-cause mortality risks, as well as specific risks for cancers, diabetes, depression, and cardiovascular disease. Perhaps the most valuable of Dr. Paffenbarger's contributions was the observation of persistent dose–response relationships, indicating optimal reductions in CHD morbidity and mortality at around 2,000 kcal of leisure physical activity per week.

> ••• *The well-controlled Harvard Alumni Health Study has consistently found a dose–response relationship between leisure physical activity and reduced risk of CHD morbidity and mortality, with an optimal weekly expenditure of about 2,000 kcal in vigorous sports.*

Framingham Heart Study. In the Framingham Heart Study—a follow-up of 1,909 men and 2,311 women who lived in Framingham, Massachusetts—a statistically significant inverse relationship was found between an index of overall job and leisure-time physical activity determined by a questionnaire and 14-year CHD mortality in men but not women (Kannel and Sorlie 1979). The relative risk of developing CHD for the least-active men 45 to 64 years of age compared with the most active was small (1.3) but statistically significant (figure 4.10).

Seven Countries Study. The Seven Countries Study involved 16 cohorts of men in seven countries who were 40 through 59 years old at the start of the study (Keys 1980). Differences between 10-year CHD incidence and mortality rates among populations were unrelated to the proportion of sedentary men in the population. Other risk factors, particularly serum cholesterol levels and

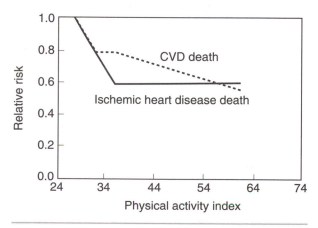

Figure 4.10 The Framingham Heart Study of men shows the relative risk of death due to cardiovascular disease versus the physical activity index.

Reprinted, by permission, from K.E. Powell, 1988, Habitual exercise and public health: An epidemiological view. In *Exercise adherence: Its impact on public health,* edited by R.K. Dishman (Champaign, IL: Human Kinetics), 30.

dietary intake of saturated fat, appeared to better explain the differences in CHD rates among countries. Only three of the seven countries showed an inverse association between physical activity (mostly occupational) and CHD, while in the others (e.g., the United States and Finland), there was no apparent association. In Finland, the country with the highest CHD incidence and mortality in the study, the 10-year follow-up revealed no difference in CHD mortality between men classified as sedentary and the most-active men. However, relatively few men were classified as sedentary in the Finnish cohorts.

Finnish Cohorts. Karvonen (1982) followed the two Finnish cohorts in the Seven Countries Study for an additional 5 years and reassessed the original 10-year data after studying in greater detail the men's physical activity habits by an extensive structured interview. Reevaluation of the original 10-year data revealed that, for men ages 50 to 69 years, CHD incidence was clearly associated with sedentary habits. Subsequent five-year CHD mortality and combined fatal and nonfatal MI rates in this age group were inversely related to physical activity status; however, the majority of men who died of CHD had already been diagnosed with CHD before the five-year follow-up. Thus it is unclear whether physical activity had a protective effect or whether the high incidence of CHD among the least-active men was related to already-present CHD.

Puerto Rico Heart Health Program. The Puerto Rico Heart Health Program (Garcia-Palmieri et al. 1982) used a physical activity rating index similar to the one used in the Framingham Study to evaluate 8,793 men, initially 45 to 65 years of age. The 8.5-year follow-up showed an inverse association between incidence of CHD events, other than angina pectoris, and physical activity (figure 4.11); the highest risk was twice as large as the lowest. Multivariate analysis to correct for confounding by other CHD risk factors confirmed that reduced physical activity contributed independently to risk of CHD. The association persisted after the data was reanalyzed to exclude CHD events in the first two and a half years to eliminate men whose low levels of physical activity might have been caused by subclinical disease.

Multiple Risk Factor Intervention Trial. The MRFIT observed over 12,000 men, initially 35 to 57 years old, who were in the upper 10% to 15% for risk of CHD based on cigarette smoking, blood pressure, and serum cholesterol. Exercise habits were estimated by a detailed interview (Minnesota Leisure Time Physical Activity Questionnaire [MLTPAQ]),

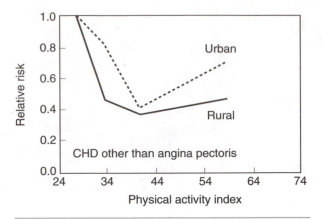

Figure 4.11 The Puerto Rico study of men shows the relative risk of cardiovascular disease other than angina pectoris versus the physical activity index.

Reprinted, by permission, from K.E. Powell, 1988, Habitual exercise and public health: An epidemiological view. In *Exercise adherence: Its impact on public health,* edited by R.K. Dishman (Champaign, IL: Human Kinetics), 30.

recalling participation in about 60 leisure-time physical activities during the preceding year (Leon et al. 1987). Frequency, duration, and intensity (in METs) of the physical activities were used to calculate total energy expenditure spent in leisure-time physical activity. After six to eight years of follow-up, there were 488 deaths. Mortality rates from all causes and from CHD among the two most-active tertiles were about 67% of the rates in the most-sedentary tertile, who averaged about 75 fewer kilocalories a day in leisure-time physical activity (figure 4.12). Mortality rates were very similar in the second and third tertiles, even though men in the most-active tertile averaged 640 kcal a day while the middle

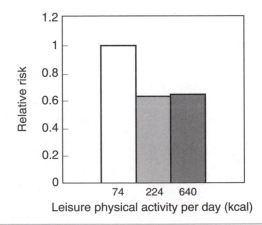

Figure 4.12 The MRFIT study shows the relative risk of cardiovascular disease versus leisure physical activity per day.

Adapted from Leon et al. 1987.

tertile had an average expenditure of about 220 kcal. This finding indicates a threshold of benefit somewhere between 75 and 220 daily kilocalories rather than a dose response, for which we would expect a further decrease in mortality rate with an increase in energy expenditure from 220 to 640 daily kilocalories. Results were unchanged after adjustment for age and other risk factors, so the reduced relative risk of mortality seen in the more-active men was independent of several confounding factors.

Sixteen years later, the men in the least-active decile, who had averaged 5 min a day of leisure-time physical activity at the beginning of the study, had 22% higher CHD death rates than men in the second to fourth least-active deciles, who had averaged about 20 min a day of mainly light- and moderate-intensity physical activity (Leon, Myers, and Connett 1997). Exercising longer than 20 min a day conferred no additional reduction in the risk of dying from CHD. Hence, even a modest amount of daily physical activity was better than being sedentary for middle-aged and older men at high risk for CHD.

Physical Fitness and Coronary Heart Disease Risk

The imprecise methods available to assess regular physical activity most likely result in an underestimation of the true magnitude of the association between all-cause and CHD mortality by misclassifying some inactive people as active and some active people as inactive. More objective measurement of fitness potentially yields a more accurate estimate of risk among middle-aged and older adults, as fitness becomes increasingly dependent on physical activity rather than genetics. Low physical fitness is associated with increased risk of CHD and CVD. The reported relative risks are generally higher (ranging from about 2.2 to 8.0) in studies that examine physical fitness than in studies that examine physical activity (approximately 2.0).

••• *Fitness, an objective measure that is a good index of changes in physical activity among middle-aged and older adults, is more strongly related to reduced CHD than are other estimates of physical activity.*

••• *The true size of the protective effect of physical activity against all-cause and CHD mortality is probably underestimated by the currently available methods used to measure physical activity, which undoubtedly misclassify some inactive people as active and some active people as inactive.*

Los Angeles Public Safety Employees

Physical fitness was estimated by the heart rate response to submaximal cycling exercise among

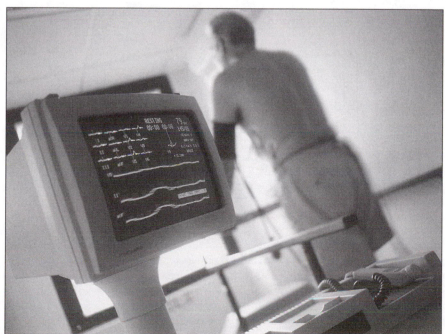
© Acestock

2,779 healthy male fire and law enforcement workers younger than 55 years in Los Angeles County, who were then followed for an average of about five years, during which 36 heart attacks occurred (Peters et al. 1983). The relative risk of heart attack after controlling for other conventional CHD risk factors was 2.2 (95% CI: 1.1–4.7) for the men who had below-average physical fitness, measured at the beginning of the study. The relative risk for men with below-average fitness was 6.6 (95% CI: 2.3–27.8) if they also had at least two of the following risk factors: high total cholesterol, elevated systolic blood pressure, or cigarette smoking.

Lipid Research Clinics Prevalence Study

Findings from the Lipid Research Clinics study indicated a strong association between cardiorespiratory fitness and CHD incidence and mortality. Ekelund et al. (1988) measured the fitness of over 3,100 healthy white men (30 to 69 years old) using a submaximal treadmill exercise test. After an average of 8.5 years, there were 45 CHD deaths. The relative risk of CHD death for men in the least-fit quartile, compared with that of the most-fit quartile, was 6.5 (95% CI: 1.5–28.7), and for CVD incidence the relative risk was 8.5 (2.0–36.7). As shown in figure 4.13, there was a striking dose–response gradient across fitness categories.

Aerobics Center Longitudinal Study

The often-cited Aerobics Center Longitudinal Study, a follow-up of over 25,000 men and 7,000 women conducted by the Cooper Institute for Aer-

obics Research in Dallas, Texas, found that mortality rates from cardiovascular disease and from all causes were lower in fit men and women than in the unfit (Blair et al. 1989). Cardiovascular fitness in this study was estimated from time on a treadmill during a maximal test protocol. The greatest difference in mortality rates was seen between the low- and moderate-fitness categories for both sexes, but there was a further reduction between the moderate- and high-fitness categories. The mortality rate for the highly fit men was about half that of the moderately fit, but the rate for the least-fit men was more than 3 times that of moderately fit men. Among women, the mortality rate for the moderately fit was 3.6 times that of the highly fit, and the low-fitness group had a mortality rate 2.5 times higher than that of the moderately fit.

Summary

Although cardiorespiratory fitness is partly explainable by genetic inheritance, a high proportion of the variation in cardiovascular fitness is explained by physical activity habits. Hence, the agreement of reduced CHD incidence among studies that measured either physical activity or fitness clearly supports the hypothesis of a causal relationship between regular physical activity and reduced risk of CHD.

Physical Activity and Fitness and Cardiovascular Disease Risk in Women

Early studies found no relationship between physical activity and CVD rates among women.

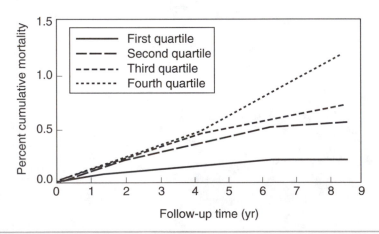

Figure 4.13 Cumulative rates of death from cardiovascular diseases in healthy men according to quartiles of exercise test heart rate. Men who were most active (first quartile) had the lowest death rate. The least-active men (fourth quartile) had nearly six times the death rate as the most-active men. Divergence of mortality curves over follow-up indicates that the effect on cardiovascular mortality is unlikely to be due to bias.

Adapted from Ekelund et al. 1988.

That was probably because of underrepresentation of women in many of the studies and inadequate measurements of physical activity in women. For example, the self-reports that were used excluded assessments of energy expenditure during child care and household chores, which were common activities for women at the time many of the early cohort studies were started. A number of more recent studies have suggested that women respond to exercise in ways similar to men and that physical activity reduces the risk of CVD in women to an extent similar to that previously shown in men.

> ••• *Recent studies have shown that women respond to exercise in ways similar to men and that physical activity reduces the risk of CVD in women to an extent similar to that in men.*

Women in Seattle

Lemaitre et al. (1995) reported results of a population-based case–control study conducted in a large Seattle health maintenance organization. The association of the risk for MI and physical activity was compared between 268 postmenopausal women who had experienced an MI between 1986 and 1991 and 925 controls matched by age and calendar year. Leisure-time physical activity was assessed by telephone interview using an instrument derived from the MLTPAQ. After adjustment for confounders, including age, diabetes, angina, family history of heart disease, cigarette smoking, alcohol intake, education, and the presence of symptoms in the month before the index date, odds ratios for women in the second, third, and fourth activity quartiles relative to the first quartile (lowest activity) were 0.52 (95% CI: 0.34–0.80), 0.40 (0.26–0.63), and 0.40 (0.25–0.63), respectively. The odds ratios for the second through fourth quartiles of energy expenditure for nonstrenuous activity—0.44 (95% CI: 0.27–0.71), 0.36 (0.22–0.59), and 0.35 (0.21–0.57), respectively—were similar to those for walking—0.38 (0.22–0.65), 0.31 (0.18–0.55), and 0.34 (0.20–0.59), respectively.

German Cardiovascular Prevention Study

The German Cardiovascular Prevention Study was a cross-sectional study of self-rated physical activity and risk for all-cause and CVD mortality among 7,689 men and 7,747 women ages 25 to 69 years surveyed from three independent national samples in Germany during 1984 to 1991 (Mensink et al. 1996). Mortality data were obtained in 1993 from federal registries, hospital records, and spouse interviews. Physical activity levels in METs were estimated for leisure time and occupational work. A conditioning activity index, which included exercise for the purpose of fitness but excluded less strenuous activities such as walking and gardening, was computed. Subjects were classified as low, moderate, or high in conditioning activity level. Men and women having high conditioning activity had more favorable risk factor levels compared with sedentary people after adjustment for age, body mass index, smoking, survey period, and socioeconomic status. Men who spent more than 2 h per week participating in sports had about one third the all-cause mortality and one fourth the CHD mortality of sedentary men. The reduction was independent of age, smoking, blood pressure, total serum cholesterol, and BMI. Results were not as clear among the women. The most-active women had total mortality that was about 30% that of the sedentary women, but that finding and results for CVD mortality among the women were statistically less reliable than for the men, mainly because there were fewer overall deaths and deaths from CVD among the women.

Iowa Women

Kushi et al. (1997) evaluated the association between physical activity assessed by a mail questionnaire and all-cause mortality in a cohort of 40,417 women living in Iowa. The women were ages 55 to 69 at baseline in 1986 and were followed for seven years. Potential confounders assessed included age, age at menarche, age at menopause, age of first live birth, parity, alcohol intake, total energy intake, cigarette smoking, use of estrogen replacement therapy, BMI (baseline and at age 18), waist-to-hip ratio, education, marital status, and history of hypertension or diabetes. After adjusting for confounders and excluding women with cancer or CHD at baseline and those who died in the first three years of follow-up, researchers found that women who participated in regular leisure-time physical activity had a 23% lower risk of mortality (RR = 0.77, 95% CI: 0.66–0.96) compared with women who did not. There was a significant trend for mortality risk to decrease with increasing participation in physical activity. Compared with those who rarely or never participated in physical activity, the relative risk was 0.76 (95% CI: 0.63–0.91) for those who participated once a week to a few times per month,

0.70 (0.58–0.85) for those who participated two to four times per week, and 0.62 (0.50–0.78) for those who participated more than four times per week. Those women who engaged in only moderate, not vigorous, physical activity as little as once per week showed a significantly reduced relative risk for mortality risk (RR = 0.78, 95% CI: 0.64–0.96).

University of Pennsylvania Alumnae

Over 1,500 female graduates of the University of Pennsylvania who were free of CVD in 1962 were questioned again in 1993 about their health (Sesso et al. 1999). During over 35,000 person-years of observation, 181 cases of CVD were identified. After adjustment for coronary risk factors, the relative risk of CVD was 33% lower (RR = 0.67, 95% CI: 0.45–1.01) for women who said they walked at least 10 blocks each day (the equivalent of 6 miles or 9.7 km each week). However, that effect was explained by lower body mass among the walkers. Only those who had a BMI less than 23 kg/m^2 were protected by walking that much.

Nurses' Health Study

In the Nurses' Health Study, 645 nonfatal heart attacks or deaths from CHD were observed among 72,488 female nurses who were from 40 to 65 years old and were free of CVD or cancer when the study began in 1986 (Manson et al. 1999). There was a strong, graded, inverse association between CHD risk and physical activity measured either as total activity (energy expended per week), walking (2.5–4.5 METs), or vigorous exercise (>6 METs). Compared with the women in the lowest quintile for weekly energy expenditure, age-adjusted relative risk for CHD decreased linearly with each increasing quintile: 0.77 (95% CI: 0.62–0.96), 0.65 (0.52–0.82), 0.54 (0.42–0.69), and 0.46 (0.36–0.60). However, only the women in the top two quintiles of total activity (the equivalent of at least 3 h of brisk walking or 1.5 h of vigorous exercise each week) had a significantly lower relative risk for CHD than the least-active quintile after making adjustments for risk factors in addition to age (smoking, BMI, menopausal status, parental history of CHD, multivitamin supplementation, alcohol use, hypertension, diabetes, hypercholesterolemia, and aspirin use) and excluding data from the first two years of the follow-up (to control for subclinical disease at study outset).

Individuals With Other Risk Factors

Perhaps the first evidence to suggest that physical activity may play an important role in re-

ducing CHD risk in individuals with other CVD risk factors came from the MRFIT (Leon et al. 1987), which indicated that physical activity significantly reduced CVD risk in men who smoked cigarettes and had high blood pressure and high serum cholesterol. Additional studies have also contributed support for this hypothesis. For example, in the Aerobic Center Longitudinal Study (Blair et al. 1996), low physical fitness was shown to be an important predictor of CHD and all-cause mortality in both smokers and nonsmokers, those with and without high cholesterol or blood pressure, and those who were considered healthy and unhealthy (as indicated by an abnormal electrocardiogram or history of CHD, stroke, hypertension, diabetes, or cancer).

> ••• *Sedentary behavior contributes substantially to the public health burden. Eliminating sedentary living would have as great or greater an impact on reducing excess mortality as eliminating other major CHD risk factors.*

The impact of physical fitness on the risk for all-cause and CHD mortality in individuals of different body sizes (normal weight: BMI ≤ 24.9 kg/m^2, overweight: BMI 25.0–29.0 kg/m^2, and obese: BMI ≥ 30.0 kg/m^2) was evaluated in the Aerobics Center Cohort (Wei et al. 1999). Results indicated that low cardiovascular fitness resulted in significant increases in the relative risk for all-cause mortality in all weight categories (normal weight: RR = 1.6, 95% CI: 1.3–2.1; overweight: RR = 1.7, 95% CI: 1.4–2.0; obese: RR = 2.3, 95% CI: 1.5–3.4). The strongest relative risk for mortality, as expected, was associated with the presence of baseline CVD (normal weight: RR = 2.3, 95% CI: 1.8–2.9; overweight: RR = 2.0, 95% CI: 1.6–2.4; obese: RR = 2.4, 95% CI: 1.7–3.5). The other risk indicators (diabetes, high cholesterol, hypertension, smoking, and low fitness) were comparable predictors of mortality in both overweight and obese men. The cardiovascular mortality rate of overweight men with any of the risk predictors other than CHD was three times higher than that of normal weight men without the risk factor, and their all-cause mortality rate was two times higher. Obese men with any of these risk predictors had CHD mortality rates five times higher and all-cause mortality rates three times higher than that of normal weight men without the risk predictors.

Hedblad et al. (1997), in a population-based cohort study conducted in the city of Malmo, Sweden, reported that physically active men who never smoked had the lowest total mortality rate and that physically inactive men who smoked had the highest mortality rate (RR = 3.6, 95% CI: 2.1–6.3, compared with active nonsmokers). The relative risk for CVD mortality was 5.5 (95% CI: 2.2–13.6) for the inactive smokers compared with the active nonsmokers. However, smokers who engaged in vigorous physical activity had a relative risk for cardiovascular mortality that was approximately 40% less than that of their sedentary counterparts. In this same cohort, Engstrom, Hedblad, and Janzon (1999) showed that vigorous physical activity was associated with a marked reduction in both all-cause (17.3 vs. 40 deaths per 1,000 person-years) and CVD mortality (6.3 vs. 21 deaths per 1,000 person-years) compared with sedentariness in 173 men with hypertension.

Physical Inactivity Compared With Other Risk Factors

In chapter 2, we introduced the concept of population attributable risk (PAR), which is an estimate of the reduction in mortality rate that might occur if all individuals with a specific risk factor (e.g., smoking, hypertension, obesity, inactivity) eliminated that factor. PAR is a theoretical calculation that depends on accurate information regarding both the relative risk for each factor and the percentage of the population exposed to the risk factor; it assumes a cause–effect association, the persistence of the risk factor into the future, and an equal distribution of potential confounding factors in the groups being compared. Even with these limitations, PAR calculations provide epidemiologists with a useful method to quantify and compare the public health burden of disease risk factors.

A number of reports have estimated the PAR for physical inactivity and compared this with the PAR for other risk factors. Based on prevalence estimates of sedentary behavior in the United States, Powell and Blair (1994) estimated the PAR for sedentary lifestyle (no leisure-time physical activity) on CHD mortality to be 16%. Using data from the Harvard Alumni Health Study, Paffenbarger et al. (1993) estimated the all-cause mortality PAR for sedentary living (<2,000 kcal/wk) at 13.2% and the PAR for no participation in moderately vigorous sport activity (≥4.5 METs)

at 12%. Thus, if men in this sample had become physically active, the all-cause mortality rate would be reduced by about 12%. In the Harvard alumni sample, the all-cause mortality PAR for low physical activity was similar to that for cigarette smoking (11.3%), hypertension (14.6%), and overweight (BMI > 26, 6.3%). Haapanen-Niemi, Vuori, and Pasanen (1999) used data from a number of population-based studies of Finnish men ages 30 to 63 to estimate PAR for sedentary behavior and other CHD risk factors for all-cause mortality. PAR for various risk factors were: cigarette smoking, 10% to 33%; high serum cholesterol, 9% to 21%; hypertension, 6% to 15%; overweight, 3% to 6%; and low leisure-time physical activity, 22% to 39%. Wei et al. (1999) used data from the Aerobics Center Longitudinal Study to compare the effects of low cardiovascular fitness with other risk indicators, including type 2 diabetes, high cholesterol, high blood pressure, and cigarette smoking. Results indicated that low fitness had a PAR for mortality that was similar to, if not larger than, those associated with the other measured risk factors. For example, in obese men (BMI ≥ 30 kg/m^2), low fitness had a PAR for all-cause mortality of 44%, which was higher than the PAR for baseline cardiovascular disease (27%), type 2 diabetes (9%), high cholesterol (18%), hypertension (4%), and cigarette smoking (9%). As might be expected, there is variability in the results of PAR estimates across studies. However, it appears that sedentary behavior contributes substantially to the public health burden and that eliminating this behavior would have as great or greater an impact on reducing excess mortality as eliminating other major CHD risk factors.

Physical Activity and Risk of Recurrent Heart Attack

Cumulative results of 22 randomized clinical trials involving 4,554 patients followed for an average of three years indicated that the odds ratios for total mortality (OR = 0.80), cardiovascular mortality (OR = 0.78), and fatal reinfarction (OR = 0.75) were lowered in groups that received exercise rehabilitation (O'Connor et al. 1989). The odds ratio for sudden death one year after exercise rehabilitation was 0.63, but exercise rehabilitation showed no protective effect against a recurrent nonfatal heart attack. Exercise rehabilitation was associated with a 20% reduction in overall mortality but did not reduce the chances of having another heart attack. Because only a few of the studies used exercise without some other type of risk-reduction treatment, it was not possible to determine whether the favorable effects resulted solely from exercise.

More recent findings from the National Exercise and Heart Disease Project, a 3-year randomized controlled trial of exercise rehabilitation among 651 men aged 30 to 64 years who previously had a myocardial infarction, indicated that each increase in exercise capacity of 1 MET after exercise training was associated with an 8% to 14% reduction in risk of CVD mortality and all-cause mortality during 19 years of follow-up, regardless of initial exercise capacity (Dorn et al. 1999).

> ••• *Exercise training after a heart attack reduces mortality risk by about 20% on average but does not appear to lower the risk of having another heart attack.*

Are the Associations Real?

The data presented previously in the chapter regarding the association between physical activity and fitness and risk of all-cause and CHD mortality were obtained from observational studies. With this study design, individuals are not randomly assigned to groups based on activity level; therefore, it cannot be assumed that high levels of physical activity or fitness cause low mortality risk. An initial step in establishing that the observed association is causal is to ensure that the observed associations are valid and not the result of some other factor, such as selection bias, loss to follow-up, problems with measurement of the independent and dependent variables, or the influence of other health factors, such as cigarette smoking, obesity, or blood pressure. Selection bias occurs when, for example, individuals with a particular genetic makeup or with undiagnosed disease are both sedentary and unfit and thus more likely to develop disease during the follow-up period. The possibility that individuals with undiagnosed disease might self-select lower physical activity or fitness, resulting in a biased observation of higher mortality in those with low activity or fitness, needs to be carefully evaluated. Protection against this type of bias in an observational study is achieved by careful initial screening of participants to try to eliminate those with diseases and by observing mortality over a long follow-up period. Individuals in the study cohort who have undiagnosed

diseases at baseline are likely to die early in the follow-up period, resulting in a cohort of healthy survivors as the length of follow-up increases. The majority of studies on activity and fitness and all-cause and CHD mortality that were discussed earlier in this chapter used what would be considered a sufficiently long follow-up period of 6 to 26 years to reduce the likelihood that the results are affected by undiagnosed disease at baseline. Additionally, many investigators do not include in their analyses mortality that occurs early in the follow-up period, thus minimizing the possibility of bias due to undiagnosed disease. Studies that find changes in physical activity or fitness associated with changes in disease risk are not likely to suffer from selection bias. For example, the results of both Paffenbarger et al. (1993) and Blair et al. (1995) indicated that individuals who changed either physical activity or physical fitness levels had a change in mortality risk in the hypothesized direction; that is, a change from low to high activity or fitness was associated with a decrease in mortality risk, and vice versa.

> ••• *A finding that changes in physical activity or fitness are associated with changes in disease risk is not likely to suffer from selection bias, even in prospective studies in which unfit participants might also have had undetected disease at study outset.*

Other factors such as loss to follow-up, misclassification of individuals' physical activity or fitness, or differences in risk characteristics other than physical activity or fitness can also lead to invalid results in a prospective cohort study. Loss to follow-up may be related to the level of physical activity or fitness and thus bias the mortality outcome. This is generally not thought to be a problem, considering that the follow-up rates reported in cohort studies on activity and fitness and mortality were 90% or higher. As discussed in chapter 3, measurement of physical activity in population studies presents a major problem. Also, most prospective studies measure physical activity only at baseline and do not consider changes in activity over the follow-up period. It is generally thought that since physical activity is measured before the mortality outcome is known, misclassification of individuals' physical activity levels would be random with respect to outcome. Random misclassification by activity level would reduce the true association between activity and mortality outcome, which means that the magnitude of the reduction in mortality associated with physical activity that is reported in the literature is most likely an underestimate.

> ••• *Because unfit participants might be less likely to volunteer for retesting, loss to follow-up may be related to the level of physical activity and fitness and thus bias the mortality outcome.*

It is also likely that individuals who are physically active or fit differ from sedentary or unfit individuals in other health habits or disease risk factors, such as cigarette smoking, alcohol intake, blood pressure, BMI, lipid profile, dietary habits, and so on, which may influence the association of physical activity or fitness with reduced mortality. Properly conducted cohort studies have statistically controlled for most, but not all, potential risk factors, and the significant association of activity and fitness with mortality persists. The adjustment of study results for other risk factors, particularly the major ones such as cholesterol, blood pressure, smoking, and obesity, is controversial. Some researchers have argued that a favorable change in a risk factor that is associated with a change in activity or fitness is part of the causal pathway through which physical activity and fitness affect mortality risk and therefore should not be controlled in the analysis.

Strength of the Evidence

Given that a valid association of physical activity and fitness with all-cause and CHD mortality exists, as the preceding sections have demonstrated, the next question to ask is: Are the observed associations causal? As outlined in chapter 2, epidemiologists apply five main criteria that, if satisfied, help establish that the observed associations are causal. These criteria, Mill's canons, are temporal sequence, strength of association, consistency of results, biological plausibility, and dose response.

Temporal Sequence

In a prospective cohort design, the independent variable (activity or fitness) is measured before the outcome occurs, thus demonstrating the appropriate temporal sequence.

Strength of Association

In their review of the literature on physical activity and CHD mortality, Powell et al. (1987) reported that the relative risk associated with inactivity varied across studies but ranged from 1.5 to 2.4, with a median of about 1.9 for all 47 determinations of relative risk obtained from these studies considered. Therefore, the risk of CHD mortality is almost twice as high for sedentary individuals as for physically active individuals. Earlier we noted that the population attributable risk of CHD mortality associated with low physical activity was as large or larger as that of other risk factors, such as cigarette smoking, high blood pressure, high serum cholesterol, and overweight.

Consistency of Results

The data about the association of activity and fitness with all-cause and CHD mortality are remarkably consistent for men and women. Most studies, even though they were conducted at different times using different methodologies and samples from different parts of the world, have yielded similar results.

Biological Plausibility

An important consideration in establishing causality is the evidence for the biological plausibility of the observed association. The association of activity and fitness with all-cause mortality is predominantly with cancer and CHD. We discuss the biological mechanism involved in the cancer–activity association in more detail in chapter 11. For now, it is sufficient to know that data from both animal and human studies show a favorable effect of physical activity on both the immune and endocrine systems that could potentially lead to a decreased risk of cancer. The biological mechanisms that explain the protective effect of physical activity against CHD are not fully known but include factors mainly related to myocardial oxygen supply and demand and myocardial electrical stability. Increased levels of HDL cholesterol, decreased body weight and blood pressure, and improved glucose tolerance are the mechanisms best supported by current scientific evidence.

Myocardial Oxygen Supply and Demand. Normal adaptations to exercise training include lowered blood lipids, which should lower the risk of atherosclerotic plaques and help maintain normal blood supply to the heart. Another common adaptation is a lowering of heart rate and blood pressure at rest and during submaximal exercise. Those factors combined (e.g., systolic blood pressure × heart rate) are an index of the metabolism (i.e., the oxygen demand) of the heart. In addition, a few postmortem necropsy studies have shown less coronary atherosclerosis or injury to the myocardium among men who had been regular exercisers. These studies include a widely publicized autopsy on famous lifelong marathon runner Clarence DeMar (Currens and White 1961) and studies in Westchester County, New York (Stamler et al. 1970); Great Britain (Morris and Crawford 1958); Israel (Mitrani, Karplus, and Bunner 1970); and Finland (Rissanen 1976). Even when the prevalence of severe coronary atherosclerosis was similar among men who had been sedentary, moderately active, or very active, physically active men had larger lumens in the coronary arteries. Moreover, physically active men were less likely to have complete occlusions of major coronary arteries and had less scarring from ischemic events and healed infarcts, even when they had advanced atherosclerosis. Experimental studies on rats and monkeys also have reported that the interior diameters of coronary arteries were larger after regular exercise (Leon 1972; Leon and Bloor 1977). Also, regular exercise reduced the severity of coronary atherosclerosis in monkeys fed a high-fat, high-cholesterol diet (Kramsch et al. 1981).

> ••• *Regular exercise lowers the oxygen demands of the heart during physical activity of a fixed intensity, thus reducing the risk of ischemia during physical work.*

Several lines of research suggest that physical activity might reduce the risk of coronary thrombosis. Decreased hematocrit resulting from an expansion of plasma volume is a hallmark response to regular physical activity. Thus, exercise training should lead to reduced viscosity (thickness) of the blood, which might reduce coagulability and platelet stickiness. Regular physical activity also might decrease platelet aggregation by changes in the metabolism of **prostaglandins.** Results from some cross-sectional, population-based studies are consistent with such views. For example, leisure-time physical activity, but not job activity, was inversely related to plasma viscosity among 3,500 men and women ages 25 to 64 years (Koenig et al. 1997), even after ad-

justment for age, cholesterol, smoking, blood pressure, and body weight for height. Strenuous exercise also was associated with lower activity of clotting factor VII in a cross-sectional study of nearly 4,000 men ages 45 to 69 years (Connelly, Cooper, and Meade 1992). Low leisure-time physical activity was associated with high levels of clotting factor VII, independently of total serum cholesterol, BMI, and insulin levels, which each were associated with higher levels of clotting factor VII (Bladbjerg, Moller, and Jespersen 1998).

Several hemostatic factors also are markers of inflammation, and recent studies suggest that the protective effects of physical activity against CVD may partly result from effects on inflammation as well as hemostasis. For example, the association between physical activity and markers of inflammation was examined in a healthy cohort of 5,888 men and women 65 or more years old in the cross-sectional Cardiovascular Health Study (Geffken et al. 2001). Blood levels of C-reactive protein, fibrinogen, white blood cells, and albumin and clotting factor VIII activity were compared among the cross section, which was divided into quartiles by self-reported physical activity. After adjustment for age, sex, race, smoking, BMI, CVD, diabetes, and hypertension, people in the highest quartile of physical activity had 19% lower concentration of C-reactive protein, 6% lower white blood cell count, 4% lower concentration of fibrinogen, and 3% less clotting factor VIII activity than people in the lowest quartile of physical activity. Further analysis suggested that the lower levels of inflammatory markers among the more-active people might be largely explained by their lower BMI and blood glucose levels.

Another, larger cross-sectional study, the National Health and Nutrition Examination Survey III (NHANES III, 1988–1994), examined the association between C-reactive protein and physical activity among 13,748 adults 20 years of age or older (Ford 2002). After adjusting for age, sex, ethnicity, education, work status, smoking, hypertension, BMI, waist-to-hip ratio, HDL-C concentration, and aspirin use, the odds ratios for elevated C-reactive protein concentration (defined as the 85th percentile or higher for each sex) were 0.98 (95% CI: 0.78–1.23), 0.85 (0.70–1.02), and 0.53 (0.40–0.71) for participants who engaged in light, moderate, and vigorous physical activity, respectively, during the previous month compared with participants who did not engage in any leisure-time physical activity.

A companion analysis of the NHANES III study examined the relationship between physical activity and elevated inflammation as indicated by a high C-reactive protein level, white blood cell count, and fibrinogen level in 3,638 apparently healthy men and women 40 years and older (Abramson and Vaccarino 2002). After adjusting for age, sex, race, education, blood pressure, HDL and LDL levels, blood glucose, BMI, waist-to-hip ratio, smoking, alcohol use, dietary fat, and vitamin C and E supplementation, the odds of having an elevated C-reactive protein level were reduced among people who were active 22 or more times per month (OR = 0.63, 95% CI: 0.43–0.93) when compared with those engaging in physical activity 0 to 3 times per month. Similar associations were seen for white blood cell count and fibrinogen levels.

Finally, in a cross-sectional study of 135 black, white, and Native American middle-aged, overweight women, plasma C-reactive protein levels decreased linearly across tertiles of cardiorespiratory fitness and increased across tertiles of BMI (LaMonte et al. 2002). After adjustment for BMI, smoking, diabetes, and estrogen use, the differences in C-reactive protein levels among fitness tertiles remained, except for the black women. Among all women, after adjusting for race and the confounders, the odds of high-risk C-reactive protein levels (>0.19 mg/dl) were 0.67 (95% CI: 0.19–2.4) among fit (>6.5 METs) versus unfit women.

In addition to those studies of physical activity, cardiorespiratory fitness levels were inversely associated with C-reactive protein levels in a sample of 722 men from the Aerobics Center Longitudinal Study after adjustments for age, body mass index, vitamin use, statin medication use, aspirin use, the presence of inflammatory disease, cardiovascular disease, diabetes, and smoking habit (Church et al. 2002).

Though those cross-sectional studies suggest that regular physical activity might have protective effects against chronic, low-grade inflammation, they lack the proper temporal sequence needed to permit an inference of cause and effect. Prospective studies have yielded similar findings, however, providing more compelling evidence of a favorable effect of physical activity on inflammation.

The relationship between physical activity and hemostatic and inflammatory variables was examined prospectively among 3,810 British men from 60 to 79 years of age who had initially been medically screened 20 years earlier (Wannamethee et al. 2002). Physical activity showed a significant inverse dose–response relationship with fibrinogen, plasma and blood viscosity, platelet count, several coagulation factors, tissue plasminogen activator antigen, white blood cell count, and C-reactive protein in men with or without CVD, even after adjustment for the possible confounders of age, BMI, smoking, and alcohol use. Men who became physically active during the 20 years since the study began had levels of the blood variables similar to those of the men who remained active throughout the 20 years, whereas the men who became inactive had levels similar to those of the men who remained inactive.

In an experimental study of the effects of exercise training on some peripheral inflammatory markers associated with endothelial dysfunction, blood levels of granulocyte-macrophage **colony stimulating factor** (GM-CSF), macrophage chemoattractant protein-1 (MCP-1), soluble intercellular adhesion molecule-1 (ICAM-1), and soluble vascular cell adhesion molecule-1 (VCAM-1) were measured before and after 12 weeks of exercise in 12 patients who had stable congestive heart disease (Adamopoulos et al. 2001). A crossover research design was used in which patients were randomly assigned first to either exercise or usual care, followed by the other condition, thus serving as their own controls. The exercise training increased the patients' maximal oxygen uptake by 13% and was accompanied by significant reductions in serum GM-CSF, MCP-1, ICAM-1, and VCAM-1. Thus, exercise training appears to favorably affect peripheral inflammatory markers of the interaction between macrophages and endothelial cells among patients with congestive heart failure.

> ••• *Exercise and habitual, moderately intense physical activity are associated with a favorable blood clotting profile and lower levels of markers for chronic low-grade inflammation that are predictors of sudden coronary death resulting from blood clots after ruptures of atheromas.*

Response to Acute Exercise   Though **acute exercise** increases blood coagulability, that effect appears to be offset by a co-occurring increase in fibrinolysis. Each of these responses increases with increasing intensity and duration of exercise (el-Sayed 1996). The increase in fibrinolysis after submaximal exercise is mainly explained by increases in tPA levels (about 40%) and tPA activity (about 150%), which return to resting levels within 30 min, and about a 25% decrease in PAI-1 activity that persists up to 1 h after exercise (e.g., DeSouza et al. 1997).

Adaptations After Chronic Exercise. Findings are not yet conclusive, but several studies suggest that **chronic exercise** diminishes increased coagulability during exercise while maintaining fibrinolytic activity. Cross-sectional population-based studies have indicated that regular, strenuous physical activity is associated with lower levels of plasma fibrinogen in young adults (Folsom et al. 1993) and middle-aged men (Connelly, Cooper, and Meade 1992). Also, physically active women have lower levels of fibrinogen, lower levels of tPA, lower PAI-1 levels and activity, but higher tPA activity than sedentary women, regardless of age (DeSouza, Jones, and Seals 1998). In a study of 700 men and nearly 800 women ages 25 to 64 years, tPA activity was 30% higher in the most-active men and 12% higher in the most-active women compared with their sedentary counterparts. PAI-1 activity was 40% and 30% lower among the most-active men and women, respectively. Those differences remained after adjustment for age, BMI, and waist-to-hip ratio but not after further adjustment for triglyceride and insulin levels (Eliasson, Asplund, and Evrin 1996).

A clinical study showed that platelet stickiness and aggregability were temporarily increased by a single session of maximal cycling exercise but were decreased at rest and after exercise following 8 weeks of cycling exercise for 30 min per day, 5 days per week, at an intensity of 60% of maximal aerobic capacity. Those training adaptations were reversed by 12 weeks of physical deconditioning (Wang, Jen, and Chen 1995). Similarly, increases in maximal power output of 12% in men and 18% in women after 9 months of exercise training were accompanied by reductions in PAI-1 levels, independent of reduced plasma triglyceride levels (Ponjee et al. 1996). Six months of exercise training that increased maximal oxygen uptake by about 20% was accompanied by a 140% increase in tPA level, a 40% increase in tPA activity, a 60% decrease in PAI-1 activity, and a 13% decrease in fibrinogen level in men ages 60 to 82 years but not in men ages 24 to 30 years (Stratton et al. 1991). Finally, a group of men already in an exercise program were divided into two groups: those with and those without CHD, matched by age and amount of physical activity (Fernhall et al. 1997). Both groups had similar increases in tPA activity and decreases in PAI-1 activity after a maximal exercise test but no changes in tPA or PAI-1 levels.

Electrical Stability of the Myocardium. Animal studies that induced myocardial ischemia by occluding a coronary artery have shown that the increased oxygen demand of the heart during acute exercise actually increases the risk of ventricular **fibrillation,** the leading cause of sudden cardiac death (Dawson, Leon, and Taylor 1979). In contrast, though, an increase in the ratio of oxygen supply to oxygen demand during exercise, which occurs after exercise training, should reduce the risk of ventricular fibrillation in people who have coronary artery disease. The reduction in sympathetic nervous system activity and catecholamine secretion during exercise of a fixed intensity, which occurs after exercise training, also should reduce myocardial irritability and the risk of ventricular fibrillation. However, exercise conditioning in CHD patients does not appear to change the frequency of irregular heartbeats originating outside the **sinoatrial node** (Laslett et al. 1983).

Dose Response

To determine whether a cause-and-effect relationship exists, it must be determined whether mortality risk decreases by a predictable dose–response pattern (e.g., linearly or curvilinearly) with increasing levels of activity or fitness, or whether there is a threshold level of activity or fitness above which further reductions in mortality risk do not occur. Though the results from many studies in the literature suggest a dose–response association between activity or fitness and all-cause and CHD mortality, a number of studies suggest a threshold effect. For example, the MRFIT study, a seven-year follow-up of 12,138 middle-aged men at high risk for CHD, noted that participation in moderate leisure-time physical activity (the middle half of the activity distribution) was associated with a 63% reduction in CHD and a 70% reduction in total mortality compared with the low-activity group. However, the mortality rates in the high- and moderate-activity groups were similar, suggesting a threshold effect for physical activity. Lindsted, Tonstad, and Kuzma (1991) reported on the association of physical activity with all-cause mortality in a 26-

year follow-up of 9,484 men who were members of the California Seventh Day Adventist Church. Physical activity was assessed using the question, "How much exercise do you get (work or play)?" Response choices were "none," "slight" (both inactive), "moderate" (moderately active), or "heavy" (highly active). Participation in moderate activity was associated with a significant reduction in both all-cause and CVD mortality, with no further benefit for high activity. A report from the Harvard Alumni Health Study on a cohort of 12,516 middle-aged and older men (mean age 57.7) also suggested a threshold effect (Sesso, Paffenbarger, and Lee 2000). In this study, physical activity was assessed using the Harvard Alumni Activity Survey at baseline. During the 16-year follow-up period (1977–1993), there were 2,135 incident cases of CHD. An L-shaped association was noted between total weekly physical activity energy expenditure and CHD risk. CHD risk was reduced by approximately 20% in the group of men with energy expenditures greater than 1,000 kcal/wk. Compared with those whose physical activity energy expenditure was less than 500 kcal/wk, the relative risks for CHD, after adjustment for age, BMI, alcohol intake, hypertension, diabetes mellitus, smoking, and premature parental death (<65 years), were 0.90 (95% CI: 0.79–1.03) for those who expended 500 to 999 kcal/wk, 0.81 (0.71–0.92) for those who expended 1,000 to 1,999 kcal/wk, 0.80 (0.69–0.93) for those who expended 2,000 to 2,999 kcal/wk, and 0.81 (0.71–0.94) for those who expended over 3,000 kcal/wk.

> ••• *Most studies agree that the reduction in CHD with increasing physical activity is linear or negatively accelerating between about 1,000 to 3,000 kcal of leisure-time physical activity each week.*

Negatively accelerating dose response and a threshold for the effect of cardiovascular fitness on risk for all-cause and CHD mortality have also been reported. For example, in the Aerobics Center Longitudinal Study cohort, Blair et al. (1989) reported a large decline in the age-adjusted mortality rate between the least-fit quintile (64.0 per 10,000 person-years) and the second quintile (25.5 per 10,000 person-years), with continuing, but lessened, additional benefit with further increases in cardiovascular fitness (27.1, 21.7, and 18.6 per 10,000 person-years for the third, fourth, and fifth quintiles, respectively). A study of 1,960

Norwegian men ages 40 to 59 measured physical fitness as total work performed on a symptom-limited cycle ergometer test and followed the men for 16 years to assess all-cause and CHD mortality (Sandvik et al. 1993). The relative risk for all-cause mortality in the most-fit group (quartile 4) compared with the least-fit group (quartile 1) was 0.54 (95% CI: 0.32–0.89) after adjustment for conventional risk factors. All-cause mortality was similar in fitness quartiles 1, 2, and 3, suggesting a threshold effect for cardiovascular fitness. The results were slightly different for CHD mortality. Here the adjusted relative risks compared with quartile 1 were 0.45 (95% CI: 0.22–0.92), 0.59 (0.28–1.22), and 0.41 (0.20–0.84) for quartiles 2, 3, and 4, respectively.

Despite the complexity of the evidence about the dose–response association between physical activity and reduced CHD, a systematic review of 31 studies (20 were prospective cohort studies) published between 1958 and August 2000 concluded that physical activity has a causal, dose–response relationship with reduced risk of CHD morbidity and mortality (Kohl 2001). In that review, 20 studies were interpreted as supporting a dose response. Three studies showed mixed results, depending on the measure of physical activity used or the way the cohort was split up for analysis. Another 8 studies either showed no association of physical activity with CHD or suggested a threshold or a U-shaped response pattern with a reduction in risk with a moderate amount of physical activity followed by increased risk with high physical activity.

What Intensity of Physical Activity Decreases Mortality Risk?

Related to the dose–response issue is the question of what intensity of physical activity is required to obtain either optimal or minimal reductions in mortality risk. To date, results of studies that have addressed the issue of physical activity and all-cause and CHD mortality have been inconsistent. A number of studies have suggested that participation in rather vigorous physical activity, generally defined as ≥6 METs, is required to see a reduction in mortality risk. For example, the early work of Morris et al. (1973, 1980) with British civil servants indicated that 30 min per day of leisure physical activity at a vigorous intensity (7.5 kcal/min) was required to achieve a decrease in CHD risk. In the U.S. railroad cohort, Slattery and Jacobs (1988) reported that intense, but not light to moderate, occupational physical activity was associated with reduced all-cause mortality. In Finnish men, Lakka et al. (1994) showed a decreased risk of MI for men who participated in conditioning physical activity (a mean of 6 METs) but not for those who participated in nonconditioning activity (a mean of 2.6 METs) or in walking or cycling to work (a mean of 4.0 METs).

Harvard Alumni Health Study

Three reports from the Harvard Alumni Health Study showed a benefit with vigorous but not with light to moderate activity. Lee, Hsieh, and Paffenbarger (1995) reported that only participation in vigorous activity (≥6 METs) was associated with a decreased risk for all-cause mortality. A report by Sesso, Paffenbarger, and Lee (2000) suggested an association between decreased CHD risk and participation in vigorous physical activity (≥6 METs), whereas participation in moderate (4–6 METs) or light (<4 METs) activity had no clear association with CHD risk. Lee and Paffenbarger (2000) reported that participation in light activity (<4 METs) was not associated with decreased all-cause mortality rates. They noted that participation in moderate activity (4–6 METs) was somewhat beneficial (although most reported relative risks for increasing level of moderate activity were not statistically significant), while participation in vigorous activity (≥6 METs) was clearly associated with deceased mortality rates.

••• Though many studies suggest that vigorous exercise is more protective against CHD than is light or moderately intense physical activity, walking has reduced risk for men and women in several studies.

In contrast to the previous reports suggesting that vigorous activity is required to decrease rates of all-cause and CHD mortality, the results from a number of studies suggest that participation in moderate-intensity activity, particularly walking, may decrease mortality risk. For example, in an early study from the Netherlands, Magnus, Matroos, and Stracklee (1979) reported that moderate-intensity physical activity, such as brisk walking, stair climbing, and gardening, if done regularly throughout the course of the year, is associated with decreased CHD risk. In the MRFIT cohort, a reduced risk of mortality was noted with increased amounts of physical activity that were primarily of light to moderate intensity. Lee and Paffenbarger (2000) showed in the Harvard alumni cohort that after adjusting for other components of physical activity, distance walked per week and number of stories climbed per week were associated with a reduced risk of mortality. The relative risk for walking more than 20 km/wk versus less than 5 km/wk was 0.84 (95% CI: 0.75–0.94), and the relative risk for climbing 35 stories or more per week versus fewer than 10 stories was 0.82 (0.75–0.94).

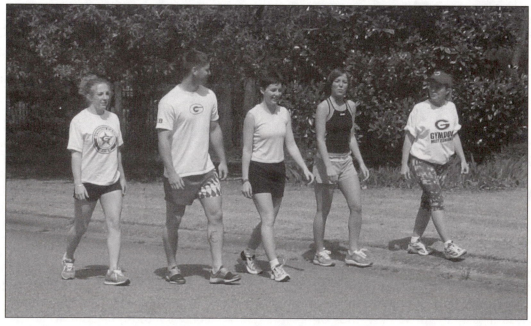

Courtesy of the author.

Seniors in Washington State

Among a group of 1,645 people ages 65 and older who were members of a health maintenance organization in the state of Washington, those who reported walking more than 4 h/wk had a 30% reduction in risk of hospitalization for cardiovascular disease during the next four years compared with those who walked less than 1 h/wk (LaCroix et al. 1996). The risk reduction was independent of age, sex, treated high blood pressure, current estrogen use, chronic disease, physical function, ethnicity, education, income, self-rated health status, smoking, alcohol use, and BMI measured at the beginning of the study, as well as whether the subject also participated in more-vigorous leisure physical activities. Walking more than 4 h/wk was not associated with reduced risk of death, however, after controlling for other risk factors and health measured at study outset.

King County, Washington

Lemaitre et al. (1999) reported on a case–control study to investigate the association between regular participation in high- and moderate-intensity physical activity and the risk for primary cardiac arrest. The physical activity habits of 333 people (ages 25 to 74 years) whose cardiac arrests occurred between 1988 and 1994 in King County, Washington, were compared with 503 age- and sex-matched controls. The spouses of the cases and controls were interviewed using an instrument derived from the MLTPAQ regarding participation in 15 high-intensity (>6 kcal/min) and 6 moderate-intensity activities. Similar odds ratios were noted for all levels of activity intensity. Using participants who performed no physical activity as the reference and controlling for age, education, diabetes, hypertension, and general health status, the odds ratio for primary cardiac arrest was 0.34 (95% CI: 0.13–0.89) for those who performed only gardening activities more than 60 min per week, 0.27 (0.11–0.67) for those who walked for exercise for more than 60 min/wk, and 0.34 (0.16–0.75) for those who engaged in any high-intensity physical activity.

Dutch Men

In a group of 800 retired Dutch men ages 64 to 84 years at study outset, 10-year death rates from total CVD (199 deaths), CHD (90 deaths), stroke (47 deaths), and all causes (373 deaths) were compared between the 30% most physically active and 30% least active (Bijnen et al. 1998). After adjustments for age, chronic diseases, ciga-rette smoking, and alcohol use at the beginning of the study, the relative risk of death from CVD and all causes was about 25% to 30% lower for the most-active men. Time spent in more-intense activities (≥ 4 kcal $\cdot$ kg^{-1} $\cdot$ h^{-1}) was more strongly associated with death from each cause except CHD than were less-intense activities, regardless of type of physical activity. Walking or cycling for 20 min at least three times per week predicted a 30% reduction in risk of both CVD and all-cause deaths, independently of other biological risk factors.

Honolulu Heart Program

Recent studies of other cohorts confirm that walking offers a substantial reduction in risk of CHD, similar to more vigorous exercise in elderly men and in middle-aged women. Results from the Honolulu Heart Program suggest that a minimal amount, or threshold, of walking is needed for a reduction in CHD risk (Hakim et al. 1999). Among 2,678 men ages 71 to 93 years in 1991 to 1993, 109 developed CHD two to four years later. In those who had been walking less than 0.25 mile (0.4 km) or between 0.25 and 1.5 miles (0.4–2.4 km) each day when the study began, the incidence rates of CHD (5.1% and 4.5%, respectively) were about twice that of men who walked more than 1.5 miles per day (2.5%). The results did not change after adjustment for age and other risk factors.

Nurses' Health Study

In a report from the Nurses' Health Study cohort, Manson et al. (1999) examined the association of total physical activity as well as vigorous and walking activity with the incidence of CHD in 72,488 apparently healthy female nurses, ages 40 to 65 years at the baseline examination in 1986. During an eight-year follow-up period, 645 incidents of either nonfatal MI or CHD death were documented. Compared with women in the lowest quintile of total physical activity, women in quintiles 2 to 5 had multivariately adjusted relative risks of CHD events of 0.88 (95% CI: 0.71–1.10), 0.81 (0.64–1.02), 0.74 (0.58–0.95), and 0.66 (0.51–0.86), respectively. Walking for exercise was also associated with a reduced risk for CHD events. Women in the highest quintile for walking, who walked about three or more hours per week at a brisk pace, had a multivariately adjusted relative risk of 0.65 (95% CI: 0.47–0.91) compared with women who walked infrequently. Walking and vigorous exercise were both associated with a reduction in CHD risk. For each 5 MET-hours per week spent in walking, the multivariately adjusted relative risk of CHD events was 0.86 (95% CI: 0.74–0.99), and for every 5 MET-hours per week spent in vigorous exercise, the multivariately adjusted relative risk of CHD events was 0.94 (95% CI: 0.89–0.99). Therefore, in this cohort of women, the risk reduction associated with vigorous exercise and walking were quite similar when the number of MET-hours spent per week were the same for both activities.

As is evident from the conflicting results presented, the optimal intensity of physical activity to reduce all-cause and CHD mortality risk remains unresolved. The lack of consistency in results across studies may largely relate to imprecision in measuring moderate physical activity, particularly walking. In addition, the available studies differ greatly in sample size, definition of outcomes, and number and types of confounders considered. The argument has also been put forth that it is difficult, if not impossible, to expend the requisite amount of energy in light to moderate activity to reduce mortality risk. It is likely that future studies, using more sophisticated physical activity assessment methods, will provide a better understanding of the optimal exercise regime to decrease mortality risk.

For example, a recent prospective analysis of data from the Health Professionals' Follow-up Study of over 44,000 U.S. men observed between 1986 to 1998 examined associations between CHD risk and the amount, type, and intensity of physical activity (Tanasescu et al. 2002). The investigators found that total physical activity, running, weight training, and rowing each was inversely and linearly related to risk of CHD, after adjustment for age, smoking, and several CHD risk factors. Running for an hour or more per week was associated with a 42% risk reduction (RR = 0.58; 95% CI: 0.44–0.77). Weight training for 30 min or more per week was associated with a 23% risk reduction (RR = 0.77; 95% CI: 0.61–0.98). Rowing for 1 h or more per week was associated with an 18% risk reduction (RR = 0.82; 95% CI: 0.68–0.99). Average exercise intensity was associated with reduced CHD risk independent of the total amount of physical activity expressed as MET-hours. The RRs (95% CIs) corresponding to moderate (4–6 METs) and high (6–12 METs) activity intensities were 0.94 (0.83–1.04) and 0.83 (0.72–0.97) compared with low activity intensity (<4 METs). A half hour per day or more of brisk walking was associated with an 18% risk reduc-

tion (RR = 0.82; 95% CI: 0.67–1.00). Walking pace was associated with reduced CHD risk independent of the number of walking hours. The investigators concluded that average exercise intensity was associated with reduced risk independent of the number of MET-hours spent in physical activity.

Summary

The U.S. Surgeon General's report on physical activity and health concluded that the evidence for a protective effect of physical activity against CHD was strong. CHD is caused by the interaction of several factors, each of which plausibly affects the etiology of atherosclerosis or its consequences. Experimental confirmation that physical inactivity directly causes CHD likely will never be obtained because the cost of population-based randomized clinical trials is too great. It is also unethical to assign individuals to a sedentary control group, given the strong and consistent evidence for a protective effect of increased physical activity against the risk for both CHD mortality and total mortality. Public health policy in the United States is already aggressively encouraging people to be more active because about 40 epidemiologic studies, many that were reviewed in this chapter, agree that leisure-time physical activity is strongly associated with lowered risks of CHD incidence and CHD mortality in both men and women regardless of age. The reduced risks are independent of most other major risk factors for CHD, but the protective effect of physical activity can also operate indirectly by positively affecting several other biological risk factors for CHD, including blood pressure, body weight, blood lipids, and factors associated with atherosclerosis and blood coagulability.

> ••• *Regular physical activity reduces CHD risk independently of other risk factors, but it can also favorably influence risk factors such as blood pressure, body weight, blood lipids, and blood clotting factors.*

Many of the studies of physical activity and mortality have been prospective and generally show that the protective effect of physical activity is not explained by poor health in sedentary individuals at baseline. Nonetheless, because many of these studies began when the participants were middle-aged, it was impossible to know with certainty whether those who were sedentary had subclinical conditions that caused both the sedentary behavior and the disease or mortality outcome.

Epidemiologic studies also suggest a dose–response relationship between physical activity and rates of CHD, but the shape of the association and quantity of physical activity that provides optimal protection against the development of CHD remain controversial. This is largely true because of the difficulty of measuring leisure-time physical activity precisely in population-based studies, the difficulty of comparing the amounts of physical activity estimated by different methods across studies, the lack of validation of self-reported physical activity with objective measures such as fitness, and the fact that very few studies have attempted to determine how much change in physical activity or fitness is associated with how much change in morbidity or mortality from CHD.

Nonetheless, there is general consensus among epidemiologists that a window of protection from CHD disease and death includes a range from about 750 to 2,000 kcal/wk of moderate-intensity (3–6 METs), dynamic, endurance exercise (such as walking or jogging about 7.5 to 20 miles, or 12 to 32 km, per week). In the absence of leisure physical activity, at least an hour of intermittent hard physical labor a week also seems to offer protection against CHD. Clinical experiments have shown that those amounts of exercise provide enough of a stimulus to increase HDL cholesterol levels and fibrinolytic factors, while helping to decrease blood pressure, triglycerides, body fat, and blood coagulability. Population studies also suggest a favorable effect of moderate physical activity on inflammatory features of atherogenesis and cardiac thrombosis. The specific effect of acute or regular physical activity on inflammation remains to be determined by experimental studies.

Whether the relationship of lowered risk of CHD with increasing levels of weekly energy expenditure or increasing physical fitness is linear is not clear. At present, most evidence supports a negatively accelerating decline in risk, where the largest reductions occur with moderate levels of activity or fitness as compared with those who are least active or fit. Risk continues to decline thereafter but to a diminishing degree. Whether the rate of energy expenditure (i.e., intensity of the physical activity) provides additional protection against CHD events and death also remains

unclear. On balance, the available evidence indicates that energy expended in vigorous exercise confers more health-protective benefits than light activity, but the actual intensity of physical activity has not been measured in epidemiologic studies and the definition of *vigorous* has varied among studies. Though based on observational rather than experimental studies, the message is clear: Something is better than nothing, but exactly how much is enough remains unclear. It is likely that the amount and intensity of regular exercise required to increase and maintain cardiorespiratory fitness would also be adequate to reduce the risks of CHD. In very sedentary and older adults, brisk walking is enough of a stimulus for fitness gains and maintenance. A few recent clinical studies have tested the hypothesis that accumulating 30 to 40 min of aerobic exercise in three or so separate sessions could have CHD benefits comparable to a single session of sustained activity of the same duration. Though early findings suggest that CHD risk factors (e.g., body fat percentage, blood lipids, and blood pressure) can be altered favorably by intermittent activity, so far no randomized controlled trials have been completed to confirm that intermittent activity affords the same degree of heart protection as sustained exercise.

Bibliography

Abramson, J.L., and V. Vaccarino. 2002. Relationship between physical activity and inflammation among apparently healthy middle-aged and older U.S. adults. *Archives of Internal Medicine* 162 (11): 1286–1292.

Adamopoulos, S., J. Parissis, C. Kroupis, M. Georgiadis, D. Karatzas, G. Karavolias, K. Koniavitou, A.J. Coats, and D.T. Kremastinos. 2001. Physical training reduces peripheral markers of inflammation in patients with chronic heart failure. *European Heart Journal* 22 (9): 791–797.

Albert C.M., J. Ma, N. Rifai, M.J. Stampfer, and P.M. Ridker. 2002. Prospective study of C-reactive protein, homocysteine, and plasma lipid levels as predictors of sudden cardiac death. *Circulation* 105: 2595–2599.

American Heart Association. 1991. *1992 heart and stroke facts.* Dallas: American Heart Association.

———. 2000. *2001 heart and stroke statistical update.* Dallas: American Heart Association.

———. 2001. *2002 heart and stroke statistical update.* Dallas: American Heart Association.

Berlin, J.A., and G.A. Colditz. 1990. A meta-analysis of physical activity in the prevention of coronary heart disease. *American Journal of Epidemiology* 132: 612–628.

Bijnen, F.C., C.J. Caspersen, E.J. Feskens, W.H. Saris, W.L. Mosterd, D. Kromhout. 1998. Physical activity and 10-year mortality from cardiovascular diseases and all causes: The Zutphen Elderly Study. *Archives of Internal Medicine* 158: 1499–1505.

Bijnen, F.C., C.J. Caspersen, and W.L. Mosterd. 1994. Physical inactivity as a risk factor for coronary heart disease:

A WHO and International Society and Federation of Cardiology position statement. *Bulletin of the World Health Organization* 72 (1): 1–4.

Bijnen, F., E. Feskens, C. Caspersen, S. Giampaoli, A. Nissinen, A. Menotti, W. Mosterd, and D. Kromhout. 1996. Physical activity and cardiovascular risk factors among elderly men in Finland, Italy, and the Netherlands. *American Journal of Epidemiology* 143: 553–661.

Bladbjerg, E.M., L. Moller, and J. Jespersen. 1998. Association of factor VII protein concentration with lifestyle factors. *Scandinavian Journal of Clinical and Laboratory Investigation* 58: 323–330.

Blair, S., E. Horton, A. Leon, I. Lee, L. Drinkwater, R. Dishman, M. Mackey, and M. Kienholz. 1996. Physical activity, nutrition, and chronic disease. *Medicine and Science in Sports and Exercise* 28 (3): 335–349.

Blair, S.N., H.W. Kohl III, C.E. Barlow, R.S. Paffenbarger Jr., L.W. Gibbons, and C.A. Macera. 1995. Changes in physical fitness and all-cause mortality: A prospective study of healthy and unhealthy men. *Journal of the American Medical Association* 273: 1093–1098.

Blair, S., H. Kohl, R. Paffenbarger, D. Clark, K. Cooper, and L. Gibbons. 1989. Physical fitness and all-cause mortality: A prospective study of healthy men and women. *Journal of the American Medical Association* 262: 2395–2401.

Blair, S.N., and M. Wei. 2000. Sedentary habits, health, and function in older women and men. *American Journal of Health Promotion* 15: 1–8.

Bouchard, C., R. Lesage, G. Lortie, J.A. Simoneau, P. Hamel, M.R. Boulay, L. Perusse, G. Theriault, and C. LeBlanc. 1986. Aerobic performance in brothers, dizygotic and monozygotic twins. *Medicine and Science in Sports and Exercise* 18: 639–646.

Brunner, D., G. Manelis, M. Modan, and S. Levin. 1974. Physical activity at work and the incidence of myocardial infarction, angina pectoris and death due to ischemic heart disease: An epidemiological study in Israeli collective statements (kibbutzim). *Journal of Chronic Diseases* 27: 217–233.

Cassell, J., S. Heyden, A.C. Bartel, B.H. Kaplan, H.A. Tyroler, J.C. Cornoni, and J.C. Hames. 1971. Occupation and physical activity and coronary heart disease. *Archives of Internal Medicine* 128: 920–928.

Centers for Disease Control and Prevention. 1999. Achievements in public health, 1900–1999: Decline in deaths from heart disease and stroke—United States, 1900–1999. *Morbidity and Mortality Weekly Report* 48 (30): 649–656.

Centers for Disease Control and Prevention. 2003. Deaths: Preliminary data for 2001. *National Vital Statistics Reports* 51 (5): 1–48.

Chapman, J.M., and F.J. Massey. 1964. The inter-relationship of serum cholesterol, hypertension, body weight and risk of coronary heart disease: Results of the first ten years' follow-up in the Los Angeles Heart Study. *Journal of Chronic Diseases* 17: 933–947.

Church, T.S., C.E. Barlow, C.P. Earnest, J.B. Kampert, E.L. Priest, and S.N. Blair. 2002. Associations between cardiorespiratory fitness and C-reactive protein in men. *Arteriosclerosis, Thrombosis, and Vascular Biology* 22: 1869–1876.

Connelly, J.B., J.A. Cooper, and T.W. Meade. 1992. Strenuous exercise, plasma fibrinogen, and factor VII activity. *British Heart Journal* 67: 351–354.

Curfman, G. 1993. The health benefits of exercise: A critical appraisal. *New England Journal of Medicine* 328 (8): 574–575.

Currens, J.H., and P.D. White. 1961. Half century of running: Clinical, physiological, and pathological findings in the case of Clarence DeMar ("Mr. Marathon"). *New England Journal of Medicine* 265: 988–993.

Dawson, A.K., A.S. Leon, and H.L. Taylor. 1979. Effect of submaximal exercise on vulnerability to fibrillation in the canine ventricle. *Circulation* 60: 798–804.

DeSouza, C.A., D.R. Dengel, M.A. Rogers, K. Cox, and R.F. Macko. 1997. Fibrinolytic responses to acute physical activity in older hypertensive men. *Journal of Applied Physiology* 82: 1765–1770.

DeSouza, C.A., P.P. Jones, and D.R. Seals. 1998. Physical activity status and adverse age-related differences in coagulation and fibrinolytic factors in women. *Arteriosclerosis, Thrombosis, and Vascular Biology* 18: 362–368.

Division of Chronic Disease Control and Community Intervention. 1993. Public health focus: Physical activity and prevention of coronary heart disease. *Journal of the American Medical Association* 279: 1529–1530.

Dorn, J., J. Naughton, D. Imamura, and M. Trevisan. 1999. Results of a multicenter randomized clinical trial of exercise and long-term survival in myocardial infarction patients: The National Exercise and Heart Disease Project (NEHDP). *Circulation* 100 (17): 1764–1769.

Easton, J. 1799. *Human longevity; recording the name, age, place of residence, and year of the decease, of 1712 persons who attained a century, & upwards, from A.D. 66 to 1799.* Salisbury, England: Author.

Ekelund, L.G., W.L. Haskell, J.L. Johnson, F.S. Whaley, M.H. Criqui, and D.S. Sheps. 1988. Physical fitness as a predictor of cardiovascular mortality in asymptomatic North American men: The Lipid Research Clinics mortality follow-up study. *New England Journal of Medicine* 319: 1379–1384.

Eliasson, M., K. Asplund, and P.E. Evrin. 1996. Regular leisure time physical activity predicts high activity of tissue plasminogen activator: The Northern Sweden MONICA Study. *International Journal of Epidemiology* 25: 1182–1188.

el-Sayed, M.S. 1996. Effects of exercise on blood coagulation, fibrinolysis, and platelet aggregation. *Sports Medicine* 22: 282–298.

Engstrom, G., B. Hedblad, and L. Janzon. 1999. Hypertensive men who exercise regularly have a lower rate of cardiovascular mortality. *Journal of Hypertension* 17: 737–742.

Epstein, L., G.T. Miller, F.W. Sitt, and J.N. Morris. 1976. Vigorous exercise in leisure-time, coronary risk factors, and resting electrocardiograms in middle-aged civil servants. *British Heart Journal* 38: 403–409.

Erikssen, G., K. Liestol, J. Bjornholt, E. Thaulow, L. Sandvik, and J. Erikssen. 1998. Changes in physical fitness and changes in mortality. *Lancet* 352: 759–762.

Fernhall, B., L.M. Szymanski, P.A. Gorman, J. Milani, D.C. Paup, and C.M. Kessler. 1997. Fibrinolytic activity is similar in physically active men with and without a history of myocardial infarction. *Arteriosclerosis, Thrombosis, and Vascular Biology* 17: 1106–1113.

Fletcher, G.F., G. Balady, S.N. Blair, J. Blumenthal, C. Caspersen, B. Chaitman, S. Epstein, E.S. Sivarajan Froelicher, V.F. Froelicher, I.L. Pina, and M.L. Pollock. 1996. Statement on exercise: Benefits and recommendations for physical activity programs for all Americans. A statement for health professionals by the Committee on Exercise and Cardiac Rehabilitation of the Council on Clinical Cardiology, American Heart Association. *Circulation* 94 (4): 857–862.

Folsom, A.R., N. Aleksic, D. Catellier, H.S. Juneja, and K.K. Wu. 2002. C-reactive protein and incident coronary heart disease in the Atherosclerosis Risk in Communities (ARIC) study. *American Heart Journal* 144 (2): 233–238.

Folsom, A.R., H.T. Qamheih, J.M. Flack, J.E. Hilner, K. Liu, B.V. Howard, and R.P. Tracy. 1993. Plasma fibrinogen: Levels and correlates in young adults. The coronary artery risk development in young adults (CARDIA) study. *American Journal of Epidemiology* 138: 1023–1036.

Ford, E.S. 2002. Does exercise reduce inflammation? Physical activity and C-reactive protein among U.S. adults. *Epidemiology* 13 (5): 561–568.

Fried, L.P., R.A. Kronmal, A.B. Newman, D.E. Bild, M.B. Mittelmark, J.F. Polak, J.A. Robbins, and J.M. Gardin. 1998. Risk factors for 5-year mortality in older adults: The Cardiovascular Health Study. *Journal of the American Medical Association* 279 (8): 585–592.

Garcia-Palmieri, M.R., R. Costas Jr., M. Cruz-Vidal, P.D. Sorlie, and R.J. Havlik. 1982. Increased physical activity: A protective factor against heart attacks in Puerto Rico. *American Journal of Cardiology* 50: 749–755.

Geffken, D., M. Cushman, G. Burke, J. Polak, P. Sakkinen, and R. Tracy. 2001. Association between physical activity and markers of inflammation in a healthy elderly population. *American Journal of Epidemiology* 153 (3): 242–250.

Haapanen-Niemi, N., I. Vuori, and M. Pasanen. 1999. Public health burden of coronary heart disease risk factors among middle-aged and elderly men. *Preventive Medicine* 28: 343–348.

Hakim, A.A., J.D. Curb, H. Petrovitch, B.L. Rodriguez, K. Yano, G.W. Ross, L.R. White, and R.D. Abbott. 1999. Effects of walking on coronary heart disease in elderly men: The Honolulu Heart Program. *Circulation* 100 (1): 9–13.

Hamsten, A. 1995. Hemostatic function and coronary artery disease. *New England Journal of Medicine* 332: 677–678.

Hedblad, O., M. Ogren, S.O. Isacsson, and L. Jansen. 1997. Reduced cardiovascular mortality risk in male smokers who are physically active. Results for a 25-year follow-up of the prospective population study of men born in 1914. *Archives of Internal Medicine* 157: 893–899.

Hellenius, M., U. Faire, B. Berglund, A. Hamsten, and I. Krakau. 1993. Diet and exercise are equally effective in reducing risk for cardiovascular disease: Results of a randomized controlled study in men with slightly to moderately raised cardiovascular risk factors. *Atherosclerosis* 103: 81–91.

Hennekens, C.H., J. Rosner, M.J. Jesse, M.E. Drolette, and F.E. Speizer. 1977. A retrospective study of physical activity and coronary deaths. *International Journal of Epidemiology* 6: 243–246.

Hinkle, L.E., L.A. Whitney, E.W. Lehman, J. Dunn, B. Benjamin, R. King, A. Plakun, and B. Flehiner. 1968. Occupation, education, and coronary heart disease. *Science* 161: 238–246.

Homocysteine Lowering Trialists' Collaboration. 1998. Lowering blood homocysteine with folic acid based supplements: Meta-analysis of randomised trials. *British Medical Journal* 316 (7135): 894–898.

Kampert, J., S.N. Blair, C.E. Barlow, and H.W. Kohl III. 1996. Physical activity, physical fitness, and all-cause and cancer mortality: A prospective study of men and women. *Annals of Epidemiology* 6: 452–457.

Kannel, W.B., and P. Sorlie. 1979. Some health benefits of physical activity: The Framingham Study. *Archives of Internal Medicine* 139: 857–861.

Karvonen, M.J. 1982. Physical activity in work and leisure time in relation to cardiovascular diseases. *Annals of Clinical Research* 14 (Suppl. 34): 118–123.

Keys, A. 1980. *Seven countries: A multivariate analysis of death and coronary disease.* Cambridge, MA: Harvard University Press.

Kipple, K.F., ed. 1993. *The Cambridge world history of human disease.* New York: Cambridge University Press.

Koenig, W., M. Sund, A. Doring, and E. Ernst. 1997. Leisure-time physical activity but not work-related physical activity is associated with decreased plasma viscosity: Results from a large population sample. *Circulation* 95: 335–341.

Kohl, H.W. III. 2001. Physical activity and cardiovascular disease: Evidence for a dose response. *Medicine and Science in Sports and Exercise* 33 (Suppl. 6): S472–S483.

Kramsch, L.M., A.J. Aspen, B.M. Abramowitz, T. Kreimendal, and W.B. Hood Jr. 1981. Reduction of coronary artherosclerosis by moderate conditioning exercise in monkeys on an atherogenic diet. *New England Journal of Medicine* 305: 1483–1489.

Kujala, U.M., J. Kaprio, S. Sarna, and M. Koskenvuo. 1998. Relationship of leisure-time physical activity and mortality: The Finnish twin cohort. *Journal of the American Medical Association* 279 (6): 440–444.

Kushi, L.H., R.M. Fee, A.R. Folsom, P.J. Mink, K.E. Anderson, and T.A. Sellers. 1997. Physical activity and mortality in postmenopausal women. *Journal of the American Medical Association* 277: 1287–1292.

LaCroix, A.Z., S.G. Leveille, J.A. Hecht, L.C. Grothaus, and E.H. Wagner. 1996. Does walking decrease the risk of cardiovascular disease hospitalizations and death in older adults? *Journal of the American Geriatric Society* 44: 113–120.

Lakka, T.A., J.M. Venalainen, R. Rauramaa, R. Slagnen, J. Tuomilehto, and J.T. Salonen. 1994. Relation of leisure-time physical activity and cardiorespiratory fitness to the risk of acute myocardial infarction in men. *New England Journal of Medicine* 330: 1549–1554.

LaMonte, M.J., J.L. Durstine, F.G. Yanowitz, T. Lim, K.D. DuBose, P. Davis, and B.E. Ainsworth. 2002. Cardiorespiratory fitness and C-reactive protein among a tri-ethnic sample of women. *Circulation* 106 (4): 403–406.

Laslett, L., P.S. Baiser, L. Palmer, and E.A. Amsterdam. 1983. Ventricular ectopy frequency and complexity not altered in exercise training in coronary disease patients. *Cardiology* 70: 284–290.

Lee, I.M., C.C. Hsieh, and R.S. Paffenbarger Jr. 1995. Exercise intensity and longevity in men. The Harvard Alumni Health Study. *Journal of the American Medical Association* 273: 1179–1184.

Lee, I.M., and R.S. Paffenbarger Jr. 1996. Do physical activity and physical fitness avert premature mortality? *Exercise and Sport Science Reviews* 24: 135–171.

Lee, I.M., and R.S. Paffenbarger Jr. 2000. Associations of light, moderate, and vigorous intensity physical activity and longevity: The Harvard Alumni Health Study. *American Journal of Epidemiology* 151: 293–299.

Lee, I.M., and R.S. Paffenbarger. 2001. Preventing coronary heart disease: The role of physical activity. *Physician and Sportsmedicine* 29 (2): 37–52.

Lee, I.M., and P.J. Skerrett. 2001. Physical activity and all-cause mortality: What is the dose–response relation? *Medicine and Science in Sports and Exercise* 33 (Suppl. 6): S459–S471.

Lemaitre, R.N., S.R. Heckbert, B.M. Psaty, and D.S. Siscovick. 1995. Leisure-time physical activity and the risk of non-fatal myocardial infarction in postmenopausal women. *Archives of Internal Medicine* 155: 2302–2308.

Lemaitre, R.N., D.S. Siscovick, T.E. Raghunathan, S. Weinmann, P. Arbogast, and D.Y. Lin. 1999. Leisure-time physical activity and the risk of primary cardiac arrest. *Archives of Internal Medicine* 159: 686–690.

Leon, A.S. 1972. Comparative cardiovascular adaptation to exercise in animals and man and its relevance to coronary heart disease. In *Comparative pathophysiology of circulatory disturbances,* edited by C.M. Bloor. New York: Plenum.

Leon, A.S., and H. Blackburn. 1977. The relationship of physical activity to coronary heart disease and life expectancy. *Annals of the New York Academy of Sciences* 301: 361–378.

Leon, A.S., and C.M. Bloor. 1977. The effects of complete and partial deconditioning on exercise-induced cardio-vascular changes in the rat. *Advances in Cardiology* 18: 81–92.

Leon, A.S., J. Connett, D.R. Jacobs Jr., and R. Rauramaa. 1987. Leisure-time physical activity levels and risk of coronary heart disease and death: The Multiple Risk Factor Intervention Trial. *Journal of the American Medical Association* 258: 2388–2395.

Leon, A.S., M.J. Myers, and J. Connett. 1997. Leisure time physical activity and the 16-year risks of mortality from coronary heart disease and all-causes in the Multiple Risk Factor Intervention Trial (MRFIT). *International Journal of Sports Medicine* 18 (Suppl. 3): S208–S215.

Libby, P., P.M. Ridker, and A. Maseri. 2002. Inflammation and atherosclerosis. *Circulation* 105: 1135–1143.

Lindsted, K.D., S. Tonstad, and J.W. Kuzma. 1991. Self-report of physical activity and patterns of mortality in Seventh-Day Adventist men. *Journal of Clinical Epidemiology* 44: 355–364.

Lloyd-Jones, D.M., M.G. Larson, A. Beiser, and D. Levy. 1999. Lifetime risk of developing coronary heart disease. *Lancet* 353 (9147): 89–92.

Magnus, K., A. Matroos, and J. Stracklee. 1979. Walking, cycling, or gardening with or without seasonal interruption in relation to acute coronary events. *American Journal of Epidemiology* 110: 724–733.

Malinow, M.R., A.G. Bostom, and R.M. Krauss. 1999. Homocysteine, diet, and cardiovascular diseases: A statement for health-care professionals from the nutrition committee, American Heart Association. *Circulation* 99: 178–182.

Manson, J.E., F.B. Hu, J.W. Rich-Edwards, G.A. Colditz, M.J. Stampfer, W.C. Willett, F.E. Speizer, and C.H. Hennekens. 1999. A prospective study of walking as compared with vigorous exercise in the prevention of coronary heart disease in women. *New England Journal of Medicine* 341 (9): 650–658.

Maresca, G., A. Di Blasio, R. Marchioli, and G. Di Minno. 1999. Measuring plasma fibrinogen to predict stroke and myocardial infarction: An update. *Arteriosclerosis, Thrombosis, and Vascular Biology* 19 (6): 1368–1377.

McCully, K.S. 1969. Vascular pathology of homocysteinemia: Implications for the pathogenesis of arteriosclerosis. *American Journal of Pathology* 56: 111–128.

McGinnis, J.M, and W.H. Foege. 1993. Actual causes of death in the United States. *Journal of the American Medical Association* 270: 2207–2212.

McGrew, R.E. 1985. *Encyclopedia of medical history.* New York: McGraw-Hill.

McQuillan, B.M., J.P. Beilby, M. Nidorf, P.L. Thompson, and J. Hung. 1999. Hyperhomocysteinemia but not the C677T mutation of methylenetetrahydrofolate reductase is an independent risk determinant of carotid wall thickening. *Circulation* 99: 2383–2388.

Menotti, A., A. Keys, C. Aravanis, H. Blackburn, A. Dontas, F. Fidanza, M.J. Karvonen, D. Kromhout, S. Nedeljkovic, A. Nissinen, et al. 1989. Seven Countries Study: First 20-year mortality data in 12 cohorts of six countries. *Annals of Medicine* 21 (3): 175–179.

Mensink, G.B., M. Deketh, M.D. Mul, A.J. Schuit, and H. Hoffmeister. 1996. Physical activity and its association with cardiovascular risk factors and mortality. *Epidemiology* 7: 391–397.

Mitrani, Y., H. Karplus, and D. Bunner. 1970. Coronary atherosclerosis in cases of traumatic death. In *Physical activity and aging,* vol. 4 of *Medicine and sport,* edited by D. Bruner and E. Jokl. Baltimore: University Park Press.

Morris, J.N., S.P.W. Chave, C. Adams, C. Sirey, L. Epstein, and D.J. Sheehan. 1973. Vigorous exercise in leisure-time and the incidence of coronary heart disease. *Lancet* 1: 333–339.

Morris, J.N., D.G. Clayton, M.G. Everitt, A.M. Semmence, and E.H. Burgess. 1990. Exercise in leisure time: Coronary attack and death rates. *British Heart Journal* 63: 325–334.

Morris, J.N., and M.D. Crawford. 1958. Coronary heart disease and physical activity of work: Evidence of a national necropsy survey. *British Medical Journal* 2: 1488–1496.

Morris, J.N., M.D. Everitt, R. Pollard, S.P.W. Chave, and A.M. Semmence. 1980. Vigorous exercise in leisure-time: Protection against coronary heart disease. *Lancet* 2: 1207–1210.

Morris, J.N., J.A. Heady, P.A.B. Raffle, C.G. Roberts, and J.W. Parks. 1953. Coronary heart disease and physical activity of work. *Lancet* 2: 1053–1057, 1111–1120.

Mortensen, J.M., T.T. Stevensen, and L.H. Whitney. 1959. Mortality due to coronary heart disease analyzed by broad occupational groups. *Archives of Industrial Health* 19: 1–4.

Multiple Risk Factor Intervention Trial Research Group. 1982. Multiple Risk Factor Intervention Trial: Risk factor changes and mortality results. *Journal of the American Medical Association* 248: 1465.

Myers, J., M. Prakash, V. Froelicher, D. Do, S. Partington, and J.E. Atwood. 2002. Exercise capacity and mortality among men referred for exercise testing. *New England Journal of Medicine* 346 (11): 793–801.

National Heart, Lung, and Blood Institute. 1998. *Morbidity and mortality: 1998 chartbook on cardiovascular, lung, and blood diseases.* Rockville, MD: U.S. Department of Health and Human Services, National Institutes of Health.

Ng-Mak, D.S., B.P. Dohrenwend, A.F. Abraido-Lanza, and J.B. Turner. 1999. A further analysis of race differences in the National Longitudinal Mortality Study. *American Journal of Public Health* 89: 1748–1751.

O'Connor, G.T., J.E. Buring, S. Yusuf, S.Z. Goldhaber, E.M. Olmstead, R.S. Paffenbarger Jr., and C.H. Hennekens. 1989. An overview of randomized trials of rehabilitation with exercise after myocardial infarction. *Circulation* 80 (2): 234–244.

Paffenbarger, R.S. Jr., and W.E. Hale. 1975. Work activity and coronary heart disease mortality. *New England Journal of Medicine* 292: 545–550.

Paffenbarger, R.S. Jr., W.W. Hale, R.J. Brand, and R.T. Hyde. 1977. Work-energy level, personal characteristics, and fatal heart attack: A birth cohort effect. *American Journal of Epidemiology* 105: 200–213.

Paffenbarger, R.S. Jr., R.T. Hyde, A.L. Wing, and C.C. Hsieh. 1986. Physical activity, all-cause mortality, and longevity of college alumni. *New England Journal of Medicine* 314: 605–613.

Paffenbarger, R.S. Jr., R.T. Hyde, A.L. Wing, I.M. Lee, D.L. Jung, and J.B. Kampert. 1993. The association of changes in physical-activity level and other lifestyle characteristics with mortality among men. *New England Journal of Medicine* 328: 538–545.

Paffenbarger, R.S. Jr., A. Wing, and R. Hyde. 1978. Physical activity as an index of heart attack risk in college alumni. *American Journal of Epidemiology* 108: 168–175.

———. 1981. Chronic disease in former college students: XVI. Physical activity as an index of heart attack risk in college alumni. *American Journal of Epidemiology* 108: 161–175.

Paul, O.M., M.H. Lepper, W.H. Phelan, G.W. Dupertuis, and G.W. Macmillan. 1963. A longitudinal study of coronary heart disease. *Circulation* 28: 20–31.

Perls, T.T., and R.C. Fretts. 1998. Why women live longer than men. *Scientific American,* June.

———. 2001. The evolution of menopause and human lifespan. *Annals of Human Biology* 28: 237–245.

Peters, R.K.L., L.D. Cady Jr., D.P. Bischoff, L. Berstein, and M.C. Pike. 1983. Physical fitness and subsequent myocardial infarction in healthy workers. *Journal of the American Medical Association* 249: 3052–3056.

Physical activity and cardiovascular health: NIH consensus Development Panel on Physical Activity and Cardiovascular Health. 1996. *Journal of the American Medical Association* 276: 241–246.

Pomrehn, P.R., R.B. Wallace, and L.F. Burmeister. 1982. Ischemic heart disease mortality in Iowa farmers. The influence of life-style. *Journal of the American Medical Association* 248: 1073–1076.

Ponjee, G.A., E.M. Janssen, J. Hermans, and J.W. van Wersch. 1996. Regular physical activity and changes in risk factors for coronary heart disease: A nine month prospective study. *European Journal of Clinical Chemistry and Clinical Biochemistry* 34: 477–483.

Powell, K.E., and S.N. Blair. 1994. The public health burdens of sedentary living habits: Theoretical but realistic estimates. *Medicine and Science in Sports and Exercise* 26: 851–856.

Powell, K.E., P.D. Thompson, C.J. Caspersen, and J.S. Kendrick. 1987. Physical activity and the incidence of coronary heart disease. *Annual Review of Public Health* 8: 253–287.

Punsar, S., and M. Karvonen. 1976. Physical activity and coronary disease in population from east and west Finland. *Advances in Cardiology* 18: 196–207.

Rifai, N., and P.M. Ridker. 2002. Inflammatory markers and coronary heart disease. *Current Opinion in Lipidemiology* 13 (4): 383–389.

Rissanen, V. 1976. Occupational physical activity and coronary artery disease: A clinicopathologic appraisal. *Advances in Cardiology* 18: 113–121.

Rose, G. 1969. Physical activity and coronary heart disease. *Proceedings of the Royal Society of Medicine* 62: 1183–1188.

Rosenman, R.H., R.J. Brand, C.D. Jenkins, M. Friedman, R. Straus, and M. Wurm. 1975. Coronary heart disease in Western Collaborative Group Study: Final follow-up experience of 8 1/2 years. *Journal of the American Medical Association* 23: 871–877.

Rosenman, R.H., M. Friedman, R. Straus, C.D. Jenkins, S.J. Zyzanski, and M. Wurm. 1970. Coronary heart disease in the Western Collaborative Group Study: A follow-up experience of 4 1/2 years. *Journal of Chronic Diseases* 28: 178–190.

Rosenman, R.H., M. Friedman, R. Straus, C.D. Jenkins, S.J. Zyzanski, and M. Wurm. 1970. Coronary heart disease in the Western Collaborative Group Study: A follow-up experience of 4 1/2 years. *Journal of Chronic Diseases* 28: 178–190.

Ross, R., and J.A. Glomset. 1976. The pathogenesis of arteriosclerosis. *New England Journal of Medicine* 295: 369, 420.

Sandvik, L., J. Erikssen, E. Thaulow, G. Erikssen, R. Mundal, and K. Rodahl. 1993. Physical fitness as a predictor of mortality among healthy, middle-aged Norwegian men. *New England Journal of Medicine* 328 (8): 533–537.

Scarabin, P.Y., M.F. Aillaud, P. Amouyel, A. Evans, G. Luc, J. Ferrieres, D. Arveiler, and I. Juhan-Vague. 1998. Associations of fibrinogen, factor VII and PAI-1 with baseline findings among 10,500 male participants in a prospective study of myocardial infarction: The PRIME Study. *Thrombosis and Haemostasis* 80 (5): 749–756.

Sesso, H.D., R.S. Paffenbarger, T. Ha, and I.M. Lee. 1999. Physical activity and cardiovascular disease risk in middle-aged and older women. *American Journal of Epidemiology* 150 (4): 408–416.

Sesso, H.D, R.S. Paffenbarger Jr., and I.M. Lee. 2000. Physical activity and coronary heart disease in men: The Harvard Alumni Health Study. *Circulation* 102: 975–980.

Shapiro, S., E. Weinblatt, C.W. Frank, and R.V. Sager. 1969. Incidence of coronary heart disease in a population insured for medical care (HIP): Myocardial infarction, angina pectoris, and possible myocardial infarction. *American Journal of Public Health* 59 (Suppl. 2): 1–101.

Siscovick, D.S., N.S. Weiss, A.P. Hallstrom, T.S. Inui, and D.R. Peterson. 1982. Physical activity and primary cardiac arrest. *Journal of the American Medical Association* 248: 3113–3117.

Slattery, M.L., and D.R. Jacobs Jr. 1988. Physical fitness and cardiovascular disease mortality: The U.S. Railroad Study. *American Journal of Epidemiology* 127: 571–580.

Spain, D.M., and V.A. Bradess. 1957. Sudden death from coronary atherosclerosis: Age, race, sex, physical activity, and alcohol. *Archives of Internal Medicine* 100: 228–231.

———. 1960. Occupational physical activity and the degree of coronary atherosclerosis in "normal" men: A postmortem study. *Circulation* 22: 239–242.

Stamler, J.D., D.M. Berkson, H.A. Lindberg, et al. 1970. Long term epidemiologic studies on the possible role of physical activity and physical fitness in the prevention of premature clinical coronary heart disease. In *Physical activity and aging,* vol. 4 of *Medicine and sports,* edited by D. Brunner and E. Jokl. Baltimore: University Park Press.

Stamler, J., H.A. Lindberg, D.M. Berkson, A. Shaffer, W. Miller, and A. Poindexter. 1960. Prevalence and incidence of coronary heart disease in strata of the labor force of a Chicago industrial corporation. *Journal of Chronic Diseases* 11: 405–420.

Stratton, J.R., W.L. Chandler, R.S. Schwartz, M.D. Cerqueira, W.C. Levy, S.E. Kahn, V.G. Larson, K.C. Cain, J.C. Beard, and I.B. Abrass. 1991. Effects of physical conditioning on fibrinolytic variables and fibrinogen in young and old healthy adults. *Circulation* 83: 1692–1697.

Szymanski, L.M., R.R. Pate, and J.L. Durstine. 1994. Effects of maximal exercise and venous occlusion on fibrinolytic activity in physically active and inactive men. *Journal of Applied Physiology* 77: 2305–2310.

Tanasescu, M., M.F. Leitzmann, E.B. Rimm, W.C. Willett, M.J. Stampfer, and F.B. Hu. 2002. Exercise type and intensity in relation to coronary heart disease in men. *Journal of the American Medical Association* 288: 1994–2000.

Taylor, H.B., H. Blackburn, A. Keys, R.W. Parlin, C. Vasquez, and T. Puchner. 1970. Five-year follow-up of employees of selected U.S. railroad companies. *Circulation* 41 (Suppl. 1): 120–139.

Taylor, H.L., E. Klepetar, A. Keys, R.W. Parlin, and H. Blackburn. 1962. Death rates among physically active and sedentary employees of the railroad industry. *American Journal of Public Health* 52: 1697–1707.

Taylor, H.L., A. Mellotti, and V. Puddu. 1970. Five year follow-up of railroad men in Italy. *Circulation* 41 (Suppl.): 111–122.

Tunstall-Pedoe, H., K. Kuulasmaa, M. Mahonen, H. Tolonen, E. Ruokokoski, and P. Amouyel. 1999. Contribution of trends in survival and coronary-event rates to changes in coronary heart disease mortality: 10-year results from 37 WHO MONICA project populations. Monitoring trends and determinants in cardiovascular disease. *Lancet* 353 (9164): 1547–1557.

U.S. Department of Health and Human Services. 1996. *Physical activity and health: A report of the surgeon general.* Atlanta: U.S. Department of Health and Human Services, Centers for Disease Control and Prevention, National Center for Chronic Disease Prevention and Health Promotion.

Wang, J.S., C.J. Jen, and H.I. Chen. 1995. Effects of exercise training and deconditioning on platelet function in men. *Arteriosclerosis, Thrombosis, and Vascular Biology* 15: 1668–1674.

Wannamethee, S.G., G.D. Lowe, P.H. Whincup, A. Rumley, M. Walker, and L. Lennon. 2002. Physical activity and hemostatic and inflammatory variables in elderly men. *Circulation* 105 (15): 1785–1790.

Wei, M., J.B. Kampert, C.E. Barlow, M.Z. Nichaman, L.W. Gibbons, R.S. Paffenbarger Jr., and S.N. Blair. 1999. Relationship between low cardiorespiratory fitness and mortality in normal-weight, overweight, and obese men. *Journal of the American Medical Association* 282: 1547–1553.

Williams, P.T., P.D. Wood, W.L. Haskell, and K. Vranizan. 1982. The effects of running mileage and duration on plasma lipoprotein levels. *Journal of the American Medical Association* 247: 2674–2679.

Willius, F.A., and T.E. Keys, eds. 1961. *Classics of cardiology : A collection of classic works on the heart and circulation with comprehensive biographic accounts of the authors : fifty-two contributions by fifty-one authors.* New York: Henry Schuman.

World Health Organization. 2003. *The World Health Report 2002: Reducing risks, promoting healthy life.* Geneva, Switzerland.

Zukel, W.J., R.H. Lewis, P.E. Enterline, R.C. Painter, and L.S. Ralston. 1959. A short-term community study of the epidemiology of coronary heart disease. *American Journal of Public Health* 49: 1630–1639.

Web Site

http://consensus.nih.gov. This site provides access to the NIH Consensus Development Program of the U.S. National Institutes of Health.

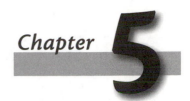

Chapter **5**

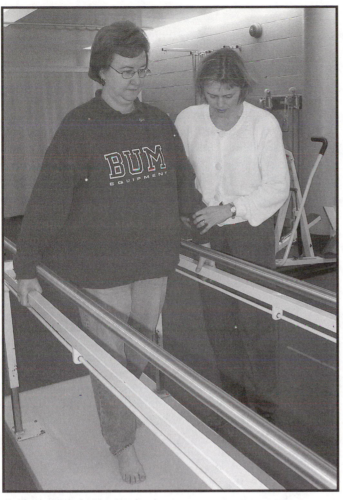

© John T. Fowler

Cerebrovascular Disease and Stroke

Apoplexy is a stroke of God's hands.
—Oxford English Dictionary, 1599

A stroke is the loss or impairment of bodily function resulting from injury or death of brain cells after insufficient blood supply. Hippocrates is credited with first describing stroke and its crippling effects. He used the Greek term *apolessein,* which means to be thunderstruck, because the disease was seen as a catastrophic, uncontrollable event of nature. Before the Renaissance of medicine in the 16th century, the *Oxford English Dictionary* defined apoplexy (from *apoplexia,* the Latin derivation of apolessein) as "a stroke of God's hands," hence the modern usage of the term *stroke* to denote a cerebrovascular accident.

> ••• *A stroke is the loss or impairment of bodily function resulting from injury or death of brain cells after insufficient blood supply.*

113

> ### Five Common Signs of Stroke
>
> - Sudden numbness or weakness of the face, arm, or leg, especially on one side of the body
> - Sudden confusion and trouble speaking or understanding
> - Sudden trouble seeing in one or both eyes
> - Sudden trouble walking, dizziness, or loss of balance or coordination
> - Sudden, severe headache with no known cause
>
> American Heart Association 2002.

See "Five Common Signs of Stroke" for warning signs. Not all of the common signs occur during a stroke. When they occur but last only a short while (e.g., a few minutes), they may indicate what is known as a **transient ischemic attack (TIA).** A TIA is not a stroke, but it can be a **prodromal** (i.e., early) **symptom;** TIAs precede about 10% of strokes and are a major risk factor for stroke. About a third of people who have had one or more TIAs subsequently have a stroke within five years. That rate is nearly 10 times greater than the rate of stroke among people of the same age and sex who have not had a TIA (American Heart Association 2002; Goldstein et al. 2001; Helgason and Wolf 1997; Mohr et al. 1997).

> ••• **When signs of a stroke occur but last only a short while (e.g., a few minutes), they may indicate a transient ischemic attack.**

Stroke is the common endpoint for cerebrovascular disease and is characterized by abrupt onset of persisting neurological symptoms that arise from injury or death of brain cells. About 75% to 80% of strokes are classified as primary ischemic or thromboembolic strokes. They result from thrombosis (clotting in a vessel) or **stenosis** (narrowing of the artery), which together account for about 70% of all strokes, or from **embolism** (occlusion of a vessel by a circulating clot or atheroma), which accounts for another 5% to 10% of strokes. The other 15% to 20% of all strokes result from bleeding in the brain and are classified as primary hemorrhagic strokes (Kelley 1998). About 5% to 10% of strokes are subarach-noid hemorrhages, which occur when a vessel on the brain's surface ruptures and bleeds into the space between the brain and the cranium. Another 10% of strokes are intracerebral hemorrhages. Both ischemic and hemorrhagic types of stroke can lead to death or permanent brain damage, but people often recover lost brain function after a mild stroke.

> ••• **From 75% to 80% of strokes result from thrombosis (clotting in a vessel), stenosis (narrowing of the artery), or embolism (e.g., occlusion of a vessel by a circulating clot or atheroma). Other cases result from bleeding in the brain.**

Magnitude of the Problem

Cerebrovascular disease kills about 4.4 million people each year worldwide, second only to coronary heart disease, which causes 6.3 million deaths (Murray and Lopez 1997). In the United States 600,000 people had strokes in 1999; 160,000 people died (American Heart Association 2002). In 1990, the worldwide incidence of first-ever stroke was higher for females (120 per 100,000) than males (110 per 100,000), and this difference between women and men was higher in developed countries, including the United States: 172 per 100,000 for females and 149 per 100,000 for males (Murray and Lopez 1997). The average age at onset also was higher for both women (72 years) and men (68 years) in developed nations than the worldwide averages for women (66 years) and men (63 years). Mortality rates from first-ever stroke worldwide are about 76 per 100,000 in males and 90 per 100,000 in females. In developed nations, those rates are about 82 per 100,000 for males and 115 per 100,000 for females.

> ••• **About a third of people who've had one or more transient ischemic attacks subsequently have a stroke within five years.**

According to the National Heart, Lung, and Blood Institute, stroke has been the third leading cause of death in the United States since 1938, following coronary heart disease and cancer. Similar to the reduction in heart attack deaths, the death rate from stroke in the United States has dropped sharply since 1950, from 89 per 100,000 to a current rate of approximately 27 per 100,000.

In addition to its contribution to total mortality, stroke is also the leading cause of adult disability in the United States. According to the National Institute of Neurological and Communicative Disorders and Stroke, nearly two thirds of the 4.5 million U.S. stroke survivors alive in 2002 were disabled in some way. Disabilities include the loss of control over bodily functions; gait problems; impaired vision, speech, or comprehension; depression; memory loss; and paralysis. The effects of stroke also place a significant burden on the survivor's family, friends, and caregivers. The annual economic burden of stroke is about $30 billion to $40 billion each year (American Heart Association 2002).

*** *According to the National Heart, Lung, and Blood Institute, stroke has been the third leading cause of death in the United States since 1938, following coronary heart disease and cancer.*

Risk Factors for Stroke

Primary risk factors for stroke, in addition to TIA, include age over 55 years, female sex, cigarette smoking, alcohol abuse, hypertension, diabetes, coronary heart disease, and **cardiac arrhythmias** (e.g., atrial fibrillation) (Sacco, Wolf, and Gorelick 1999). In the WHO MONICA project, 12,224 strokes occurred in 18 populations in 11 countries during a three-year period in men and women ages 35 to 64. Smoking and high blood pressure accounted for 21% of stroke incidence in men and 42% in women (Stegmayr et al. 1997).

Obesity, hypercholesterolemia, and physical inactivity are considered secondary contributing risk factors to stroke (Goldstein et al. 2001). The primary risk factors, discussed in the preceding paragraph, have been clearly implicated in the pathogenesis of atherosclerosis. The secondary risk factors are equally important but are not as directly linked to the development of atherosclerosis. The risk of recurrent stroke during the first year after an ischemic stroke is about 10%, which increases to about 50% after five years (Sacco et al. 1982). Most of the major risk factors for first stroke, with the exception of age, race, and sex, are either correctable or modifiable in all age groups by hygienic behaviors or medical

Selected Risk Factors for Stroke

- *Age.* Stroke risk doubles each decade after age 55. Two thirds of strokes occur in people older than 65 years.

- *Sex.* Women have slightly higher stroke risk and are more likely to die from a stroke than men, but men die sooner than women from other causes, so there are more female (2.3 million) than male (2.2 million) stroke survivors in the United States.

- *Race.* Blacks have twice the risk of stroke of other Americans, possibly because they have more of the other key risk factors.

- *Atrial fibrillation.* Irregular contraction of the heart's atria causes an irregular heartbeat, which can lead to pooling of blood in the heart and contribute to clot formation and ischemic stroke.

- *Coronary heart disease.* Atherosclerosis underlies both coronary artery disease and carotid artery disease and is thus a main cause of ischemic stroke. Hence, people with coronary heart disease are at increased risk of stroke.

treatment. Figure 5.1 depicts the relative risk associated with the major uncontrollable and medical risk factors for stroke. The following section describes the association between the modifiable risk factors (hypertension, smoking, alcohol abuse, hypercholesterolemia, diabetes, and obesity) and stroke risk in more detail.

Hypertension

Hypertension is the primary risk factor for the development of stroke (Kannel et al. 1970), and stroke is a common consequence for people with hypertension. In the Framingham Heart Study, men with hypertension (over 160/95 mmHg) were about four times more likely to suffer a stroke than those who were normotensive (Kannel 1999; Kannel et al. 1970). In the Nurses' Health Study, the relative risk for stroke in women with hypertension was 4.2 compared with their normotensive counterparts (Fiebach et al. 1989). The elevated risk of stroke in these women occurred at all levels of BMI. Hence, hypertension appears to be an independent risk factor for stroke in middle-aged women. Even among young adults,

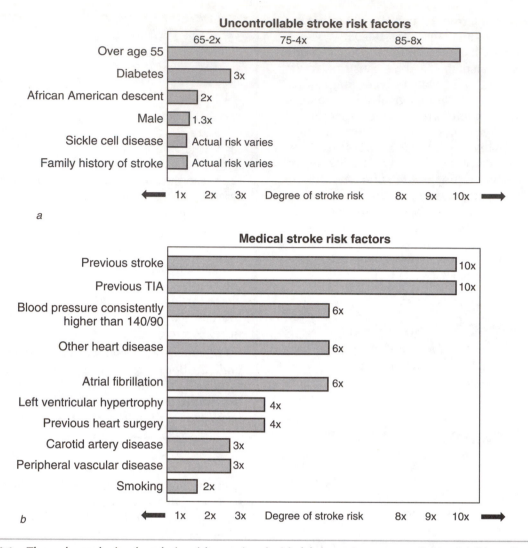

Figure 5.1   These charts depict the relative risk associated with (a) the major uncontrollable and (b) medical risk factors for stroke.

Adapted with permission of National Stroke Association, 2000. Available: www.stroke.org.

the odds ratio of stroke was five times higher among those with hypertension (You et al. 1997). Effective control of hypertension appears to reduce the risk of stroke by about 40%.

Smoking

The risk of stroke is greater in persons who smoke, increases with the number of cigarettes smoked, and is lower among those who have given up smoking compared with current smokers. Mechanisms linking the components of tobacco smoke with arterial damage and the subsequent development of atherosclerosis have been identified. The Framingham Heart Study, for example, found about a 60% increase in the relative risk for stroke

in female smokers compared with nonsmokers, independent of several other risk factors (Wolf et al. 1988). In eastern Finland, a decline in the prevalence of hypertension and smoking accounted for about 29% of the subsequent decline in stroke incidence during an eight-year follow-up of two population cohorts of men and women ages 30 to 59 years (Tuomilehto et al. 1991).

Alcohol Abuse

Alcohol consumption has been shown to both increase and decrease the risk for stroke. A prospective study of female nurses in the United States showed that among middle-aged women, moderate alcohol consumption decreased the risk of ischemic stroke (Stampfer et al. 1988). However, a report on the Honolulu Heart Program cohort showed that even light drinking in men significantly increased the risk of hemorrhagic stroke (Donahue et al. 1986). Despite the mixed evidence, it is generally accepted that moderate alcohol consumption may reduce the risk of thrombosis associated with atherosclerosis and ischemic stroke. If that effect is explainable by anticoagulability of blood, it paradoxically could pose a risk for hemorrhagic stroke because of a blood-thinning effect. This hypothesis would be consistent with the effects of drugs that inhibit platelet aggregation (e.g., aspirin) and can reduce recurrent cerebrovascular accidents among people with CVD (Algra and van Gijn 1996; Antiplatelet Trialists' Collaboration 1994). However, aspirin is not recommended for the primary prevention of stroke because 325 to 500 mg daily has an unclear effect on reducing ischemic stroke and can double the risk of hemorrhagic stroke (Peto et al. 1988; Steering Committee of the Physicians' Health Study Research Group 1989).

Hypercholesterolemia

Elevated blood cholesterol has been associated only moderately with an increased risk for stroke. However, clinical trials have shown that statin drugs used to lower cholesterol have reduced the thickening of the carotid artery wall (Hodis et al. 1996) and reduced the frequency of strokes by about 30% (Cholesterol and Recurrent Events Trial Investigators 1996).

Obesity and Diabetes Mellitus

Overweight, as measured by BMI, is also an independent risk factor for stroke in both men and women (Lindenstrom, Boysen, and Nyboe 1993a, 1993b). Data from the Third National Health and Nutrition Examination Survey (NHANES III) and the Framingham Heart Study indicate that the lifetime risk of stroke is elevated among middle-aged men and women who are obese (i.e., BMI > 30; Thompson et al. 1999). Among young adults, the odds ratio of stroke is nearly 12 times higher among those with diabetes (You et al. 1997), possibly explainable by microvascular disease.

*** *Among young adults, the odds ratio of stroke is nearly 12 times higher among those with diabetes.*

Etiology of Stroke

Much of the pathophysiology of stroke involves atherosclerotic disease and hemostatic dysfunction similar to that of coronary heart disease, discussed in chapter 4. The physiological mechanisms of stroke are classified as embolic, lacunar (i.e., brain cavities resulting from decreased perfusion in small, deep vessels), or thrombotic depending on the presence of risk factors for stroke and preexisting medical conditions (Mohr et al. 1997).

Embolic Stroke

Precipitating factors for embolic stroke include atrial fibrillation, sinoatrial disorder, recent myocardial infarction, bacterial endocarditis (inflammation of the heart), cardiac tumors, and valve disorders. Stroke occurs within weeks after about 2% of heart attacks, mainly from circulating clots from the wall of the left ventricle or from an atherosclerotic blood vessel. Medical risk factors for left ventricular thrombosis are large infarctions, dilation of the left ventricle (usually from congestive heart failure), and atrial fibrillation. Atherosclerotic plaques in the aortic arch are a main source of atherothrombosis (Vahedi and Amarenco 2000).

Lacunar: Reduced Perfusion

Stroke that results from reduced perfusion occurs with severe stenosis (greater than 70% narrowing) of the carotid and basilar arteries and with stenosis of small arteries deep in the brain. Inflammation from infections can also cause arterial stenosis. Strokes are commonly reported in patients with bacterial or tuberculous meningitis, cerebral cysticercosis (a cyst formed by tapeworm larvae), fungal infection, and herpes zoster (i.e., shingles). Lacunar infarcts result mainly from blockage of small arteries deep in the brain by small atherosclerotic plaques, cholesterol embolism, clots resulting from rheumatic heart disease or endocarditis, and arteriosclerosis of the cerebral arteries.

Thrombotic Stroke

Precipitating conditions for thrombotic stroke involve mainly abnormal regulation of hemostatic factors, such as anticlotting proteins, and of the fibrinolytic system that can occur at any age (see chapter 4). Genetic defects in regulatory hemostatic proteins are common in people who have vessel clots in their 20s or 30s. However, a causal link between hemostatic disease and stroke has not yet been established.

Physical Activity and Stroke Risk: The Evidence

A lack of physical activity appears to be associated with increased risk for stroke; however, the evidence for the association between inactivity and stroke is not entirely clear. This uncertainty was expressed in the conclusions of the U.S. Surgeon General's report on physical activity and health (U.S. Department of Health and Human Services 1996). A recent review of 15 major studies corroborated the conclusions of that report (Kohl 2001). Only four of these studies focused on women. Thirteen were prospective cohort studies with observation periods ranging from 5 to 26 years. About half the studies showed a statistically significant reduction in the rate of stroke or stroke death among active compared with less-active people after controlling for confounders. Only six studies showed evidence of a linear dose–response reduction in risk with increasing physical activity. Table 5.1 summarizes key prospective cohort studies that examined the effect of leisure-time physical activity on stroke risk.

TABLE 5.1 KEY PROSPECTIVE COHORT STUDIES OF PHYSICAL ACTIVITY AND STROKE RISK

Study	Cohort	Years of observation	Results
Kannel and Sorlie 1979	1,909 Framingham men 35–64 years old	14	Lower stroke risk, but not after adjustment for confounders
Paffenbarger et al. 1984	16,936 Harvard alumni 34–68 years old	About 16	Linear reduction in stroke death after adjusting for age, smoking, and hypertension
Harmsen et al. 1990	7,495 Swedish men 47–55 years old	About 12	No association with stroke death
Lindsted et al. 1991	9,484 men ≥ 30 years old	26	No association with stroke death
Wannamethee and Shaper 1992	7,735 British men 40–59 years old	8.5	Linear reduction in stroke and stroke death after adjusting for coronary heart disease
Abbott et al. 1994	7,530 Hawaiian and Japanese men 45–68 years old	22	No association in men 45–54 years old; linear reduction in stroke for men 55–68 years old
Kiely et al. 1994	4 Framingham cohorts of men and women 35–69 years old and 49–83 years old	18–32	No association in men or women 35–69 years old after adjusting for confounders; linear reduction in stroke and stroke death in men 49–83 years old
Rosengren and Wilhelmsen 1997	7,142 men 47–55 years old	20	No association with stroke death after adjusting for confounders
Bijnen et al. 1998	802 Dutch men 64–84 years old	10	No association with stroke death after adjusting for age, smoking, and alcohol use
Lee and Paffenbarger 1998	11,130 Harvard alumni, mean age 58 years	13	No association with stroke or stroke death after adjusting for confounders
Evenson et al. 1999	Multiracial sample of 8,296 women and 6,279 men 45–64 years old	7	No association with stroke or stroke death after adjusting for confounders
Hu et al. 2000	72,488 female nurses 40–55 years old	8	Linear reduction in ischemic stroke after adjusting for confounders; increased activity reduced risk by 29%. No association with hemorrhagic stroke.

Modified from Kohl 2001.

> ••• *A lack of physical activity appears to be associated with increased risk for stroke; however, the evidence for the association is not entirely clear.*

Case–Control Studies

The following sections describe two case–control studies that have assessed the association between physical activity and stroke. The evidence of a cause-and-effect association is also evaluated.

Birmingham, England

In one case–control study, 125 men and women ages 35 to 74 who had suffered a first stroke and 198 controls matched by age and sex were recruited over a two-year period from 11 general medical practices in west Birmingham, England (Shinton and Sagar 1993). The patients and controls were divided into groups by whether they reported engaging or not engaging in regular vigorous exercise (e.g., digging, running, swimming, cycling, tennis, squash, and keeping fit) during youth (ages 15 to 25), early middle age (ages 25 to 40), and late middle age (aged 40 to 55). When disability after the stroke prevented a response, the closest relative or friend of the subject was interviewed. Figure 5.2 shows that a history of vigorous exercise during ages 15 to 25 (odds ratio adjusted for age and sex: 0.33, 95% confidence interval [CI]: 0.20–0.60) and increasing years of participation in vigorous exercise between the ages of 15 and 55 was associated with

an increasing reduction in the rate of stroke. This effect was independent of potential risk factors, including race, social class, peak BMI, subscapular skinfold thickness, cigarette smoking, alcohol consumption, dietary intake of saturated fat, family history of stroke, and histories of hypertension, diabetes mellitus, and cardiac ischemia. Among the 65 cases and 169 controls who were free of cardiac ischemia, peripheral vascular disease, and poor health, recent vigorous exercise and walking protected against stroke: the odds ratios were 0.41 (95% CI: 0.20–1.0) for recent vigorous exercise and 0.30 (0.10–0.70) for recent walking. The study suggested a dose–response relationship between more years of participation in vigorous exercise and decreased risk of stroke that was independent of other risk factors and consistent between sexes.

Northern Manhattan Stroke Study

The Northern Manhattan Stroke Study was a case–control study designed to investigate the association between leisure-time physical activity and ischemic stroke in an urban, multiethnic population (Sacco et al. 1998). Case subjects had experienced a first ischemic stroke, and for every case, two control subjects matched by age, sex, and race were recruited through random-digit dialing. Physical activity was assessed through a standardized in-person interview regarding the frequency and duration of 14 separate activities during the two weeks prior to the interview. Over a 30-month period, 369 case and 678 control subjects were enrolled. Their mean age was 70 years; 57% were women, 18% white, 30% black, and 52% Hispanic.

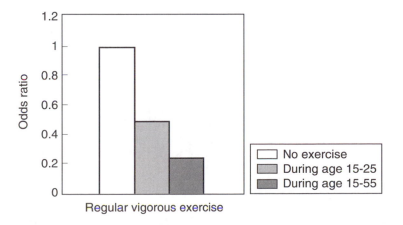

Figure 5.2 Physical activity and recurrent stroke in Birmingham, England. The numbers are adjusted for race, social class, peak BMI, skinfold thickness, smoking, alcohol consumption, dietary saturated fat, family history of stroke, and histories of hypertension, diabetes mellitus, and cardiac ischemia.

Adapted from Shinton and Sagar 1993.

Results indicated that leisure-time physical activity is associated with a significantly reduced risk of stroke after adjustment for cardiac disease, peripheral vascular disease, hypertension, diabetes, smoking, alcohol use, obesity, medical reasons for limited activity, education, and season of enrollment. The protective effects of physical activity were observed in both younger and older groups, in men and women, and in whites, blacks, and Hispanics. Figure 5.3 shows a dose response for both intensity and duration of physical activity, regardless of age, sex, or ethnicity. Light- to moderate-intensity activities had an odds ratio of 0.39 (95% CI: 0.26–0.58), and heavy activity had an odds ratio of 0.23 (0.10–0.54). Duration of less than 2 h per week had an odds ratio of 0.42 (0.14–0.70), less than 5 h per week 0.35 (0.25–0.45), and more than 5 h per week 0.31 (0.25–0.59). Hence, there was a small linear gradient of decreased risk with increasing time spent in activity each week.

Prospective Studies

The following sections describe some of the major prospective cohort studies that have assessed the association between physical activity and stroke.

Finnish Cohort

Beginning in 1972, Salonen, Puska, and Tuomilehto (1982) followed a randomly selected population sample from eastern Finland for seven years. Physical activity at work and during leisure time were recorded for 3,978 men and 3,688 women.

During the seven-year follow-up, 71 men and 56 women had a stroke. After controlling for age, total serum cholesterol, diastolic blood pressure, height, weight, and smoking, low physical activity at work was associated with a relative risk for stroke of 1.6 in men and 1.7 in women. The study showed an appropriate temporal sequence, independence of several confounders, and a moderately strong association between reduced occupational physical activity and increased stroke risk that was consistent between sexes.

Harvard Alumni Health Study

In the Harvard alumni cohort, the incidence of stroke was inversely related to self-reported weekly energy expenditure (figure 5.4; Paffenbarger et al. 1984). The stroke incidence rate for subjects expending less than 500 kcal each week was 6.5 per 10,000 person-years of observation, for those expending 500 to 1,999 kcal each week it was 5.2, and for those expending more than 2,000 kcal each week it was 2.4.

British Men

Physical activity levels were measured among 7,630 British men ages 40 to 59, sampled randomly from general medical practices in 24 towns in England, Wales, and Scotland (Wannamethee and Shaper 1992). During a 9.5-year follow-up, 128 men suffered a major stroke. After statistical adjustment for age, social class, smoking, alcohol consumption, BMI, systolic blood pressure, and prevalence of ischemic heart disease or prior strokes, men who engaged in moderate activity and vigorous activity had 30% and 60% lower

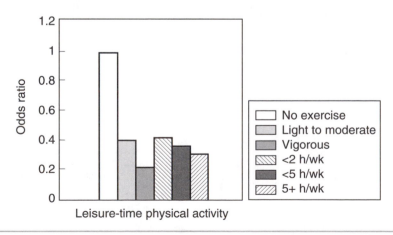

Figure 5.3 Physical activity and ischemic stroke in the Northern Manhattan Stroke Study includes 369 cases of first stroke, 678 controls, mean age of 70 years, 57% women, 52% Hispanic, 30% black, 18% white, and matched on age, sex, and race.

Adapted from Sacco et al. 1998.

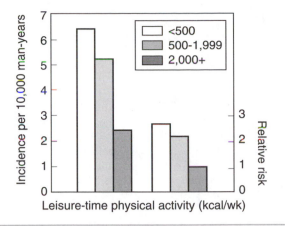

Figure 5.4   Physical activity and stroke in the Harvard Alumni Study cohort includes rates and relative risks of first stroke for more than 10,000 men who entered college in 1916–1950. Follow-ups were done in the 1960s and 1978. Study was independent of blood pressure, age, smoking, body weight, and family history of CVD.

Adapted from Paffenbarger et al. 1984.

rates of stroke, respectively, compared with inactive men. The continued reduction in relative risk with increasing intensity of physical activity indicated a dose–response relationship.

Framingham Cohort

In a follow-up of the Framingham cohort, men and women were categorized into tertiles according to physical activity level (Kiely et al. 1994). Participants reporting medium or high levels of physical activity were compared with those reporting low levels of physical activity. The association between physical activity and the rate of stroke was analyzed twice over a 32-year follow-up period: first at 50 years of age among 1,897 men and 2,299 women, and again when the remaining 1,361 men and 1,862 women were 63 to 64 years old. Among the men, physical activity (independent of age, systolic blood pressure, serum cholesterol, number of cigarettes smoked per day, glucose intolerance, total vital capacity, BMI, left ventricular hypertrophy, atrial fibrillation, vascular disease, history of congestive heart failure, history of ischemic heart disease, and occupation) was associated with a reduced risk for stroke. The lowest relative risk, 0.40 (95% CI: 0.24–0.69), was found among older men in the medium activity tertile. The highest level of physical activity did not confer an additional reduction in risk beyond that of the medium level. Physical activity level was not associated with a reduced risk of stroke among women in this cohort.

Honolulu Heart Study

The Honolulu Heart Study classified 7,530 Hawaiian men of Japanese descent 45 to 68 years old as inactive, partially active, or active based on self-reports of 24-h physical activity at the time of study enrollment (Abbott et al. 1994). Risk of stroke during 22 years of follow-up was examined separately in younger (45 to 54 years) and older (55 to 68 years) men. Among the older men, the inactive men had a relative risk of 3.7 (95% CI: 1.3–10.4) for hemorrhagic stroke compared with active men; this risk was independent of hypertension, diabetes mellitus, and left ventricular hypertrophy. In older men who did not smoke cigarettes, the relative risk of thromboembolic stroke among inactive men was 2.8 compared with active men. The relative risk of partially active older men was 2.4 (95% CI: 1.0–5.7) compared with those who were active. Hence, an independent dose–response relationship was observed between increasing physical activity levels and decreasing risk for thromboembolic stroke. No associations were found between risk of stroke and either physical activity level or smoking in men ages 45 to 54, for whom the prevalence of stroke is low compared with older men.

NHANES I Cohort

As part of the NHANES I epidemiologic follow-up study, 5,081 whites and 771 blacks 45 to 74 years of age who initially had no history of stroke were reassessed twice during a 12-year follow-up after initial measurements taken from 1971 to 1975 (Gillum, Mussolino, and Ingram 1996). Participants rated their levels of habitual physical activity, both recreational and nonrecreational, as low, moderate, or high. They were also categorized based on resting pulse rate. There were 249 cases of stroke among the white women, 270 among the white men, and 104 among the black men and women combined. The incidence of stroke was highest among those who were least active, regardless of sex or race. In addition, among white women ages 65 to 74, low nonrecreational physical activity was independently associated with an increased risk of stroke (RR = 1.82, 95% CI: 1.10–3.02) after adjusting for age, smoking, history of diabetes, history of heart disease, education, systolic blood pressure, total serum cholesterol, BMI, and hemoglobin concentration. Similar associations between low recreational physical activity and increased risk of stroke were seen for white men and for black men and women. A dose–response relationship between activity level and reduced stroke incidence was observed among white women. Similarly, a linear relationship was found between resting pulse rate and increased risk of stroke in blacks but not in whites. The study provided evidence for a consistent reduction in risk of stroke among middle-aged and older adults regardless of sex, age, and race.

Atherosclerosis Risk in Communities Study

More recently, ischemic stroke incidence in more than 14,000 adults ages 45 to 64 years without history of stroke or CHD at study outset was observed for about seven years (Evenson et al. 1999). The risk ratios were about 0.80 to 0.90 (95% CI: 0.6–1.26) in the highest quartile of sport and leisure physical activity compared with the lowest quartile, after adjustment for age, sex, race, smoking, and education. These nonsignificant and modest reductions in risk were further diluted after adjustment for hypertension, diabetes, fibrinogen levels, and BMI, suggesting that the influence of physical activity on the risk of ischemic stroke is not direct but may operate indirectly through other key risk factors for stroke.

Physicians' Health Study Cohort

Lee et al. (1999) reported results from an 11-year follow-up of a Physicians' Health Study cohort of 21,823 men ages 40 to 80 years who were free of self-reported myocardial infarction, stroke, transient ischemic attack, and cancer at baseline. During the follow-up period, 533 cases of stroke were reported. Physical activity level was measured in the baseline examination as the frequency of exercise vigorous enough to work up a sweat. Results are shown in figure 5.5. After adjustment for age, smoking, alcohol intake, history of angina, and parental history of myocardial infarction, the relative risks of total stroke associated with vigorous exercise less than once a week, once a week, two to four times a week, and five or more times a week at baseline were 1.00 (reference group), 0.79 (95% CI: 0.61–1.03), 0.80 (0.65–0.99), and 0.79 (0.61–1.03), respectively; p = 0.04 for this trend. However, when the results were adjusted for potential mediators of the association between physical activity and stroke, such as BMI, history of hypertension, high cholesterol, and diabetes mellitus, the corresponding relative risks for total stroke were 1.00 (reference group), 0.81 (0.61–1.07), 0.88 (0.70–1.10), and 0.86 (0.65–1.13), respectively; p = 0.25 for this trend. The authors concluded that exercise vigorous

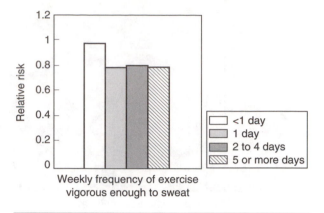

Figure 5.5   Physical activity and stroke in the U.S. Physician's Health Study cohort includes relative risk of stroke among 21,823 men 40 to 80 years of age and 533 cases of stroke during 11 years of follow-up. Study was independent of age, smoking, alcohol intake, history of angina, and parental history of MI, and not independent of hypertension, BMI, high cholesterol, and diabetes.
Adapted from Lee et al. 1999.

enough to work up a sweat was associated with a decreased risk of stroke in men and that this association was mediated by beneficial effects of physical activity on body weight, blood pressure, serum cholesterol, and glucose tolerance.

Icelandic Men

Agnarsson et al. (1999) reported on a study of 4,484 men ages 40 to 80 years at baseline who were followed for approximately 11 years, during which 249 cases of stroke were identified. At baseline, participants responded to questions in a yes/no format about participation in regular physical activity during age periods 20 to 29, 30 to 39, 40 to 49, and 50 to 59 years. Those who responded affirmatively were asked to report the number of hours per week and the type of physical activity in which they participated. Results indicated that after adjusting for other known stroke risk factors, leisure-time physical activity maintained after 40 years of age was associated with a reduced stroke risk: the relative risk was 0.69 (95% CI: 0.47–1.01) for total stroke and 0.62 (0.40–0.97) for ischemic stroke.

Nurses' Health Study Cohort

In this study, 407 incident cases of stroke were observed during eight years of follow-up among 72,488 female nurses ages 40 to 65 years who were free from cardiovascular disease and cancer at baseline in 1986 and who completed physical activity questionnaires in 1986, 1988, and 1992 (Hu et al. 2000). Results indicated that after controlling for age, BMI, history of hypertension, and other covariates, increasing levels of physical activity were inversely associated with the risk for both total and ischemic stroke (figure 5.6). Relative risks for total stroke from the lowest to highest quintile of physical activity were, respectively, 1.0 (reference), 0.98 (95% CI: 0.75–1.29), 0.82 (0.61–1.10), 0.74 (0.54–1.01), and 0.66 (0.47–0.91); *p* for trend = 0.005. Relative risks for ischemic stroke were 1.0 (reference), 0.87 (0.62–1.23), 0.83 (0.58–1.19), 0.76 (0.52–1.11), and 0.52 (0.33–0.80); *p* for trend = 0.003. Walking for exercise was also associated with reduced risk for total stroke. Relative risks for total stroke from lowest to highest quintile of walking (in METs) were, respectively, 1.0, 0.76 (0.56–1.04), 0.78 (0.56–1.07), 0.70 (0.52–0.95), and 0.66 (0.48–0.91); *p* for trend = 0.01. The respective relative risks of ischemic stroke were 1.0, 0.77 (0.52–1.13), 0.75 (0.50–1.12), 0.69 (0.47–1.01), and 0.60 (0.39–0.90); *p* for trend = 0.02. These results suggest that, for women, participation in physical activity, including moderate-intensity activity such as walking, results in a reduction in risk for both total and ischemic stroke in a dose–response manner.

Strength of the Evidence

As described earlier, before determining whether an association between a risk factor and disease is causal, it is important to determine that the observed association is valid and not the result of selection bias, loss to follow-up, problems of measuring the independent and dependent variables, or other health factors. In general, both the case–control and prospective studies on physical activity and stroke risk have been well conducted and have used follow-up periods of sufficient length to reduce the effect on the results of undiagnosed disease at entry to the study and to ensure an adequate number of stroke events for analysis. The physical activity assessment methods used in these studies vary considerably, from simply asking the frequency of exercise-induced sweating to the use of more detailed activity histories. There is undoubtedly some degree of misclassification of physical activity using these methods that would potentially bias the results toward finding no association between physical activity and stroke risk. The independence of the association between physical activity and stroke risk is open to question. Though several studies have shown a significant association of physical activity with stroke risk after adjustment for other major stroke risk factors, others have not. Additionally, no studies to date have examined the association between physical fitness and stroke risk or the association between changes in physical activity or physical fitness and changes in stroke risk.

Although there is a considerably smaller amount of data on the association of physical activity with stroke risk than on its association with reduced risk of heart disease, about half the

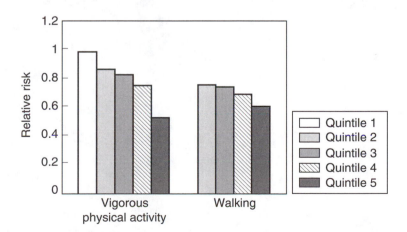

Figure 5.6   Physical activity and stroke in the Nurses' Health Study cohort includes 72,488 women free of CVD in 1986, age range of 40 to 65 years, 407 incident cases of stroke during eight years of follow-up. Study was independent of age, BMI, and history of hypertension.

Adapted from Hu et al. 2000.

published studies on physical activity and stroke suggest a protective effect of physical activity, especially for ischemic stroke. In this section we evaluate the consistency, strength of association, temporal sequence, dose response, and biological plausibility of the evidence.

Temporal Sequence

Ten of the 12 studies included in our review used a prospective design in which the independent variable, physical activity, was assessed prior to knowledge of the outcome, stroke incidence. Therefore, these studies satisfy the criteria of temporal sequence.

Strength of Association

The degree of risk reduction for stroke associated with participation in physical activity is generally strong and relatively consistent among studies. The risk reduction observed is typically in the range of 30% to 60%.

Consistency

Though not all studies agree, most have shown that the risk of ischemic stroke among people who are physically active is less than that of their sedentary counterparts after adjustment for other stroke risk factors. Consistent results have been shown across different ages and ethnic groups, in both sexes, and in both Americans and Europeans.

Dose Response

Evidence for a dose-gradient reduction in stroke risk with increasing weekly energy expenditure or higher intensity of physical activity is less clear than for coronary heart disease. Some studies showed a dose–response gradient of reduced stroke with increasing physical activity. Others showed a threshold effect; a certain minimum level of activity was associated with protection against stroke, but further increases in activity showed no greater decrease in risk. Three prospective cohort studies of leisure-time physical activity suggested an inverted-U relationship, in which a reduction in stroke risk was apparent only at moderate amounts of physical activity. The Northern Manhattan Stroke Study reported a dose–response relationship between both intensity and duration of leisure physical activity and stroke risk that was consistent among ages, sexes, and races. The Nurses' Health Study also indicated a dose response to both total physical activity and walking for exercise. On balance, it appears that more physical activity each week confers more protection against ischemic stroke, regardless of whether the intensity of the activity is moderate or vigorous.

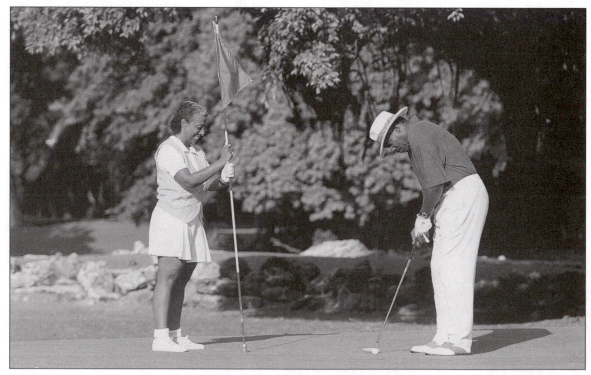

© Digital Vision

Biological Plausibility

A possible explanation for the generally positive association between physical activity and reduced rate of ischemic stroke is that physical activity reduces risk of developing atherosclerosis and thrombosis. Ischemic stroke involves a pathophysiology similar to atherosclerotic disease, and arterial thrombosis develops similarly to coronary heart disease. Hence, the benefits of physical activity on reducing clotting risk, reducing blood lipids, and increasing HDL could explain a reduction in the risk of developing ischemic cerebrovascular disease.

Indeed, evidence is emerging that cardiorespiratory fitness may play a role in retarding the progression of carotid atherosclerosis in middle-aged men. Recently, the association of cardiorespiratory fitness and the progression of early carotid atherosclerosis was examined in a four-year follow-up study of 854 Finnish men 42 to 60 years of age (Lakka et al. 2001). After adjustments for age and cigarette smoking, there were inverse relationships between maximal aerobic capacity and surface roughness and thickness of the intima of the carotid artery and plaque height measured by ultrasonography. Those inverse associations were weakened but remained after additional adjustment for systolic blood pressure, serum levels of apolipoprotein B (a risk factor for atherosclerosis), diabetes, and plasma fibrinogen levels. Men in the lowest quartile of maximal aerobic capacity ($26 \text{ ml} \cdot \text{kg}^{-1} \cdot \text{min}^{-1}$) had twice the increase in mean thickness of the carotid artery intima and 31% greater increase in surface roughness compared with men in the highest quartile of maximal aerobic capacity ($>36 \text{ ml} \cdot \text{kg}^{-1} \cdot \text{min}^{-1}$).

It is also possible that regular physical activity helps protect against stroke mortality by mitigating brain cell damage after a stroke. Convincing evidence from studies of rodents shows that moderate physical activity has a neurotropic effect on neurons in several brain regions (Cotman and Berchtold 2002) and reduces brain damage (Wang, Yang, and Yu 2001) and mortality rate (Ang et al. 2003; Stummer et al. 1994) after stroke.

Summary

The U.S. Surgeon General's report on physical activity and health (U.S. Department of Health and Human Services 1996) concluded that the evidence for a protective effect of physical activity against stroke was as yet unclear. About half of the dozen or so prospective studies showed a reduced risk of ischemic stroke in physically active individuals, regardless of age, sex, and ethnicity, compared with their sedentary counterparts after adjustment for other stroke risk factors. It appears that increased physical activity is associated with a reduced risk of atherosclerosis and blood clotting. Thus, an association between physical activity and decreased risk of ischemic stroke might be expected. Given that the incidence of stroke is relatively low, the association between activity and stroke can be evaluated only in large cohort studies, where the measures of physical activity often are not very precise and often do not allow an evaluation of a dose–response association. Better physical activity assessment techniques are necessary to describe more clearly the intensity and duration of physical activity associated with optimal reduction in stroke risk. Also, many studies did not classify the type of stroke, which is important because the mechanisms by which physical activity might protect against stroke could differ according to whether stroke results from ischemia, reduced perfusion, or embolism.

Bibliography

Abbott, R.D., B.L. Rodriguez, C.M. Burchfiel, and J.D. Curb. 1994. Physical activity in older middle-aged men and reduced risk of stroke: The Honolulu Heart Program. *American Journal of Epidemiology* 139: 881–893.

Agnarsson, U., G. Thorgeirsson, H. Sigvaldason, and N. Sigfusson. 1999. Effects of leisure-time physical activity and ventilatory function on risk for stroke in men: The Reykjavik Study. *Annals of Internal Medicine* 130: 987–990.

Algra, A., and J. van Gijn. 1996. Aspirin at any dose above 30 mg offers only modest protection after cerebral ischaemia. *Journal of Neurological and Neurosurgical Psychiatry* 60 (2): 197–199.

Amarenco, P., A. Cohen, C. Tzourio, B. Bertrand, M. Hommel, G. Besson, C. Chauvel, P.J. Touboul, and M.G. Bousser. 1994. Atherosclerotic disease of the aortic arch and the risk of ischemic stroke. *New England Journal of Medicine* 331: 1474–1479.

American Heart Association. 1998. *1999 heart and stroke statistical update.* Dallas: American Heart Association.

———. 2002. *Heart and stroke statistical update.* Dallas: American Heart Association.

Ang, E.T., P.T. Wong, S. Moochhala, and Y.K. Ng. 2003. Neuroprotection associated with running: Is it a result of increased endogenous neurotrophic factors? *Neuroscience* 118: 335–345.

Antiplatelet Trialists' Collaboration. 1994. Collaborative overview of randomised trials of antiplatelet therapy: I. Prevention of death, myocardial infarction, and stroke by prolonged antiplatelet therapy in various categories of patients. *British Medical Journal* 308 (6921): 81–106. Erratum, *British Medical Journal* 308 (6943): 1540.

Barnett, H.J.M., J.P. Mohr, B.M. Stein, and F.M. Yatsu, eds. 1992. *Stroke: Pathophysiology, diagnosis, and management.* 2nd ed. New York: Churchill Livingstone.

Bijnen, F.C., C.J. Caspersen, E.J. Feskens, W.H. Saris, W.L. Mosterd, and D. Kromhout. 1998. Physical activity and 10-year mortality from cardiovascular diseases and all causes: The Zutphen Elderly Study. *Archives of Internal Medicine* 158 (14): 1499–1505.

Blair, S.H., C.L. Wells, R.D. Weathers, and R.S. Paffenbarger. 1994. Chronic disease: The physical activity dose–response controversy. In *Advances in exercise adherence,* edited by R.K. Dishman, pp. 31–54. Champaign, IL: Human Kinetics.

Cholesterol and Recurrent Events Trial Investigators. 1996. The effect of pravastatin on coronary events after myocardial infarction in patients with average cholesterol levels. *New England Journal of Medicine* 335 (14): 1001–1009.

Cotman, C.W., and N.C. Berchtold. 2002. Exercise: A behavioral intervention to enhance brain health and plasticity. *Trends in Neurosciences* 25: 295–301.

Donahue, R.P., R.D. Abbott, D.M. Reed, and K. Yano. 1986. Alcohol and hemorrhagic stroke: The Honolulu Heart Program. *Journal of the American Medical Association* 255: 2311–2314.

Evenson, K.R., W.D. Rosamond, J. Cai, J.F. Toole, R.G. Hutchinson, E. Shahar, and A.R. Folsom. 1999. Physical activity and ischemic stroke risk: The Atherosclerosis Risk in Communities Study. *Stroke* 30: 1333–1339.

Fiebach, N.H., P.R. Hebert, M.J. Stampfer, G.A. Colditz, W.C. Willett, and B. Rosner. 1989. A prospective study of high blood pressure and cardiovascular disease in women. *American Journal of Epidemiology* 130: 646–654.

Gillum, R.F., M.E. Mussolino, and D.D. Ingram. 1996. Physical activity and stroke incidence in women and men: The NHANES I epidemiological follow-up study. *American Journal of Epidemiology* 143: 860–869.

Goldstein, L.B., R. Adams, K. Becker, C.D. Furberg, P.B. Gorelick, G. Hademenos, M. Hill, G. Howard, V.J. Howard, B. Jacobs, et al. 2001. Primary prevention of ischemic stroke: A statement for healthcare professionals from the Stroke Council of the American Heart Association. *Circulation* 103: 163–182.

Hardman, A.E. 1996. Exercise in the prevention of atherosclerotic, metabolic and hypertensive diseases: A review. *Journal of Sports Sciences* 14: 201–218.

Harmsen, P., A. Rosengren, A. Tsipogianni, and L. Wilhelmsen. 1990. Risk factors for stroke in middle-aged men in Goteborg, Sweden. *Stroke* 21: 223–229.

Helgason, C.M., and P.A. Wolf. 1997. American Heart Association Prevention Conference IV. Prevention and rehabilitation of stroke. Executive summary. *Circulation* 96 (2): 701–717.

Higgins, M., W. Kannel, R. Garrison, J. Pinsky, and J. Stokes. 1988. Hazards of obesity: The Framingham experience. *Acta Medica Scandinavica* 723: 23–36.

Hodis, H.N., W.J. Mack, L. LaBree, R.H. Selzer, C. Liu, P. Alaupovic, H. Kwong-Fu, and S.P. Azen. 1996. Reduction in carotid arterial wall thickness using lovastatin and dietary therapy: A randomized clinical trial. *Annals of Internal Medicine* 124 (6): 548–556.

Hu, F.B., M.J. Stampfer, G.A. Coldwitz, A. Ascherio, K.M. Rexrode, W.C. Willett, and J.E. Manson. 2000. Physical activity and risk of stroke in women. *Journal of the American Medical Association* 283: 2961–2967.

Hypertension Detection and Follow-Up Program Cooperative Group. 1979. Five-year findings of the hypertension detection and follow-up program: I. Reduction in mortality in persons with high blood pressure, including mild hypertension. *Journal of the American Medical Association* 242 (23): 2562–2571.

Kannel, W.B. 1999. Historic perspectives on the relative contributions of diastolic and systolic blood pressure elevation to cardiovascular risk profile. *American Heart Journal* 138 (3 Pt 2): 205–210.

Kannel, W.B., and P. Sorlie. 1979. Some health benefits of physical activity: The Framingham Study. *Archives of Internal Medicine* 139: 857–861.

Kannel, W.B., P.A. Wolf, J. Verter, and P.M. McNamara. 1970. Epidemiologic assessment of the role of blood pressure in stroke: The Framingham Study. *Journal of the American Medical Association* 214: 301–310.

Kelley, R.E. 1998. Stroke prevention and intervention. *Postgraduate Medicine* 103 (2): 43–62.

Kiely, D.K., P.A. Wolf, L.A. Cupples, A.S. Beiser, and W.B. Kannel. 1994. Physical activity and stroke risk: The Framingham Study. *American Journal of Epidemiology* 140: 860–869.

Kohl, H.W. III. 2001. Physical activity and cardiovascular disease: Evidence for a dose response. *Medicine and Science in Sports and Exercise* 33 (Suppl. 6): S472–S483.

Lakka, T.A., J.A. Laukkanen, R. Rauramaa, R. Salonen, H.M. Lakka, G.A. Kaplan, and J.T. Salonen. 2001. Cardiorespiratory fitness and the progression of carotid atherosclerosis in middle-aged men. *Annals of Internal Medicine* 134 (1): 12–20.

Lee, I.M., C.H. Hennekens, K. Berger, J.E. Bering, and J.E. Manson. 1999. Exercise and stroke risk in male physicians. *Stroke* 1: 1–6.

Lee, I.M., and R.S. Paffenbarger Jr. 1998. Physical activity and stroke incidence: The Harvard Alumni Health Study. *Stroke* 29: 2049–2054.

Lee, I.M., and P.J. Skerrett. 2001. Physical activity and all-cause mortality: What is the dose–response relation? *Medicine and Science in Sports and Exercise* 33 (Suppl. 6): S459–S470.

Lindenstrom, E., G. Boysen, and J. Nyboe. 1993a. Lifestyle factors and risk of cerebrovascular disease in women: The Copenhagen City Heart Study. *Stroke* 24: 1468–1472.

———. 1993b. Risk factors for stroke in Copenhagen, Denmark: II. Lifestyle factors. *Neuroepidemiology* 12: 43–50.

Lindsted, K.D., S. Tonstad, and J.W. Kuzma. 1991. Self-report of physical activity and patterns of mortality in Seventh Day Adventist men. *Journal of Clinical Epidemiology* 44: 355–364.

Mohr, J.P., G.W. Albers, P. Amarenco, V.L. Babikian, J. Biller, R.L. Brey, B. Coull, J.D. Easton, C.R. Gomez, C.M. Helgason, et al. 1997. American Heart Association Prevention Conference. IV. Prevention and rehabilitation of stroke. Etiology of stroke. *Stroke* 28 (7): 1501–1506.

Murray, C.J., and A.D. Lopez. 1997. Mortality by cause for eight regions of the world: Global Burden of Disease Study. *Lancet* 349 (9061): 1269–1276.

Paffenbarger, R.S. Jr., R.T. Hyde, A.L. Wing, and C.H. Steinmetz. 1984. A natural history of athleticism and cardiovascular health. *Journal of the American Medical Association* 252: 491–495.

Peto, R., R. Gray, R. Collins, K. Wheatley, C. Hennekens, K. Jamrozik, C. Warlow, B. Hafner, E. Thompson, S. Norton, et al. 1988. Randomised trial of prophylactic daily aspirin in British male doctors. *British Medical Journal (Clinical Research Edition)* 296 (6618): 313–316.

Rosengren, A., and L. Wilhelmsen. 1997. Physical activity protects against coronary death and deaths from all causes in middle-aged men: Evidence from a 20-year follow-up of the primary prevention study in Goteborg. *Annals of Epidemiology* 7: 69–75.

Sacco, R., R. Gan, B. Boden-Albala, F. Lin, D. Kargman, A. Hauser, S. Shea, and M. Paik. 1998. Leisure-time physical activity and ischemic stroke: The Northern Manhattan Stroke Study. *Stroke* 29: 380–387.

Sacco, R.L., P.A. Wolf, and P.B. Gorelick. 1999. Risk factors and their management for stroke prevention: Outlook for 1999 and beyond. *Neurology* 53 (7 Suppl. 4): S15–S24.

Sacco, R.L., P.A. Wolf, W.B. Kannel, and P.M. McNamara. 1982. Survival and recurrence following stroke: The Framingham Study. *Stroke* 13 (3): 290–295.

Salonen, J.T., P. Puska, and J. Tuomilehto. 1982. Physical activity and risk of myocardial infarction, cerebral stroke, and death: A longitudinal study in Eastern Finland. *American Journal of Epidemiology* 115: 526–537.

Shinton, R., and G. Sagar. 1993. Lifelong exercise and stroke. *British Medical Journal* 307: 231–234.

Stampfer, M.J., G.A. Colditz, W.C. Willett, F.E. Speizer, and C.H. Hennekens. 1988. A prospective study of moderate alcohol consumption and the risk of coronary disease and stroke in women. *New England Journal of Medicine* 319: 267–273.

Steering Committee of the Physicians' Health Study Research Group. 1989. Final report on the aspirin component of the ongoing Physicians' Health Study. *New England Journal of Medicine* 321 (3): 129–135.

Stegmayr, B., K. Asplund, K. Kuulasmaa, A.M. Rajakangas, P. Thorvaldsen, and J. Tuomilehto. 1997. Stroke incidence and mortality correlated to stroke risk factors in the WHO MONICA Project: An ecological study of 18 populations. *Stroke* 28 (7): 1367–1374.

Stummer, W., K. Weber, B. Tranmer, A. Baethmann, and O. Kempski. 1994. Reduced mortality and brain damage after locomotor activity in gerbil forebrain ischemia. *Stroke* 25: 1862–1869.

Thompson, D., J. Edelsberg, G.A. Colditz, A.P. Bird, and G. Oster. 1999. Lifetime health and economic consequences of obesity. *Archives of Internal Medicine* 159: 2177–2183.

Tuomilehto, J., R. Bonity, Q. Stewart, A. Nissinen, and J.T. Salonen. 1991. Hypertension, cigarette smoking and the decline in stroke incidence in eastern Finland. *Stroke* 22: 7–11.

U.S. Department of Health and Human Services. 1996. *Physical activity and health: A report of the Surgeon General.* Atlanta: U.S. Department of Health and Human Services, Centers for Disease Control and Prevention, National Center for Chronic Disease Prevention and Health Promotion.

Vahedi, K., and P. Amarenco. 2000. Cardiac causes of stroke. *Current Treatment Options in Neurology* 2: 305–318.

Wang, R.Y., Y.R. Yang, and S.M. Yu. 2001. Protective effects of treadmill training on infarction in rats. *Brain Research* 922: 140–143.

Wannamethee, G., and A.G. Shaper. 1992. Physical activity in British middle aged men. *British Medical Journal* 304: 597–601.

Wolf, P.A., R.B. D'Agostino, W.B. Kannel, R. Bonita, and A.J. Belanger. 1988. Cigarette smoking as a risk factor for stroke: The Framingham Study. *Journal of the American Medical Association* 259: 1025–1029.

You, R.X., J.J. McNeil, H.M. O'Malley, S.M. Davis, A.G. Thrift, and G.A. Donnan. 1997. Risk factors for stroke due to cerebral infarction in young adults. *Stroke* 28: 1913–1918.

Web Sites

www.americanheart.org. This is the site of the American Heart Association, which provides the Heart and Stroke Statistical Update annually for the United States.

www.strokeassociation.org. This is the site of the American Stroke Association, a division of the American Heart Association, that disseminates information about the prevention and treatment of stroke to the public and to health professionals.

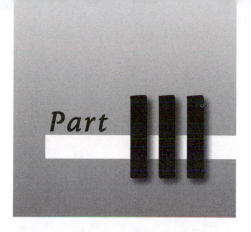

Part **III**

PHYSICAL ACTIVITY AND RISK FACTORS

A key objective of physical activity epidemiology is to determine whether physical activity exerts a protective effect on all-cause and cardiovascular disease mortality that is independent of other risk factors, such as hypertension, hyperlipidemia, and obesity. However, adjustment to control the confounding influences of such risk factors on mortality risk reduction might underestimate the protective effects of physical activity by obscuring its indirect influence on reducing risk factors that are biologically involved in the pathogenesis of CVD and other causes of premature death, such as diabetes and cancer. Moreover, hypertension, hyperlipidemia, and obesity are regarded as diseases in themselves, in addition to being key risk factors for all-cause and CVD mortality. Hence, it is doubly important to determine whether physical activity has healthful effects by altering these conditions in positive ways. The chapters in this part describe population-based studies and clinical experiments that provide evidence that physical activity and exercise play a role in the primary and secondary prevention of mild hypertension, hyperlipidemia, and obesity.

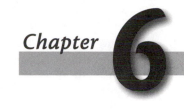

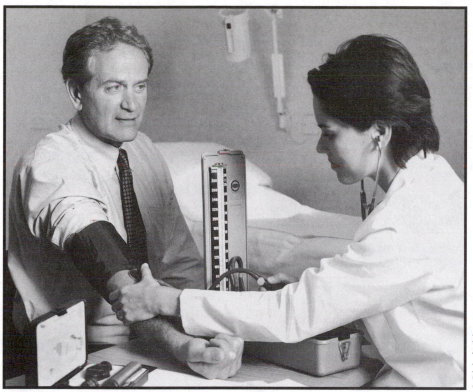

Chapter 6

© Digital Vision

Physical Activity and Hypertension

The pulses of the ventricles are felt in the arteries, to wit, the distension produced by the jet of blood.

—William Harvey (1578–1657), On the Motion of the Heart and Blood in Animals

Hypertension is a major risk factor for coronary heart disease and stroke. Though ancient physicians observed "hardening of the pulse" 2,000 years ago and hypertension has been recognized as a disease since the 1600s, a British theologian and science hobbiest named Stephen Hales was the first person to measure blood pressure (Ruskin 1956). In 1733, he placed a brass pipe in the carotid artery of a horse and attached the pipe to a flexible goose's trachea, which then was connected to a 12-foot-tall (3.7-m) glass tube. As his horse bled to death, the blood rose in the tube more than 9 feet (2.7 m). One hundred fifty years later, the first sphygmo-

manometer was invented by Ritter von Basch. In 1905, Russian Nikolai Sergeyevich Korotkoff used a stethoscope to detect an arterial pulse during inflation of a blood pressure cuff, leading to the use of what are now known as Korotkoff sounds to determine the blood pressures that correspond with the systolic and diastolic phases of the heartbeat (Wain 1970).

The measurement of blood pressure has a long history, but recognition of diseases associated with high blood pressure is relatively new. Until about the 1940s, high blood pressure was often referred to as benign essential hypertension, indicating a condition of unknown origin and little consequence for health. The Joint National Committee on Prevention, Detection, Evaluation, and Treatment of High Blood Pressure has defined hypertension as a systolic blood pressure of 140 mmHg or greater or diastolic blood pressure of 90 mmHg or greater or as taking antihypertensive medication (Joint National Committee 2003). Severity of hypertension is further categorized with the classification system shown in table 6.1.

TABLE 6.1 CLASSIFICATION OF BLOOD PRESSURE FOR ADULTS AGES 18 YEARS AND OLDER

Category	Systolic, mmHg	Diastolic, mmHg
Normal	<120	<80
Prehypertension	120–139	80–89
Stage 1 hypertension	140–159	90–99
Stage 2 hypertension	≥160	≥100

••• *Until about the 1940s, high blood pressure was often referred to as benign essential hypertension, indicating a condition of unknown origin and little consequence for health.*

Primary or essential hypertension, in which the cause is unknown or unpredictable, accounts for 90% to 95% of hypertension cases. Most cases of secondary hypertension, in which the cause is known, result from renal nephritis; hypersecretion of corticosteroids from the adrenal gland, including hyperaldosteronism; pheochromocytoma (a tumor in the **adrenal medulla,** which leads to hyperse-

cretion of **catecholamines**); or malfunction of the renin–angiotensin–aldosterone system.

••• *Primary or essential hypertension, in which the cause is unknown or unpredictable, accounts for 90% to 95% of hypertension cases.*

Magnitude of the Problem

Though mortality rates from coronary heart disease and stroke have declined during the past 25 years, the prevalence of hypertension has remained high at about 50 million Americans (American Heart Association 2002; National Center for Health Statistics 1997) (figure 6.1). During 30 years of prospective observation of participants in the Framingham Heart Study, two out of three middle-aged (45- to 54-year-old) people developed hypertension (Kannel, Garrison, and Dannenberg 1993). A recent analysis of data from the Third National Health and Nutrition Examination Survey (NHANES III) conducted from 1999 to 2000 estimated that the prevalence of high blood pressure has increased to 28.7% of U.S. adults 18 years and older (about 58 million people) (Hajjar and Kotchen 2003).

According to NHANES III, the total prevalence of hypertension among U.S. men and women ages 18 to 74 years is about 20%, representing about 43 million noninstitutionalized adults. Another 13 million had been diagnosed as having hypertension by a health professional but didn't meet the Joint National Committee criteria for hypertension (Burt, Whelton et al. 1995). The prevalence of hypertension is disproportionately higher among

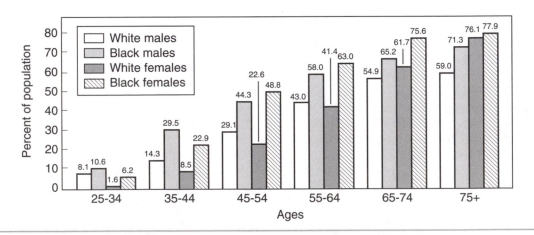

Figure 6.1 High blood pressure in Americans over 25 years of age by age, sex, and race.

Reprinted from *American Journal of Hypertension*, Vol. 13, M. Wolz et al., "Statement from the national high blood pressure education program: Prevalence of hypertension," pp. 103–104, Copyright 2000, with permission from *American Journal of Hypertension*.

older people and African Americans. About 50% of white men and women and about 75% of black men and women ages 60 to 74 years have hypertension (Burt, Cutler et al. 1995). About 10% to 15% of hypertension occurs in children or youths, and 70% of those cases are mild hypertension. The annual costs associated with hypertension in the United States are estimated to be $37 billion, with antihypertensive drug costs of $15.5 billion accounting for nearly half that amount (American Heart Association 2002).

NHANES III showed that the prevalence of hypertension declined from 1960 to 1991 but rose again from a prevalence of about 25% among adults in 1991 to nearly 29% in 2000, an increase of about 8 million people. The Framingham Heart Study has estimated that the prevalence of stage 1 or 2 hypertension (>160/95 mmHg) has declined by two thirds during the past 40 years. Some of that decline, however, can be explained by more people today having their hypertension normalized by antihypertensive medication. According to National Ambulatory Medical Care Surveys (National Center for Health Statistics 1995), hypertension was the most frequent principal diagnosis for patients visiting U.S. office-based physicians from 1980 to 1995. Hypertension accounted for 3.2% of all visits to office-based physicians in 1995, who mentioned at least one antihypertensive drug in nearly 80% of those visits (Nelson and Knapp 2000).

••• *According to NHANES III, the total prevalence of hypertension among U.S. men and women ages 18 to 74 years is about 20%, about 43 million noninstitutionalized adults.*

Drug Treatment of Hypertension

Top 5 drugs	% of total hypertension prescriptions
Diuretics	12%
SNS receptor blockers	8%
ACE inhibitor or SNS receptor blockers	18%
Calcium channel blocker	21%
Combined ACE inhibitor, plus SNS receptor blocker, plus diuretic	7%

Data from Nelson and Knapp 2000.

Treating Hypertension

Ancient physicians observed that dietary salt "hardened the pulse" nearly 2,000 years before the methods to measure blood pressure in humans were developed. Most of the drugs used to treat hypertension were developed in response to clinical observations that led to an evolving understanding of the etiology of hypertension. Drugs that block **sympathetic nervous system (SNS)** ganglions or deplete catecholamines were developed in the 1940s after it was observed that surgical lesioning of sympathetic nerves successfully lowered blood pressure. Diuretics were developed in the 1950s after a low-sodium diet was found to lower blood pressure in some people. Renin was discovered in the kidneys in the late 1800s and found to be elevated in some people with high blood pressure, but the development of **angiotensin-converting enzyme (ACE)** inhibitors didn't occur until the 1980s.

History of Hypertension Treatment

1940s
- Thiocyanates
- Ganglion-blocking agents
- Catecholamine depletors (*Rauwolfia* derivatives)

1950s
- Vasodilators (hydralazine)
- Peripheral sympathetic inhibitors (guanethidine)
- Monoamine oxidase inhibitors
- Diuretics

1960s
- Central α_2-agonists (SNS inhibitors)
- β-adrenergic inhibitors

1970s
- α-adrenergic inhibitors
- Alpha-beta-blockers

1980s
- ACE inhibitors
- Calcium channel blockers

1990s
- **Angiotensin II** receptor antagonists

2000s
- Gene therapy
- Physical activity?

Adapted from Moser 1997.

Though drugs have high efficacy for managing hypertension and generally reducing mortality rates, it is often difficult to find the right combination for best effect, and hypertensive drugs haven't reduced mortality for white women in some studies (Anastos et al. 1991). Also, popular antihypertension drugs have serious side effects. For example, a recent randomized controlled trial conducted in the United States and Canada that included over 33,000 men and women aged 55 years or older with hypertension found that, compared with patients taking a diuretic, other patients had serious adverse events during a 5-year follow-up after taking the following drugs: an alpha-adrenergic blocking drug increased the incidence of heart attacks and strokes by 25%; a calcium channel blocker increased risk of heart failure by 38%; an ACE inhibitor increased risk of stroke by 15% and risk of heart failure by 19% (Furberg et al. 2002). For mild to moderate high blood pressure, frontline treatment often focuses on low risk interventions including weight loss, reduction of dietary salt, and increased physical activity.

Lifestyle Modifications for Primary Prevention of Hypertension

- Maintain normal body weight for adults (BMI: 18.5–24.9 kg/m^2)
- Reduce dietary sodium intake to no more than 100 mmol/d (approximately 6 g of sodium chloride or 2.4 g of sodium per day)
- Engage in regular aerobic physical activity such as brisk walking (at least 30 min per day, most days of the week)
- Limit alcohol consumption to no more than 1 oz (30 ml) of ethanol (e.g., 24 oz [720 ml] of beer, 10 oz [300 ml] of wine, or 2 oz [60 ml] of 100-proof whiskey) per day in most men and to no more than 0.5 oz (15 ml) of ethanol per day in women and lighter-weight persons
- Maintain adequate intake of dietary potassium (>90 mmol [3,500 mg] per day)
- Consume a diet that is rich in fruits and vegetables and in low-fat dairy products with a reduced content of saturated and total fat

Source: National High Blood Pressure Education Program (Whelton et al. 2002).

In addition to age and race, high body fat, insulin resistance, dietary sodium, and alcohol use are known risk factors for hypertension (Fletcher and Bulpitt 1994). Thus, **primary prevention** of hypertension focuses on lifestyle changes, including decreasing salt intake, increasing potassium intake, losing weight, reducing stress, and increasing physical activity. About a decade ago, the Preventive Services Task Force appointed by the U.S. Office of Disease Prevention and Health Promotion concluded that the evidence was strong and independent of other risk factors that inactive men and women had about a one third to a one half greater risk of developing hypertension than active or fit people (Harris et al. 1989). That conclusion was based on observations of just two cohorts, the Harvard alumni and the Aerobics Center Longitudinal Study, but other evidence agrees with that early view.

Hypertension Etiology

Theories about circulation have their origins in the writings of Hippocrates, who thought arteries carried blood but veins carried air, and Galen, who showed that arteries and veins each carried blood. Galen, though, believed that blood flowed from and to the heart in separate arterial and venous systems. It was not until 1616 that the British physician William Harvey concluded that blood circulation was a closed circuit, with capillaries connecting arteries and veins.

The basic determinants of blood pressure are described by Poiseuille's law, which states that laminar blood flow ($\dot{Q}$) through a vessel is limited by the difference in pressure along the length of the vessel (ΔP), the radius of the vessel (r), the viscosity of the blood (η), and vessel length (l) according to the following equation:

$$\dot{Q} = \frac{\Delta P \pi r^4}{8 \eta l}$$

Simplifying and solving the equation for pressure, we can determine that blood pressure is the algebraic product of blood flow (i.e., cardiac output) and **total peripheral resistance (TPR)** to flow. In practical terms, a person's blood pressure depends on the volume of blood, its rate of flow, and especially the diameter of blood vessels. Hypertension develops from an abnormal elevation in one or all of the factors that influence blood flow or resistance to flow, and the specific mechanisms that alter blood flow or resistance vary with age, race, and body composition.

> ••• *Blood pressure is the algebraic product of blood flow (i.e., cardiac output) and total peripheral resistance to flow.*

Autonomic Nervous System

Though the osmolality (i.e., concentrations of ions such as sodium) of the blood, **mineralocorticosteroids** such as aldosterone, and hemodynamic factors such as blood volume and viscosity influence blood pressure, so does the **autonomic nervous system (ANS).** The neurotransmitter **norepinephrine** (also called **noradrenaline**), released from sympathetic nerves, and the hormone **epinephrine** (also called **adrenaline**), secreted from the medulla of the adrenal gland, bind with **adrenergic receptors** (or adrenoreceptors) on cells of the heart to increase its rate and force of contraction, on the kidneys, and on smooth muscle cells in blood vessels, which then constrict to increase peripheral resistance. Hence, blood pressure increases during activity of the sympathetic nervous system (figure 6.2). A necessary step between the binding of norepinephrine or epinephrine (the "first messengers") with an adrenoreceptor and the contraction of muscle cells is activation of a "second messenger," cyclic AMP, which regulates calcium channels that govern depolarization of the muscle cell (figure 6.3). Several drugs used to treat hypertension either inhibit sympathetic nerve activity (e.g., an α_2-agonist like clonidine), block β-adrenoreceptor binding (e.g., propranolol), or block calcium channels (e.g., verapamil).

In contrast to actions of the sympathetic nervous system, the neurotransmitter **acetylcholine,** released from the vagus nerve of the **parasympathetic nervous system,** binds with cholinergic receptors on the heart and blood vessels to slow the heart and relax muscle cells, thus lowering blood pressure, and on the kidneys. Systolic and diastolic blood pressures consequently depend on the balance of waxing and waning activity of the sympathetic and parasympathetic branches of the autonomic nervous system. An imbalance in favor of greater sympathetic activation can increase blood pressure by increasing cardiac output and total peripheral resistance through direct actions on the heart and blood vessels or indirectly through the kidney by altering the regulation of the renin–angiotensin–aldosterone system. A key action of acetylcholine's binding with blood vessels is the release of vascular releasing factors, such as nitric oxide, which are derived from endothelial cells that line blood vessels.

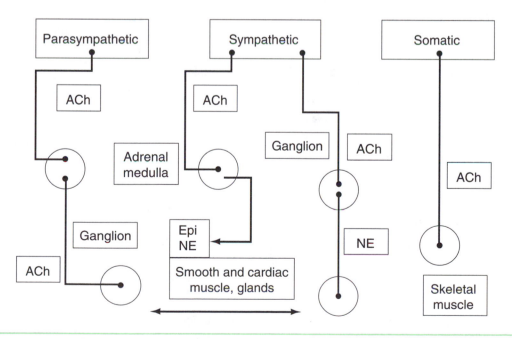

Figure 6.2   Autonomic nerves.

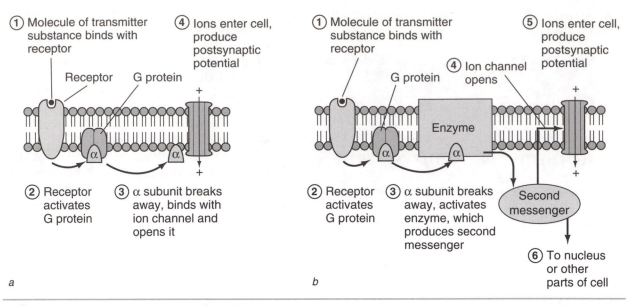

Figure 6.3   A **receptor** can open an ion channel (a) directly or (b) indirectly by a second messenger.

From N.R. Carlson *Physiology of Behavior* 5/E © 1994. Published by Allyn and Bacon, Boston, MA. Copyright © 1994 by Pearson Education. Reprinted by permission of the publisher.

Physical Activity and Reduced Hypertension Risk: The Evidence

Both population-based epidemiologic studies and clinical experiments provide substantial evidence that moderate-intensity physical activity is associated with primary prevention and **secondary prevention** (i.e., treatment) of mild hypertension. The following sections describe that evidence and evaluate its strength for demonstrating causality.

> ••• *Both population-based epidemiologic studies and clinical experiments provide substantial evidence that moderate-intensity physical activity is associated with primary prevention and treatment of mild hypertension.*

Cross-Sectional Studies

The following cross-sectional studies examined the association of physical activity and risk of hypertension.

North Carolina

The relationship of physical activity to hypertension was examined in a cross-sectional study of 1,751 African American adults ages 20 to 50 years who lived in Pitt County, North Carolina (Ainsworth et al. 1991). Hypertension was defined as a diastolic pressure of 90 mmHg or higher or current use of antihypertensive medication. Sixty-five percent of women and 44% of men were classified as sedentary. Being sedentary was not associated with the prevalence of hypertension in men, but the odds ratio of hypertension for sedentary women (26% had hypertension) was 1.3 times that of active women (20% had hypertension). After adjustment for age, BMI, alcohol use, and waist-to-hip ratio, this odds ratio was 1.6.

Southern California

Nearly 650 white women ages 50 to 89 years living in Southern California were classified according to self-reported leisure-time physical activity into the categories light (58%), moderate (24%), heavy (6%), or no (12%) physical activity (P.D. Reaven, Barrett-Conner, and Edelstein 1991). The active and inactive women did not differ in alcohol or cigarette use or prevalence of coronary heart disease or diabetes, but the active women were younger, lighter for their height, and had lower insulin levels. Age-adjusted systolic and diastolic blood pressures in the women who reported no physical activity were about 13 mmHg and 6 mmHg higher, respectively, than in women who reported heavy leisure physical activity during the past two weeks. After adjustments for age, BMI, and insulin levels, there was an overall linear trend for lower blood pressures with higher levels of physical activity.

Seventh Day Adventists

Among 114 African American Seventh Day Adventists about 55 years old, those who reported at least 20 min of vigorous exercise two or more times per week (mean four days a week) were classified as exercisers, and those who exercised once a week or less were classified as nonexercisers (Melby, Goldflies, and Hyner 1991). The groups had the same dietary intake of nutrients, but exercisers had lower BMI, waist circumference, and triceps skinfold thickness. After adjustment for age and sex, systolic and diastolic blood pressures were about 10 mmHg and 4 mmHg lower, respectively, among exercisers than among nonexercisers. After adjustment for the anthropometric differences, systolic blood pressure was still about 8 mmHg lower in the exercisers. Forty-two percent of the nonexercisers were diagnosed as hypertensive by a physician and were taking blood pressure medicine, compared with 20% of the exercisers.

Prospective Cohort Studies

The following prospective cohort studies examined the association of physical activity and risk of hypertension. Prospective studies help estab-lish the temporal sequence of activity or inactivity and subsequent hypertension.

Aerobics Center Longitudinal Study (ACLS)

Nearly 5,000 men and over 1,200 women 20 to 65 years old who had a medical examination and treadmill fitness test at the Cooper Clinic in Dallas between 1970 and 1981 later responded to a mail survey about their health in 1982 (Blair et al. 1984). People were classified as low or high in physical fitness according to their time to reach exhaustion during the treadmill test. During an average of four years of follow-up observation, 240 people developed high blood pressure, defined as greater than 140/90 mmHg. The relative risk for developing hypertension was 1.5 for the low-fitness group after adjustment for age, BMI, sex, and baseline blood pressure (figure 6.4). People in the low-fitness category who had high normal systolic pressures (between 130 to 139 mmHg) and diastolic pressures (between 85 to 89 mmHg) had more than 10 times the risk of developing hypertension than those who were highly fit and had normal pressures (below 120/85 mmHg).

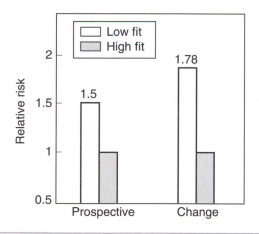

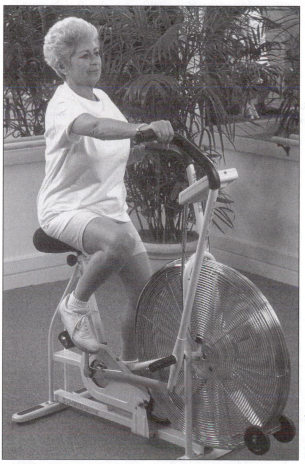

Figure 6.4 Fitness and hypertension in the Aerobics Center Longitudinal Study includes 4,800 men and 1,200 women aged 20 to 65 years, treadmill time in 1970 to 1980, followed by approximately four years, and 240 became hypertensive. Results included relative risk for low fit 1.50. The relative risk was 1.78 for those who remained low fit compared to those who remained or became high fit.

Adapted from Blair et al. 1984.

© SportsChrome

Of those people in the ACLS cohort, 1,300 had a second clinic exam between 1970 and 1981. Hence, the association between altered fitness from the time of the first test until the second and changes in blood pressure could be examined. People who moved from the low-fitness group to the high-fitness group during that time had about half the risk of developing hypertension of those whose fitness remained low.

Harvard Alumni Health Study

About 15,000 male graduates of Harvard who entered college during the years 1916 to 1950 and were judged to have normal blood pressures at that time completed a questionnaire in 1962 or 1966, when they were 35 to 74 years old, and again in 1972, for a 6- to 10-year period of observation (Paffenbarger et al. 1983). During that time, the standard definition for hypertension was a systolic pressure of at least 160 mmHg or a diastolic pressure of at least 90 mmHg or both. Two thirds of the men reported that they expended less than 2,000 kcal per week in leisure-time physical activity. After adjustment for age, those men had a 30% greater risk of developing hypertension than those who reported expending more than 2,000 kcal each week. In addition, the men who did not participate in vigorous recreational sports had a 35% higher risk of developing hypertension than those who were vigorously active. Those relative risks were independent of age, BMI over 36, a gain in BMI since college of at least 5, at least one hypertensive parent, and at least one parent with coronary heart disease.

A later analysis of nearly 17,000 Harvard male alumni from 1962 to 1985 found an inverse association between participation in vigorous recreational sports during middle age and the risk of developing hypertension that was independent of BMI, weight gain, or parental hypertension (Paffenbarger et al. 1991). In another analysis between 1977 and 1988, there were 885 cases of hypertension among 6,390 men observed for 72,544 person-years. Moderately vigorous sports participation led to a reduced risk of hypertension, but walking, stair climbing, and light sports did not alter that risk (Paffenbarger and Lee 1997). Being overweight, parental hypertension, alcohol use, or cigarette use increased the risk of hypertension. The combination of all these factors accounted for one quarter to one half of the new cases of hypertension. Those men who became active in vigorous sports between the 1960s and 1977 (Paffenbarger and Lee 1997) had a lower incidence of hypertension, independent

of overweight, smoking, or alcohol use. The intensity of physical activity reduced the risk of hypertension more than total energy expenditure.

University of Pennsylvania Alumni

Another study involving college alumni followed men who attended the University of Pennsylvania between the years 1931 and 1940 (Paffenbarger, Thorne, and Wing 1968). The time span between college and completion of a 1962 questionnaire was between 22 and 31 years. During this time, 9% of the 7,685 subjects developed hypertension diagnosed by a physician. They were between 20 and 60 years old at the time of diagnosis. Activity level was assessed as less than or more than 5 h of sports participation per week. About 40% of those surveyed reported that they spent less than 5 h per week playing sports. They had a 30% higher age-adjusted risk of developing hypertension than men who spent 5 h or more in sports each week. However, systolic pressure over 130 mmHg (RR = 2.7), diastolic pressure over 80 mmHg (RR = 2.2), and parental history of hypertension (RR = 1.7) were better predictors of hypertension.

In a later analysis of the Penn cohort, nearly 740 of 5,500 men developed hypertension between 1962 and 1985 (Paffenbarger et al. 1991). Participation in sports during college did not alter the incidence rate of hypertension. Neither did walking, stair climbing, or light recreational sports during middle age. However, participation in vigorous recreational sports in middle age reduced hypertension, independent of overweight, gain in weight, or history of parental hypertension. Vigorous sports did not reduce the death rate among those who had hypertension, but overweight and smoking increased their death rate.

Iowa Women

The two-year incidence of hypertension was examined in a cohort of nearly 42,000 women ages 55 to 69 years living in Iowa (Folsom et al. 1990). The relative risk of developing hypertension was 30% higher among women in the lowest third of leisure-time physical activity than the most-active upper third of the women sampled. However, that risk reduction was not independent of the lower BMI, lower waist-to-hip ratio, less smoking, and younger age of the most-active women.

The Northwestern Trial

Two groups of about 200 men and women ages 30 to 44 who were at high risk of developing hypertension (with high normal diastolic pressure, overweight, with resting heart rate $\geq$ 80, or any combination of these) were observed for about five years (Stamler et al. 1989). One group was observed without intervention, while the other was instructed about changing their lifestyles by (a) decreasing overweight by at least 4.5 kg (10 lb) or 5%, (b) decreasing sodium intake to no more than 1,800 mg per day, (c) decreasing alcohol use to no more than two drinks a day, and (d) increasing moderate physical activity to 30 min at an intensity of 70% to 75% of maximum heart rate, three days each week.

The incidence of hypertension in the control group was twice that of the experimental intervention group (19.2% vs. 8.8%). About 75% of the intervention group reported an increase in physical activity and had increased fitness. Because several behaviors were changed at once, the study did not demonstrate an independent effect of exercise on the incidence of hypertension, but it did show the efficacy of nonpharmacologic interventions in people at high risk for developing hypertension.

Physical Activity and Treatment of Hypertension: The Evidence

A review of 25 clinical studies completed by 1988 concluded that regular exercise is effective for reducing systolic blood pressure by about 11 mmHg and diastolic blood pressure by about 8 mmHg in men and women with mild hypertension (figure 6.5; Hagberg 1990).

Collectively, the reductions in mild hypertension observed in those studies differed according to several factors. People with mild hypertension benefited more than those diagnosed with severe hypertension or those with normal blood pressures. Women had larger reductions (–19/–14 mmHg) than men (–7/–5 mmHg). The drop in systolic blood pressure was less in heavier people, but the reductions after exercise training were independent of weight change. The decreases in blood pressures were smaller when exercise intensity was higher. Drops in pressure were not consistent among studies when the intensity of exercise exceeded 75% of aerobic capacity. The reductions in diastolic blood pressure were greater the longer the exercise training program lasted. The reductions in blood pressure after exercise training were similar to or larger than other nonpharmacologic treatments of mild hypertension (Gordon et al. 1990).

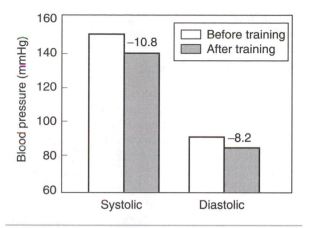

Figure 6.5 Cumulative results of 25 clinical studies on chronic exercise and mild hypertension.
Adapted from Hagberg 1990.

Subsequent research showed that men with severe hypertension can also benefit from moderately intense exercise. After 16 weeks of cycling exercise for 45 min three days a week at an intensity of about 75% of maximum heart rate, African American men who had blood pressures over 180/110 mmHg when not medicated reduced their medicated diastolic pressure from 89 to 83 mmHg and reduced the size and thickness of their left ventricles (Kokkinos et al. 1995). (An enlarged left ventricle with thickened walls is a common side effect of chronic hypertension.)

> ••• *A more recent analysis of results from more than 40 randomized controlled trials showed average reductions in systolic/diastolic blood pressure of about 7/6 mmHg among people with hypertension and about 3/2 mmHg among normotensives (Fagard 2001).*

Strength of the Evidence

When judged by the criteria of Mill's canons, the evidence is moderately strong that leisure-time physical activity is independently associated with reduced risk of developing hypertension and is effective in reducing blood pressure among adults who have mild hypertension.

Temporal Sequence

Large prospective cohort studies, which demonstrate the appropriate temporal sequence, have shown lowered risk of developing hypertension among people who are physically active.

Strength of Association

The cumulative evidence from about a dozen observational studies using both cross-sectional and prospective cohort designs shows a 30% to 50% reduction in the risk of developing hypertension when active adults are compared with sedentary peers. Results from more than 40 randomized controlled trials have shown average reductions in systolic/diastolic blood pressure of about 7/6 mmHg among people with hypertension and about 3/2 mmHg among normotensives (Fagard 2001).

Consistency

The majority of evidence has come from studies of white men of European ancestry. Nonetheless, a sufficient number of studies have been conducted with women and people of non-European ethnicities to suggest that physical activity reduces blood pressure equally regardless of age, sex, or ethnicity.

Dose Response

A recent quantitative review of the cumulative evidence about aerobic or endurance physical activity and lowered blood pressure focused on dose response and included 44 studies involving 2,674 adults (65% were men) published through 1999 (Fagard 2001). Fifty-two outcomes were evaluated for normotensive participants, and 16 outcomes were available for hypertensive groups. The review concluded that there was no convincing evidence of a dose response to exercise training. Exercise intensities ranging from 40% to 70% of aerobic capacity, lasting between 30 min and 1 h, and repeated three to five times each week for at least four weeks were equally associated with reduced blood pressure. Likewise, weekly energy expenditure during exercise was unrelated to the magnitude of blood pressure reductions.

••• *There is no clear evidence of a dose response to exercise training for lowering blood pressure. Exercise intensities ranging between 40% to 70% of exercise capacity, lasting between 30 min and 1 h, and repeated three to five times each week for at least four weeks appear equally effective for reducing blood pressure.*

Biological Plausibility

Systolic/diastolic blood pressures can be temporarily lowered by about 19/8 mmHg in hypertensive people and 9/4 mmHg in normotensive people 2 to 4 h after a single session of moderately intense (>35% of maximal heart rate) running, walking, cycling, or swimming (Kenney and Seals 1993). Whether this acute hypotensive effect of exercise explains part of the long-term effects of regular exercise on lowering blood pressure is not known. However, it is likely that some of the same mechanisms that regulate blood pressure during and after exercise are altered by long-term physical activity habits. Because the hemodynamic profiles of people diagnosed with hypertension can vary, it is important to consider whether the effects of physical activity on cardiac output and total peripheral resistance differ in the primary and secondary prevention of hypertension.

In cardiogenic, or hyperdynamic, hypertension, which is usually seen in young people with borderline hypertension, resting cardiac output can be elevated by 10% to 20% despite normal total peripheral resistance (Weir 1991). Among older adults, hypertension is more commonly accompanied by decreased cardiac output but increased total peripheral vascular resistance. The suggested mechanisms for these changes are a decrease in maximum heart rate (i.e., a chronotropic response) and vascular stiffening and changes in central nervous system regulation of blood pressure that accompany aging. There seems to be a correlation between increasing age and increasing systolic blood pressure in both men and women. The same relationship is seen with diastolic blood pressure until ages 50 to 60. After those ages, diastolic pressure typically levels off in men and women or declines slightly in men (Fletcher and Bulpitt 1994).

African Americans typically have increased total peripheral resistance, decreased cardiac output, decreased renin production, and normal or expanded plasma volume compared with white people (Pickering 1994). People who are obese tend to have a high cardiac output, expanded plasma volume, increased sympathetic nervous system activity, and normal or slightly decreased peripheral resistance (Weir 1991).

••• *Evidence indicates that exercise training can decrease resting blood pressure by reducing basal cardiac output or total peripheral resistance.*

> ## Exercise and Hypertension: Plausible Mechanisms
>
> ### Decreased cardiac output
>
> Decreased SNS nerve activity?
>
> Increased cardiac **vagal tone?**
>
> Decreased resting catecholamine levels?
>
> Decreased β_1-**receptors?**
>
> Increased α_2-**receptors?**
>
> Renal effects: increased sodium excretion?
>
> ### Decreased total peripheral resistance
>
> Decreased SNS nerve activity?
>
> Decreased resting catecholamine levels?
>
> Increased α_2-receptors?
>
> Decreased α_1-**receptors?**
>
> Decreased insulin?
>
> Endothelial relaxers?

Cardiac Output

Cardiac output is the product of the stroke volume of the heart and heart rate, so a reduction in cardiac output must be explained by a reduction in one or both of those factors. In people with normal blood pressure, a common adaptation after exercise training is a reduced resting heart rate but a compensatory increase in stroke volume so that cardiac output is unchanged. The increased stroke volume results mainly from increased plasma volume and venous return to the left heart. A different response to chronic exercise may result for people with hypertension. Some studies have observed no change in heart rate, despite reduced blood pressure after exercise training (Krotkiewski et al. 1979). That outcome might be explained by a reduction in plasma volume, which has been observed after 10 weeks of exercise training in obese people with hypertension (Weir 1991).

Total Peripheral Resistance

Changes in total peripheral resistance (TPR) in response to acute exercise have been studied in both normotensive and hypertensive patients. Cleroux et al. (1992) reported that a 27% reduction in TPR and a 20% reduction in plasma norepinephrine accompanied postexercise hypotension in people with mild hypertension who exercised for 30 min at an intensity of 50% $\dot{V}O_2$max. The ef-

fect continued for up to 90 min after cessation of exercise, despite a 30% increase in cardiac output after exercise. A common finding in a number of studies is a reduction in plasma norepinephrine levels, suggesting reduced sympathetic nervous system activity with exercise training (Arakawa 1993). This could favorably affect cardiac output as well as peripheral resistance.

> ••• *When judged by the criteria of Mill's canons, the evidence is moderately strong that leisure-time physical activity is independently associated with reduced risk of developing hypertension and is effective in reducing blood pressure among adults who have mild hypertension.*

One study showed that people with hypertension had about 30% lower levels of taurine than did normotensive peers (Arakawa 1993). Taurine is an amino acid that has antihypertensive properties and is found in high concentrations in the myocardium, brain, and skeletal muscle. Exercise training three times a week for 10 weeks at an intensity of 40% to 60% $\dot{V}O_2$max increased serum taurine concentrations by 26% in Japanese men and women with hypertension, with accompanying reductions in plasma levels of norepinephrine and blood pressure (Tanabe et al. 1989).

Insulin

Insulin resistance and hyperinsulinemia have also been implicated in the development of hypertension. People with hypertension are commonly insulin resistant, hyperinsulinemic, and hyperglycemic, whether the hypertension is treated or not. There seems to be a direct relationship between plasma insulin concentration and blood pressure, and hyperinsulinemia has been shown to precede development of hypertension (G.M. Reaven 1988). It appears that blood pressure can be regulated by changes in insulin metabolism, thus explaining why weight loss, which enhances insulin sensitivity and decreases plasma insulin levels, can decrease blood pressure in those with hypertension (Gilders, Voner, and Dudley 1989). Also, blood pressure was decreased in obese patients after exercise training without any change in weight, but only in those who were hyperinsulinemic before training (Kiyonaga et al. 1985). The mechanism explaining the relationship between hyperinsulinemia and blood pressure may be related to increased sympathetic nervous system activity in obese as well as nonobese people or to promotion of sodium reabsorption by the renal tubes that leads to increased plasma volume (G.M. Reaven 1995). It is possible that one mechanism of preventing hypertension with exercise is preventing obesity, as obesity is related to insulin resistance and has been shown to be an independent direct risk factor for cardiovascular disease and primary hypertension.

Stress Reactivity

Several prospective studies have shown that exaggerated blood pressure responses during the cold pressor test (i.e., submersion of the hand or foot in ice water) predicts the development of hypertension, but others have not (e.g., Carroll et al. 1996; Kasagi 1994; Menkes et al. 1989). Those studies did not control cardiorespiratory fitness, which is inversely related to the risk of future hypertension (Blair et al. 1984). Several studies have shown that cardiorespiratory fitness level mitigates the increases in systolic blood pressures (Dishman, Jackson, and Nakamura 2002; Dishman et al. 2003; Jackson and Dishman 2002) during the cold pressor among women but not men and suggest that fitness is associated with altered vascular responses (Jackson and Dishman 2002) or either blunted sympathetic, or augmented parasympathetic, nervous system responses during some types of stress.

Though there are several potential mechanisms whereby exercise might help reduce or prevent high blood pressure, it is not yet clear which of those mechanisms are most reliably affected by physical activity or whether the same mechanisms that reduce blood pressure in hypertensive people also prevent hypertension in people with normal blood pressure.

Summary of the Evidence

Longitudinal and cross-sectional studies have demonstrated the protective effects of exercise training and physical fitness on the primary and secondary prevention of hypertension. Those effects typically are independent of age and body mass. However, diet was not well controlled in many studies, mainly because of the impracticality of measuring diet in population studies that last many years. Also, population studies have not provided enough evidence to draw conclusions about whether there is a dose–response relationship between physical activity and primary prevention of hypertension. Often, only one level of physical fitness or physical activity was reported. Clinical studies of treatment of mild

hypertension have suggested an inverse relationship between intensity of exercise, expressed as a percentage of $\dot{V}O_2max$, and reduced blood pressure after exercise training. Reductions in systolic and diastolic pressure were more reliable when the intensity of the exercise was below about 75% of aerobic power. Reductions in diastolic pressure were larger when the length of the training program was longer. Some experimental studies do not show a positive effect of exercise training on blood pressure (Blumenthal, Siegel, and Appelbaum 1991; Gilders, Voner, and Dudley 1989). However, lack of an antihypertensive effect of exercise does not necessarily imply lack of a preventive effect. On balance, it appears that regular physical activity of moderate intensity offers some protection against primary hypertension (American College of Sports Medicine 1993). This type of exercise training should be considered one of the nonpharmacologic methods for prevention of hypertension.

Summary

On balance, epidemiologic and clinical studies have shown that regular physical activity has potential for reducing or preventing mild hypertension. Clinical studies have the advantage of experimental control, but it is difficult to separate the independent effects of physical activity from those of dietary and weight changes in many studies, especially as hypertension, hyperlipidemia, and obesity are intricately related to each other. Also, it is virtually impossible to prevent fat loss during increased physical activity without increasing caloric intake, which can influence hypertension and hyperlipidemia if micronutrients also change with the altered food intake. Nonetheless, many studies have indicated that much of the benefit of moderate physical activity appears sufficiently independent, consistent, temporally logical, and biologically plausible to support the current public health position that physical activity represents an effective adjuvant in the prevention and treatment of hypertension. At present, evidence does not support a linear dose–response gradient for typical middle-aged or older adults who have been sedentary and embark on a new physical activity program. Some emerging evidence suggests that a dose response may exist among recreational runners who perform at a level substantially above that likely to be a feasible goal for people who currently are sedentary, who constitute a large part of the population of the United States and other countries. Randomized controlled trials of exercise training among people diagnosed with stage 1 hypertension show an average reduction in resting systolic blood pressure of about 7 mmHg for systolic blood pressure and 6 mmHg for diastolic blood pressure (Fagard 2001). Reductions of this magnitude are potentially important for public health, as population-based evidence in the United States has estimated that a 5 mmHg reduction of systolic blood pressure would be accompanied by a 14% reduction in the population risk of stroke mortality, a 9% reduction in CHD mortality, and a 7% reduction in all-cause mortality (Whelton et al. 2002).

Bibliography

Ainsworth, B.E., N.L. Keenan, D.S. Strogatz, J.M. Garrett, and S.A. James. 1991. Physical activity and hypertension in black adults: The Pitt County study. *American Journal of Public Health* 81: 1477–1479.

American College of Sports Medicine. 1993. American College of Sports Medicine position stand: Physical activity, physical fitness, and hypertension. *Medicine and Science in Sports and Exercise* 25: i–x.

American Heart Association. 2002. *Heart and stroke statistical update*. Dallas: American Heart Association.

Anastos, K., P. Charney, R.A. Charon, E. Cohen, C.Y. Jones, C. Marte, D.M. Swiderski, M.E. Wheat, and S. Williams. 1991. Hypertension in women: What is really known? The Women's Caucus, Working Group on Women's Health of the Society of General Internal Medicine. *Annals of Internal Medicine* 115 (4): 287–293.

Arakawa, K. 1993. Antihypertensive mechanisms of exercise. *Journal of Hypertension* 11: 223–229.

Blair, S.N., N.N. Goodyear, L.W. Gibbons, and K.H. Cooper. 1984. Physical fitness and incidence of hypertension in healthy normotensive men and women. *Journal of the American Medical Association* 252: 487–490.

Blumenthal, J.A., W.C. Siegel, and M. Appelbaum. 1991. Failure of exercise to reduce blood pressure in patients with mild hypertension: Results of a randomized controlled trial. *Journal of the American Medical Association* 266 (15): 2098–2104.

Burt, V.L., J.A. Cutler, M. Higgins, M.J. Horan, D. Labarthe, P. Whelton, C. Brown, and E.J. Roccella. 1995. Trends in the prevalence, awareness, treatment, and control of hypertension in the adult US population. Data from the health examination surveys, 1960 to 1991. *Hypertension* 26: 60–69.

Burt, V.L., P. Whelton, E.J. Roccella, C. Brown, J.A. Cutler, M. Higgins, M.J. Horan, and D. Labarthe. 1995. Prevalence of hypertension in the US adult population. Results from the Third National Health and Nutrition Examination Survey, 1988-1991. *Hypertension* 25: 305–313.

Carlson, N. 1994. *Physiology and behavior*. 5th ed. Boston: Allyn & Bacon.

Carroll, D., G.D. Smith, D. Sheffield, G. Willemsen, P.M. Sweetnam, J.E. Gallacher, and P.C. Elwood. 1996. Blood pressure reactions to the cold pressor test and the prediction of future blood pressure status: Data from the Caerphilly study. *Journal of Human Hypertension* 10: 777–780.

Cleroux, J., N. Kouame, A. Nadeau, D. Coulombe, and Y. Lacourciere. 1992. Aftereffects of exercise on regional and systemic hemodynamics in hypertension. *Hypertension* 19: 183–191.

Dishman, R.K., E.M. Jackson, and Y. Nakamura. 2002. Influence of fitness and gender on blood pressure responses during active or passive stress. *Psychophysiology* 39: 568–576.

Dishman, R.K., Y. Nakamura, E.M. Jackson, and C.A. Ray. 2003. Blood pressure and muscle sympathetic nerve activity during cold pressor stress: Fitness and gender. *Psychophysiology* 40: 370–380.

Fagard, R.H. 2001. Exercise characteristics and the blood pressure response to dynamic physical training. *Medicine and Science in Sports and Exercise* 33 (Suppl. 6): S484–S492.

Fletcher, A., and C. Bulpitt. 1994. Epidemiology of hypertension in the elderly. *Journal of Hypertension* 12 (Suppl. 6): S3–S5.

Folsom, A.R., R.J. Prineas, S.A. Kaye, and R.G. Munger. 1990. Incidence of hypertension and stroke in relation to body fat distribution and other risk factors in older women. *Stroke* 21 (5): 701–706.

Furberg, C.D., J.T. Wright Jr., B.R. Davis, J.A. Cutler, M. Alderman, H. Black, W. Cushman, R. Grimm, L.J. Haywood, F. Leenen, et al. 2002. Major outcomes in high-risk hypertensive patients randomized to angiotensin-converting enzyme inhibitor or calcium channel blocker vs diuretic: The Antihypertensive and Lipid-Lowering Treatment to Prevent Heart Attack Trial (ALLHAT). *Journal of the American Medical Association* 288: 2981–2997.

Gilders, R.M., C. Voner, and G.A. Dudley. 1989. Endurance training and blood pressure in normotensive and hypertensive adults. *Medicine and Science in Sports and Exercise* 21: 629–636.

Gordon, N.F., C.B. Scott, W.J. Wilkinson, J.J. Duncan, and S.N. Blair. 1990. Exercise and mild essential hypertension: Recommendations for adults. *Sports Medicine* 10 (6): 390–404.

Haffner, S.M., E. Ferrannini, H.P. Hazuda, and M.P. Stern. 1992. Clustering of cardiovascular risk factors in confirmed prehypertensive individuals. *Hypertension* 20: 38–45.

Hagberg, J.M. 1990. Exercise, fitness, and hypertension. In *Exercise, fitness, and health: A consensus of current knowledge*, edited by C. Bouchard, R.J. Shephard, T. Stephens, J.R. Sutton, and B.D. McPherson, pp. 455–466. Champaign, IL: Human Kinetics.

Hajjar, I., and T.A. Kotchen. 2003. Trends in prevalence, awareness, treatment, and control of hypertension in the United States, 1988–2000. *Journal of the American Medical Association* 290: 199–206.

Harris, S.S., C.J. Caspersen, G.H. DeFriese, and E.H. Estes Jr. 1989. Physical activity counseling for healthy adults as a primary preventive intervention in the clinical setting: Report for the U.S. Preventive Services Task Force. *Journal of the American Medical Association* 261: 3588–3598.

Hubert, H.B., M. Feinleib, P.M. McNamara, and W.P. Castelli. 1983. Obesity as an independent risk factor for cardiovascular disease: A 26 year follow-up of participants in the Framingham Heart Study. *Circulation* 67: 968–977.

Jackson, E.M., and R.K. Dishman. 2002. Hemodynamic responses to stress among black women: Fitness and parental hypertension. *Medicine and Science in Sports and Exercise* 34: 1097–1104.

Joint National Committee on Prevention, Detection, Evaluation, and Treatment of High Blood Pressure. 2003. The seventh report of the Joint National Committee on Prevention, Detection, Evaluation, and Treatment of High Blood Pressure. U.S. Department of Health and Human Services. NIH Publication No. 03-5233. Bethesda, MD: NHLBI.

Kannel, W.B., R.J. Garrison, and A.L. Dannenberg. 1993. Secular blood pressure trends in normotensive persons: The Framingham study. *American Heart Journal* 125: 1154–1158.

Kasagi, F. 1994. Prognostic value of the cold pressor test for hypertension based on 28-year follow-up. *Hiroshima Journal of Medical Sciences* 43 (3): 93–103.

Kenney, M.J., and D.R. Seals. 1993. Postexercise hypotension: Key features, mechanisms, and clinical significance. *Hypertension* 22 (5): 653–664.

Kiyonaga, A., K. Arakawa, H. Tanaka, and M. Shindo. 1985. Blood pressure and humoral response to aerobic exercise. *Hypertension* 7: 125–131.

Kokkinos, P.F., P. Narayan, J.A. Colleran, A. Pittaras, A. Notargiacomo, D. Reda, and V. Papademetriou. 1995. Effects of regular exercise on blood pressure and left ventricular hypertrophy in African-American men with severe hypertension. *New England Journal of Medicine* 333 (22): 1462–1467.

Krotkiewski, M., K. Mandroukas, L. Sjostrom, L. Sullivan, H. Wetterqvist, and P. Bjorntorp. 1979. Effects of long-term physical training on body fat, metabolism, and blood pressure in obesity. *Metabolism* 28: 650–658.

Lyons, S.A., and R.J. Petrucelli. 1987. *Medicine: An illustrated history.* New York: Abradale Press.

Melby, C.L., D.G. Goldflies, and G.C. Hyner. 1991. Blood pressure and anthropometric differences in regularly exercising and nonexercising black adults. *Clinical and Experimental Hypertension* A13: 1233–1248.

Menkes, M.S., K.A. Matthews, D.S. Krantz, U. Lundberg, L.A. Mead, B. Qaqish, K. Liang, C.B. Thomas, and T.A. Pearson. 1989. Cardiovascular reactivity to the cold pressor test as a predictor of hypertension. *Hypertension* 14: 524–530.

Moser, M. 1997. Evolution of the treatment of hypertension from the 1940s to JNC V. *American Journal of Hypertension* 10: 2S–8S.

National Center for Health Statistics. 1997. *Health: United States, 1996.* Hyattsville, MD: U.S. Public Health Service.

National Center for Health Statistics. 1995. *National Ambulatory Medical Care Survey summaries: 1995. Advance data from vital health statistics.* Publication No. 286. Hyattsville, MD: National Center for Health Statistics.

Nelson, C.R., and D.A. Knapp. 2000. Trends in antihypertensive drug therapy of ambulatory patients by US office-based physicians. *Hypertension* 36: 600–603.

Paffenbarger, R.S. Jr. 1982. Energy imbalance and hypertension risk. In *Diet and exercise: Synergisms in health maintenance,* edited by P.L. White and T. Mondeika, pp. 115–125. Chicago: American Medical Association.

Paffenbarger, R.S. Jr., D.L. Jung, R.W. Leung, and R.T. Hyde. 1991. Physical activity and hypertension: An epidemiological view. *Annals of Medicine* 23: 319–327.

Paffenbarger, R.S. Jr., and I.M. Lee. 1997. Intensity of physical activity related to incidence of hypertension and all-cause mortality: An epidemiological view. *Blood Pressure Monitoring* 2 (3): 115–123.

Paffenbarger, R.S. Jr., M.C. Thorne, and A.L. Wing. 1968. Chronic disease in former college students: VIII. Charac-teristics in youth predisposing to hypertension in later years. *American Journal of Epidemiology* 88: 25–32.

Paffenbarger, R.S., A.L. Wing, R.T. Hyde, and D.L. Jung. 1983. Physical activity and incidence of hypertension in college alumni. *American Journal of Epidemiology* 117: 245–257.

Pickering, T.G. 1994. Hypertension in blacks. *Current Opinion in Nephrology and Hypertension* 3: 207–212.

Reaven, G.M. 1988. Role of insulin resistance in human disease. *Diabetes* 37: 1595–1607.

———. 1995. Are insulin resistance and/or compensatory hyperinsulinemia involved in the etiology and clinical course of patients with hypertension? *International Journal of Obesity* 19 (Suppl. 1): S2–S5.

Reaven, P.D., E. Barrett-Conner, and S. Edelstein. 1991. Relation between leisure-time physical activity and blood pressure in older women. *Circulation* 83: 559–565.

Rosenthal, M., W.L. Haskell, R. Solomon, A. Widstrom, and G.M. Reaven. 1983. Demonstration of a relationship between level of physical training and insulin stimulated glucose utilization in normal humans. *Diabetes* 32: 408–411.

Ruskin, A. 1956. *Classics in arterial hypertension.* Springfield, IL: Charles C Thomas.

Stamler, J., R. Stamler, and J.D. Neaton. 1993. Blood pressure, systolic and diastolic, and cardiovascular risks: U.S. population data. *Archives of Internal Medicine* 153: 598–615.

Stamler, R., J. Stamler, F.C. Gosch, J. Civinelli, J. Fishman, P. McKeever, A. McDonald, and A.R. Dyer. 1989. Primary prevention of hypertension by nutritional hygienic means: Final report of a randomized clinical trial. *Journal of the American Medical Association* 262: 1801–1807.

Tanabe, Y., H. Urata, A. Kiyonaga, M. Ikeda, H. Tanaka, M. Shindo, and K. Arakawa. 1989. Changes in serum concentrations of taurine and other amino acids in clinical antihypertensive exercise therapy. *Clinical and Experimental Hypertension* A11: 149–165.

Wain, H. 1970. *A history of medicine.* Springfield, IL: Charles C Thomas.

Weir, M.R. 1991. Impact of age, race, and obesity on hypertensive mechanisms and therapy. *American Journal of Medicine* 90 (Suppl. 5A): 3S–14S.

Whelton, P.K., J. He, L.J. Appel, J.A. Cutler, S. Havas, T.A. Kotchen, E.J. Roccella, R. Stout, C. Vallbona, M.C. Winston, and J. Karimbakas. 2002. Primary prevention of hypertension: Clinical and public health advisory from The National High Blood Pressure Education Program. *Journal of the American Medical Association* 288: 1882–1888.

Wolz, M., J. Cutler, E.J. Roccella, F. Rohde, T. Thom, and V. Burt. 2000. Statement from the National High Blood Pressure Education Program: Prevalence of hypertension. *American Journal of Hypertension* 13: 103–104.

Web Site

www.nhlbi.nih.gov/health/prof/heart/index.htm. Cardiovascular disease information for health professionals provided by the National Heart, Lung, and Blood Institute of the National Institutes of Health.

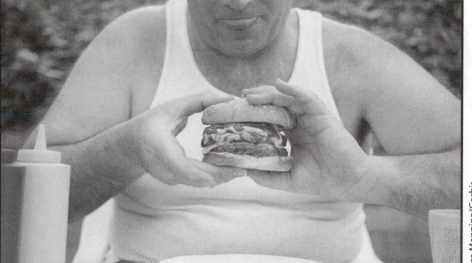

© Lawrence Manning/Corbis

Physical Activity and Hyperlipidemia

Their heart is as fat as grease.

—*Psalms 119:70*

Cholesterol is a waxy substance found in all cell membranes, including those in the brain, nerves, muscle, skin, liver, intestines, and heart. Small amounts of cholesterol are needed to produce many hormones, vitamin D, and the bile acids that help digest fat. Too much cholesterol in the blood contributes to atherosclerosis, the disease process that hardens and blocks arteries and leads to CHD and ischemic stroke. **Hypercholesterolemia** commonly refers to levels of total serum cholesterol that exceed the population average of 200 mg/dl among adults. After describing hyperlipidemia and its impact on public health, this chapter presents the evidence that physical activity is associated with lowered blood lipids, decreased **low-density lipoprotein cholesterol** (**LDL-C,** the "bad" cholesterol), and increased **high-density lipoprotein cholesterol** (**HDL-C,** the "good" cholesterol), changes that can help explain part of the protective effect that physical activity confers against cardiovascular disease and mortality.

Total Cholesterol and CHD Risk: Framingham Heart Study	
Cholesterol (mg/dl)	**Relative risk**
300	3.0
260	2.0
235	1.4 (average level of CHD cases)
225	1.0 (average)
220	0.95 (average level of people without CHD)
200	0.90
185	0.80
150	Likely protection threshold against CHD

••• *An estimated 102.3 million American adults have total blood cholesterol levels of 200 mg/dl and higher, which is above desirable levels. Of these, 41.3 million have levels of 240 mg/dl or higher, which is considered high risk for heart disease (American Heart Association 2002).*

Lipoprotein fractions, which transport cholesterol, are better predictors of CHD risk. A low level of HDL-C ($\leq$40 mg/dl) is a major risk factor for CHD; the incidence of CHD is about 18% among people having an HDL-C level below 25 mg/dl. Average levels of HDL-C are 40 to 50 mg/dl in men and 50 to 60 mg/dl in women. As a general rule, a 1% change from average in HDL-C is accompanied by about a 3% change in CHD risk, but a high ratio of total serum cholesterol to HDL-C is a better predictor of increased risk than is either component alone.

HDL and CHD Risk: Framingham Heart Study

HDL (mg/dl)	RELATIVE RISK	
	Men	Women
25	2.00	—
30	1.80	—
35	1.50	—
40	1.22	1.94
45	1.00	1.55
50	0.82	1.25
55	0.67	1.00
60	0.55	0.80
65	0.45	0.64
70	—	0.52
75	Protection threshold against CHD?	

High levels of LDL-C (>160 mg/dl) and triglycerides (>200 mg/dl) also are associated with a high risk of CHD. Generally, an LDL-C level less than 130 mg/dl is predictive of a total cholesterol of less than 200 mg/dl and is normal, LDL-C levels of 130 to 159 mg/dl are considered borderline risk, and levels greater than 160 mg/dl are predictive

HDL Ratios and CHD Risk: Framingham Heart Study

RR	Total/HDL	LDL/HDL
MEN		
0.50	3.43	1.00
1.00	4.97	3.55
2.00	9.55	6.35
3.00	24.00	8.00
WOMEN		
0.50	3.27	1.47
1.00	4.44	3.22
2.00	7.05	5.00
3.00	11.04	6.14

of a total cholesterol greater than 240 mg/dl and are regarded as high risk. High blood levels of triglycerides elevate the risk of CHD in men by 32% and women by 76% independently of HDL-C levels (Hokanson and Austin 1996). The incidence of CHD is about 12.5% among individuals with triglyceride levels above 145 mg/dl. Table 7.1 gives guidelines for determining hyperlipidemia from the National Cholesterol Education Program.

TABLE 7.1 NATIONAL CHOLESTEROL EDUCATION PROGRAM GUIDELINES FOR HYPERCHOLESTEROLEMIA

Total cholesterol (mg/dl):
Optimal < 200; borderline high 200–239; high $\geq$ 240

LDL-C (mg/dl):
Optimal < 100; near optimal 100–129; borderline high 130–159; high 160–189; very high $\geq$ 190

Triglycerides (mg/dl):
Normal < 150; borderline high 150–199; high 200–499; very high $\geq$ 500

HDL-C (mg/dl):
Low < 40; high > 60

Values are based on blood levels after fasting.

Third Report of the National Cholesterol Education Program Expert Panel on Detection, Evaluation, and Treatment of High Blood Cholesterol in Adults (Adult Treatment Panel III). National Cholesterol Education Program; National Heart, Lung, and Blood Institute; National Institutes of Health. NIH Publication No. 01-3670. May 2001.

Magnitude of the Problem

Estimates from NHANES III and the National Center for Health Statistics show that about 41 million U.S. adults have high CHD and stroke risk because they have total cholesterol levels of 240 mg/dl or higher. Another 61 million have borderline high levels between 200 and 240. Ten percent of youths 12 to 19 years of age have levels over 200 mg/dl. About 18% of men and 20% of white Americans 20 to 74 years old have levels of 240 mg/dl or higher. Compared with whites, high cholesterol is about 10% to 15% less prevalent among African Americans and Mexican Americans and about 50% to 60% less prevalent among Native Americans. Nonetheless, those ethnic groups have elevated CHD risk from other factors (American Heart Association 2002).

Figures 7.1 and 7.2 show the prevalence rates of high LDL-C and low HDL-C among Americans ages 20 and older by sex and selected racial and ethnic groups.

What Are Lipoproteins?

Cholesterol and other fats (i.e., lipids) are not soluble in water, so they are carried in the blood by binding with proteins. Such lipoproteins include triglycerides, **chylomicrons,** LDL, and HDL; they differ in their relative composition of cholesterol, lipids, **phospholipids,** and proteins. They also differ in size and density such that higher concentrations of lipids are found

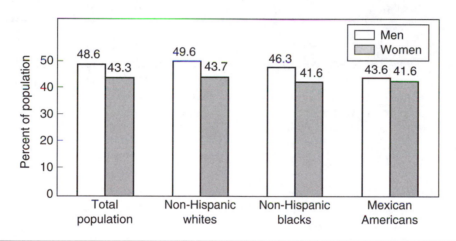

Figure 7.1   Age-adjusted prevalence of Americans age 20 and older with LDL cholesterol of 130 mg/dl or higher by race/ethnicity and sex. United States: 1988–1994.

American Heart Association 2002.

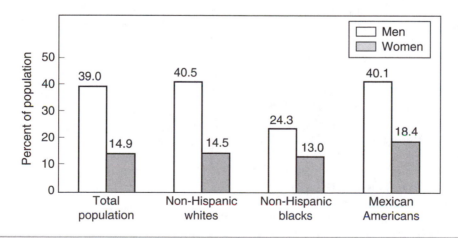

Figure 7.2   Age-adjusted prevalence of Americans age 20 and older with HDL cholesterol of 40 mg/dl or lower by race/ethnicity and sex. United States: 1988–1994.

American Heart Association 2002.

TABLE 7.2 CHARACTERISTICS OF LIPOPROTEINS				
Characteristic	HDL	LDL	VLDL	Chylomicrons
Density (g/ml)	1.21–1.06	1.06–1.006	1.006–0.95	<0.95
Size (Å)	50–100	215–220	300–800	400–10,000
Lipid (% of total)	~50%	~75%	~90%	~98%
Triglyceride	4–10	10	50–70	85–95
Cholesterol	25–35	45–60	10–20	2–10
Phospholipid	30–50	20–30	10–20	4–12
Major apoprotein	A-I, A-II	B	B, C-III, E	A-I, A-II, E
Source: Major	Intestine	Plasma	Liver	Intestine
Minor	Liver		Intestine	

in lipoprotein molecules that are larger and less dense (table 7.2).

Triglyceride is the major form of biological fat; it is formed when a glycerol molecule is esterified by three fatty acid molecules. (An ester is formed by removing water between the hydroxyl groups of an alcohol and an acid.) Dietary triglycerides make up about 98% of chylomicrons, which are formed in the intestines and enter the blood circulation via the lymphatic duct. Triglycerides are hydrolyzed (i.e., split by water) into glycerol and fatty acids by the enzyme **lipoprotein lipase (LPL)** for use in cellular oxidative respiration (e.g., as fuel during muscle contraction). LPL is found in the capillary endothelium of the heart, skeletal muscle, and adipose tissue. Its **hydrolysis** (the splitting of a compound with water) of triglycerides helps to clear chylomicrons from blood circulation. Chylomicron remnants that remain after hydrolysis can be atherogenic, but LPL can reduce the adhesion of chylomicron remnants to endothelial cells and promote their re-esterification in the liver. **Very low density lipoprotein cholesterol (VLDL-C)** is mainly responsible for the transport of nonhydrolyzed triglycerides synthesized in liver cells to adipose cells for storage. After depositing some of its triglycerides in adipose cells, VLDL cholesterol is converted into LDL cholesterol (Tortora and Grabowski 1993). LDL cholesterol is the main transporter of cholesterol in the blood. HDL-C removes cholesterol from extrahepatic (outside the liver) tissue by the process of **reverse cholesterol transport.** Reverse transport involves

esterification and storage of cholesterol in the core of the HDL molecule by the enzyme **lecithin: cholesterol acyltransferase (LCAT),** which is regulated by a protein named apolipoprotein A-1 (or apo A-1). The transfer of cholesterol ester from newly formed HDL-C (which is designated HDL3) to LDL-C, VLDL-C, and chylomicrons in exchange for triglycerides is regulated by **cholesterol ester transfer protein (CETP).** The ultimate fate of the less dense forms, HDL2 and HDL1, is metabolism in the liver, which is regulated by **hepatic lipoprotein lipase (HPL),** or resynthesis, which is regulated by the enzyme acyl-CoA:cholesterol acyltransferase (ACAT).

Triglycerides

Triglycerides are the most abundant lipids in the human body. They consist of a glycerol molecule combined with three fatty acids. High levels of triglycerides are closely associated with hypercholesterolemia and can be used to predict VLDL levels by assuming that VLDL = triglycerides/5. Levels of VLDL exceeding 40 mg/dl indicate lipoproteinemia. Levels of LDL-C can be estimated using Friedewald's equation: LDL-C = Total cholesterol − HDL − VLDL.

HDL Structure and Function

High-density lipoprotein cholesterol (HDL-C) consists of a family of molecules that range in density from approximately 1.06 to 1.21 g/ml. HDL-C has a high phospholipid content relative to other lipoproteins in the blood. The majority of HDL-C phospholipid is **lecithin,** which yields two fatty acid molecules after hydrolysis. HDL-C also has the largest surface area, about 80% greater than other lipoproteins in the blood. HDL-C molecules are classified according to increasing density into three subclasses or fractions: HDL1, HDL2, and HDL3 (Eisenberg 1984). The most abundant fractions are HDL2 and HDL3. There are several major differences between the HDL-C fractions (Eisenberg 1984). First, the core diameter of the particle increases from HDL3 to HDL1. The core of HDL1 is about 50% larger than HDL3, and the cholesterol ester content and triglyceride content of HDL1 is three to four times greater than HDL3. HDL2 has about twice the surface area of HDL3 and 50% more protein (**apoproteins** [apo] A, C, and E) than HDL3. HDL1 has less protein than HDL2, but the protein is of only one class, apo E. HDL1 has the most apo E of any HDL fraction.

HDL-C Formation

There are three main sources of new HDL-C molecules: (1) secretion from the liver or small intestine; (2) lipid and protein fragments from the hydrolysis of other lipoproteins rich in triglycerides, such as VLDL and chylomicrons; and (3) from chemical interactions between phospholipids and apoproteins. New HDL-C molecules secreted by the liver are disk shaped (Hamilton et al. 1976) and contain surface apo E, C, and A-1 proteins, in that order of density (Marsh 1976). In contrast, in HDL-C in the blood, apo A-1 is most predominant and apo E is least predominant. The discrepancy probably results from the actions of the enzyme LCAT on new HDL-C molecules (Eisenberg 1984). In contrast to the liver, the intestine secretes new HDL-C molecules that have high apo A-1.

A second source of new HDL-C is from hydrolyzed chylomicrons and VLDL (Shepherd and Packard 1989; Winkler and Marsh 1989). The molecules that are shed during lipolysis from the surface of chylomicrons and VLDL contain apo A-1, apo C, phospholipids, and free cholesterol (Eisenberg 1976; Tall and Small 1978) and interact with LCAT.

The third source of new HDL-C is the binding of unbound apoproteins, especially apo A-1, and phospholipids in the plasma (Eisenberg 1984). Apo A-1 is the key in all three types of new HDL-C formation. Both the liver and intestine secrete

apo A-1 at about the same rate (Wu and Windmueller 1979). Apo A-1 is the main coenzyme for LCAT reactions and is essential for the formation of other HDL-C fractions. The pool of free, secreted apo A-1 can be transformed into new HDL-C, excreted in urine, or absorbed into low-density lipoproteins (Eisenberg 1984). Apo A-1 also regulates the removal of excess cholesterol from tissues outside the liver (Barbaras et al. 1986; Mahlberg and Rothblat 1992).

HDL3 Formation

Formation of a spherical HDL3 molecule from new HDL-C depends on the activity of LCAT (Norum 1984). In the plasma, LCAT binds to the new HDL-C and a lower-density lipoprotein and catalyzes the esterification of free cholesterol. The esterification involves the transfer of a free fatty acid from a phospholipid (lecithin) located on the shell of an HDL-C molecule to another cholesterol molecule (Norum 1984). The esterified cholesterol is hydrophobic (i.e., repels water molecules) and moves to the core of the HDL-C molecule. The esterified cholesterol leaves a gap, or space, on the surface of the HDL-C molecule, which is filled by cholesterol from cell membranes, such as endothelial cells, or from other lipoproteins (Tall and Small 1978; Eisenberg 1984; Tall 1990). The transfer of cholesterol from other lipoproteins or cell surfaces to HDL-C is the first part of the reverse cholesterol transport mediated by HDL-C. Over time, the core of the new HDL-C enlarges and the molecule becomes HDL3.

HDL2 Formation

As HDL3 accumulates cholesterol esters, its diameter increases and its density decreases. The addition of esterified cholesterol to the core of HDL3 also increases the surface region of HDL3, thus being transformed to HDL2. As the surface region of the HDL-C increases, it is able to accept more apoproteins, in particular, apo A-1.

An important characteristic of HDL2 is the capacity to transfer cholesterol ester to LDL-C directly (Eisenberg 1984) or to exchange it for triglycerides in VLDL-C and chylomicrons through the action of CETP (Tall 1986). The CETP reaction depends on the apoproteins present on the surface of the lipoproteins. The magnitude of the transfer, though, is determined by the relative proportions of cholesterol ester and triglyceride in the lipoproteins and is proportional to the surface area of the lipoproteins (Deckelbaum et al.

1982). The exchange of cholesterol ester for triglyceride by the CETP reaction reduces the HDL2 core content of cholesterol. After more CETP and LCAT reactions, HDL2 is transformed into a larger, less dense HDL1 molecule, which contains mainly triglycerides and apo E absorbed from VLDL and chylomicrons (figure 7.3; Daerr and Greten 1982).

Risk Factors

Only 1 in 500 people has the genetic form of hypercholesterolemia known as the heterozygous familial type. Hence, almost everyone has some control over whether blood cholesterol or its components rise to the level that exaggerates risk for CHD. Though nearly 70% of the variation in blood cholesterol level is explained by endogenous production by the liver, dietary intake of cholesterol from meats, poultry, fish, seafood, and dairy products explains most of the fluctuation in each person's serum cholesterol level. Fruits, vegetables, grains, nuts, and seeds have no cholesterol. Though the national goal for dietary cholesterol is less than 300 mg per day, the

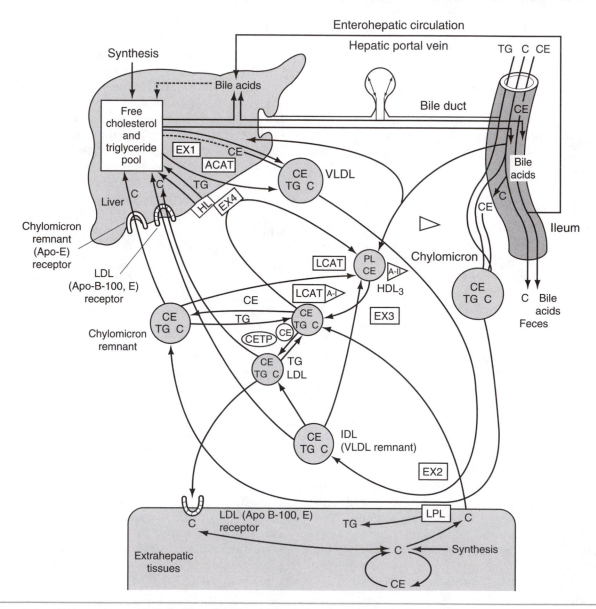

Figure 7.3 Lipoprotein metabolism. Plausible sites whereby exercise might increase HDL-C levels are noted for LCAT and HPL activity at the liver (EX1 and EX4); LCAT, CETP, and apoproteins regulating reverse transport by HDL-C (EX3); and the activity of LPL (EX2).

Reprinted, by permission, from J.L. Durstine and W.L. Haskell, 1994, "Effects of exercise training on plasma lipids and lipoproteins," *Exercise and Sport Sciences Reviews* 22: 477-521, with adaptation, by permission, from Murray et al., 1990, *Harper's Biochemistry*, 22nd ed. (New York: Appleton & Lange), 255.

average American daily intake is 450 mg among men and 320 mg among women.

Cigarette smoking, diabetes mellitus, obesity, alcohol, androgenic and anti-inflammatory steroids, and emotional stress also negatively influence blood lipid levels, especially increasing triglyceride and LDL-C levels (table 7.3). Obesity and cigarette smoking reduce HDL-C. Total cholesterol, LDL-C, and triglyceride levels are elevated in people with diabetes mellitus, but levels tend to normalize when blood glucose levels are controlled (Conti and Tonnessen 1992).

TABLE 7.3	WHAT INFLUENCES LIPOPROTEINS?
Sex	Total is lower and HDL-C is higher in pre-menopausal women.
Age	Total increases and HDL decreases with age.
% Body fat	Total and LDL-C are higher, but HDL-C is lower, among overweight and obese people.
Diet	Total, LDL-C, and triglycerides are higher with fat and cholesterol intake.
Diabetes	Total, LDL-C, and triglycerides are elevated, but normalized when glucose is controlled.
Alcohol	Moderate use increases HDL-C.
Smoking	HDL-C decreases.
Steroids	HDL-C decreases.
Stress	Total increases and HDL-C decreases.
Exercise	HDL-C increases and triglycerides decrease.

Sex and Estrogen

Before menopause, women usually have total cholesterol levels that are lower than those of men of the same age. As women and men get older, until about 60 to 65 years of age, their blood cholesterol levels rise. In women, menopause often causes an increase in LDL cholesterol and a decrease in HDL cholesterol, and after the age of 50, women often have higher total cholesterol levels than men of the same age. Some women may benefit from hormone replacement therapy (also called estrogen replacement therapy) after menopause because estrogen lowers LDL and raises HDL.

Alcohol Use

Alcohol intake increases HDL cholesterol but does not lower LDL cholesterol. However, drinking too much alcohol can damage the liver and heart muscle and lead to high blood pressure and elevated triglycerides, so alcoholic beverages should not be used as a way to prevent heart disease.

••• *Studies among people with heart disease have shown that lowering blood cholesterol can reduce the risk of dying from heart disease, having a nonfatal heart attack, and needing bypass surgery or angioplasty.*

Drug Treatment

When proper diet, regular physical activity, and weight loss aren't sufficient to lower high blood lipids, cholesterol drugs are the treatment of choice. This is especially the case when the following CHD risk factors are present:

- Age: 45 years or older for men, 55 years or older (or after menopause without estrogen replacement therapy) for women
- Family history: CHD before age 55 in a father, a brother, or a son or before age 65 in a mother, a sister, or a daughter
- Tobacco smoking or living or working every day with people who smoke
- Hypertension: Blood pressure of 140/90 mmHg or higher
- HDL-C lower than 40 mg/dl
- Diabetes: Fasting blood sugar level of 126 mg/dl or higher

The drugs commonly used to lower LDL-C levels include the **statin** drugs (e.g., lovastatin, pravastatin, and simvastatin), which lower LDL levels by inhibiting an enzyme named HMG CoA reductase, and bile acid sequestrants (e.g., cholestyramine, colestipol), or nicotinic acid (i.e., niacin), which is preferred for patients with triglycerides over 250 mg/dl because bile acid sequestrants can elevate triglycerides. Other popular drugs used to lower triglycerides include gemfibrozil, probucol, and clofibrate. Combination therapy is often used in patients with extreme hyperlipidemia, but this requires careful monitoring because of the increased occurrence of side effects such as constipation, stomach pain, and cramping (National Heart, Lung, and Blood Institute 2002).

Cholesterol Therapy

LDL cholesterol	Level for drug consideration	Goal of therapy
No CHD and fewer than 2 CHD risk factors	190 mg/dl or higher*	Less than 130 mg/dl
No CHD but 2 or more CHD risk factors	160 mg/dl or higher*	Less than 130 mg/dl
Diagnosis of CHD	130 mg/dl or higher**	100 mg/dl or less

* In men less than 35 years old and premenopausal women with levels of 190 to 219 mg/dl, drug therapy should be delayed except in high-risk patients (e.g., those with diabetes).

**In CHD patients with levels of 100 to 129 mg/dl, drug treatment depends on the clinical judgment of the physician.

Drug therapy may not be appropriate for some patients who meet the preceding criteria, including the elderly.

National Cholesterol Education Program (National Heart, Lung, and Blood Institute 2002).

••• *Studies among people without heart disease have shown that lowering blood cholesterol can reduce the risk of developing heart disease, including heart attacks and deaths related to heart disease. This is true for those with high blood cholesterol levels and even for those with average levels.*

Hyperlipidemia Etiology

Dietary intake of cholesterol and fat has a strong influence on blood levels of cholesterol and lipids, even when a person's synthesis and metabolism of lipoproteins are normal. Cholesterol-lowering drugs are designed to alter various aspects of the synthesis and metabolism of lipoproteins. Likewise, it is believed that regular physical activity has metabolic effects, in addition to promoting weight loss, that can positively affect the regulatory physiology of lipid and cholesterol. The most consistent and fully studied effects of regular exercise on cholesterol fractions are a decrease in triglycerides and an increase in HDL-C, with a somewhat smaller lowering of LDL-C. To help understand how those effects might be biologically plausible, it is necessary to understand the basic physiology of lipoproteins, especially the metabolism of HDL-C.

••• *A 10% decrease in total blood cholesterol levels may result in an estimated 30% reduction in the incidence of coronary heart disease.*

The risk of heart attack in both men and women overall is highest at lower HDL-C levels and higher total blood cholesterol levels. However, people with lower levels of HDL-C (37 mg/dl or lower in men and 47 mg/dl or lower in women) are at a high risk, regardless of their total blood cholesterol levels. Conversely, those with high levels of total blood cholesterol have a lower risk of heart attack when they also have higher levels of HDL-C (53 mg/dl or greater in men and 67 mg/dl or greater in women).

HDL-C Metabolism

Though hydrolysis of HDL-C is regulated by hepatic lipase activity, the concentration of HDL2 in plasma is regulated by lipoprotein lipase (LPL). The primary fate of HDL2 is the hydrolysis of its triglyceride and phospholipid content by hepatic lipase (Eisenberg 1984; Shepherd and Packard 1989; Durstine and Haskell 1994). The net effect of hepatic lipase is the conversion of HDL2 back to HDL-C in the liver. Increased activity of LPL increases the hydrolysis of VLDL and chylomicrons, increasing the formation of lower-density lipoprotein remnants, which can be cleared by the liver or can yield cholesterol more easily to HDL-C (Eisenberg 1984; Eisenberg and Deckelbaum 1989). LCAT and LPL activity may exert a protective effect against atherosclerosis, beyond that of increasing HDL2 molecules, by reducing blood levels of triglycerides and cholesterol. LPL also can attach to chylomicron remnants that remain after triglycerides are hydrolyzed to fatty acids for cell fuel and aid the uptake of these remnants by the liver. This is important because chylomicron remnants can penetrate endothelial cells and contribute to atherogenesis, just as cholesterol fragments can.

The protective effect of decreased hepatic lipase activity against atherosclerosis is more difficult to understand. Hepatic lipase hydrolyzes triglyceride and phospholipid from HDL2 and returns an HDL3 molecule back into the circulation. In addition, hepatic lipase may also remove HDL-C from the circulation via the **phospholipase** activity of hepatic lipase (Tall 1990). Decreasing hepatic lipase activity causes an increase in HDL2 molecules, but an elevated HDL2 fraction alone would not necessarily exert a protective effect against atherosclerosis. However, apo A-1 is required for the uptake of cholesterol by HDL-C (Barbaras et al. 1986; Mahlberg and Rothblat 1992). Hepatic lipase causes the release of apo A-1 (Melchior et al. 1994). Thus, decreasing hepatic lipase activity can enhance the capacity of HDL-C to extract cholesterol from extrahepatic tissue and from other lipoproteins. Also, a reduction in hepatic lipase reduces hydrolysis of HDL2, so HDL2 molecules can become larger HDL1 molecules, which contain primarily apo E. HDL1 molecules, then, would be cleared by apo B-100/E or apo E receptors in the liver.

> ••• *For sedentary people, it appears that moderate physical activity, such as brisk walking 8 to 15 miles a week for six to nine months, increases HDL levels and lowers triglyceride levels in the blood. Among recreational runners (i.e., those who run 15–60 miles, or 24–97 km, a week), HDL levels are higher in those who run faster, regardless of distance.*

Physical Activity and Lipoprotein Levels: The Evidence

Most of the studies of physical activity and lipoproteins done so far, including the earliest in 1957, were clinical studies of exercise training among people with normal or borderline high cholesterol levels. Those studies mainly involved white men and have limited application to the general population of people at risk for CHD. Though prospective cohort studies have not yet been reported, several observational, population-based studies and about 30 randomized controlled trials have been published in the past 15 years. Summaries of some of these studies and some specific examples follow.

Cross-Sectional Clinical and Population-Based Studies

In cross-sectional comparisons of small, clinical samples, male and female endurance athletes of the same age had 20% to 30% higher levels of HDL-C than untrained peers, and a dose–response relationship was seen between more physical activity and greater HDL-C (Durstine and Haskell 1994). However, moderate intensities of exercise were not as effective for increasing HDL-C in young and middle-aged women as in men.

Weekly running distance was associated with HDL-C and other blood lipid levels among nearly

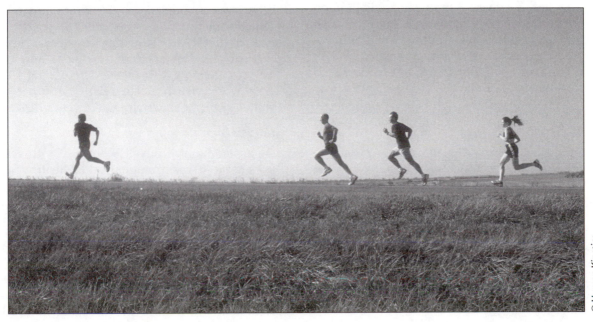

© Human Kinetics

3,000 healthy, nonsmoking men ages 30 to 64 years (Kokkinos et al. 1995). After adjustments for BMI and alcohol consumption, there was an increase in HDL-C of about 0.3 mg/dl for each mile run. LDL-C and triglyceride levels were positively associated with BMI and inversely correlated with the distance run per week, the frequency of exercise per week, and the duration of the exercise sessions. Those who ran 11 to 14 miles (17.7–22.5 km) per week had 11% higher HDL-C and 8% lower LDL-C compared with nonrunners. Higher HDL-C levels were observed among men who ran 7 to 14 miles (11.3–22.5 km) per week at paces of 10 to 11 min per mile (about 6–7 min/km).

Marathon Study

Leisure-time physical activity was quantified from self-reports of the past year in 537 healthy men ages 20 to 60 years (Marrugat et al. 1996). After adjustments for age, alcohol consumption, smoking, and BMI, each 100 kcal expended per day in leisure-time physical activity at an intensity greater than 7 kcal/min during the previous year was associated with an increase of 2.09 mg/dl (0.054 mmol/L) in HDL-C. Intensities of 9.5 to 12 kcal/min were associated with lower levels of total cholesterol, non-HDL cholesterol, and triglycerides. Better physical fitness was associated with physical activities requiring at least 5 kcal/min. There was a threshold in the intensity of exercise associated with serum lipid profile (7 kcal/min) and physical fitness (5 kcal/min).

Boston Area Health Study

A case–control study of 340 patients (266 men, 74 women) who survived a first myocardial infarction were matched with 340 controls by sex, age, and place of residence (O'Connor et al. 1995). Total energy expenditure was not associated with blood lipids or apolipoproteins, but moderate to vigorous participation in recreational sports was directly related to HDL-C and HDL2.

Strong Heart Study

Total physical activity (leisure plus occupational) and blood lipoproteins were studied in about 4,500 American Indian men and women ages 45 to 74 years who were selected from 13 communities in Arizona, Oklahoma, and the Dakotas (Yurgalevitch et al. 1998). Among diabetic men and nondiabetic men and women, physical activity was associated positively with levels of apo A-1, after controlling for several other factors, such as age, BMI, smoking, alcohol use, and waist-to-hip ratio.

U.S. Work-Site Study

The association of strength training and blood lipids was examined among 8,500 working men with a mean age of 40 years (Tucker and Silvester 1996). After adjustment for smoking, alcohol use, BMI, age, and other types of physical activity, the odds ratio of hypercholesterolemia among men who spent 4 to 7 h each week strength training was half that observed in nonlifters. Spending less than 4 h a week in strength training conferred no protection against high cholesterol levels.

Aerobics Center Longitudinal Study

In contrast, another study suggested that strength is associated with unfavorable lipid profiles. A cross-sectional analysis in the Aerobics Center Longitudinal Study examined the association between muscular strength and serum lipid and lipoprotein status in a group of 1,193 women and 5,460 men (Kohl et al. 1992). After adjustments for age, body composition, and cardiovascular fitness, there was no association between muscular strength and total cholesterol or LDL-C for either men or women. However, triglycerides were higher in stronger men, who also had lower HDL-C. The findings suggest that strength is associated with a less favorable lipid profile. However, most of the people studied were not involved in regular resistance training, so other unknown factors common to inherent muscular strength and lipids, or other factors not controlled in the study, probably explain the findings.

Postmenopausal Women

The association between physical activity and HDL-C was examined in 255 white postmenopausal women with a mean age of 58 years (Cauley et al. 1986). After adjusting for several factors, physical activity was independently and positively associated with higher HDL-C and HDL2. There was a nearly linear relationship between frequency of sport activity and level of HDL2.

Spanish Men

The association of physical activity with serum apo A protein was examined in 332 healthy Spanish men ages 20 to 60 years (Martin et al. 1999). Among men with a family history of CHD, the odds of having above-average levels of apo A of men who expended more than 300 kcal each day in leisure physical activity was less than 15% that of men who expended less than 300 kcal a day. The results suggest that regular daily physical activity is helpful for controlling apo A protein levels in men who have a family history of CHD.

Exercise Training and Lipoprotein Levels: The Evidence

Clinical studies have examined the effects of exercise training on cholesterol and blood lipid levels from as early as 1957. Since then, around half of the more than 70 studies of men and women have reported an association of aerobic or resistance exercise with decreased triglycerides and increased HDL-C. Results have generally been more favorable among men, possibly because estrogen appears to influence lipid metabolism in women. Fluctuations in sex hormone levels in women during the menstrual cycle produce variations in blood lipoprotein levels that must be considered in studies on premenopausal women. The effects on LDL-C and total cholesterol have been less consistent.

A recent review examined 51 exercise training studies published since 1987 involving about 4,700 adults (60% were men) ages 18 to 80 years (mean age 47 years; Leon and Sanchez 2001). The studies lasted at least 12 weeks and consisted mainly of structured group exercise among healthy, sedentary white people; a few studies monitored lifestyle or home exercise or used resistance exercise. Twenty-eight of the studies were randomized control trials. Only nine studies involved people with high total cholesterol levels (>240 mg/dl). There were just two studies of African Americans and two studies of Asians. Generally, the exercise intensities were moderate to vigorous, with weekly energy expenditures ranging from about 500 kcal to 4,800 kcal. The most consistent outcome of physical activity, independent of dietary intervention, was a mean increase in HDL-C of about 5%. Decreases in LDL-C (about 5%) and triglycerides (about 4%) were less consistently seen, and total cholesterol was unchanged by exercise training. Those changes were independent of the age or sex of the participants and the weekly energy expenditure. Only a handful of studies used more than one intensity of exercise, so there was not enough evidence to judge whether a dose response occurred with increasing exercise intensity.

In most of the studies, diets were not manipulated, and weight loss on average was negligible (mean less than 1 kg, ranging from no loss to a 7.2-kg loss) after exercise. Fifteen studies of overweight or obese people combined exercise and dietary restriction. In these studies, weight loss ranged from 7 to 18 kg, so changes in lipoproteins in those people could have been confounded or moderated by weight loss.

Randomized Clinical Trials

The cumulative results of 31 randomized clinical trials of aerobic or resistance exercise training conducted for at least four weeks and involving over 1,800 participants with and without hyperlipidemia indicate that aerobic exercise training led to small but statistically significant decreases of about 0.10 mmol/L (3.8 mg/dl) each in total cholesterol, LDL-C, and triglycerides and an increase in HDL-C of 0.05 mmol/L (1.9 mg/dl; Halbert et al. 1999). An exercise frequency exceeding three times a week was not more beneficial. The evidence for the effects of resistance exercise training was inconclusive.

Averaging the results from studies conducted on very different types of people using different types and amounts of exercise prevents strong conclusions about the efficacy of exercise for altering blood lipids in specific circumstances. Even so, it is still informative to examine some individual studies that represent some of those differing circumstances.

Aerobic Exercise Training

The effects of endurance exercise training on plasma lipoprotein lipids were determined in 10 men aged 46 to 62 years with coronary artery disease who maintained body weight and their diets during the study (Heath et al. 1983). Training increased $\dot{V}O_2$max by 30% and HDL-C by 11%, while reducing plasma cholesterol by 8%, LDL-C by 9%, and triglycerides by 13%. Changes in LDL-C and $\dot{V}O_2$max were inversely correlated (r = –0.73), while the changes in LDL-C and HDL-C each were correlated inversely with the levels measured before training. Thus, the authors concluded that protective effects of exercise against atherogenic risk seemed to be the result of a training effect, since they correlated best with changes in $\dot{V}O_2$max and were greatest in patients who initially had low $\dot{V}O_2$max, high LDL-C, and low HDL-C levels.

Stanford, California. In a randomized study, 48 sedentary, healthy men ages 30 to 55 were assigned to a running program that lasted a year, while another 33 remained sedentary (Wood et al. 1983). The group of runners increased their cardiorespiratory fitness and lost body fat, but the changes in lipoprotein levels were not statistically different from the controls. However, the 25 men who ran an average of at least 8 miles

(12.9 km) per week had an increase in HDL-C of 4.4 mg/dl and an increase in HDL2 of 3.3 mg/dl. Increases in HDL-C and HDL2 and decreases in LDL-C were directly related to weekly running distance. Because lost body fat also was related to increased HDL-C, part of the effects of running on HDL might have been explained by fat loss.

In another Stanford study, the effects of exercise and of the National Cholesterol Education Program (NCEP) diet, which restricts fat and cholesterol, were studied in 180 postmenopausal women ages 45 to 64 years and nearly 200 men ages 30 to 64 years who had below-average levels of HDL-C (<60 mg/dl in women, <44 mg/dl in men) and elevated LDL-C (125–210 mg/dl in women, 125–190 mg/dl in men; Stefanick et al. 1998). They were randomly assigned to aerobic exercise, the NCEP diet, diet plus exercise, or a control group that received no intervention. After a year, dietary intake of fat and cholesterol, as well as body weight, decreased in both women and men in both the diet group and the diet-plus-exercise group. HDL-C, triglyceride levels, and the ratio of total cholesterol to HDL-C were not affected by diet or exercise. However, LDL-C was reduced by 14.5 mg/dl among women and 20 mg/dl among men in the diet-plus-exercise group. The diet did not change LDL-C in either women or men unless they also participated in exercise.

The effects of weight loss by dieting or by running on apo A-1, apo A-2, and HDL were studied in sedentary, moderately overweight men randomly assigned to three groups: (1) running about 10 miles (16 km) a week without reducing caloric intake, (2) eating about 350 fewer kilocalories each day, and (3) no change in eating or exercise habits (Williams et al. 1992). After one year, body weight was reduced by 7 kg in dieters and 4 kg in runners. The runners and dieters each had a decrease in HDL3 and an increase in HDL2. The runners also had increases in plasma apo A-1 levels. However, when the lipoprotein changes were adjusted for how much weight was lost, they disappeared, so the favorable effects of exercise were not independent of weight loss.

Overweight Men. Changes in total cholesterol, HDL-C, LDL-C, and triglycerides were examined in 51 sedentary, overweight men after nine months of endurance exercise training (treadmill walking, jogging, and stationary cycling) consisting of 45 min at 70% to 80% of maximal oxygen uptake three days each week (about 1,000 kcal/wk). The men had normal total cholesterol levels but were on the American Heart Association Step I Diet

to lose weight. To determine whether genetic factors influenced the outcome, the men were classified according to their isoform of the apo E regulatory protein for lipid metabolism: apo E2 (n = 6), apo E3 (n = 33), or apo E4 (n = 12). The men of all genotypes had similar age, body weight and composition, and plasma lipoprotein and lipid profiles at the beginning of the study. Men with the apo E2 genotype had a larger mean increase in plasma HDL-C and HDL2-C with exercise training than the other two groups (HDL-C was 8 mg/dl, 3 mg/dl, and 2 mg/dl for the apo E2, E3, and E4 groups, respectively; HDL2-C was 5, 1, and 1 mg/dl, respectively). That effect remained even after adjusting for body weight changes. Though based on a very small group of men, these findings suggest that the gene for apo E—which regulates uptake of LDL by extrahepatic tissues, uptake of chylomicron remnants by the liver, and, to a lesser extent, the function of HDL-C molecules—may moderate the effects of exercise training on HDL-C responses.

Premenopausal Women. Duncan, Gordon, and Scott (1991) studied 102 sedentary premenopausal women to determine the effects of 24 weeks of walking. Three groups of subjects walked the same distance five days per week, but their speeds differed; the groups walked 3 miles (4.8 km) in 36, 45, or 60 min by week 14 and thereafter. Figure 7.4 shows that aerobic fitness increased in a dose–response manner; however, increases in HDL-C were similar among the three groups and did not follow a dose-dependent pattern with increasing walking speed.

In contrast, 50 healthy middle-aged women (mean age, 50 years) were randomly assigned to 12 weeks of walking and jogging or 12 weeks of resistance exercise (Blumenthal et al. 1991). Peak oxygen uptake was increased by 18%, from 26.7 to 31.4 ml · kg^{-1} · min^{-1}, after aerobic exercise but unchanged after resistance training. Both exercise groups had small reductions in total cholesterol and HDL-C, increases in apo A-1, and no change in triglycerides. Because both premenopausal and postmenopausal women were included, it was not possible to determine whether the exercise responses were independent of reproductive hormone status.

Forty obese women (BMI = 33) ages 21 to 60 years (mean = 43) participated in a 16-week randomized control trial that combined a low-fat 1,200-kcal diet with either a structured step aerobics exercise training program or a moderate lifestyle physical activity program (weekly energy

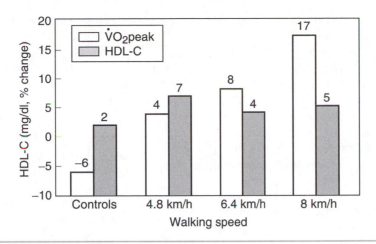

Figure 7.4　An HDL dose response? Study included premenopausal women who walked 5 days per week for 24 weeks. Adapted from Duncan, Gordon, and Scott 1991.

cost of about 1,500 kcal; Andersen et al. 1999). Changes in body weight, body composition, cardiovascular risk profiles, and physical fitness were compared after 16 weeks and one year later. Mean (± SD) 16-week weight losses were about 8 (± 4) for both groups. A year later, the aerobic group had regained 1.6 kg on average, while the lifestyle activity group regained half that amount, 0.8 (± 4.6) kg. Reductions in triglyceride (16%) and total cholesterol (10%) levels were seen after 16 weeks of the weight-loss program regardless of the type of exercise but returned to near the initial levels a year later. Both forms of exercise seemed equivalent and would have accounted for about 40% of the weight loss after 16 weeks. However because they each were combined with diet, it wasn't possible to directly determine the relative importance of exercise compared with the diet for reducing the cholesterol and triglyceride levels.

Postmenopausal Women.　Seals and colleagues (1984) reported that six months of high-intensity endurance training resulted in increased HDL-C and decreased triglyceride levels in elderly women. Other evidence suggests that estrogen replacement optimizes the effects of regular exercise on blood lipids in postmenopausal women. Lindheim and colleagues (1994) studied the effects of a six-month moderate exercise program with and without oral estrogen replacement on blood lipid and lipoprotein levels in postmenopausal women. One hundred healthy, sedentary, postmenopausal women ages 42 to 59 were randomly assigned to one of the following four groups: exercise, estrogen replacement, exercise

and estrogen replacement, and a control group that received neither estrogen nor exercise. Exercise consisted of treadmill walking or cycling for about 30 min at least three times a week. Women in the exercise group had a 5% decrease in total cholesterol and a 10% decrease in LDL-C. The exercise group had a 20% reduction in triglycerides but no change in HDL-C. However, both the sedentary and the exercising groups that got estrogen therapy had a nearly 10% increase in HDL-C levels.

African American Men With Hypertension.　Sufficiently intense exercise also can improve lipid metabolism in patients with hypertension. Thirty-six African American men ages 35 to 76 years with essential hypertension were randomly assigned to no exercise or to cycling exercise at 60% to 80% of maximum heart rate, three times per week for 16 weeks (Kokkinos et al. 1998). Peak oxygen uptake in the exercise group improved nearly 10%, but body weight was unchanged. Though changes in HDL-C among the exercisers did not exceed those in the control group, they nonetheless were greater in men who exercised at higher intensities. Ten men who exercised at 75% of maximal heart rate or higher had a 10% increase (from 42 to 46 mg/dl) in HDL-C. Thus, low- to moderate-intensity aerobic exercise might not provide a sufficient stimulus to alter blood lipid levels in African American men with severe hypertension.

HERITAGE Family Study.　Recent evidence suggests that the impact of aerobic exercise training on blood lipids is independent of changes in cardiorespiratory fitness and is more related to energy expenditure and reduced body fat (Katzmarzyk et al. 2001). Men (77 black and 218 white) and women (131 black and 224 white) ages 17 to 65 years participated in five months of endurance cycling training that led to a 17.5% increase in maximal oxygen uptake and a 3.3% decrease in body fat mass. After controlling for age, the change in fitness was unrelated to changes in blood lipids, regardless of race. In contrast, changes in fat mass among men were correlated inversely with changes in HDL-C and HDL2-C and positively with the ratio of total cholesterol to HDL; among women they were correlated positively with total cholesterol, LDL-C, and the ratio of total cholesterol to HDL. Hence, the changes in blood lipids after endurance exercise training were unrelated to changes in cardiorespiratory fitness but were related to changes in body fat mass. This suggests that the metabolic influences of physical activity on blood lipids depend more on energy expenditure or fat loss than on fitness changes.

Available evidence supports the hypothesis that endurance exercise training at both moderate and vigorous intensities has a favorable influence on the blood lipid profile. The most frequently observed change is an increase in the HDL-C. It is estimated that for every 1 mg/dl increase in HDL-C, the risk of a coronary heart disease event is reduced by 3% in men and about 4% in women. Reduction in total blood cholesterol, LDL-C, and triglycerides also may occur with endurance exercise. In general, a 1% reduction in LDL-C is associated with a 2% to 3% lower risk of heart disease.

Resistance Exercise Training

Studies of the effects of resistance exercise training on blood lipoprotein levels have produced conflicting results. Most cross-sectional studies have reported a reduced HDL-C level or an elevated total cholesterol-to-HDL ratio in resistance-trained athletes compared with endurance-trained athletes. Because of selection biases in many of these studies, there has been poor control for other factors that might influence lipids and lipoproteins, such as age, body composition, diet, and anabolic or androgenic steroid use.

In contrast, most clinical studies found that resistance exercise training led to favorable changes in lipoprotein and lipid levels. However, many of those studies had no control group and took a single blood sample before and after training. Many also studied people with normal levels of lipoproteins and lipids and did not verify that diet was controlled during the exercise training (Hurley 1989). When those factors are controlled, resistance exercise training does not appear to alter lipoprotein or lipid levels among individuals who have hypercholesterolemia.

Men at Risk.   Changes in lipoprotein and lipid levels and activity of lipoprotein lipase and hepatic lipase were examined in 16 untrained, middle-aged men who had high total cholesterol (about 230 mg/dl), high LDL-C (140 mg/dl), high triglycerides (190 mg/dl), low HDL-C (35 mg/dl), and two or more other risk factors for CHD (Kokkinos et al. 1991). At least two blood samples were taken on separate days before the exercise began. After 20 weeks of resistance exercise training, the exercisers had a 50% increase in upper-body strength, a 37% increase in lower-body strength, and no change in $\dot{V}O_2$max or percent body fat. There also were no changes in blood levels of triglycerides, total cholesterol, HDL-C, and LDL-C or in the activity of lipoprotein lipase and hepatic lipase. Though diet was reportedly not changed, possible effects of smoking, alcohol use, and blood glucose or insulin levels were not controlled in this study.

Premenopausal Women.   Twenty-four healthy but sedentary premenopausal women with normal levels of cholesterol and lipoproteins were randomly assigned either to participating in 45- to 50-min resistance exercise sessions at 85% of one-repetition maximum (1RM) three days a week or to remaining sedentary (Prabhakaran et al. 1999). After 14 weeks, the exercisers had increased their strength, lost body fat, and decreased total cholesterol from 180 to 164 mg/dl, LDL-C from 115 to 99 mg/dl, and the ratio of total cholesterol to HDL-C from 4.2 to 3.6. Triglycerides and HDL-C were not changed by the resistance exercise training.

Obese Women.   Sixteen sedentary obese women ages 22 to 57 years performed three sets of six to eight repetitions at 60% to 70% of 1RM three times a week. Six others remained sedentary (Manning et al. 1991). The women reported that their diets remained unchanged. After 12 weeks, body weight, BMI, and caloric intake remained unchanged. Though strength increased by 58%, blood levels of total cholesterol, HDL-C, LDL-C, triglycerides, apo A-1, and apo B-100 and the ratio of total cholesterol to HDL-C were unchanged. Apo B is the primary apoprotein constituent of LDL cholesterol. Thus, resistance exercise training in the absence of body fat loss does not appear to alter lipoprotein levels among sedentary obese women. Though six of the women were postmenopausal, their lipoprotein levels at the beginning of the study were not different from those of the younger women, so it was unlikely that estrogen status affected the studies outcomes. However, the levels of total cholesterol (200 mg/dl), HDL-C (59 mg/dl), LDL-C (120 mg/dl), and triglycerides (110 mg/dl) were normal at the beginning of the study, so there was little room for improvement regardless of the intervention used.

Strength of the Evidence

The overall evidence is encouraging that regular aerobic or endurance exercise can improve lipoprotein profiles (Durstine and Thompson 2001).

Temporal Sequence

The population-based observational studies have so far been limited to cross-sectional studies, which lack the proper sequence to establish causality: physical activity measurements before lipid outcome measurements.

Strength of Association

The cumulative evidence from about 30 randomized controlled trials indicates that aerobic and endurance exercise training increases HDL-C by about 5%. Similar reductions of about 5% for LDL-C and 4% for triglycerides have been reported, but in fewer studies and less consistently than for HDL-C levels. A few population-based cross-sectional studies have shown similar effects, but prospective cohort studies have not yet been reported.

Consistency

Improvements in lipoprotein profiles after exercise generally have been similar for both men and women regardless of age. Though results have been encouraging for ethnic minorities, the vast majority of studies have been conducted on white men of European ancestry. People with lower HDL-C levels before exercise training had greater increases after exercise, but fewer than 10 studies examined the effects of exercise among people with high cholesterol. Those studies used varying methods. Hence, it is premature to determine whether the benefits of exercise have been underestimated or whether they occur reliably in people who have hyperlipidemia.

Dose Response

Though a few observational studies of recreational runners have reported a linear increase in HDL-C and linear reductions in LDL-C and triglycerides with increasing weekly running distance and with faster running pace, there have not been enough randomized controlled trials comparing different intensities to determine experimentally whether a dose response exists. Based on the collective evidence, it appears that aerobic or endurance exercise expending between 500 and 5,000 kcal each week for at least 12 weeks and conducted at moderate or vigorous intensities yields similar changes in lipoproteins. Changes do not appear to depend on changes in fitness.

Biological Plausibility

The blood lipid improvements most consistently reported with exercise are increased HDL cholesterol (mainly HDL2) and decreased triglycerides. One mechanism by which exercise is responsible for lowered triglycerides and increased HDL cholesterol is the increased use of triglycerides as energy during prolonged exercise. The enzyme LPL, found in extrahepatic tissues, is responsible for breaking down triglycerides into fatty acids that are then used as fuel during prolonged exercise at moderate intensities. As triglycerides are hydrolyzed, VLDL molecules shrink and lose surface cholesterol to HDL molecules for reverse transport to the liver for excretion as bile salts (Gibbons and Mitchell 1995). Gene transcription, protein synthesis, and activity of LPL have been shown to persist for up to 48 h after acute endurance exercise (Ferguson et al. 1998; Seip et al. 1997). Increased LPL activity after exercise might explain the blunting effect of acute exercise on postprandial lipemia (i.e., high triglycerides after a meal). A recent quantitative review of the evidence accumulated from 555 people in 29 studies indicated that people who exercise before a meal have an attenuation of the triglyceride increase after a meal of one half standard deviation, regardless of their sex or age, the type of meal, or the intensity, duration, or timing of the exercise (Stewart and Cureton 2003).

A second mechanism by which exercise increases HDL cholesterol is through another enzyme called lecithin:cholesterol acyltransferase (LCAT). It is known that exercise increases LCAT activity. LCAT is responsible for transferring free fatty acids in the blood and esterification of cholesterol to yield HDL2 cholesterol. However, LCAT is not a rate-limiting enzyme, so increased LCAT activity after exercise may merely indicate higher lipid availability as a result of increased LPL activity. A third mechanism thought to be responsible for the increase in HDL cholesterol levels with exercise involves the decreased activity of yet another enzyme, hepatic lipase. Hepatic lipase, an enzyme found in the liver, is responsible for HDL2 catabolism. Exercise can decrease the activity of hepatic lipase. This results in less HDL cholesterol catabolism, leading to more HDL-C remaining in the blood.

Several studies also indicate that regular exercise can favorably affect apo A-1, which regulates the activity of LCAT; apo B-100, which regulates LDL receptors; and levels of cholesterol ester transfer protein (CETP), which regulates the transfer of cholesterol ester from HDL molecules to other lipoproteins for reverse transport of cholesterol from extrahepatic tissues. It is not yet established whether exercise training affects CETP activity. Table 7.4 summarizes changes in lipoprotein enzyme changes that accompany exercise.

Summary

The American Heart Association and the World Health Organization have concluded that high levels of total cholesterol, LDL cholesterol, and triglycerides and low levels of HDL cholesterol are primary risk factors for developing coronary heart disease and atherosclerosis. Though weight loss, reduced dietary fat and cholesterol, and the statin drugs remain the frontline interventions for the primary and secondary preven-

tion of hypercholesterolemia, physical activity also is recommended. Randomized controlled trials and a few cross-sectional, population-based studies have generally agreed that physical activity can help increase HDL-C levels and decrease LDL-C and triglyceride levels. Those effects appear to be largely independent of age, sex, and weight loss. Though the biological mechanisms are not fully understood, physical activity has a favorable effect on several features of fat and cholesterol metabolism, including increases in regulatory apoproteins, CETP, and enzymes such as LPL and LCAT.

Bibliography

American College of Sports Medicine. 1993. *The American College of Sports Medicine's resource manual for guidelines for exercise testing and prescription.* 2nd edition. Philadelphia: Lea and Febiger.

American Heart Association. 2002. *Heart and stroke statistical update.* Dallas: American Heart Association.

Andersen, R.E., T.A. Wadden, S.J. Bartlett, B. Zemel, T.J. Verde, and S.C. Franckowiak. 1999. Effects of lifestyle activity vs. structured aerobic exercise in obese women: A randomized trial. *Journal of the American Medical Association* 281 (4): 375–376.

Anderson, D.W., A.V. Nichols, S.S. Pan, and F.T. Lindgren. 1978. High lipoprotein distribution: Resolution and determination of three major components in a normal population sample. *Atherosclerosis* 29: 161–179.

Backer, J.M., and E.A. Dawidowicz. 1981. Mechanism of cholesterol exchange between phospholipid vesicles. *Biochemistry* 20 (13): 3805–3810.

Ball, M., and J. Mann. 1994. *Lipids and heart disease: A guide for the primary care team.* 2nd edition. New York: Oxford University Press.

Barbaras, R., P. Grimaldi, R. Negrel, and G. Ailhaud. 1986. Characterization of high-density lipoprotein binding and cholesterol efflux in cultured mouse adipose cells. *Biochimica et Biophysica Acta* 888: 143–156.

Bisgaier, C.L., and R.M. Glickman. 1983. Intestinal synthesis, secretion, and transport of lipoproteins. *Annual Review of Physiology* 45: 625–636.

TABLE 7.4	LIPOPROTEIN ENZYME CHANGES THAT ACCOMPANY EXERCISE	
Enzyme	**Single exercise bout**	**Exercise training**
LPL activity	Increased ~4 h after exercise	Increased
HL activity	Unchanged	Unchanged except with weight loss
LCAT activity	Increased or unchanged	Increased or unchanged
CETP activity	Not studied	Increased or unchanged
CETP mass	Increased	Increased

Adapted from Durstine and Thompson 2001.

Blumenthal, J.A., K. Matthews, M. Fredrikson, N. Rifai, S. Schniebolk, D. German, J. Steege, and J. Rodin. 1991. Effects of exercise training on cardiovascular function and plasma lipid, lipoprotein, and apolipoprotein concentrations in premenopausal and postmenopausal women. *Arteriosclerosis and Thrombosis* 11: 912–917.

Cauley, J.A., R.E. LaPorte, R.B. Sandler, T.J. Orchard, C.W. Slemenda, and A.M. Petrini. 1986. The relationship of physical activity to high density lipoprotein cholesterol in postmenopausal women. *Journal of Chronic Diseases* 39 (9): 687–697.

Chajek, T., L. Aron, and C.J. Fielding. 1980. Interaction of lecithin:cholesterol acyltransferase and cholesteryl ester transfer protein in the transport of cholesteryl ester into sphingomyelin liposomes. *Biochemistry* 19: 3673–3677.

Conti, C.R., and D. Tonnessen. 1992. *Heart disease and high cholesterol: Beating the odds.* Reading, MA: Addison-Wesley.

Daerr, W.H., and H. Greten. 1982. In vitro modulation of the distribution of normal human plasma high density lipoprotein subfractions through the lecithin:cholesterol acyltransferase reaction. *Biochimica et Biophysica Acta* 710 (2): 128–133.

Deckelbaum, R.J., S. Eisenberg, Y. Oschry, E. Butbul, I. Sharon, and T. Olivecrona. 1982. Reversible modification of human plasma low density lipoproteins toward triglyceride-rich precursors. *Journal of Biological Chemistry* 257: 6509–6517.

Deckelbaum, R.J., S. Eisenberg, Y. Oschry, E. Granot, I. Sharon, and G. Bengtsson-Olivecrona. 1986. Conversion of human plasma high density lipoprotein-2 to high density lipoprotein-3. *Journal of Biological Chemistry* 261: 5201–5208.

Deckelbaum, R.J., T. Olivecrona, and S. Eisenberg. 1984. Plasma lipoproteins in hyperlipidemia: Roles of neutral lipid exchange and lipase. In *Treatment of hyperlipoproteinemia,* edited by L.A. Carlson and A.G. Olsson, pp. 85–93. New York: Raven Press.

Duncan, J.J., N.F. Gordon, and C.B. Scott. 1991. Women walking for health and fitness. How much is enough? *Journal of the American Medical Association* 266 (23): 3295–3299.

Durstine, J.L., and W.L. Haskell. 1994. Effects of exercise training on plasma lipids and lipoproteins. *Exercise and Sport Sciences Reviews* 22: 477–521.

Durstine, J.L., and P.D. Thompson. 2001. Exercise in the treatment of lipid disorders. *Cardiology Clinics* 19: 471–488.

Eisenberg, S. 1976. Metabolism of very low density lipoprotein. In *Lipoprotein metabolism,* edited by H. Greten, pp. 32–43. Heidlberg: Springer-Verlag.

———. 1984. High density lipoprotein metabolism. *Journal of Lipid Research* 25: 1017–1058.

Eisenberg, S., and R. Deckelbaum. 1989. Intravascular lipoprotein remodelling: Neutral lipid transfer proteins. In *Human plasma lipoproteins,* edited by J.C. Fruchart and J. Shepherd. New York: de Gruyter.

Ferguson, M.A., N.L. Alderson, S.G. Trost, D.A. Essig, J.R. Burke, and J.L. Durstine. 1998. Effects of four different single exercise sessions on lipids, lipoproteins, and lipoprotein lipase. *Journal of Applied Physiology* 85: 1169–1174.

Fielding, C.J., and P.E. Fielding. 1981. Regulation of human plasma lecithin:cholesterol acyltransferase activity by lipoprotein acceptor cholesteryl ester content. *Journal of Biological Chemistry* 256: 2102–2104.

Fielding, P.E., and C.J. Fielding. 1980. A cholesteryl ester transfer complex in human plasma. *Proceedings of the National Academy of Sciences* 77: 3327–3330.

Gibbons, L.W., and T.L. Mitchell. 1995. HDL cholesterol and exercise. *Your Patient and Fitness* 9 (4): 6–13.

Green, P.H.R., and R.M. Glickman. 1981. Intestinal lipoprotein metabolism. *Journal of Lipid Research* 22: 1153–1173.

Hagberg, J.M., R.E. Ferrell, L.I. Katzel, D.R. Dengel, J.D. Sorkin, and A.P. Goldberg. 1999. Apolipoprotein E genotype and exercise training–induced increases in plasma high-density lipoprotein (HDL)- and HDL2-cholesterol levels in overweight men. *Metabolism* 48 (8): 943–945.

Halbert, J.A., C.A. Silagy, P. Finucane, R.T. Withers, and P.A. Hamdorf. 1999. Exercise training and blood lipids in hyperlipidemic and normolipidemic adults: A meta-analysis of randomized, controlled trials. *European Journal of Clinical Nutrition* 53: 514–522.

Hamilton, R.L., M.C. Williams, C.J. Fielding, and R.J. Havel. 1976. Discoidal bilayer structure of nascent high density lipoproteins from perfused rat liver. *Journal of Clinical Investigation* 58: 667–680.

Haskell, W.L. 1984. The influence of exercise on the concentrations of triglyceride and cholesterol in human plasma. In *Exercise and sport sciences reviews,* edited by R.L. Terjung, pp. 205–244. Lexington, MA: D.C. Heath.

Heath, G.W., A.A Ehsani, J.M. Hagberg, J.M. Hinderliter, and A.P. Goldberg. 1983. Exercise training improves lipoprotein lipid profiles in patients with coronary artery disease. *American Heart Journal* 105 (6): 889–895.

Hokanson, J.E., and M.A. Austin. 1996. Plasma triglyceride is a risk factor for cardiovascular disease independent of high-density lipoprotein cholesterol: A meta-analysis of population-based prospective studies. *Journal of Cardiovascular Risk* 3: 213–219.

Horowitz, B.S., I.J. Goldberg, J. Merab, T.M. Vanni, R. Ramakrishnan, and H.N. Ginsberg. 1993. Increased plasma and renal clearance of an exchangeable pool of apolipoprotein A-1 in subjects with low levels of high density lipoprotein cholesterol. *Journal of Clinical Investigation* 91: 1743–1752.

Hurley, B.F. 1989. Effects of resistive training on lipoprotein-lipid profiles: A comparison to aerobic exercise training. *Medicine and Science in Sports and Exercise* 6: 689–693.

Katzmarzyk, P.T., A.S. Leon, T. Rankinen, T. Gagnon, J.S. Skinner, J.H. Wilmore, D.C. Rao, and C. Bouchard. 2001. Changes in blood lipids consequent to aerobic exercise training related to changes in body fatness and aerobic fitness. *Metabolism* 50: 841–848.

Kekki, M. 1980. Lipoprotein–lipase action determining plasma high density lipoprotein cholesterol level in adult normolipaemics. *Atherosclerosis* 37: 143–150.

Kohl, H.W. III, N.F. Gordon, C.B. Scott, H. Vaandrager, and S.N. Blair. 1992. Musculoskeletal strength and serum lipid levels in men and women. *Medicine and Science in Sports and Exercise* 24: 1080–1087.

Kokkinos, P.F., J.C. Holland, P. Narayan, J.A. Colleran, C.O. Dotson, and V. Papademetriou. 1995. Miles run per week and high-density lipoprotein cholesterol levels in healthy, middle-aged men. *Archives of Internal Medicine* 155 (4): 415–420.

Kokkinos, P.F., B.F. Hurley, M.A. Smutok, C. Farmer, C. Reece, R. Shulman, C. Charabogos, J. Patterson, S. Will, J. Devane-Bell, and A.P. Goldberg. 1991. Strength training does not improve lipoprotein–lipid profiles in men at risk for CHD. *Medicine and Science in Sports and Exercise* 23 (10): 1134–1139.

Kokkinos, P.F., P. Narayan, J. Colleran, R.D. Fletcher, R. Lakshman, and V. Papademetriou. 1998. Effects of moderate intensity exercise on serum lipids in African-American men with severe systemic hypertension. *American Journal of Cardiology* 81 (6): 732–735.

Leon, A.S., and O.A. Sanchez. 2001. Response of blood lipids to exercise training alone or combined with dietary intervention. *Medicine and Science in Sports and Exercise* 33 (Suppl. 6): S502–S515.

Lindheim, S.R., M. Notelovitz, E.B. Feldman, S. Larsen, F.Y. Khan, and R.A. Lobo. 1994. The independent effects of exercise and estrogen on lipids and lipoproteins in postmenopausal women. *Obstetrics and Gynecology* 83 (2): 167–171.

Mahlberg, F.H., and G.H. Rothblat. 1992. Cellular cholesterol efflux. *Journal of Biological Chemistry* 267: 4541–4550.

Mahley, R.W., and T.L. Innearity. 1983. Lipoprotein receptors and cholesterol homeostasis. *Biochimica et Biophysica Acta* 737: 197–222.

Manning, J.M., C.R. Dooly-Manning, K. White, I. Kampa, S. Silas, M. Kesselhaut, and M. Ruoff. 1991. Effects of a resistive training program on lipoprotein-lipid levels in obese women. *Medicine and Science in Sports and Exercise* 23: 1222–1226.

Marrugat, J., R. Elosau, M. Covas, L. Molina, J. Rubies-Prat, and the Marathon investigators. 1996. Amount and intensity of physical activity, physical fitness, and serum lipids in men. *American Journal of Epidemiology* 143 (6): 562–569.

Marsh, J.B. 1976. Apoproteins of the lipoproteins in a nonrecirculating perfusate of rat liver. *Journal of Lipid Research* 17: 85–90.

Martin, S., R. Elosua, M.I. Covas, M. Pavesi, J. Vila, and J. Marrugat. 1999. Relationship of lipoprotein(a) levels to physical activity and family history of coronary heart disease. *American Journal of Public Health* 89: 383–385.

McGoon, M.D. 1993. *Mayo Clinic heart book.* New York: Morrow.

Melchior, G.W., C.K. Castle, R.W. Murray, W.L. Blake, D.M. Dinh, and K.R. Marotti. 1994. Apolipoprotein A-1 metabolism in cholesterol ester transfer protein transgenic mice. *Journal of Biological Chemistry* 269: 8044–8051.

National Center for Health Statistics. 1995. *Health: United States.* Hyattsville, MD: Public Health Service.

National Heart, Lung, and Blood Institute. September 2002. Third report of the National Cholesterol Education Program expert panel on the detection, evaluation, and treatment of high blood cholesterol levels in adults (Adult Treatment Panel III), National Cholesterol Education Program, National Heart, Lung, and Blood Institute, National Institutes of Health, Publication No. 02-5215.

Norum, K.R. 1984. Familial lecithin:cholesterol acyltransferase deficiency. In *Clinical and metabolic aspects of high density lipoproteins,* edited by N.E. Miller and G.J. Miller, pp. 297–318. Amsterdam: Elsevier.

O'Connor, G.T., C.H. Hennekens, W.C. Willett, S.Z. Goldhaber, R.S. Paffenbarger Jr., J.L. Breslow, I.M. Lee, and J.E. Buring. 1995. Physical exercise and reduced risk of nonfatal myocardial infarction. *American Journal of Epidemiology* 142 (11): 1147–1156.

Oschry, Y., and S. Eisenberg. 1982. Rat plasma lipoproteins: Re-evaluation of a lipoprotein system in an animal devoid of cholesteryl ester transfer activity. *Journal of Lipid Research* 23: 1099–1106.

Prabhakaran, B., E.A. Dowling, J.D. Branch, D.P. Swain, and B.C. Leutholtz. 1999. Effect of 14 weeks of resistance training on lipid profile and body fat percentage in premenopausal women. *British Journal of Sports Medicine* 33: 190–195.

Seals, D.R., J.M. Hagberg, B.F. Hurley, A.A. Ehsani, and J.O. Holloszy. 1984. Endurance training in older men and women. I. Cardiovascular responses to exercise. *Journal of*

Applied Physiology: Respiratory, Environmental & Exercise Physiology 57 (4): 1024–1029.

Seip, R.L., K. Mair, T.G. Cole, and C.F. Semenkovich. 1997. Induction of human skeletal muscle lipoprotein lipase gene expression by short-term exercise is transient. *American Journal of Physiology* 272 (2 Pt 1): E255–E261.

Shepherd, J., and C.J. Packard. 1989. Lipoprotein metabolism. In *Human plasma lipoproteins,* edited by J.C. Fruchart and J. Shepherd. New York: de Gruyter.

Shepherd, J., C.J. Packard, J.M. Stewart, B.D. Vallance, T.D.V. Lawrie, and H.G. Morgan. 1980. The relationship between the cholesterol content and subfraction distribution of plasma high-density lipoproteins. *Clinica Chimica Acta* 101: 57–62.

Stefanick, M.L., S. Mackey, M. Sheehan, N. Ellsworth, W.L. Haskell, and P.D. Wood. 1998. Effects of diet and exercise in men and postmenopausal women with low levels of HDL cholesterol and high levels of LDL cholesterol. *New England Journal of Medicine* 339: 12–20.

Stewart, D.J., and K.J. Cureton. 2003. Effects of prior exercise on post-prandial lipemia: A quantitative review. *Metabolism* 52: 418–424.

Tall, A.R. 1986. Plasma lipid transfer proteins. *Journal of Lipid Research* 27: 361–367.

———. 1990. Plasma high density lipoproteins. *Journal of Clinical Investigation* 86: 379–384.

Tall, A.R., and D.S. Small. 1978. Plasma high density lipoproteins. *New England Journal of Medicine* 299: 1232–1236.

Tortora, G.J., and S.R. Grabowski. 1993. *Principles of anatomy and physiology.* 7th edition. New York: Harper-Collins College.

Tran, Z.V., A. Weltman, G.V. Glass, and D.P. Mood. 1983. The effects of exercise on blood lipids and lipoproteins: A meta-analysis of studies. *Medicine and Science in Sports and Exercise* 15 (5): 393–402.

Tucker, L.A., and L.J. Silvester. 1996. Strength training and hypercholesterolemia: An epidemiological study of 8499 employed men. *American Journal of Health Promotion* 11 (1): 35–41.

Williams, P.T., R.M. Krauss, K.M. Vranizan, J.J. Albers, and P.D. Wood. 1992. Effects of weight-loss by exercise and by diet on apolipoproteins A-I and A-II and the particle-size distribution of high-density lipoproteins in men. *Metabolism* 41 (4): 441–449.

Williams, P.T., M.L. Stefanick, K.M. Vranizan, and P.D. Wood. 1994. The effects of weight loss by exercise or by dieting on plasma high-density lipoprotein (HDL) levels in men with low, intermediate, and normal-to-high HDL at baseline. *Metabolism* 43 (7): 917–924.

Windmueller, H.G., and A.L. Wu. 1981. Biosynthesis of plasma apolipoproteins by rat small intestine without dietary or biliary fat. *Journal of Biological Chemistry* 256: 3013–3016.

Winkler, K.E., and J.B. Marsh. 1989. Characterization of nascent high density lipoprotein subfractions from perfusates of rat liver. *Journal of Lipid Research* 30: 979–996.

Wood, P.D., W.L. Haskell, S.N. Blair, P.T. Williams, R.M. Krauss, F.T. Lindgren, J.J. Albers, P.H. Ho, and J.W. Farquhar. 1983. Increased exercise level and plasma lipoprotein concentrations: A one-year, randomized, controlled study in sedentary, middle-aged men. *Metabolism* 32: 31–39.

Wu, A.L., and H.G. Windmueller. 1979. Relative contributions by liver and intestine to individual plasma apolipoproteins in the rat. *Journal of Biological Chemistry* 254: 7316–7322.

Yurgalevitch, S.M., A.M. Kriska, T.K. Welty, O. Go, D.C. Robbins, and B.V. Howard. 1998. Physical activity and lipids and lipoproteins in American Indians ages 45–74. *Medicine and Science in Sports and Exercise* 30: 543–549.

Web Sites

www.americanheart.org. Official Web site of the American Heart Association. Provides information and links to the public and professionals about lipoproteins and cardiovascular disease.

www.nhlbi.nih.gov/chd/. Site of the National Cholesterol Education Program maintained by the National Heart, Lung, and Blood Institute of the National Institutes of Health.

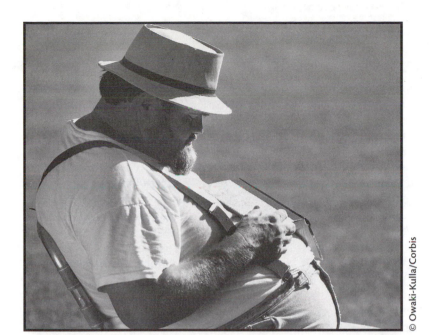

© Owaki-Kulla/Corbis

 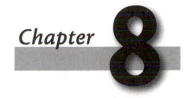

Physical Activity and Obesity

I am resolved to grow fat, and look young till forty.

—*John Dryden (1631–1700), The Maiden Queen, Act III, Scene 1*

What have I done to merit these cruel sufferings? Many things; you have ate and drank too freely, and too much indulged those legs of yours in their indolence . . . the quantity of meat and drink proper for a man, who takes a reasonable degree of exercise, would be too much for another, who never takes any.

—*Benjamin Franklin (1706–1790), Dialogue Between Franklin and the Gout*
Midnight, 22 October, 1780 (Matthews 1914)

Overweight and **obesity** are characterized by excess body fat resulting from a positive energy balance (i.e., an energy intake greater than energy expenditure). Although being overweight was socially valued during the economic austerity of 17th-century Europe, as portrayed by the English dramatist John Dryden in the quotation that opens this chapter, it has become a 21st-century burden to the public health of developed nations. The U.S. National Institutes of Health (NIH) regard obesity as a chronic disease that develops from an interaction of a person's genotype, the environment, and the person's dietary and physical inactivity habits (National Heart, Lung, and Blood Institute 1998). In contrast to underfeeding, which quickly leads to vulnerability to infectious diseases or conditions such as diarrhea that can result in permanent mental and physical impairment or death, excess weight gain manifests its health risks during adulthood, contributing to chronic but reversible diseases. People who are overweight or obese have higher risks of developing hypertension, hypercholesterolemia, type 2 diabetes, coronary heart disease (CHD), stroke, gallbladder disease, osteoarthritis, and cancers of the uterus, prostate, breast, and colon. Based on cumulative data from the National Health and Nutrition Examination Survey III and the Framingham Heart Study, moderately obese (BMI > 32.5 kg/m^2), middle-aged men and women have about double the risk of hypertension, triple the risk of type 2 diabetes, and a 1-year reduction in life expectancy compared with their non-obese peers (Thompson et al. 1999). After adjusting for other risk factors, the risk of type 2 diabetes among U.S. adults aged 18 to 44 years increases by 6% for each 5 to 8 pounds of body mass (Hillier and Pedula 2001). According to data from the Behavioral Risk Factor Surveillance System maintained by the Centers for Disease Control and Prevention, obese U.S. adults with a BMI of 40 or higher have about seven times higher risk of diabetes, six times higher risk of hypertension, double the risk of high cholesterol, and four times the risk of self-rated fair or poor health compared to adults with normal weight (Mokdad et al. 2003).

Obesity cost the United States 12% of the annual national health care budget during the late 1990s, $118 billion, more than double the $47 billion attributable to smoking. After cigarette smoking, obesity and overweight are the second leading cause of preventable death in the United States. The number of annual deaths in the United States among adults aged 18 years or older attributable to obesity in 1991 was estimated to be approximately 280,000 (Allison et al. 1999). An estimated 300,000 deaths in the United States in 1990 were attributed each year to poor diets and physical inactivity, behaviors that contribute to obesity (McGinnis and Foege 1993).

Magnitude of the Problem

According to a recent summary of statistics from the World Health Organization, the United Nations, and individual nations, there now are 1.1 billion people worldwide who are overweight (Gardner and Halweil 2000). This is the first time in recorded history that the number of people who are overweight equals the number of people who are underfed and underweight. Paradoxically, the prevalence of overweight and obesity is increasing rapidly in developing nations as well as in already developed nations. For example, in Brazil and Colombia, where poverty leads to underfeeding in a large portion of the population, 36% and 41%, respectively, of the population is overweight. The National Center for Health Statistics estimates that in the United States 55% of adults 20 years or older are overweight, including the more than 20% of adults who are considered obese (Mokdad et al. 1999, 2000, 2003; figure 8.1), and 13% of youths are overweight or obese (figure 8.2). A majority of the populations of Russia, the United Kingdom, and Germany also are overweight.

The prevalence of overweight and obesity in the United States has increased steadily during the past 40 years. Just 10 years ago, only 12% of Americans were classified as obese. Figure 8.3 illustrates the marked increase in the prevalence of obesity in the United States from 1991 to 2000. Estimates from the Behavioral Risk Factor Surveillance System maintained by the Centers for Disease Control and Prevention indicate that the prevalence of adult obesity in the United States is reaching epidemic status, increasing from 19.8% to 20.9% between 2000 and 2001 (Mokdad et al. 2003), an increase of nearly 6% in a single year.

The ongoing National Health and Nutrition Examination Survey (NHANES), a series of cross-

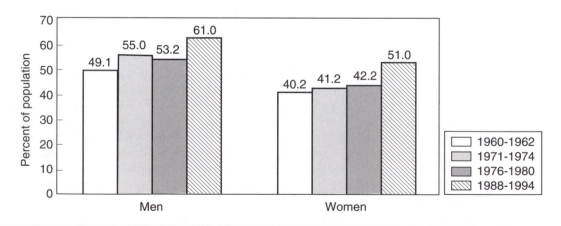

Figure 8.1   Age-adjusted prevalence of overweight in Americans ages 20 to 74 by sex and survey. United States: 1960–1962, 1971–1974, 1976–1980, and 1988–1994.

American Heart Association 2002.

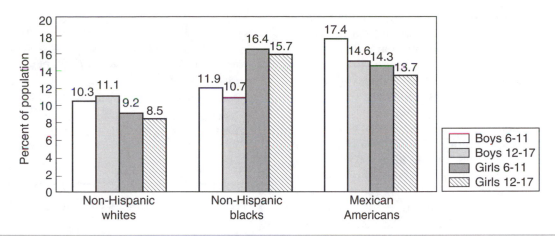

Figure 8.2   Prevalence of overweight in children and adolescents by sex, age, and race/ethnicity. United States: 1988–1994.
American Heart Association 2002.

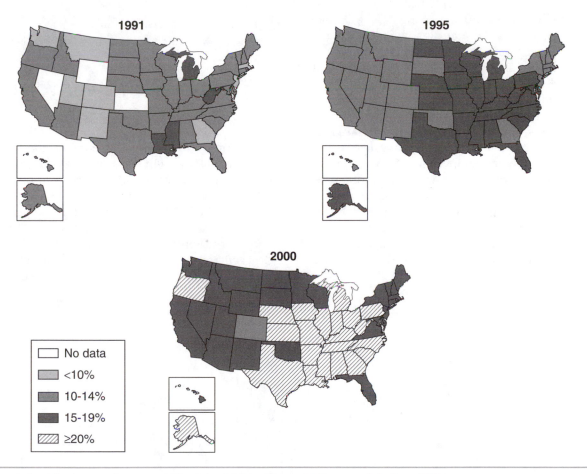

Figure 8.3   Obesity trends among U.S. adults. BMI ≥ 30, or ~30 lb overweight for a 5'4" woman.
Data from A.H. Mokdad et al., 1999, 2001.

sectional national surveys conducted every five years or so since 1960 and now conducted yearly, estimated that during the period from 1976 to 1980 about 24% of men and 27% of women were 20% or more above desirable weight based on 1983 Metropolitan Life Insurance Company actuarial height and weight tables. **Desirable weight** on those tables is the weight that predicts normal life expectancy according to body frame, age, and sex. In the period between 1988 and 1991, those rates had increased by nearly 30%, up to 31.3% of men and 34.1% of women (Kuczmarski 1992; Kuczmarski et al. 1994; Williamson 1993). Thus, compared with past surveys, adults had gained about 3.6 kg of body weight.

The National Longitudinal Survey of Youth, a prospective cohort study of 8,270 children aged 4 to 12 years conducted from 1986 to 1998 reported steady increases in the prevalence of overweight (defined as greater than the 95th percentile of age- and sex-specific BMI) during that time, doubling the prevalence rates to 21.5% in African American, 21.8% in Hispanic, and rising by half to 12.3% in white youth (Strauss and Pollack 2001). According to the National Health and Nutrition Examination Survey (NHANES), the prevalence rate of over-weight in youth was 10.4% among 2 to 5 year olds, 15.3% among 6 to 11 year olds, and 15.5% among 12 to 19 year olds in 1999 to 2000 compared to rates of 7.2%, 11.3%, and 10.5%, respectively, in 1988 to 1994. Gains were comparatively largest among non-Hispanic black and Mexican American adolescents (Ogden et al. 2002).

The rates of overweight and obesity are high-est in groups of people who have less formal education and lower income and in some mi-nority groups, especially American Indians and African American and Mexican American wom-en, where they approach 50% (figure 8.4). It is discouraging that the U.S. population steadily lost ground, failing to meet the *Healthy People 2000* objective that only 20% of the population be overweight.

> ••• *Fifty-five percent of adults and 13% of youths in the United States are overweight or obese; the prevalence of adult obesity has doubled to 23% in the past decade. The economic burden of obesity is $118 billion a year, 12% of the national health care budget.*

Health Risks of Obesity

Hypertension	Gallbladder disease
Hypercholesterolemia	Osteoarthritis
Type 2 diabetes	Cancer (uterus, prostate, breast, colon)
Coronary heart disease	Stroke

Treatment of Overweight and Obesity

Preventing and treating obesity is challenging. The average weight loss in dietary interven-tions with people who are obese is about 10 kg (22 lb) over an average period of 18 weeks; two thirds of the loss is maintained for one year, but pretreatment weight is regained within three to five years (Foreyt and Goodrich 1994). The only drug currently approved by the Food and Drug Administration (FDA) for long-term use in the

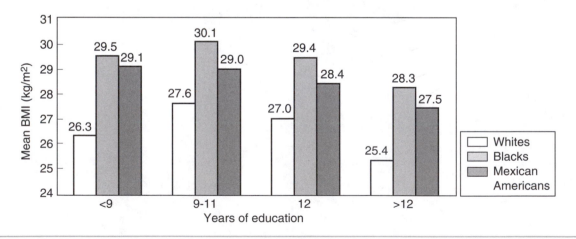

Figure 8.4   Mean BMI for women ages 25 to 64 by education and race/ethnicity. United States: 1988–1994.

Reprinted, by permission, from M.A. Winkleby et al. 1998, "Third national health and nutrition examination survey, 1988-1994," *Journal of the American Medical Association* 280: 356-362.

treatment of obesity is sibutramine. Approval of orlistat is pending. The use of the serotonin agonists dexfenfluramine and fenfluramine, alone or combined with the stimulant phentermine, is not recommended by the FDA because of evidence suggesting increased risk of pulmonary hypotension and valvular heart disease.

The NIH expert panel on obesity and overweight (National Heart, Lung, and Blood Institute 1998) reached these conclusions:

• Physical activity is a clinically accepted approach to weight loss, as are low-calorie diets and lower-fat diets, behavior therapy, pharmacotherapy, surgery, and combinations of these techniques.

• For most overweight people, the initial goal of a prudent weight-loss program is to lose about 10% of weight over a period of six months. Among people with BMIs in the range of 27 to 35, that goal can be achieved by a decrease of 300 to 500 kcal per day, which will result in weight losses of about 0.5 to 1 lb (0.2–0.5 kg) per week. For obese people with BMIs over 35, deficits of up to 500 to 1,000 kcal per day are required to achieve those goals. After six months, the rate of weight loss usually declines, and weight tends to stabilize at a plateau because of the resulting reduction in basal metabolic rate that accompanies the lower body mass.

• Lost weight is usually regained unless a weight maintenance program consisting of dietary therapy, physical activity, and behavior therapy is continued indefinitely. After six months of successful weight loss, efforts to maintain weight loss should be undertaken.

> ••• *Without sustained physical activity, the average weight loss after dieting among people who are obese is about 10 kg (22 lb); one third is gained back within a year, and nearly all is gained back within three to five years.*

Assessing and Defining Overweight and Obesity

Though the most accurate methods of assessing body fat require laboratory equipment, Quetelet's **body mass index (BMI)** and relative weight are the standard methods used to estimate overweight and obesity in epidemiologic studies. Relative weight is calculated by dividing body weight by the midpoint of desirable weight for a person judged to have a medium frame as recommended in the 1959 or 1983 Metropolitan Life tables. For many years, a body weight of 20% or more above desirable body weight was viewed as the threshold for health risk. That equates to a body mass index of 27.8 for men and 27.3 for women (Kuczmarski 1992). More recently, the NIH defined people as overweight when BMI is in the range of 25 to 29.9 kg/m² and as obese when BMI equals or exceeds 30 kg/m² (National Heart, Lung, and Blood Institute 1998). Hence, someone can be overweight but not obese, but an obese person is also overweight. Obesity is further categorized as class I (BMI, 30–34.9), class II (BMI, 35–39.9), and class III (BMI, equal to or greater than 40). Weight classifications by BMI are shown in table 8.1. Table 8.2 converts selected heights and weights to BMI. For example, a BMI of 30 equates to being about 30 lb (13.6 kg) overweight.

TABLE 8.1 CLASSIFICATION OF OVERWEIGHT AND OBESITY BY BMI

	Obesity class	BMI (kg/m²)
Underweight		<18.5
Normal		18.5–24.9
Overweight		25.0–29.9
Obesity	I	30.0–34.9
	II	35.0–39.9
Extreme obesity	III	≥40

National Institutes of Health 1998.

Patterning of Body Fat and Disease Risk

Excess fat in the abdomen out of proportion to total body fat is another risk factor of chronic diseases associated with obesity. **Waist circumference** is positively correlated with abdominal fat content and provides a clinically acceptable measurement for assessing a patient's abdominal fat content before and during weight-loss treatment. Girth at the waist greater than 102 cm (40 in.) for men and 88 cm (35 in.) for

TABLE 8.2 SELECTED BMI UNITS CATEGORIZED BY INCHES (CM) AND POUNDS (KG)			
	BMI 25 kg/m²	BMI 27 kg/m²	BMI 30 kg/m²
HEIGHT IN INCHES (CM)	**BODY WEIGHT IN POUNDS (KG)**		
58 (147.32)	119 (53.98)	129 (58.51)	143 (64.86)
59 (149.86)	124 (56.25)	133 (60.33)	148 (67.13)
60 (152.40)	128 (58.06)	138 (62.60)	153 (69.40)
61 (154.94)	132 (59.87)	143 (64.86)	158 (71.67)
62 (157.48)	136 (61.69)	147 (66.68)	164 (74.39)
63 (160.02)	141 (63.96)	152 (68.95)	169 (76.66)
64 (162.56)	145 (65.77)	157 (71.22)	174 (78.93)
65 (165.10)	150 (68.04)	162 (73.48)	180 (81.65)
66 (167.64)	155 (70.31)	167 (75.75)	186 (84.37)
67 (170.18)	159 (72.12)	172 (78.02)	191 (86.64)
68 (172.72)	164 (74.39)	177 (80.29)	197 (89.36)
69 (175.26)	169 (76.66)	182 (82.56)	203 (92.08)
70 (177.80)	174 (78.93)	188 (85.28)	207 (93.90)
71 (180.34)	179 (81.19)	193 (87.54)	215 (97.52)
72 (182.88)	184 (83.46)	199 (90.27)	221 (100.25)
73 (185.42)	189 (85.73)	204 (92.53)	227 (102.97)
74 (187.96)	194 (86.00)	210 (95.26)	233 (105.69)
75 (190.50)	200 (90.72)	216 (97.98)	240 (108.86)
76 (193.04)	205 (92.99)	221 (100.25)	246 (111.59)

Metric conversion formula = weight (kg)/height (m)²

Example of BMI calculation:

A person who weighs 78.93 kg and is 177 cm tall has a BMI of 25:

weight (78.93 kg)/height (1.77 m)² = 25

Nonmetric conversion formula = [weight (lb)/height (in.)²] × 704.5

Example of BMI calculation:

A person who weighs 154 lb and is 68 in. (or 5'8") tall has a BMI of 25:

[weight (154 lb)/height (68 in.)²] × 704.5 = 25

women is considered risky. Table 8.3 illustrates the additive risk of increased abdominal fat to the risk of BMI in the development of obesity-associated diseases in adults with a BMI of 25 to 34.9 kg/m². Waist circumference does not add to the accuracy of predicting disease risk in people who have a BMI of 35 kg/m² or more.

More recently, the disease risk associated with the ratio of waist-to-hip girths has been established. This **waist-to-hip ratio** predicts the patterning of visceral fat. Excess fat above the waist, so-called androidal fat, increases risk for CHD more than does excess fat below the waist, so-called gynoidal fat. The American Heart Association (2001) suggests that the desirable waist-to-hip ratio is less than 1.00 for men and less than 0.80 for women.

Some evidence indicates that extra fat stored above the waist indicates high visceral fat, which is believed to be more biologically active, that is, more readily mobilized from **adipose** cells into the bloodstream, where it can contribute to atherosclerosis. Other evidence indicates that trunk fat increases risk for CHD independently of serum lipids. For example, in the Paris Prospective Study, subcutaneous fat distribution and incidence of CHD was examined among 6,718 men ages 42 to 53 after a follow-up period of 6.6 years (Ducimetiere, Richard, and Cambien 1986). Fat distribution was described as the measurement

TABLE 8.3   CLASSIFICATION OF OVERWEIGHT AND OBESITY BY BMI, WAIST CIRCUMFERENCE, AND ASSOCIATED DISEASE RISKS

	BMI (kg/m²)	Obesity class	DISEASE RISK RELATIVE TO NORMAL WEIGHT AND WAIST CIRCUMFERENCE	
			Men ≤102 cm (≤40 in.) Women ≤88 cm (≤35 in.)	>102 cm (>40 in.) >88 cm (>35 in.)
Underweight	<18.5		—	—
Normal	18.5–24.9		—	—
Overweight	25.0–29.9		Increased	High
Obesity	30.0–34.9	I	High	Very high
	35.0–39.9	II	Very high	Very high
Extreme obesity	≥40	III	Extremely high	Extremely high

National Institutes of Health 1998.

of 13 skinfold thicknesses (5 on the trunk, 4 at the triceps level, 4 at midthigh). The trunk measurements were correlated with BMI ($r \approx 0.50$) but were better predictors of MI and angina pectoris, independent of their moderate correlations with systolic blood pressure, serum cholesterol, and serum triglycerides.

Precise measurement of the percentage of body mass that is fat and its regional distribution requires laboratory measurements that estimate the four tissue components that constitute body mass: water, mineral, protein, and fat. Body fat cannot be measured directly, so it is calculated from estimates of mineral content of bone, body water, and body density. Most commonly, mineral content is measured by dual X-ray absorptiometry (DXA), body water is measured by dilution with deuterium, and body density is measured by underwater weighing. Based on the relative portions of these four components measured directly in cadavers, predictive equations have been developed that have a standard accuracy for estimating body fat percentage of ±2% to ±3%, compared with ±5% to ±7% for BMI. Improved technology has increased the accuracy of assessment of adipose distribution and regional adiposity and can be used to validate the accuracy of girth or other anthropometric measures that are feasible to use with large numbers of people in population-based studies of disease risk and in smaller clinical trials designed to change total or regional body fatness. However, these techniques have yet to be used in large population-

based studies to determine whether they provide better estimates of CHD morbidity and mortality than do BMI and waist girth measurements.

The Consensus About Obesity

In 1995, the National Heart, Lung, and Blood Institute's Obesity Education Initiative and the National Institute of Diabetes and Digestive and Kidney Diseases assembled an expert panel charged with the identification, evaluation, and treatment of overweight and obesity in adults. Their guidelines appeared in 1998 and were based on a review of 236 studies of randomized clinical trials indexed by the National Library of Medicine from January 1980 to September 1997 (National Heart, Lung, and Blood Institute 1998). These studies lasted at least four months, with the exception of a few three-month studies of dietary therapy and pharmacotherapy. Long-term outcomes from the studies were followed for a year or longer.

These are some main conclusions of the review:

• Treatment of overweight is recommended only when patients have two or more risk factors or a high waist circumference. Treatment should focus on altering dietary and physical activity patterns to prevent development of obesity and to produce moderate weight loss.

• Cardiovascular risk factors among obese people do not differ from those of normal weight.

• Obese people who have at least three major CHD risk factors usually require medical treatment aimed at risk reduction. Their CHD risk is increased further if they are physically inactive and have high serum triglycerides (>200 mg/dl), though the increased risk has not been quantified.

• There is strong evidence that weight loss among people who are overweight or obese reduces risk factors for diabetes and cardiovascular disease (CVD). Weight loss reduces blood pressure in both hypertensive and nonhypertensive overweight individuals, reduces serum triglycerides, increases HDL cholesterol, and somewhat reduces total serum cholesterol and LDL cholesterol. Weight loss reduces blood glucose levels in overweight and obese people with and without diabetes and can reduce glycosylated hemoglobin (HbA1c) in people with type 2 diabetes.

Though obesity is considered a disease, there is controversy about whether it is an independent cause of premature death or whether it is deadly because of the constellation of risk factors for mortality that accompanies it. For example, the co-occurrence of obesity with diabetes, hypertension, and hyperlipidemia defines **metabolic syndrome X,** which constitutes an absolute risk for CHD and cardiovascular mortality. The age-adjusted prevalence of metabolic syndrome among men and women aged 20 years or older estimated from NHANES III was nearly 24%, about 47 million people (Ford et al. 2002). The prevalence rate was highest among Mexican Americans (32%). Though rates were similar for men and women averaged across ethnic groups, African American women had about a 57% higher prevalence and Mexican American women had about a 26% higher prevalence than did their male counterparts.

People who are overweight or obese usually are less physically active than are people of normal weight. A debate has recently arisen over whether overweight or physical inactivity is the more important risk factor for health. That debate is discussed in detail in the next section because accumulating evidence suggests that overweight but not obese adults who are fit have less health risk than do people who are of normal weight but unfit.

> ••• *Adults who are overweight but fit have less health risk than do people who are of normal weight but unfit.*

Metabolic Syndrome X

Metabolic syndrome X is the co-occurrence of obesity (especially visceral adiposity) with diabetes, hypertension, and hyperlipidemia, a constellation of risk factors of coronary heart disease and cardiovascular mortality. It is defined as three or more of the following:

• Waist circumference greater than 102 cm in men and 88 cm in women

• Serum triglyceride level of at least 150 mg/dl (1.69 mmol/L)

• High-density lipoprotein cholesterol level less than 40 mg/dl (1.04 mmol/L) in men and 50 mg/dl (1.29 mmol/L) in women

• Blood pressure of at least 130/85 mmHg

• Serum glucose level of at least 110 mg/dl (6.1 mmol/L)

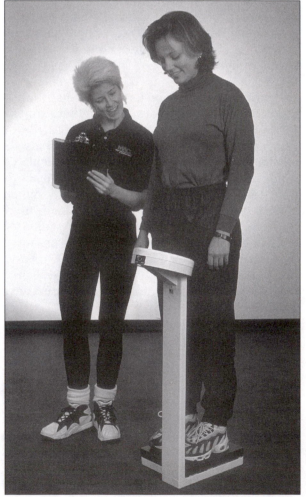

© SportsChrome

Are Overweight and Obesity Risk Factors Independent of Physical Activity?

Large-scale randomized clinical trials have not been conducted to determine whether weight loss among people who are obese reduces mortality. Neither have such studies been done for physical inactivity. Dr. Glenn Gaesser (1996, 2002), an exercise physiologist at the University of Virginia, challenged the consensus view that being fat is life-threatening and being thin guarantees health. He proposed that any person can have good health regardless of body weight by achieving and maintaining metabolic fitness, which we defined in chapter 3. In contrast to the NIH expert panel's consensus (National Heart, Lung, and Blood Institute 1998), Gaesser argued that the scientific evidence is not sufficiently strong to conclude that overweight and obesity are directly responsible for early death. A brief discussion of that evidence follows for CHD, hyperlipidemia, hypertension, and type 2 diabetes. Later, we introduce newer evidence from the Aerobics Center Longitudinal Study in Dallas that supports the hypothesis that mortality among the overweight is cut about in half among fit compared to unfit adults.

Coronary Heart Disease

Though many cross-sectional studies agreed that the prevalence of obesity is associated with primary risk factors for coronary heart disease (CHD), there is less agreement among observational cohort studies that obesity predicts CHD independently of other risk factors for CHD (NIH Development Panel on the Health Implications of Obesity 1985). Some prospective studies, including the influential Framingham Heart Study (Hubert et al. 1983), showed a positive linear association between body weight and CHD risk. In contrast, other studies reported a negative association, J- or U-shaped associations, no association, or a threshold (Barrett-Connor 1985). That lack of agreement is not easily explained by differing study methods, differing prevalence or ranges of obesity, or differing risk factors in the groups of people studied. Thus, though there are biologically plausible reasons that obesity might cause atherosclerosis, the conclusion that obesity directly causes CHD may be premature because it is based largely on studies that poorly establish temporal sequence. Also, most studies using both autopsy and angiography—including the International Atherosclerosis Project, which collected necropsy data from about 23,000 deceased people from 14 countries (Anonymous 1968)—have shown that obesity is not related to degree of atherosclerosis (Patel, Eggen, and Strong 1980; Warnes and Roberts 1984). Indeed, a study of about 4,500 elderly men and women found less atherosclerosis among people with higher body weights (Applegate, Hughes, and Zwagg 1991).

Hyperlipidemia

Whether obesity directly increases hyperlipidemia has not been established. Metabolic syndrome X among people who are obese is believed to evolve from insulin resistance among genetically predisposed people. An association between obesity and hyperlipidemia has not been demonstrated after controlling for hyperglycemia, hyperinsulinemia, and diet. Perhaps the best evidence that change in body weight leads to corresponding changes in serum cholesterol and triglycerides was provided by the Veterans Administration Normative Aging Study, which observed 1,400 men for about 12 years (Borkan 1986). Change in weight predicted change in lipids after adjustment for baseline age, initial levels of lipids, and smoking status. However, the predictive relationship was not strong and was not computed independently of diet, glycemic status, or physical activity.

Hypertension

Weight loss is often accompanied by reductions in blood pressure among people who are obese (Cambien et al. 1985; Dustan 1985). Obese people commonly have an elevated cardiac output and expanded blood volume measured at rest. Among the obese who are normotensive, peripheral vascular resistance is lower than normal. The association between weight and high blood pressure has been explained by two main hypotheses. One idea is that genetics and environment might affect both traits simultaneously or that a common factor links the two disorders. A second idea is that excess weight might have a direct influence on blood pressure. However, how obesity would cause hypertension in the absence of hyperlipidemia, hyperinsulinemia, and hyperglycemia has not yet been determined.

••• *Moderate physical activity can help lower blood pressure among overweight and obese people even when they do not lose weight.*

The epidemiologic evidence for a causal relationship between obesity and hypertension has been inconsistent. Results from the Framingham Heart Study indicated that weight loss was associated with improvements in blood pressure, but it was also associated with higher prevalence and incidence of CVD and higher death rates (Higgins et al. 1993). Having low weight at the outset of the study and maintaining that weight was the most predictive of blood pressure control and reduced risk of CVD morbidity and death. Similarly, two prospective observational studies of men in France suggested that increases in BMI were related to decreased CVD death, despite the higher blood pressures among men with high BMI (Cambien et al. 1985), but the use of antihypertensive medications was not controlled in those studies. It is possible that the overweight men had better medical control of their hypertension, despite its higher absolute level.

Type 2 Diabetes

Higher levels of adiposity contribute to insulin resistance in muscle, liver, and adipose cells, apparently because the hypertrophy of fat cells impairs insulin receptor function. However, studies that increased subjects' physical activity and altered their diet indicate that obesity is not directly responsible for the increased CVD related to diabetes (Barnard, Jung, and Inkeles 1994; Barnard et al. 1992). In those studies, serum levels of glucose and lipids usually were normalized without changes in body weight. Thus, for people who are overweight but not obese, decreased insulin resistance in muscle and the liver appears to explain improved glucose tolerance (Berdanier 1995). Chapter 9 on diabetes describes the evidence that physical activity, which has a low prevalence among obese people, is associated with improved glucose tolerance independently of weight loss, probably resulting from the insulin-like effect of muscle contraction and a subsequent increase in the insulin sensitivity of skeletal muscle.

> ••• *High body fat contributes to impaired glucose tolerance and diabetes risk by impairing insulin receptor function in muscle, liver, and fat cells. Physical activity can improve insulin sensitivity and glucose tolerance in people who are overweight or obese.*

With the exclusion of extreme obesity, overweight and obesity should be viewed as a product of the lifestyle habits of overeating and inadequate physical activity. Physical activity or increased fitness can also modify the impact of overweight and moderate obesity on several cardiovascular risk factors and all-cause mortality.

Fat But Fit?

A few well-controlled prospective cohort studies showed that people can be overweight yet healthy if they are also physically fit or physically active.

Lipid Research Clinics Mortality Study

In the Lipid Research Clinics Mortality Study, 4,276 men ages 30 to 69 years were observed for an average of 8.5 years (Ekelund et al. 1988). Fitness was determined by time to exhaustion and submaximal heart rate during treadmill walking. BMI was not an independent risk factor for mortality. However, among the lowest levels of physical fitness, the relative risks were 2.7 to 3.0 for CVD deaths and 2.8 to 3.2 for CHD deaths after adjusting for age, systolic blood pressure, high-density lipoproteins, glucose level, smoking, resting heart rate, regular physical activity, and BMI.

Aerobics Center Longitudinal Study

The most convincing evidence for a positive health benefit of fitness, independent of fatness, has come from the Cooper Clinic cohort in Dallas. In those analyses, the association of fitness with reduced risk of CVD and all-cause mortality was independent of overweight (Lee, Blair, and Jackson 1999; Wei et al. 1999).

Risks of developing CVD and mortality were compared among men and women at three fitness levels determined by a maximal effort treadmill test: low (the 20% least fit), moderate (the middle 40%), and high fitness (the 40% most fit). A BMI of 27.0 or greater was used to define overweight. The relative risk (RR) of CVD for the low-fit male group was 1.7 after adjustment for all other variables studied (age, exam date, smoking, cholesterol, family history, abnormal electrocardiogram, chronic illness, and BMI). The corresponding RR for all-cause death was 1.5 after adjustment for the same variables. For the overweight men and women, the RR for CVD and all-cause death after adjustment for the other risk factors did not differ from those who had normal weight.

Women with a BMI over 25 kg/m² had the same RR as those with BMIs in the 22 to 25 range if they had a high level of fitness. In contrast, those with the highest fitness level and the lowest BMI (<20 kg/m²) had half the RR for all-cause death compared with heavier women of the same fitness level. Findings generally were similar among men. The highest RRs were in men with the lowest BMIs, regardless of fitness level. The RR for all-cause death among men having moderate or high fitness was reduced about the same whether BMI was 20 to 25 or over 25.

Hence, overweight was not an independent risk for CVD or premature death in the Dallas cohort. Moreover, being moderately or highly fit conferred protection against CVD and premature death regardless of the level of overweight. Figure 8.5 shows results of eight years of follow-up of nearly 22,000 men, ages 30 to 83, from the Dallas cohort. The RR of all-cause and CVD mortality among low-fit men was twice that of fit men, whether BMI indicated normal weight or overweight (>27.8).

Nonetheless, the comparisons between fitness and BMI in the Dallas cohort were not adjusted for smoking, cancer, and other risk factors that might explain high mortality among people with low BMIs. Indeed, it is believed that such factors account for a falsely elevated estimate of risk among low-weight people. For example, several population studies have reported that the age-adjusted relationship between BMI and mortality is described by a J shape, such that risk is elevated at the lowest BMI, lower around normal BMI, and elevated even more at high BMI. The elevated risk at the lowest BMI may be explained by other factors that cause disease and may contribute to low weight, such as smoking and cancer.

Harvard Alumni Health Study

Results from the nearly 17,000 male Harvard alumni ages 34 to 74 indicated that being physically active can reduce risk of death even in the presence of obesity (Paffenbarger et al. 1986). The Harvard Alumni Health Study looked for relationships between mortality from all causes and known mortality risk factors. The 25% to 33% reduction in all-cause deaths among men who expended at least 2,000 kcal per week was still present regardless of smoking, high BMI, or gains in body weight during the years of follow-up. Higher BMI was associated with an age-adjusted reduction in RR of approximately 20% to 25%, except in the case of extreme overweight, which reduced RR only by 5%. Low net weight gain since the college years was associated with a 33% increase in RR, though that finding might be explained by smoking or wasting diseases such as cancer, which were not controlled for.

Nurses' Health Study

About 115,000 women ages 30 to 55 without CVD or cancer at the beginning of the study were followed for 16 years (Manson et al. 1995). Of the 4,700 deaths during that time, about 880 were from CVD and nearly 2,600 were from cancer. The J-shaped pattern of mortality across the range of BMI disappeared when women who had never smoked were excluded from analysis. Then the risk for mortality increased linearly with each increment in BMI. Nonetheless, mortality was not elevated markedly (RR = 1.6) until BMI reached 27, which was at the 65th percentile. When BMI exceeded 29 (the 75th percentile), RR was a little more than 2.0. At that level and higher, about half the deaths could be explained by obesity. However, 98% of the women in the Nurses' Health Study were white, so the results are not generalizable to men and other races.

Adjustments for the higher levels of vigorous physical activity reported by the lower-weight women did not alter the high risk among women with BMIs over 27. Nonetheless, it was not possible to determine from the study whether there was much variation in physical activity among the overweight women, so the role of physical activity in explaining increasing risk as BMI increased beyond 27 was unclear.

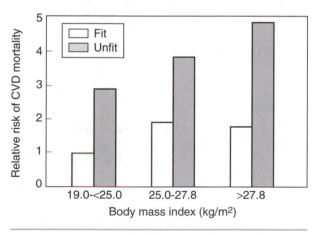

Figure 8.5 Aerobics Center Longitudinal Study with 21,856 men followed for approximately eight years.

Adapted from Lee, Jackson, and Blair 1998; Lee, Blair, and Jackson 1999.

Yo-Yo Weight Cycling a No-No?

The paradox of the increasing prevalence of obesity in the United States is the increasing number of adults engaging in voluntary weight loss during the same period (Serdula et al. 1999; Williamson et al. 1992). In the 1950s and the early 1960s, only 7% of men and 14% of women were trying to lose weight, whereas in 1989, a national survey indicated that approximately 25% of men and 40% of women were trying to lose weight. The average man wanted to lose 30 lb (13.6 kg) and weighed 178 lb (80.7 kg). The average woman wanted to lose 31 lb (14.1 kg) and weighed 133 lb (60.3 kg). These trends were seen regardless of age, sex, and ethnicity. Most overweight individuals who are attempting to lose weight are not successful, especially in the long term. This means that a large majority of the adult population engages in weight cycling.

The Multiple Risk Factor Intervention Trial (MRFIT) assessed the morbidity and mortality implications of weight change (Blair et al. 1993; Leon et al. 1987). MRFIT was a randomized multicenter primary prevention trial designed to assess whether multifactor intervention would reduce CHD mortality. Subjects were in the upper 10% to 15% of risk for CHD. In keeping with the studies discussed previously, low levels of leisure-time physical activity, determined by questionnaire, were associated with an increased risk of mortality. The primary measure of weight variability was the intrapersonal (i.e., within each person) standard deviation of weight, which was determined during clinic visits over the six- to seven-year period of the study. The weight variability index was subsequently divided into quartiles. The relative risk for all-cause mortality in the fourth quartile was 1.64 compared with the first quartile. Cardiovascular death showed a similar pattern; however, this pattern was not shown in the heaviest men. This study concluded that greater weight variability was associated with greater risk for CVD and all-cause mortality in some types of high-risk men.

> ••• *Regular physical activity can help offset the weight fluctuations, loss of nonfat body mass, and subsequent health risk of restrictive yo-yo dieting.*

This finding was also supported by the Normative Aging Study (Borkan 1986). After controlling for initial values of the given risk factor, weight, age, and smoking status, the change in weight remained a significant predictor of other CHD risk factors. These findings were not supported by the National Task Force on the Prevention and Treatment of Obesity (1994). The conclusion from this committee's review of the literature was that the adverse evidence was not strong enough to override the potential benefits of moderate weight loss in obese individuals. In addition, they concluded that data from studies that, like the MRFIT, indicated a link between weight change and increased disease risk and mortality did not adequately control for intentional or unintentional weight loss. Translated into practice, this means that the adverse affects of weight cycling should not discourage obese individuals from taking efforts to reduce their body weight.

The Problems of Fad Diets

The U.S. population, especially white women, appear obsessed with weight-loss approaches that promise quick loss without exercise. Popular diets include ketogenic, liquid protein, and very low calorie diets. High-protein diets rely on fat mobilization, which increases the formation of ketone bodies and can contribute to acidosis, dehydration, electrolyte imbalance, and excessive excretion of potassium, all of which can contribute to cardiac arrhythmias, liver problems, and kidney malfunction. Ketogenic diets emphasize carbohydrate restriction in the belief that restriction of dietary carbohydrates forces the body to metabolize more stored fat as the primary energy fuel. However, this can result in loss of muscle tissue rather than fat mass because the body uses its protein as a primary fuel to maintain blood glucose. Regular exercise can help offset the wasting effect of severe caloric restriction (Mole et al. 1989).

Liquid high-protein diets can be even more dangerous. During their peak popularity in the 1970s, the Food and Drug Administration attributed 58 sudden deaths to complications associated with the use of liquid high-protein diets for rapid weight loss (McArdle, Katch, and Katch 1991). Sixteen deaths occurred among obese women who had no history of heart disease but died of sudden cardiac death after losing an average of 37.6 kg during periods of time ranging from two to eight months.

The starvation diet, or very low calorie diet, is medically recommended for people suffering from class II and III obesity, those whose body mass is 40% to 50% fat and whose health is acutely at risk. Though very low calorie diets appear to help people sustain their dieting attempts, like high-protein diets, they result in more loss of lean tissue and water from muscle than of fat mass.

Etiology of Overweight and Obesity: Set Point or Settling Point?

Weight gain resulting from excess storage of fat is ultimately explained by an intake of calories that exceeds those expended. However, the physiological mechanisms that govern the metabolic balance of food consumption and energy extraction with the energy costs of basal metabolism, digestion, and physical exertion are complex and incompletely understood. Moreover, the factors that influence the behaviors of eating and physical activity, which determine energy balance and gains or loss of body fat, are even less well understood. Two common theories about the etiology of overweight and obesity, set point and settling point, address how physical activity can play a role in the treatment or prevention of overweight and obesity. The concept of reasonable weight provides an alternative view of weight goals for obese people.

Set Point Theory

Set point theory hypothesizes that the body has an internal control mechanism, that is, a set point, located in the lateral hypothalamus of the brain, that regulates metabolism to maintain a certain level of body fat. Though evidence in rats has supported the **theory,** there is no scientific consensus that such a metabolic set point exists in humans for fat maintenance. Though weight losses after the use of stimulant drugs, nicotine, and exercise seem consistent with the concept of an altered set point, these effects can also be explained by the alteration of basal metabolism in ways that do not require a change in the set point.

Studies using mainly dietary restriction have shown that weight loss is accompanied by a decrease in fat-free body mass and basal energy expenditure (Sum et al. 1994). Severe caloric restriction has been shown to depress resting metabolism by as much as 45% (McArdle, Katch,

and Katch 1991). If dietary restriction is chosen as the main weight-loss approach, a prudent program should

1. meet nutritional needs by providing a balance of the major food groups,
2. emphasize gradual rather than rapid weight loss,
3. accommodate the dieter's habits and taste preferences and avoid rigid rituals,
4. minimize hunger and fatigue while providing at least 1,200 to 1,500 kcal per day,
5. enhance health and facilitate positive changes in lifestyle and problematic eating habits, and
6. require physician approval if the dieter is older than 35 and also intends to markedly increase physical activity (Wardlaw, Insel, and Seyler 1992).

Settling Point Theory

Interventions designed to alter diet and reduce weight have used principles of behavior therapy with modest success, particularly among the obese (Foreyt and Goodrich 1993). The most successful weight-loss programs incorporate physical activity (Pavlou, Krey, and Steffee 1989; Perri et al. 1986). The **settling point theory** was proposed by obesity researcher James Hill of the University of Colorado to help explain why overweight and obesity are more than problems of metabolism (Hill, Pagliassotti, and Peters 1994). His idea is that weight loss and gain in most humans are more related to the patterns of diet and physical activity that they "settle" into as habits based on the interaction of their genetic dispositions, learning, and environmental cues to behavior. Evidence suggests that obese people are more sensitive to food-related stimuli in the social and physical environment, which influence their energy intake, than to the stimuli for energy expenditure.

> ••• *The idea of a settling point recognizes that overweight and obesity are more than metabolic problems for most overweight and obese people. People who have settled into weight-gain habits appear more sensitive to food-related cues than opportunities for physical activity.*

Reasonable Weight

Also recognizing the importance of behavioral factors and a person's history in implementing a successful weight-loss or -maintenance program, Yale psychologist and weight-loss expert Kelly Brownell has popularized the notion of **reasonable weight** rather than "desirable" weight (Wilfley and Brownell 1994). His view is that desirable weight has been judged by normative (i.e., averaged among many people) weights associated with risks for disease and mortality rather than the impact of weight gain on individuals, their unique histories, and the circumstances that contribute to their settling point and to their likelihood of successful maintenance of weight loss.

What Is a Reasonable Weight Goal?

Clinical questions:

Is there a history of excess weight in your parents or grandparents?

What is the lowest weight you have maintained as an adult for at least one year?

What is the largest size of clothes you would say, "I look pretty good considering where I have been?"

At what weight would you wear these clothes?

What does a friend or family member of your age and frame weigh who looks "normal" to you?

At what weight can you live with the required changes in eating and exercise?

Wilfley and Brownell 1994.

Physical Activity and Overweight or Obesity: The Evidence

There is scientific consensus that physical activity plays an important role in the treatment of overweight and obesity. Though most studies of physical activity and obesity are clinical studies of weight loss, a few well-controlled prospective cohort studies agree that physical activity or changes in cardiorespiratory fitness help minimize weight gain during early and middle adulthood.

Observational Population-Based Studies

A review of 11 prospective cohort studies and 1 cross-sectional study concluded that physical activity or increased fitness measured by maximal treadmill endurance is associated with minimizing weight gain or a reduction in the risk of large weight gains (e.g., 5–10 kg) among adults over periods ranging from 2 to 10 years (DiPietro 1999).

> ••• *Physical activity contributes to weight loss and helps minimize the weight gain that commonly occurs as people age.*

Though the studies used different methods to measure physical activity, different definitions of weight change, and poor control of confounders such as smoking and diet that also affect weight change, they generally agreed that being physically active has potential efficacy as an intervention for slowing the weight gain commonly associated with aging during the early and middle adult years. However, low physical activity can be both a cause and a consequence of weight gain. More prospective studies with several measures of both physical activity and body weight over time are needed to fully describe the temporal relationship between physical activity and weight change in the general population.

Finnish Cohort

Predictors of weight gain were studied for an average of about five and a half years in 12,669 Finnish adults who were examined twice during that period (Rissanen et al. 1991). Risk factors associated with the prevalence of obesity (BMI $\geq$ 30 kg/m^2) were also examined in another cross-sectional survey of 5,673 adults. The risk of gaining 5 kg or more was elevated in people with little leisure-time physical activity, as well as in those with a low level of education, chronic diseases, or heavy alcohol use. Having children and calorie consumption also predicted weight gain in women. The prevalence of obesity was inversely associated with the level of education and physical activity and positively associated with alcohol consumption in men and parity in women.

NHANES I Follow-Up Study

Data from the 1982 to 1984 epidemiologic follow-up to the NHANES I survey (conducted from 1971 to 1975) were used to examine the relationship between leisure physical activity level (low, medium, or high) and weight change among a representative U.S. sample of 3,515 men and 5,810 women ages 25 to 74 years (Williamson et al. 1993). A low level of physical activity reported in the follow-up survey was strongly related to major weight gain. The relative risk of major weight gain (>13 kg) for the lowest physical activity category in the follow-up survey compared with the high-activity category was 3.1 (95% confidence interval [CI]: 1.6–6.0) for men and 3.8 (2.3–6.5) for women. Also, the relative risk for people who reported low physical activity at both the initial and follow-up surveys was 2.3 (0.9–5.8) in men and 7.1 (2.2–23.3) in women.

Nurses' Health Study

Among a cohort of 121,700 women, the mean two-year weight gain among 1,476 women who stopped smoking was 3 kg compared to 0.6 kg among 7,832 women who continued smoking (Kawachi et al. 1996). Women who had smoked up to a pack of cigarettes a day and quit without changing their physical activity levels gained an average of 2.3 kg more (95% CI: 1.9–2.6) than women who continued smoking. By comparison, women who quit smoking but increased their physical activity by 8 to 16 MET-hours per week gained 1.8 kg (95% CI: 1.0–2.5); weight gain was only 1.3 kg (0.7–1.9) in women who increased exercise by more than 16 MET-hours per week.

The CARDIA Study

Weight change was studied prospectively over seven years in a U.S. cohort of black and white men (N = 1,823) and women (N = 2,083) ages 18 to 30 years (Lewis et al. 1997). Weight increased an average of 5.2 kg (SE = 0.2, n = 811) in white women, 8.5 kg (SE = 0.3, n = 882) in black women, 4.8 kg (SE = 1.0, n = 711) in black men, and 2.6 kg (SE = 0.8, n = 944) in white men. Decreased physical fitness was strongly associated with weight gain in both sexes. Each 1-min decrease in maximal treadmill endurance time predicted a 1.5-kg weight gain for men and a 2.1-kg gain for women.

U.S. Male Health Professionals

The influences of habitual physical activity, TV watching, smoking, and diet on weight change were observed over four years in 19,478 men ages 40 to 75 in 1986, who were free of cancer, coronary heart disease, stroke, and diabetes (Coakley et al. 1998). Weight gain was adjusted for initial age, hypertension, and hypercholesterolemia. Middle-aged men who increased their vigorous physical activity, decreased TV viewing, and stopped eating between meals lost an average weight of 1.4 kg (95% CI: 1.6–1.1 kg), compared with a weight gain of 1.4 kg in the total cohort. The prevalence of obesity among middle-aged men was lowest among those who maintained a relatively high level of vigorous physical activity, compared with those who were relatively sedentary. Each 1.5-h increase in weekly vigorous physical activity predicted a 2-kg weight loss in men ages 45 to 54.

Aerobics Center Longitudinal Study

Change in fitness was used as an index of physical activity among 4,599 men and 724 women (mean age 43 years) who had three or more measurements of body weight and fitness (maximal treadmill endurance time) between 1970 and 1994 (DiPietro et al. 1998). Change in fitness between the first two measurements (after about 2 years) predicted weight gain or loss over the average period of 7.5 years between the first and last measurements of body weight. During that time, men gained an average of 0.6 kg, and women gained an average of 1.5 kg. However, there was wide variation in weight change (the standard deviation was about 5 kg) that was linearly dependent on the changes in fitness. Among both men and women, each minute of improved treadmill endurance reduced weight gain by 0.6 kg, reduced the risk of a weight gain of 5 kg or more by 14% in men and 9% in women, and reduced the risk of a weight gain of 10 kg or more by 21% in both men and women.

Exercise Training Studies

Although physical activity has great potential efficacy for reducing body fat mass, studies have found that its actual effectiveness is small. Among normal-weight men and women, exercise training studies that followed the American College of Sports Medicine (ACSM) guidelines for increasing or maintaining cardiorespiratory fitness found that on average body weight was lowered by 1.5 kg (3.3 lb) and fat mass was lowered by 2.2% (ACSM 1983). People's body mass and fat mass responses to exercise training vary. Even between identical twins tested under strict control of diet and exercise, the variation in fat mass loss is about 20%. Nonetheless, there is a general consensus among researchers on weight loss that physical activity is the most variable of the components of energy balance and that it appears to be the best single predictor of success in maintaining weight loss. That is a key fact, especially when contrasted with the ineffectiveness of dieting for sustaining weight loss in most people.

Treating Moderate Obesity

- Food intake is weakly related to obesity in population-based studies.

- Physical activity usually has an inverse association with body mass and fatness.

- Physical activity is the most variable component of energy balance.

- Physical inactivity contributes to obesity, and obesity in turn contributes to physical inactivity.

Shah and Jeffery 1991.

Restricting Caloric Intake and Increasing Physical Activity

Food restriction produces a decline in basal energy expenditure that accompanies the decline in body weight. Basal metabolic rate (BMR) and the thermic effect of food are reduced during food restriction. BMR declines as total mass and fat-free mass decline. Because physical activity, especially resistance exercise, can decrease the percentage of body mass that is fat while increasing fat-free mass, it has the potential to retard the reduction in BMR common during restrictive diets. Initial body fat influences the changes in **body composition** after chronic exercise. People with more body fat have some protection against the loss of fat-free mass during early weight loss. They lose only about 0.25 kg of fat-free mass for each kilogram of body weight lost (Forbes 1992).

There is a consensus that an exercise program cannot prevent some loss of fat-free mass during substantial weight loss, even when caloric intake is maintained at the level prior to beginning the exercise program. Exercise can lead to a small gain in fat-free mass as body fat is reduced. This occurs when body weight is not changed after the exercise program. Hence, people who desire to increase or maintain fat-free mass during an exercise program must have a diet of sufficient calories to balance the increased energy expenditure.

Lost body weight is usually regained when diets are used alone, but diet combined with increased exercise seems to yield better maintenance of weight loss, as long as the exercise program is maintained after the diet ends. Figure 8.6 illustrates the results of an eight-week diet among obese adults (Pavlou, Krey, and Steffee 1989). Not only was exercise as effective as diet for weight loss, but adding an exercise program

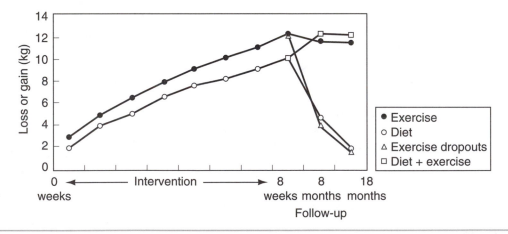

Figure 8.6   Study on moderately obese people illustrates that not only was exercise as effective for weight loss as an eight-week diet among adults, but adding an exercise program at the end of a diet prevented participants from regaining weight later.

Adapted from Pavlou, Krey, and Steffee 1989.

at the end of the diet also prevented participants from regaining weight 8 and 18 months later.

Exercise is recognized as perhaps the most important predictor of long-term success in weight maintenance. Kayman, Bruvold, and Stern (1990) compared formerly obese women who had lost weight and kept it off with obese women who had lost weight but regained it. Figure 8.7 shows that of the maintainers, 92% exercised regularly (a minimum of three times a week for more than 30 min). Only 34% of the women who regained their weight reported regular exercise.

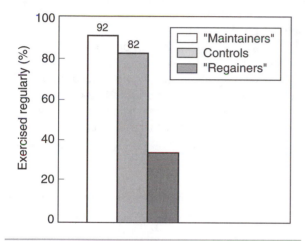

Figure 8.7 Exercise and weight maintenance.
Data from Kayman et al., 1990.

Strength of the Evidence

Temporal Sequence

About a dozen prospective cohort studies agreed that increases in physical activity or fitness (defined as increased maximal treadmill endurance) predict weight loss or an attenuation of weight gain over periods of 2 to 10 years.

Strength of Association

A recent quantitative review evaluated 22 nonrandomized and 9 randomized clinical trials published between 1966 and 2000 that studied the effect of exercise training on weight or fat loss (Ross and Janssen 2001). Twenty short-term studies lasting four months or less increased energy expenditure by an average of 2,200 kcal/wk and reported mean reductions in body weight of 0.18 kg/wk and fat weight of 0.21 kg/wk. Eleven long-term studies lasting 6.5 months or more increased energy expenditure by an average of

1,100 kcal/wk and reported mean reductions in body weight of 0.06 kg/wk and fat weight of 0.06 kg/wk.

Consistency

Though limited in number, population-based observational studies that included men and women or nationally representative cohorts indicated that increased physical activity or fitness (defined as maximal treadmill endurance) predict attenuation of weight gain, regardless of age, sex, and race or nationality. Similarly, randomized controlled trials have shown that exercise training contributes to weight and fat loss in both men and women regardless of race, though more men than women have been studied and most studies were limited to white people of European descent.

Dose Response

The aforementioned review by Ross and Janssen (2001) concluded that fat loss was linearly dependent on the amount of energy expenditure in the short-term studies but not the long-term studies. The weight loss during the short-term studies was about 85% of what would be predicted based on energy expenditure, assuming a controlled diet. In contrast, weight loss was just 30% of that expected in the long-term studies, suggesting poor adherence by the participants to either the prescribed physical activity or the prescribed diet. Only three studies of women had them expend more than 1,500 kcal/wk, so it was not clear whether the dose response occurred in women. Also, studies generally did not compare results between men and women or among people of different races.

Biological Plausibility

Energy expenditure can be increased by increasing BMR, the energy cost of muscular work, the thermic effect of food digestion, and the thermic effect of exercise. BMR constitutes 60% to 75% of daily energy expenditure. Thermic effects of food digestion and physical activity and the direct energy cost of physical activity constitute the remaining 25% to 40% (Poehlman and Melby 1998). BMR is the energy needed to maintain cell life at rest. It depends on age, sex, genetic factors, and fat-free mass. There is scientific consensus that a single session of exercise has two major acute effects on energy expenditure.

Recommendations for Weight Loss

The American College of Sports Medicine recommends that the minimum amount of physical activity needed to reduce total body mass and fat mass is three exercise sessions per week for 10 to 20 weeks of at least 20 min duration that expend 300 kcal each session (ACSM 1983). Greater frequency and duration at low to moderate intensity are needed for bigger effects, which indicates a dose response. For example, it is expected that exercise three to four days per week for six months at 45% to 55% of $\dot{V}O_2$max would lead to a weight loss comparable to exercise five to six days per week for three months at 75% of $\dot{V}O_2$max. Dietary restriction (1,250 kcal daily) and exercise are potentially the most effective. The ACSM recently updated its recommendations for weight loss and maintenance to include a reduction in dietary energy intake of 500 to 1,000 kcal per day and a minimum of 150 min of moderate intensity exercise each week (Jakicic et al. 2001). The new recommendations by the ACSM also state that there may be further increases in weight loss and better maintenance of weight loss by increasing physical activity to 200 to 300 kcal per week.

Recently the Food and Nutrition Board of the Institute of Medicine, which has provided health policy advice to the National Academy of Sciences of the United States for the past 60 years, recommended that adults and children spend at least 1 h each day participating in moderately intense physical activity in order to maintain optimal cardiovascular health regardless of body weight (Couzin 2002). The recommendation of 1 h a day of total physical activity is based on studies that estimated the average amount of energy expended daily by people who maintain a health body weight.

First, energy expenditure during exercise can be elevated to 2 to 20 times basal metabolism, depending on the duration and intensity of the exercise. This effect contributes to an increase in total daily energy expenditure unless the added exercise is followed by a compensatory and equivalent decline in physical activity during the rest of the day.

Second, energy expenditure does not return to preexercise basal levels immediately after exercise ends. The period of postexercise elevation in BMR can be a few minutes or 24 h, depending on the intensity and duration of the exercise (Hill, Drougas, and Peters 1994). For example, light exercise (30 min at one third of aerobic capacity) causes a postexercise increase in energy expenditure of about 10 extra kilocalories during the 10 min after exercise ends, whereas heavy exercise (65–90 min at two thirds of aerobic capacity) increases postexercise energy expenditure by about 130 extra kilocalories over a period of 24 h (Poehlman 1989).

Regular Physical Activity

Most investigators have found that aerobic exercise training in nonobese individuals has little effect on BMR. This is not surprising because training in nonobese subjects generally has a

How Does Exercise Help People Lose Body Fat?

- Increases energy expenditure
- Retards loss of muscle mass, hence maintaining BMR
- Increases metabolic rate during and after exercise
- Possibly increases SNS activity in people who have abnormally low tonic activity of the sympathetic nervous system (i.e., hypostress syndrome)
- Possibly suppresses appetite acutely after exercise; however, overall appetite tends to increase with chronic increases in physical activity
- Offsets effects of weight cycling (yo-yo dieting)
- Positive psychological effects that help people adhere to dietary or exercise programs

Adapted from Grilo, Brownell, and Stunkard 1993.

very small effect on fat-free mass, the major determinant of BMR. Other studies have found that exercise can affect BMR independently of effects on body composition, although those effects varied widely. There is also no agreement among studies whether chronic exercise affects the thermic effect of food. Oddly, very little is known about the effects of a chronic exercise program on total daily energy expenditure. It would seem that exercise should increase the total amount of physical activity of sedentary individuals, but it is possible that the added physical exertion may actually reduce their spontaneous activity and therefore also decrease their overall physical activity in a 24-h period. It is unclear whether exercise training alters the energy cost—that is, the economy—of completing a specific type of physical activity. Does a person expend fewer calories completing the same amount of work after becoming trained? Such an increase in economy does seem to occur during activities that do not require postural support of the body weight, such as cycling exercise. It is possible that regular exercise might also improve energy economy during weight-bearing activities such as walking, running, and games, where improvements in the skills of gait or timing of limb movements could decrease the energy costs of the activity (Hill, Drougas, and Peters 1994).

Resistance Exercise

Studies have shown that weight training led to reductions in body fat only slightly less than those produced by aerobic exercise and that weight training also produced more substantial increases in fat-free mass, which may have the added benefit of increasing energy expenditure (Poehlman and Melby 1998). Exercise might increase BMR by increasing fat-free body mass or BMR per unit of fat-free mass (i.e., of cells other than fat). Because the energy needs of internal organs exceed that of skeletal muscle, it remains unclear whether increases in muscle mass explain the increase in BMR reported after resistance exercise training. In one study, BMR was increased by about 10%, or 180 kcal per day, 15 h after a session of resistance exercise (Melby, Scholl, and Bullough 1993).

The mean increase in BMR after resistance exercise training programs, aggregated from 12 studies of nearly 400 people, was about three quarters of a standard deviation, which is moderately large and approximates an extra 50 to 75 kcal per day. That average was influenced by larger effects from four studies that lasted more than a year. Seven of the studies compared BMR per unit of fat-free mass, which indicates cell metabolism of nonfat tissues. Among those studies, the effect of resistance exercise training was smaller, about one quarter of a standard deviation. Hence, it appears that most of the increased BMR after resistance exercise training is explained by increased fat-free mass, not increased protein turnover of nonfat cells at rest.

> ••• **Resistance exercise training can increase basal metabolic rate by an extra 50 to 75 kcal on average. Most of the increase is explained by increased nonfat body mass, not by extra use of protein as fuel.**

A possible explanation for an increase in BMR after resistance exercise is increased protein synthesis after an exercise session (Booth and Watson 1985). Myofibrillar protein levels are elevated after resistance exercise training, but their role in increased BMR is unclear. One study, which used a measure of metabolic turnover of the amino acid leucine, reported that the energy cost of protein turnover was about 20% of BMR, about 350 kcal per day (Welle and Nair 1990).

Barriers to Exercise Among People Who Are Obese

Psychological barriers

- Past negative experiences
- Teasing by peers
- Poor physical performance
- Being picked last for teams
- Feeling inadequate in exercise or sport
- Lack of confidence about exercise
- Lack of knowledge gained from experience
- Shame of being watched during exercise

Physical barriers

- Burden of excess weight
- Low level of fitness

Grilo, Brownell, and Stunkard 1993.

Metabolic Fitness

The potential importance of the concept of metabolic fitness introduced in chapter 3 is highlighted by the high failure rates of dietary weight loss programs and the clinical and epidemiologic evidence in favor of physical activity for maintaining weight loss and reducing the health risks that accompany overweight and obesity. It is also recommended that all individuals, regardless of BMI, pursue at least a moderate level of daily physical activity in addition to a prudent diet low in fat, high in complex carbohydrates, and moderate in total calories.

Physical activity reduces obesity-related risks for CHD, hypertension, hyperlipidemia, and type 2 diabetes independently of body weight loss. Moreover, as insulin resistance appears to be a key catalyst that induces the cascade of risks associated with metabolic syndrome X, the demonstrated protective role of physical activity against impaired glucose tolerance assumes special importance for people who are overweight. Improvements in diet and physical activity patterns can improve health outcomes independent of weight loss. Increased physical activity and better nutrition have been shown to normalize glucose and lipid blood profiles in the absence of significant weight loss in many individuals. The mechanism responsible for this metabolic change is an increased insulin sensitivity because of an **up-regulation** of receptors on muscle and liver cells. In addition, the insulin-like effect of exercise increases blood glucose clearance in the absence of insulin because of the action of the glucose transporter GLUT4.

The Ultimate Goal: Weight Loss or Risk Reduction?

Most individuals judge the success of diet and exercise by scale weight. Rates of weight loss with a successful program average approximately 1 kg per week, which is viewed by many as frustratingly slow progress. Hence, the high dropout rate of nearly 50% within the first six months of a weight loss or exercise program. A change from preoccupation with scale weight to healthful management of blood pressure, blood glucose, and blood lipid levels through a prudent diet and regular physical activity in pursuit of moderate physical fitness is perhaps a more important health goal for most people who are overweight but not obese.

Maximize Exercise by People Who Are Obese

- Be sensitive to psychological barriers
- Be sensitive to physical barriers
- De-emphasize exercise intensity
- Emphasize increasing self-confidence about exercising
- Emphasize regularity and enjoyment, not amount and type, of exercise
- Start at an amount suited to the person's initial fitness level
- Define routine physical activities, such as walking, climbing, pushing, carrying, and digging, as exercise
- Emphasize staying active rather than focusing on minor issues (e.g., whether it is better to exercise before or after a meal)
- Consider the person's stage of life and stage of readiness for exercise
- Consider the person's culture, ethnicity, sex, and age
- Consider the person's social support network

Wilfley and Brownell 1994.

Summary

Overweight and obesity have reached pandemic status in the United States and several other developed nations. Despite scientific debate about their independent effects on mortality, general consensus remains that people who are overweight or obese have increased risk of developing hypertension, hypercholesterolemia, type 2 diabetes, CHD, stroke, gallbladder disease, osteoarthritis, and cancers of the uterus, prostate, breast, and colon. The co-occurrence of obesity with diabetes, hypertension, and hypercholesterolemia defines metabolic syndrome X, which constitutes an absolute risk for coronary artery disease and premature death. An estimated 300,000 deaths in the United States are attributed each year to obesity resulting from overeating and physical inactivity.

This chapter described the evidence that physical activity, as the most variable aspect of energy balance, has great potential for helping people avoid becoming overweight and obese. Though the effects of exercise training on weight loss are often modest, they can be similar to the effects of dieting. The best methods for losing weight and maintaining weight loss over the long term include prudent reduction in caloric intake and increased physical activity, including resistance exercise. Finally, an above-average level of cardiorespiratory fitness substantially reduces the risk of mortality among people who are overweight.

On balance, epidemiologic and clinical studies have shown that regular physical activity has potential for reducing the primary and secondary risk of becoming overweight or obese. Clinical studies have the advantage of experimental control in most instances, but it is difficult to separate the independent effects of physical activity from those of dietary and weight changes in many studies, especially as hypertension, hyperlipidemia, and obesity are intricately related to each other. Also, it is impossible to prevent fat loss during increased physical activity without increasing caloric intake, which can influence hypertension and hyperlipidemia if nutrients change with altered food intake. Nonetheless, many studies have indicated that much of the benefit of moderate physical activity appears to be sufficiently strong, consistent, temporally logical, and biologically plausible to support the current public health position that physical activity represents an effective adjuvant in the prevention and treatment of overweight and obesity. At present, evidence does not support a linear dose–response gradient between the intensity of exercise and fat reduction among typical middle-aged or older adults who have been sedentary and embark on a new physical activity program. Weight and fat loss are linearly related to total energy expenditure from increased physical activity in programs that last about four months or less. However, that relationship is lost in longer-lasting programs, probably because people have difficulty in adhering to a diet and exercise program for long periods of time. Some emerging evidence suggests that a dose response to exercise intensity may exist among recreational runners who perform at a level substantially above that likely to be a feasible goal for people who currently are sedentary, who constitute a large part of the population of the United States and other countries.

In sum, not only does regular physical activity independently reduce the risk of all-cause and CVD mortality, it also can help protect against CVD indirectly by favorably affecting the major risk factors hypertension, hyperlipidemia, and obesity. Those factors also pose elevated risk for other prevalent and deadly diseases such as type 2 diabetes and cancer. The evidence that physical activity reduces risk of those diseases is addressed in subsequent chapters of this book.

Bibliography

Allison, D.B., K.R. Fontaine, J.E. Manson, J. Stevens, and T.B. VanItallie. 1999. Annual deaths attributable to obesity in the United States. *Journal of the American Medical Association* 282: 1530–1538.

American College of Sports Medicine. 1983. Proper and improper weight loss programs. *Medicine and Science in Sports and Exercise* 15 (1): ix–xiii.

American Heart Association. 2001. *2002 heart and stroke statistical update.* Dallas: American Heart Association.

Anonymous. 1968. General findings of the International Atherosclerosis Project. *Laboratory Investigation* 18 (5): 498–502.

Applegate, W.B., J.P. Hughes, and R.V. Zwagg. 1991. Case–control study of coronary heart disease risk factors in the elderly. *Journal of Clinical Epidemiology* 44: 409–415.

Barnard, R.J., T. Jung, and S.B. Inkeles. 1994. Diet and exercise in the treatment of NIDDM. *Diabetes Care* 17: 1469–1471.

Barnard, R.J., E.J. Ugianskis, D. Martin, and S.B. Inkeles. 1992. Role of diet and exercise in the management of hyperinsulinemia and associated atherosclerotic risk factors. *American Journal of Cardiology* 69: 440–444.

Barrett-Connor, E. 1985. Obesity, atherosclerosis, and coronary artery disease. *Annals of Internal Medicine* 103: 1010–1019.

Berdanier, C.D. 1995. Carbohydrates. In *Advanced nutrition: Macronutrients,* pp. 160–208. Boca Raton, FL: CRC Press.

Blair, S.N., J.B. Kampert, H.W. Kohl, C.E. Barlow, C.A. Macera, R.S. Paffenbarger, and L.W. Gibbons. 1996. Influences of cardiorespiratory fitness and other precursors on cardiovascular disease and all-cause mortality in men and women. *Journal of the American Medical Association* 276: 205–210.

Blair, S.N., J. Shaten, K. Brownell, G. Collins, and L. Lissner. 1993. Body weight change, all-cause mortality, and cause-specific mortality in the Multiple Risk Factor Intervention Trial. *Annals of Internal Medicine* 117: 749–757.

Booth, F.W., and P.A. Watson. 1985. Control of adaptations in protein levels in response to exercise. *Federation Proceedings* 44: 2293–2300.

Borkan, G.A. 1986. Body weight and coronary disease risk: Patterns of risk factor change associated with long-term weight change. *American Journal of Epidemiology* 124: 410–419.

Bouchard, C., and S.N. Blair. 1999. Introductory comments to the consensus on physical activity and obesity. *Medicine and Science in Sports and Exercise* 31 (Suppl. 11): S502–S508.

Cambien, F., J.M. Chretien, P. Ducimetiere, L. Guize, and J.L. Richard. 1985. Is the relationship between blood pressure and cardiovascular risk dependent on body mass index? *American Journal of Epidemiology* 122: 434–442.

Cambien, F., J.M. Warnet, E. Eschwege, A. Jacqueson, J.L. Richard, and G. Rosselin. 1987. Body mass, blood pressure, glucose, and lipids: Does plasma insulin explain their relationships? *Arteriosclerosis* 7 (2): 197–202.

Centers for Disease Control and Prevention. 2002. *National diabetes fact sheet: General information and national estimates on diabetes in the United States, 2000.* Atlanta: U.S. Department of Health and Human Services, Centers for Disease Control and Prevention.

Coakley, E.H., E.B. Rimm, G. Colditz, I. Kawachi, and W. Willett. 1998. Predictors of weight change in men: Results from the Health Professionals Follow-Up Study. *International Journal of Obesity and Related Metabolic Disorders* 22 (2): 89–96.

Couzin, J. 2002. Nutrition research. IOM panel weighs in on diet and health. *Science* 297 (5588): 1788–1789.

DiPietro, L. 1999. Physical activity in the prevention of obesity: Current evidence and research issues. *Medicine and Science in Sports and Exercise* 31 (11 Suppl.): S542–S546.

DiPietro, L., H.W. Kohl III, C.E. Barlow, and S.N. Blair. 1998. Improvements in cardiorespiratory fitness attenuate age-related weight gain in healthy men and women: The Aerobics Center Longitudinal Study. *International Journal of Obesity and Related Metabolic Disorders* 22 (1): 55–62.

Ducimetiere, P., J. Richard, and F. Cambien. 1986. The pattern of subcutaneous fat distribution in middle-aged men and the risk of coronary heart disease: The Paris Prospective Study. *International Journal of Obesity* 10 (3): 229–240.

Dustan, H.P. 1985. Obesity and hypertension. *Annals of Internal Medicine* 103: 1047–1049.

Ekelund, L.G., W.L. Haskell, J.L. Johnson, F.S. Whaley, M.H. Criqui, and D.S. Sheps. 1988. Physical fitness as a predictor of cardiovascular mortality in asymptomatic North American men. *New England Journal of Medicine* 319: 1379–1384.

Forbes, G.B. 1992. Exercise and lean weight: The influence of body weight. *Nutrition Reviews* 50 (6): 157–161.

Ford, E.S., W.H. Giles, and W.H. Dietz. 2002. Prevalence of the metabolic syndrome among US adults: Findings from the third National Health and Nutrition Examination Survey. *Journal of the American Medical Association* 287: 356–359.

Foreyt, J.P., and G.K. Goodrich. 1993. Evidence for success of behavior modification in weight loss and control. *Annals of Internal Medicine* 119: 698–701.

———. 1994. Impact of behavior therapy on weight loss. *American Journal of Health Promotion* 8: 466–468.

Gaesser, G.A. 2002. *Big fat lies: The truth about your weight and your health.* Updated edition. Carlsbad, CA: Gürze Books.

Gaesser, G.A. 1996. Obesity a killer disease? A closer look at the evidence. In *Big fat lies,* pp. 59–78. New York: Ballantine.

Gardner, G., and B. Halweil. 2000. *Underfed and overfed: The global epidemic of malnutrition.* Washington, DC: Worldwatch Institute.

Gibbons, L.W., S.N. Blair, K.H. Cooper, and M. Smith. 1983. Association between coronary heart disease risk factors and physical fitness in healthy adult women. *Circulation* 67: 977–983.

Grilo, C.M., K.D. Brownell, and A.J. Stunkard. 1993. The metabolic and psychological importance of exercise in weight control. In *Obesity: Theory and therapy,* 2nd edition, edited by A.J. Stunkard and T. Wadden, pp. 253–273. New York: Raven Press.

Higgins, M., R.D. D'Agostino, W. Kannel, and J. Cobb. 1993. Benefits and adverse effects of weight loss: Observations from the Framingham study. *Annals of Internal Medicine* 119: 758–763.

Hill, J.O., H.J. Drougas, and J.C. Peters. 1994. Physical activity, fitness, and moderate obesity. In *Exercise, fitness, and health: A consensus of current knowledge,* edited by C. Bouchard, R.J. Shephard, T. Stephens, J.R. Sutton, and B.D. McPherson, pp. 684–695. Champaign, IL: Human Kinetics.

Hill, J.O., M.J. Pagliassotti, and J.C. Peters. 1994. Nongenetic determinants of obesity and fat topography. In *Genetic determinants of obesity,* edited by C. Bouchard, pp. 35–48. Boca Raton, FL: CRC Press, Inc.

Hillier, T.A., and K.L. Pedula. 2001. Characteristics of an adult population with newly diagnosed type 2 diabetes. *Diabetes Care* 24: 1522–1527.

Hubert, H.B., M. Feinleib, P.M. McNamara, and W.P. Castelli. 1983. Obesity as an independent risk factor for cardiovascular disease: A 26-year follow-up of participants in the Framingham Heart Study. *Circulation* 67: 968–976.

Jakicic, J.M. 2002. The role of physical activity in prevention and treatment of body weight gain in adults. *Journal of Nutrition* 132: 3826S–3829S.

Jakicic, J.M. 1998. Treating obesity with exercise. *Physician and Sportsmedicine* 12 (4): 13–20.

Jakicic, J.M., K. Clark, E. Coleman, J.E. Donnelly, J. Foreyt, E. Melanson, J. Volek, and S.L. Volpe. 2001. American College of Sports Medicine position stand. Appropriate intervention strategies for weight loss and prevention of weight regain for adults. *Medicine and Science in Sports and Exercise* 33: 2145–2156.

Kawachi, I., R.J. Troisi, A.G. Rotnitzky, E.H. Coakley, and G.A. Colditz. 1996. Can physical activity minimize weight gain in women after smoking cessation? *American Journal of Public Health* 86 (7): 999–1004.

Kayman, S., W. Bruvold, and J.S. Stern. 1990. Maintenance and relapse after weight loss in women: Behavioral aspects. *American Journal of Clinical Nutrition* 52: 800–807.

Kuczmarski, R.J. 1992. Prevalence of overweight and weight gain in the United States. *American Journal of Clinical Nutrition* 55 (Suppl. 2): 495S–502S.

Kuczmarski, R.J., K.M. Flegal, S.M. Campbell, and C.L. Johnson. 1994. Increasing prevalence of overweight among U.S. adults. *Journal of the American Medical Association* 272: 205–211.

Lee, C.D., S.N. Blair, and A.S. Jackson. 1999. Cardiorespiratory fitness, body composition, and all-cause and cardiovascular disease mortality in men. *American Journal of Clinical Nutrition* 69 (3): 373–380.

Lee, C.D., A.S. Jackson, and S.N. Blair. 1998. US weight guidelines: Is it also important to consider cardiorespiratory fitness? *International Journal of Obesity and Related Metabolic Disorders* 22 (Suppl. 2): S2–S7.

Leon, A.S., J. Connett, D.R. Jacobs, and R. Rauramaa. 1987. Leisure-time physical activity levels and risk of coronary heart disease and death. *Journal of the American Medical Association* 258: 2388–2395.

Lewis, C.E., D.E. Smith, D.D. Wallace, O.D. Williams, D.E. Bild, and D.R. Jacobs Jr. 1997. Seven-year trends in body weight and associations with lifestyle and behavioral characteristics in black and white young adults: The CARDIA study. *American Journal of Public Health* 87 (4): 635–642.

Manson, J.E., W.C. Willet, M.J. Stampfer, G.A. Colditz, D.J. Hunter, S.E. Hankinson, C.H. Hennekens, and F.E. Spetzer. 1995. Body weight and mortality among women. *New England Journal of Medicine* 333: 677–685.

Matthews, B., ed. 1914. Dialogue between Franklin and the gout. *The Oxford Book of American Essays.* New York: Oxford University Press.

McArdle, W.D., F.I. Katch, and V.L. Katch. 1991. *Exercise physiology: Energy, nutrition and human performance.* 3rd edition. Philadelphia: Lea and Febiger.

McGinnis, J.M., and W.H. Foege. 1993. Actual causes of death in the United States. *Journal of the American Medical Association* 270: 2207–2212.

Melby, C.L., C. Scholl, and R.C. Bullough. 1993. Effect of acute resistance exercise on postexercise energy expenditure and resting metabolic rate. *Journal of Applied Physiology* 75: 1847–1853.

Mokdad, A.H., E.S. Ford, B.A. Bowman, W.H. Dietz, F. Vinicor, V.S. Bales, and J.S. Marks. 2003. Prevalence of obesity, diabetes, and obesity-related health risk factors, 2001. *Journal of the American Medical Association* 289: 76–79.

Mokdad, A.H., M.K. Serdula, W.H. Dietz, B.A. Bowman, J.S. Marks, and J.P. Koplan. 1999. The spread of the obesity epidemic in the United States, 1991–1998. *Journal of the American Medical Association* 282 (16): 1519–1522.

———. 2000. The continuing epidemic of obesity in the United States. *Journal of the American Medical Association* 284 (13): 1650–1651.

Mole, P.A., J.S. Stern, C.L. Schultz, E.M. Bernauer, and B.J. Holcomb. 1989. Exercise reverses depressed metabolic rate produced by severe caloric restriction. *Medicine and Science in Sports and Exercise* 21: 29–33.

National Heart, Lung, and Blood Institute of the National Institutes of Health. 1998. *Clinical guidelines on the identification, evaluation, and treatment of overweight and obesity in adults: The evidence report.* NIH Publication No. 98-408. Bethesda, MD: National Institutes of Health.

National Institutes of Health Development Panel on the Health Implications of Obesity. 1985. Health implications of obesity. *Annals of Internal Medicine* 103: 1073–1077.

National Task Force on the Prevention and Treatment of Obesity. 1994. Weight cycling. *Journal of the American Medical Association* 272: 1196–1201.

Ogden, C.L., K.M. Flegal, M.D. Carroll, and C.L. Johnson. 2002. Prevalence and trends in overweight among US children and adolescents, 1999–2000. *Journal of the American Medical Association* 288: 1728–1732.

Paffenbarger, R.S., R.T. Hyde, A.L. Wing, and C.C. Hsieh. 1986. Physical activity, all-cause mortality, and longevity of college alumni. *New England Journal of Medicine* 314: 605–613.

Patel, Y.C., D.A. Eggen, and J.P. Strong. 1980. Obesity, smoking and atherosclerosis. *Atherosclerosis* 36: 481–490.

Pavlou, K.N., S. Krey, and W.P. Steffee. 1989. Exercise as an adjunct to weight loss and maintenance in moderately obese subjects. *American Journal of Clinical Nutrition* 49: 1115–1123.

Perri, M.G., W.G. Macadoo, D.A. Mcallister, J.B. Lauer, and D.Z. Yancey. 1986. Enhancing the efficacy of behavior therapy for obesity: Effects of aerobic exercise and a multicomponent maintenance program. *Journal of Consulting and Clinical Psychology* 54: 670–675.

Poehlman, E.T. 1989. A review: Exercise and its influence on resting energy metabolism in man. *Medicine and Science in Sports and Exercise* 21: 515–525.

Poehlman, E.T., and C.L. Melby. 1998. Resistance training and energy balance. *International Journal of Sport Nutrition* 8: 143–159.

Rissanen, A.M., M. Heliovaara, P. Knekt, A. Reunanen, and A. Aromaa. 1991. Determinants of weight gain and overweight in adult Finns. *European Journal of Clinical Nutrition* 45 (9): 419–430.

Ross, R., and I. Janssen. 2001. Physical activity, total and regional obesity: Dose–response considerations. *Medicine and Science in Sports and Exercise* 33 (6 Suppl.): S521–S527.

Serdula, M.K., A.H. Mokdad, D.F. Williamson, D.A. Galuska, J.M. Mendlein, and G.W. Heath. 1999. Prevalence of attempting weight loss and strategies for controlling weight. *Journal of the American Medical Association* 282: 1353–1358.

Shah, M., and R.W. Jeffery. 1991. Is obesity due to overeating and inactivity, or to a defective metabolic rate? A review. *Annals of Behavioral Medicine* 13 (2): 73–81.

Strauss, R.S., and H.A. Pollack. 2001. Epidemic increase in childhood overweight, 1986–1998. *Journal of the American Medical Association* 286: 2845–2848.

Sum, C.F., K.W. Wang, D.C. Choo, C.E. Tan, A.C. Fok, and E.H. Tan. 1994. The effect of a 5-month supervised program of physical activity on anthropometric indices, fat-free mass, and resting energy expenditure in obese male military recruits. *Metabolism* 43: 1148–1152.

Thompson, D., J. Edelsberg, G.A. Colditz, A.P. Bird, and G. Oster. 1999. Lifetime health and economic consequences of obesity. *Archives of Internal Medicine* 159: 2177–2183.

U.S. Department of Health and Human Services. 1988. *The Surgeon General's report on nutrition and health.* DHHS Publication No. 88-50210. Washington, DC: U.S. Government Printing Office.

Van Itallie, T.B. 1985. Health implications of overweight and obesity in the United States. *Annals of Internal Medicine* 103: 983–988.

Wadden, T.A., and A.J. Stunkard. 1985. Social and psychological consequences of obesity. *Annals of Internal Medicine* 103: 1062–1067.

Wardlaw, G.M., P.M. Insel, and M.F. Seyler. 1992. Weight control. In *Contemporary nutrition: Issues and insights,* pp. 336–373. St. Louis: Mosby Year Book.

Warnes, C.A., and W.C. Roberts. 1984. The heart in massive (more than 300 pounds or 136 kilograms) obesity: Analysis of 12 patients studied at necropsy. *American Journal of Cardiology* 54: 1087–1091.

Wei, M., J.B. Kampert, C.E. Barlow, M.Z. Nichaman, L.W. Gibbons, R.S. Paffenbarger Jr., and S.N. Blair. 1999. Relationship between low cardiorespiratory fitness and mortality in normal-weight, overweight, and obese men. *Journal of the American Medical Association* 282: 1547–1553.

Weinsier, R.L., R.J. Fuchs, T.D. Kay, J.H. Triebwasser, and M.C. Lancaster. 1976. Body fat: Its relationship to coronary heart disease, blood pressure, lipids and other risk factors measured in a large male population. *American Journal of Medicine* 61: 815–823.

Welle, S., and K.S. Nair. 1990. Relationship of resting metabolic rate to body composition and protein turnover. *American Journal of Physiology* 258: E990–E998.

Wilfley, D.E., and K.D. Brownell. 1994. Physical activity and diet in weight loss. In *Advances in exercise adherence,* edited by R.K. Dishman, pp. 351–383. Champaign, IL: Human Kinetics.

Williamson, D.F. 1993. Descriptive epidemiology of body weight and weight change in U.S. adults. *Annals of Internal Medicine* 119 (7 Pt. 2): 646–649.

Williamson, D.F., J. Madans, R.F. Anda, J.C. Kleinman, H.S. Kahn, and T. Byers. 1993. Recreational physical activity and 10-year weight change in a U.S. national cohort. *International Journal of Obesity* 17: 279–286.

Williamson, D.F., M.K. Serdula, R.F. Anda, A. Levy, and T. Byers. 1992. Weight loss attempts in adults: Goals, duration, and rate of weight loss. *American Journal of Public Health* 82: 1251–1257.

Winkleby, M.A., H.C. Kraemer, D.K. Ahn, and A.N. Varady. 1998. Ethnic and socioeconomic differences in cardiovascular risk factors for women from the Third National Health and Nutrition Examination Survey, 1988–1994. *Journal of the American Medical Association* 280: 356–362.

Web Sites

www.nhlbi.nih.gov/health/prof/heart/index.htm. Cardiovascular disease information for health professionals provided by the National Heart, Lung, and Blood Institute of the National Institutes of Health.

www.cdc.gov/nccdphp/dnpa. Home page of the Division of Nutrition and Physical Activity of the National Center for Chronic Disease Prevention and Health Promotion.

www.nhlbi.nih.gov/guidelines/obesity/ob_home.htm. NIH *Clinical Guidelines on the Identification, Evaluation, and Treatment of Overweight and Obesity in Adults.*

www.iotf.org. Home of the International Obesity Task Force.

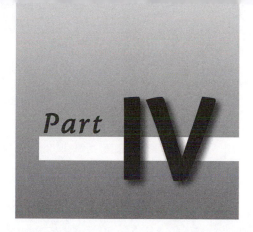

Part **IV**

PHYSICAL ACTIVITY AND CHRONIC DISEASES

The chapters in this section deal with two chronic diseases that are increasing in prevalence worldwide but nonetheless are underdiagnosed: type 2 diabetes and osteoporosis. Recent data compiled by the World Health Organization show that between 120 and 140 million people suffer from diabetes mellitus worldwide, and that this number might double by the year 2025. Much of this increase is predicted to occur in developing countries, resulting from an aging population, unhealthy diets, obesity, and a sedentary lifestyle. In the United States, diabetes is the leading cause of adult blindness, end-stage kidney failure, and nontraumatic amputations. Diabetes is the seventh leading cause of death in the United States, and it increases the risk of CHD, hypertension, and stroke two to four times. The first chapter in this section discusses the clear evidence that physical activity can help reduce the risk of type 2 diabetes.

The prevalence of osteoporosis is also increasing, especially among women of European descent. Twenty percent of U.S. women 50 years old or older who are non-Hispanic white or Asian have osteoporosis. It is predicted that more than 52 million women and men 50 years old or older in the United States will have low bone mass or osteoporosis by the year 2010. By 2020 the prevalence is expected to be 61 million. The public health impact of this trend is perhaps most clearly seen in the increased risk of fractures among people with low bone mass. For example, a woman's risk of hip fracture is equal to her combined risk of breast, uterine, and ovarian cancer, and about one in five people who fracture a hip, most after age 75, dies in the year following the fracture; 50% of the survivors become dependent on others for care. Though part of the increasing risk of osteoporosis and fractures can be explained by increased longevity, which leads to more older people, it is also becoming clear that physical inactivity contributes to bone loss and that some types of vigorous exercise that load bones with mechanical stress can promote peak bone mass in adolescents and young adults and retard the bone loss that accompanies aging.

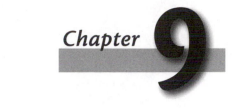

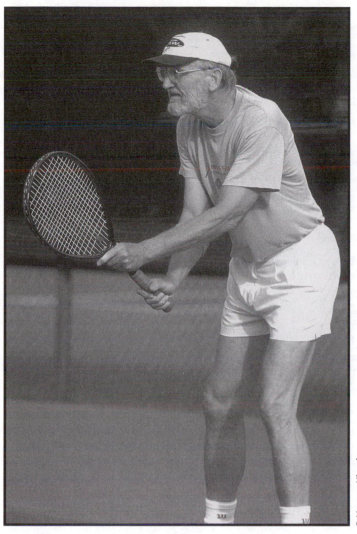

Chapter 9

© Human Kinetics

Physical Activity and Diabetes

A melting of the flesh and limbs to urine.

—*Aretaeus of Cappodocia,* A.D. *150*

Diabetes mellitus is a chronic disease caused by a deficiency in the production of insulin or its use to transport glucose from the blood into other tissues. The result is excess glucose in the blood, **hyperglycemia,** which is toxic. Diabetes is the leading cause of adult blindness, end-stage kidney failure, and nontraumatic amputations in the United States. It increases the risk of CHD, hypertension, and stroke two to four times. The economic burden of diabetes in the United States is great, about $98 billion each year: $44 billion in direct health care costs and another $54 billion for disability ($37 billion) and premature death ($17 billion) (American Diabetes Association 1998). Expressed per patient, the lifetime costs of the medical complications of diabetes have been estimated at about $47,000, with the following proportional costs: diseases of large blood vessels (52%), kidney (21%), peripheral nerves (17%), and retina of the eye (10%) (Caro, Ward, and O'Brien 2002).

The hallmark symptoms of diabetes are excessive secretion of urine (polyuria), persistent thirst (polydipsia), weight loss, and chronic fatigue or apathy. Hindu writings around 1500 B.C. first described a baffling disease that caused intense thirst and excessive urine excretion. It was first noticed when ants and flies were drawn to the urine of people suffering from diabetes. The term *diabetes,* from the Greek words for siphon, *dia*—meaning through—and *bainen*—to go—was first used around 250 B.C. to indicate that urine excretion seemed to be greater than the amount of fluids that sufferers could take in. The Latin word *mellitus* (sweetened with honey) was added later to describe the sweet urine. About A.D. 150, Greek physicians wrote how diabetes "melted the flesh" (Gordon 1960). In 1798, the English physician John Rollo was the first to detect excessive sugar in the blood of diabetics. Though centuries earlier, Greco-Roman physicians had prescribed exercise for the treatment of diabetes, Rollo ironically recommended bed rest. This chapter describes diabetes and its public health impact and then presents strong evidence that the Greeks were right and Rollo was wrong about exercise for diabetes.

Magnitude of the Problem

Recent data compiled from the MONICA project of the World Health Organization (WHO) show that between 120 million and 140 million people suffer from diabetes mellitus worldwide and that this number will double by the year 2025 if contemporary trends of increasing obesity and inactivity persist (WHO 1998). Much of this increase is predicted to occur in developing countries, resulting from an aging population, unhealthy diets, obesity, and sedentary lifestyles.

According to estimates by the U.S. Centers for Disease Control and Prevention, nearly 17 million American adults say they have been told by a doctor that they have diabetes (Mokdad et al. 2003), but another 35% of people who have diabetes haven't yet been diagnosed (Centers for Disease Control and Prevention 2002). Approximately 800,000 new cases of diabetes are diagnosed annually in the United States. The number of persons diagnosed with diabetes increased sixfold, from 1.6 million in 1958 to 10 million in 1997. According to the Behavioral Risk Factor Surveillance System, the prevalence of diagnosed diabetes in U.S. adults increased from 6.5% in 1998 to 6.9% in 1999 (Mokdad et al. 2001), a 6% increase in a single year. The rate continues to grow. From 2000 to 2001, prevalence increased from an estimated 7.3% to 7.9%, an 8% increase (Mokdad et al. 2003). Diabetes is the nation's sixth leading killer and was responsible for more than 71,000 deaths in the United States in 2001; two thirds were from cardiovascular disease (Centers for Disease Control and Prevention 2003). Diabetes and its complications occur among Americans of all ages and racial and ethnic groups, but the elderly and certain racial and ethnic groups are more commonly affected by the disease (figure 9.1). About 18% of Americans 65 years of age and older have diabetes.

Demographics of Diabetes

The Centers for Disease Control and Prevention (Centers for Disease Control and Prevention 2002; Mokdad et al. 2003) estimates that in 2000 the prevalence of diabetes in the United States was about 9.8 million women, 6.9 million men, 151,000 children (less than 20 years of age), and 7.0 million older adults (65 years of age or older). The prevalence of diabetes mellitus among Hispanic/Latino Americans is 10.2%; among non-Hispanic blacks, 13.0%; among non-Hispanic whites, 7.8%; and among American Indians and Alaska Natives who receive care from the Indian Health Service (IHS), 15.1%. The prevalence of diabetes among American Indians and Alaska natives is the highest of any cultural group in the United States, approaching 50% among women among certain tribal groups. The prevalence of type 2 diabetes is more than doubled among black and Mexican American women ages 25 to 64 who have not completed high school. Table 9.1 shows this disproportionate prevalence among U.S. minorities.

Type 2 Diabetes: Demographics

Increasing Incidence

Elderly and minorities in United States

African Americans

Hispanic Americans

Native Americans

Asian and Pacific Island Americans

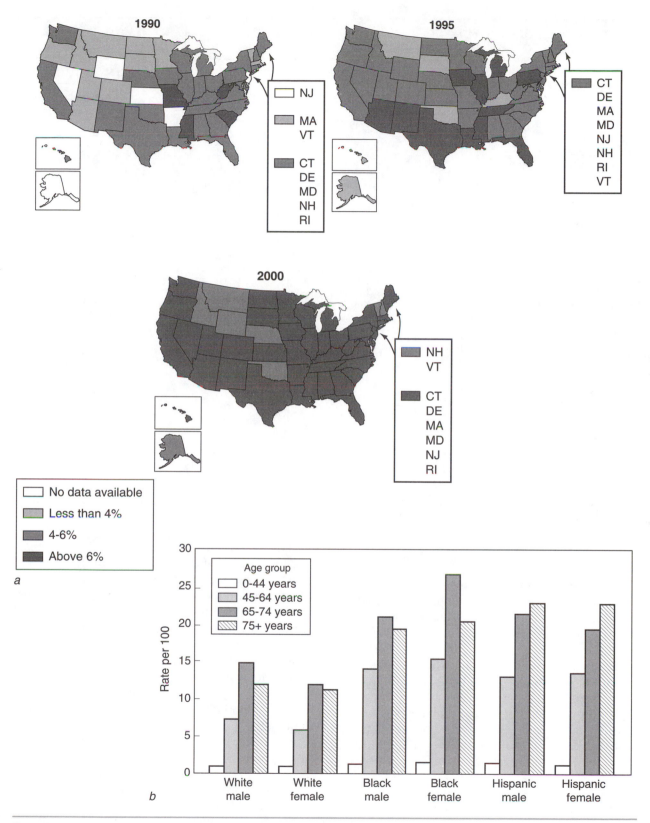

Figure 9.1 (a) Percentage of adults with diagnosed diabetes. (b) Age-specific prevalence of diagnosed diabetes, by race/ethnicity and sex. United States, 1999.

CDC. Behavioral Risk Factor Surveillance System.

TABLE 9.1   PREVALENCE OF DIABETES MELLITUS IN THE AGE RANGE 30–64 YEARS IN THE UNITED STATES STUDY POPULATIONS OF THE WHO MONICA PROJECT

ETHNIC GROUP/POPULATION	MEN		WOMEN	
	Crude rate (%)	Age-adjusted rate (%)	Crude rate (%)	Age-adjusted rate (%)
Indians Pima and Papago, AZ	47.6	49.4	48.9	51.1
Non-Hispanic white				
NHANES II	5.2	5.0	7.3	7.2
San Luis Valley, CO	3.8	2.9	4.5	2.9
Rancho Bernardo, CA	9.0	3.2	5.3	4.6
San Antonio, TX				
Middle income	9.3	8.4	10.5	7.8
Upper income	4.5	4.4	2.6	2.5
Non-Hispanic black				
NHANES II	7.9	8.5	13.0	12.1
Hispanic				
NHANES				
Mexican (Southwest)	11.1	14.0	12.4	14.2
Cuban (Miami)	11.9	11.8	4.4	4.5
Puerto Rican (New York)	14.6	17.8	9.6	12.8
San Luis Valley, CO	9.6	6.9	10.6	8.6
San Antonio, TX				
Low income	16.1	14.6	21.1	19.0
Middle income	14.7	16.7	10.3	12.1
Upper income	6.2	7.2	4.0	4.5

Reprinted, by permission, from World Health Organization, 2002. Available: http://www.who.int/ncd/dia/databases2.htm#t2.

Clinical Features

There are two principal forms of diabetes: **type 1,** also known as insulin-dependent diabetes mellitus (IDDM) or juvenile diabetes, and **type 2,** also known as non-insulin-dependent diabetes mellitus (NIDDM). In type 1 diabetes, the pancreas fails to produce insulin, which is essential for survival. This form develops most frequently in children and adolescents but is being increasingly noted later in life. Type 2 diabetes is much more common and accounts for about 90% of all diabetes cases worldwide. In the United States, about 80% of all cases of diabetes are type 2 (about 8% of all adults, or 12 million to 13 million adults). Type 2 diabetes occurs mostly in adults over age 40 and results from insulin insensitivity—that is, poor transport of insulin from the blood into the cell. About 20% of cases of type 2 diabetes occur after age 65 and another 25% occur after age 85. About half of the cases

of type 2 diabetes can normalize after weight reduction from increased physical activity and diet, and the remaining half can normalize after an increase in dietary carbohydrates that have a low glycemic index (e.g., fruits, vegetables, and pasta, which do not cause blood glucose levels to spike). The focus of this chapter is on type 2 diabetes because it is highly preventable by diet, weight loss, and physical activity. Though some evidence suggests that physical activity can help manage blood glucose levels in people with type 1 diabetes, there are special safety concerns regarding exercise by people with type 1 diabetes (e.g., preventing hypoglycemia and injuries to extremities because of microcirculation problems) that are appropriate for a book on clinical medicine rather than epidemiology.

Insulin, discovered by Canadians Frederick Banting and Charles Best in 1921, is a hormone produced by beta cells located in the islets of Langerhans of the pancreas (so named for the

German medical student, Paul Langerhans, who discovered them in 1869). Insulin regulates blood glucose and is required by all tissues except the brain and intestines (but mainly by muscle, liver, and adipose cells) for glucose to be transported from the blood across the cell membrane. Deficiencies in the normal production of insulin or in its transport into cells leads to hyperglycemia and **ketosis,** which damages tissues, especially the blood vessels and nerves.

> ••• *About 80% of diabetes cases in the United States and 90% worldwide are non-insulin-dependent, or type 2, which results from the development of insensitivity of muscle and fat cells to insulin, leading to high blood glucose levels. Increased physical activity and weight loss can normalize blood glucose in 50% of the cases.*

Normal blood glucose is 80 to 100 mg/dl post-absorptively (i.e., well after the last meal has been digested) and is normally elevated post-prandially (i.e., after a meal). In unregulated diabetics, blood glucose typically is about 300 to 400 mg/dl but can be as high as 1,000 mg/dl. When blood glucose is over 180 to 200 mg/dl, there is sugar exudate (i.e., overflow) into urine. The most common tests to measure blood glucose levels are oral glucose tolerance tests and blood glucose tests. Both tests are done after people have fasted for 8 to 12 h. The oral test involves measuring the change in blood glucose levels 2 h after a glucose drink. The blood glucose test is done without any additional glucose load to the blood. The goal of diabetes treatment is to lower fasting blood glucose after an oral glucose tolerance test to below 140 mg/dl, to lower postprandial glucose below 175 mg/dl, and to lower glycosylated hemoglobin (HbA1c) below 8%. Poor control of diabetes is judged as **impaired fasting glucose** levels higher than 200 mg/dl, postprandial glucose higher than 235 mg/dl, and HbA1c greater than 10%. Diet and exercise are useful for normalizing blood glucose levels between 140 and 235 mg/dl.

Health Burden of Diabetes

Chronic complications of uncontrolled diabetes include coronary heart disease, nerve diseases, blindness, kidney failure, and amputation of the limbs. Cardiovascular disease is two to four times more common among persons with diabetes, the risk of stroke is two to four times higher, 60% to 65% of people with diabetes have high blood pressure, and 60% to 70% have mild to severe diabetic nerve damage. Nearly 75% of the deaths among diabetics living in economically developed nations can be attributed to heart or blood vessel disease. Also, premenopausal women with diabetes do not have the same degree of protection against coronary heart disease as other women their age.

• *Diabetic neuropathy.* About half the people with diabetes have diabetic neuropathy, which can result in loss of sensations in limbs. Diabetes is a common cause of impotence in men. Nerve damage and poor circulation to the limbs causes tissue damage in the extremities, especially the foot, which can lead to ulceration. Diabetes is the leading cause of nontraumatic amputation of lower limbs.

• *Diabetic retinopathy.* Diabetic retinopathy results from damage to the small blood vessels in the eye and is a leading cause of blindness and visual disability. On average, about 2% of people with diabetes go blind, and 10% have vision problems after 15 years of diabetes. The risks of glaucoma and cataracts are increased among diabetics.

Glucose Diagnostic Criteria

Oral glucose tolerance test	Blood glucose test
Normal: <140 mg/dl	Normal: <110 mg/dl
Impaired glucose tolerance: 140–199 mg/dl	Impaired glucose tolerance: 110–125 mg/dl
Diabetes: ≥200 mg/dl	Diabetes: ≥126 mg/dl

• *Renal disease.* The risk of kidney failure is directly related to the severity and duration of diabetes and is retarded by controlling blood glucose levels, blood pressure, and restricting protein in the diet.

• *Complications in pregnancy.* The risks for birth defects and prenatal mortality are increased among women who have diabetes. **Gestational diabetes** (temporary glucose elevations during pregnancy among nondiabetic women) also increases the risks of pregnancy.

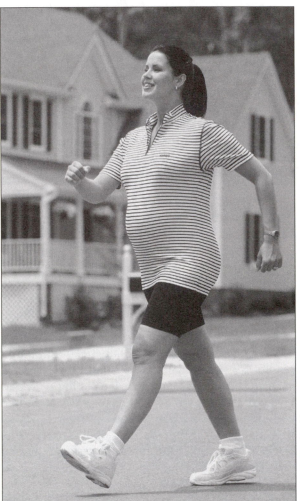

© Ariel Skelley/Corbis

Risk Factors

Diabetes mellitus is a hereditary disease. Certain genetic markers are known to indicate risk of developing type 1 diabetes, but such markers have not been determined as yet for type 2 diabetes, though it is strongly familial. Several plausible

risk factors for diabetes can be modified, especially by weight reduction and increased physical activity, to help primary and secondary prevention.

Reducing obesity has been estimated to reduce the risk of type 2 diabetes by 50% to 75% and increase physical activity by 30% to 50% (Manson and Spelsberg 1994). In contrast, the protective benefits of changing diet to decrease saturated fat and increase carbohydrate and fiber are not conclusive. Randomized clinical trials have not been conducted to confirm experimentally that changing body weight, fat distribution, diet, or physical activity independently decreases the risk of type 2 diabetes.

Etiology of Type 2 Diabetes

Around 1813 the French physiologist Claude Bernard concluded that diabetes was a disease caused by abnormal metabolism of glycogen. Today it is understood that the pathogenesis of type 2 diabetes begins with some degree of insulin resistance, mainly in skeletal muscle (figure 9.2). Compensatory initial responses include increased glucose output from the liver, followed by hyperinsulinemia in response to increased blood glucose. If high insulin levels compensate for the insulin resistance, the person maintains normal glucose tolerance; otherwise, early stages of progressive **impaired glucose tolerance (IGT)** begin. Type 2 diabetes develops in about 40% to 50% of patients with IGT; the rate of progression to overt disease is about 1% to 5% each year after developing IGT. The transition from IGT to diabetes occurs when insulin resistance becomes severe and is associated with elevated basal hepatic glucose output and subsequently a marked deterioration of insulin secretion—that is, beta cell dysfunction. Studies have found a 50% reduction in beta cell mass in people with type 2 diabetes. Also, the secretion of proinsulin (the biologically inactive precursor of insulin) is increased relative to insulin.

> ••• *Nearly half of people with IGT develop type 2 diabetes within 5 to 20 years. The most effective treatment for reducing the progression of IGT into diabetes is weight loss by diet and increased physical activity.*

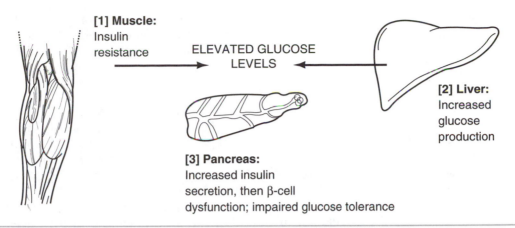

[1] Muscle:
Insulin
resistance

ELEVATED GLUCOSE
LEVELS

[2] Liver:
Increased
glucose
production

[3] Pancreas:
Increased insulin
secretion, then β-cell
dysfunction; impaired glucose tolerance

Figure 9.2 Pathogenesis of type 2 diabetes.

Clinical Tests for Diabetes

• *Glucose tolerance test:* Detects elevated serum glucose usually 2 h after oral ingestion of typically 75 mg of glucose. A positive test indicates inadequate insulin response or insulin insensitivity, but this test is not always accurate because it is influenced by preexamination diet.

• *Home glucose monitoring:* Usually done over four to seven days and is more reliable than a glucose tolerance test.

• *Glycosylated hemoglobin:* Measures the binding of glucose with the iron in red blood cells—that is, glycosylated hemoglobin (HbA1c). This is the most accurate test because it is not affected by acute plasma changes and is related to long-term exposure of red blood cells to glucose during their 120-day life span in the circulation.

Interventions for Type 2 Diabetes

Body weight control

Diet: saturated fat < 10% of calories, increased carbohydrate and fiber

Insulin or hypoglycemic drugs

Exercise

Effects of Physical Activity on Diabetes Risk: The Evidence

Exercise appears to have been first recommended to treat diabetes by an Indian physician named Sushruta around 600 B.C. It also was recommended by the Roman physician and philosopher Celsus at the beginning of the first millennium. Greco-Roman physicians were still prescribing exercise around A.D. 1000 for diabetic patients, but they preferred horseback riding because they incorrectly believed it reduced urination through the mild friction between rider and horse. A tradition of exercise treatment persisted until the latter part of the 18th century, when the British physician John Rollo recommended bed rest as the preferred treatment. The true role of exercise, though, in the primary and secondary prevention of type 2 diabetes has only emerged during the past decade or so (American College of Sports Medicine 2000).

Physical activity could potentially contribute to primary (reducing initial occurrence), secondary (reversal), and tertiary (delay of medical complications) prevention and treatment of diabetes (King and Kriska 1992). Metabolic studies suggest that the major effect of physical activity is improved glucose transport and insulin sensitivity, some of which may be indirect effects of weight loss (Goodyear and Kahn 1998). Therefore, it may have the greatest benefit in primary prevention and in early treatment of diabetes. Cross-sectional and prospective population-based studies have provided evidence consistent with such a protective benefit. There is also some evidence that exercise positively influences metabolic control of glucose and the prevention or delay of chronic medical complications in patients with type 2 diabetes.

Cross-Sectional Studies

Several studies have observed whether a decline in physical activity resulting from naturally occurring changes in culture are associated with increased risk for type 2 diabetes. Some populations that have traditionally led physically active lifestyles become sedentary after their society becomes more urban. In South Pacific island cultures, Zimmet and colleagues (1990) found a significant association between an abandonment of traditional lifestyles, which were physically demanding, in favor of more sedentary lifestyles with an increased incidence of type 2 diabetes mellitus.

Other studies observed individuals who migrated from a rural region to a more urban region. Individuals from a population subgroup who migrated were compared with individuals who remained in their homeland. For example, Kawate and colleagues (1979) found that type 2 diabetes was twice as prevalent among Japanese immigrants to the United States as among those who remained in Japan. Both types of studies have assumed that the adoption of a more urban lifestyle leads to increased risk of diabetes because of a decrease in physical activity. Of course, the effects of dietary changes are often difficult to isolate from the effects of urbanization.

Kiribati

A population-based survey of 2,938 Micronesians living on the Pacific islands of the Republic of Kiribati found that the age-adjusted prevalence of type 2 diabetes was nearly three times as high in urban as in rural samples (King et al. 1984). The rural population was leaner and engaged in more physical activity. The higher prevalence of diabetes among the urban sample was not fully explainable by greater obesity. Among women, obesity, urbanization, and physical inactivity were each independently associated with higher rates of diabetes.

A later study was extended to include Melanesians and Indians in Fiji and Melanesians in Vanuatu (Taylor et al. 1992). Urban participants were more obese than rural ones and had higher prevalence rates of diabetes. Rural participants were leaner, suffered less from diabetes, and had greater total energy intakes than urban dwellers. Rural people ate a greater proportion of carbohydrates, while urban people ate proportionally more protein and fat. Rural participants in all three studies had higher levels of physical activity.

Mauritius

The island nation of Mauritius, located in the southwest Indian Ocean, has a high prevalence of type 2 diabetes among all of its ethnic groups (Hindu and Muslim Indians, African-origin Creoles, and Chinese). These high rates of this disease among groups who differ in ethnic and genetic backgrounds illustrate the importance of environmental factors in the development of type 2 diabetes and provide a unique population in which to study behaviors that add to risk. A random sample of 4,658 Asian, Indian, Creole, and Chinese adults ages 25 to 74 years were categorized as active or inactive based on an interview conducted in 1987 about leisure and occupational physical activity. People with diabetes were excluded. Fasting glucose levels and 2-h plasma glucose and serum insulin levels after a glucose tolerance test were lower in active subjects of both sexes, independently of BMI and waist-to-hip ratio. In a subsequent study of Mauritius, total physical activity was associated with lower 2-h blood glucose levels after a glucose tolerance test among middle-aged Hindu, Creole, Chinese, and Muslim males and among Hindu and Creole females, even after adjusting for BMI, waist-to-hip ratio, age, and family history of type 2 diabetes (Pereira et al. 1995).

Pima Indians

The Pima Indians have the highest known incidence of type 2 diabetes in the United States. Among 1,054 Pima Indians ages 15 to 59 years who lived in Arizona, current (during the most recent calendar year) and lifetime leisure plus occupational physical activity were measured by questionnaire (Kriska et al. 1993). Current physical activity was inversely associated with fasting glucose levels and 2-h glucose levels after a glucose tolerance test. Active people also had lower BMIs and waist-to-thigh ratios in most sex-and-age groups, even when diabetic subjects were excluded. After adjustments for age, BMI, and waist-to-thigh ratio, 2-h glucose levels were still lower among men who were physically active, and people who reported low levels of lifetime physical activity had a higher rate of diabetes. In both males and females, the age-adjusted prevalence of type 2 diabetes was lower among people classified in the middle and top leisure physical activity groups than among those who had the lowest level of leisure physical activity during the past year.

Prospective Cohort Studies

The following section examines several different prospective cohort studies.

University of Pennsylvania Alumni Study

Nearly 6,000 male alumni of the University of Pennsylvania were observed for 14 years. A dose-dependent reduction in risk of developing type 2 diabetes mellitus was associated with higher levels of leisure-time physical activity (Helmrich et al. 1991). Figure 9.3 shows that the age-adjusted risk of type 2 diabetes decreased by 6% for each 500 kcal/wk increase in leisure-time physical activity up to 3,500 kcal/wk. The risk reduction remained after adjustments for obesity, hypertension, and parental history of diabetes.

Physicians' Health Study

Over 21,000 male U.S. physicians ages 40 to 84 years who initially were free of diabetes mellitus, myocardial infarction, cerebrovascular disease, and cancer were observed for five years after determining their initial level of self-reported frequency of vigorous exercise and other risk factors (Manson et al. 1992). During 105,141 person-years of follow-up, 285 new cases of type 2 diabetes were reported. The age-adjusted incidence was 369 cases per 100,000 person-years in men who were active less than once a week and 214 cases

per 100,000 person-years in those who exercised at least five times a week. Men who exercised at least once per week had an age-adjusted relative risk (RR) that was one third less than the risk of those who were physically inactive. The age-adjusted RR of diabetes decreased with increasing frequency of exercise: 0.77 for once weekly, 0.62 for two to four times per week, and 0.58 for five or more times per week. The protective effect of physical activity remained after adjustments for age, smoking, hypertension, and BMI. Though the overall protective effects of physical activity were independent of BMI, the association of exercise with reduced risk of type 2 diabetes was especially strong among overweight men.

Nurses' Health Study

Approximately 87,000 female U.S. nurses were observed for eight years, during which 1,300 new cases of type 2 diabetes were confirmed (Manson et al. 1991). Women who had engaged in at least one vigorous activity per week had an age-adjusted relative risk that was one third lower than women who had not participated in at least one vigorous activity. Figure 9.4 shows that when adjusted for BMI, the risk reduction conferred by vigorous activity was cut in half, to a relative risk of 0.84. Nonetheless, this reduced risk was still significantly different from women who had not exercised at least once per week. No dose response was observed, though. Up to five days each week of vigorous activity was no more beneficial than one day. When just the first two

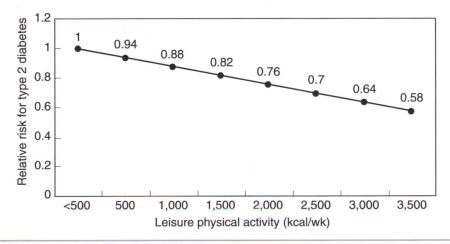

Figure 9.3 University of Pennsylvania Alumni Study examining leisure physical activity with relative risk for type 2 diabetes. The study included 5,990 males followed for 14 years with age-adjusted risk for type 2 diabetes decreased by 6% for each 500 kcal/wk increase in leisure-time physical activity up to 3,500 kcal/wk.

Adapted from Helmrich et al. 1991.

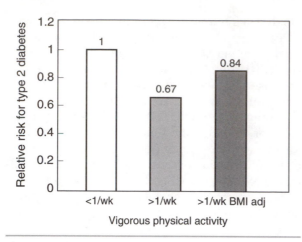

Figure 9.4 U.S. Nurses' Health Study examining vigorous physical activity with relative risk for type 2 diabetes. The study included 87,253 women followed for eight years. The relative risk is independent of weekly frequency of activity, age, BMI, and family history.

Adapted from Manson et al. 1991.

years of the study were analyzed, a period that was closer to when physical activity levels were measured, the age-adjusted RR of those who exercised was 0.5, and age- and BMI-adjusted RR was 0.69. In general, the protective effects of physical activity were seen in obese and normal-weight women and remained regardless of age and family history of diabetes.

Nurses' Health Study

This is an ongoing prospective cohort study that obtained survey reports of physical activity from women located in 11 U.S. states in 1986, with updates in 1988 and 1992 (Hu et al. 1999). A total of 70,102 female nurses ages 40 to 65 years who did not have diabetes or heart disease in 1986 were observed for eight years. The risk of developing type 2 diabetes during that time was categorized according to quintiles of MET-hours spent per week on each of eight common physical activities, including walking. During the eight years of follow-up, 1,419 new cases of type 2 diabetes were diagnosed. After adjusting for age, smoking, alcohol use, history of hypertension, history of high cholesterol, and other covariates, there was a linear reduction in the relative risks of developing type 2 diabetes from the least active to the most active quintiles of physical activity: 1.0, 0.77, 0.75, 0.62, and 0.54. That trend was attenuated, but remained significant, after adjusting for BMI: 1.0, 0.84, 0.87, 0.77, and 0.74. Among the women who were not vigorously active, the RR

of type 2 diabetes was reduced by 25% to 40% for women in the top three quintiles of weekly energy expended by walking compared with the lowest quintiles; those reductions were attenuated to 20% to 25% after adjusting for BMI. Though faster walking pace was independently related to reduced risk, similar energy expenditures from walking and vigorous physical activity were associated with similar reductions in the risk of type 2 diabetes.

Aerobics Center Longitudinal Study (ACLS)

The interaction among cardiorespiratory fitness, blood glucose levels, and mortality risk was examined in the ACLS (Kohl et al. 1992). Nearly 9,000 men were observed for approximately eight years. Age-adjusted death rates increased with higher initial levels of fasting blood glucose. Age-adjusted RR of death from all causes was elevated in the lower-fitness group across all levels of blood glucose (RR ranged from 1.80 to 3.42). The RR for death was higher in the least fit compared with the most fit across all levels of fasting glucose levels (<6.4 mmol/L, RR = 1.38; 6.4–7.8 mmol/L, RR = 1.61; >7.8 mmol/L, RR = 1.92). The study suggested that the risk of early death increases with less favorable blood glucose levels and that improved fitness levels might reduce the all-cause mortality associated with impaired carbohydrate metabolism.

Malmo, Sweden

Among nearly 7,000 men ages 47 to 49 who were screened for diabetes, over 4,600 men without diabetes were given an oral glucose tolerance test and a submaximal $\dot{V}O_2$ test of cardiorespiratory fitness (Eriksson and Lindgarde 1996). During the next six years, 116 men developed type 2 diabetes. Those men had 11% higher mean BMIs, more family history of diabetes (31% vs. 18%), 16% lower mean physical activity, 16% lower mean estimated maximal oxygen uptake, and nearly three times higher mean 2-h insulin levels after the glucose tolerance test. Men with higher physical fitness had lower 2-h insulin response to the glucose tolerance test. Hyperinsulinemia, BMI, and fasting blood glucose level were independent risk factors for type 2 diabetes. Among 278 men who had impaired glucose tolerance at baseline, 44 developed type 2 diabetes, which was predicted only by fasting glucose levels. Both physical fitness and the level of physical activity were associated with lowered risk of developing type 2 diabetes.

British Men

A cohort of 5,159 men ages 40 to 59 years with no history of coronary heart disease, type 2 diabetes, or stroke were selected from general medical practices in 18 British towns (Wannamethee, Shaper, and Alberti 2000). During an average follow-up period of 16.8 years, there were 196 new cases of type 2 diabetes. After adjustment for potential confounders (lifestyle characteristics and preexisting disease), physical activity was inversely related to risk of type 2 diabetes, blood insulin levels, and γ-glutamyltransferase level, a marker of insulin resistance in the liver. Adjustment for insulin and γ-glutamyltransferase level explained most of the reduction in risk of type 2 diabetes associated with physical activity, suggesting that physical activity reduces risk of type 2 diabetes mainly by improving insulin sensitivity (Heath et al. 1983).

Clinical Studies

Several studies conducted in the late 1980s and early 1990s examined the combined benefits of diet and physical activity on blood glucose levels among type 2 diabetics or people with IGT. The Zuni Diabetes Project was initiated in 1983 to reduce rates of obesity and provide primary and secondary prevention of type 2 diabetes. After two years of follow-up, diabetic participants in an exercise program compared with diabetic nonparticipants experienced weight loss, a drop in fasting blood glucose values, and reductions in the use of hypoglycemic medications (Heath et al. 1991). Barnard and colleagues (1992) investigated the role of diet and exercise on three different groups: 13 type 2 diabetics, 29 individuals with IGT, and 30 individuals with normal insulin and glucose levels. After 26 days, only the type 2 diabetics showed improvements in insulin levels and BMI. Although the independent effects of exercise could not be determined from those of diet because the treatments were combined, the study demonstrates that people's initial disease status can influence the outcomes of diet and exercise intervention.

Vanninen and colleagues (1992) investigated the secondary prevention of type 2 diabetes with a one-year intervention that consisted of a diet plus exercise in 80 men and women with type 2 diabetes. Fasting plasma insulin levels were lowered in both men and women. The women also had lowered fasting blood glucose and HbA1c levels. However, the women lost more weight than the men, and it is not possible to determine the independent effects of exercise and diet because they were combined into a single intervention. Other large-scale clinical trials, including two randomized controlled studies, have confirmed the benefits of increased physical activity and weight loss in reducing the progression of IGT to diabetes.

Malmo, Sweden

From the Malmo cohort of 7,000 men (discussed earlier in this chapter), 40 who had early-stage type 2 diabetes mellitus and 180 with IGT participated in a six-month intervention consisting of dietary treatment, increased physical activity, or both, followed by annual check-ups for five years (Eriksson and Lindgarde 1991). After the intervention, body weight was reduced by 2.3% to 3.7%, maximal oxygen uptake was increased by 10% to 14%, and glucose tolerance was normalized in more than half the men who initially had IGT. Men who initially had IGT but participated in the clinical exercise program had half the relative risk of developing type 2 diabetes compared with matched patients who received standard care but remained sedentary. More than half the diabetic patients were in remission after a mean follow-up of six years. Improvement in glucose tolerance was associated with both weight reduction and increased fitness, and mortality was a third lower than the rest of the cohort who were not treated.

Da Qing, China, Randomized Controlled Trial

Physical activity was included in a randomized controlled study that compared diet with exercise for reducing the development of diabetes among adults in Da Qing, China, who had IGT (Pan et al. 1997). Nearly 111,000 men and women from 33 health care clinics in the city of Da Qing were screened for IGT and type 2 diabetes. The 577 patients classified as having IGT were randomly assigned by clinic either to a control group or to one of three active treatment groups: diet only, exercise only, or diet plus exercise. Follow-up examinations were conducted at two-year intervals over a six-year period to identify subjects who developed type 2 diabetes. After six years of follow-up, those who exercised had half the rate of diabetes (8 cases per 100 person-years of observation) of those who maintained their normal physical activity levels (16 cases per 100 person-years). The cumulative incidence of diabetes at six years was 67.7% (95% CI: 59.8–

75.2) in the control group compared with 43.8% (35.5–52.3) in the diet group, 41.1% (33.4–49.4) in the exercise group, and 46.0% (37.3–54.7) in the diet-plus-exercise group ($p < 0.05$). All the intervention groups had lower rates of diabetes than the control group, independently of whether participants were lean or overweight (BMI $\geq$ 25 kg/m²). After adjusting for baseline BMI and fasting glucose, the risks of diabetes were reduced by 31%, 46%, and 42% in the diet, exercise, and diet-plus-exercise treatments, respectively. Hence, exercise was as effective as diet alone for reducing the six-year risk of diabetes in people with IGT.

U.S. Diabetes Prevention Program

The U.S. Diabetes Prevention Program was a randomized clinical trial of 3,234 adults ages 25 to 85 years (mean age 51) from 27 medical centers across the United States; it cost over $174 million (Knowler et al. 2002). Forty-five percent of the participants were ethnic minorities. All had IGT as measured by an oral glucose tolerance test, and all were overweight, with a mean BMI of 34. They were randomly assigned for three years to one of three groups: (1) lifestyle change aiming to reduce weight by 7% through a low-fat diet and exercising 150 min per week, (2) treatment with the oral hypoglycemic (i.e., reduces blood sugar) drug metformin (850 mg twice a day) plus information on diet and exercise, or (3) a control group that took a placebo pill and also received information about diet and exercise. Figure 9.5 shows the results; after an average of three years, 29% of the placebo group had developed diabe-

tes, while 22% of the metformin group and just 14% of the exercise and diet group developed diabetes. The relative risks depicted are based on crude incidence rates of 11, 7.8, and 4.8 cases per 100 person-years for the placebo, metformin, and the diet plus exercise groups, respectively. The diet and exercise led to an average weight loss of 15 lb (6.8 kg) in the first year of the study, or 7% of the group's initial average BMI; a 5% weight loss was maintained throughout the three years of the intervention. The lifestyle intervention was effective in men and women and all ethnic groups, including people 60 years old and older. The drug was effective, too, but not in older people and those who were less overweight.

Resistance Exercise

The effects of heavy-resistance weight training three days per week for 10 weeks were studied in eight 31-year-old men with type 1 (insulin-dependent) diabetes (Durak, Jovanovic-Peterson, and Peterson 1990). A randomized crossover design was used, whereby the same people underwent both an exercise treatment and a no-treatment control period and were tested before and after each. Strength increased in the squat (93.6%) and bench press (58%), while both self-monitored blood glucose and glycosylated hemoglobin (HbA1c) decreased, by 10% (from 7.85 mmol/L to 7.05 mmol/L) and 16% (from 6.9 mmol/L to 5.8 mmol/L), respectively.

Strength of the Evidence

Temporal Sequence

A substantial number of cross-sectional studies that lack the proper temporal sequence have been succeeded by a growing number of prospective cohort studies lasting 4 to 16 years and randomized controlled trials lasting from 3 months to 6 years. All these studies agreed that physical activity reduces risk of type 2 diabetes and improves glucose control in people with IGT or type 2 diabetes.

Strength of Association

A limited number of prospective cohort studies and randomized controlled trials consistently agree that regular, vigorous physical activity is associated with a 25% to 50% reduction in the risk of the development of type 2 diabetes. A larger number of nonrandomized and randomized controlled clinical trials show increases of

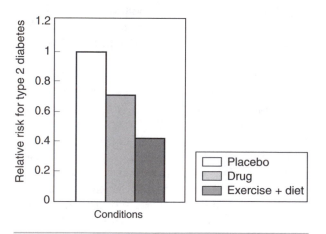

Figure 9.5 Relative risk of type 2 diabetes in people with IGT assigned to a glucostatic drug or exercise and diet compared to a placebo group.

Data from Knowler et al. 2002.

about 10% on average (ranging from 5% to 50%) in glucose tolerance in people with IGT and a 0.5% to 1% reduction in glycosylated hemoglobin in people with type 2 diabetes.

Consistency

The cross-sectional, prospective cohort, and randomized clinical trials that examined physical activity and risk of type 2 diabetes included samples of men and women from several nations who represented diverse racial and ethnic groups. There is good agreement that physical activity reduces the risk of type 2 diabetes in middle-aged and older men and women, including those who have IGT, regardless of initial fitness level, race, or ethnic background.

Dose Response

There are not enough controlled clinical studies to permit a clear consensus about the amount or intensity of physical activity that improved glucose control among people with type 2 diabetes (Kelley and Goodpaster 2001). However, clinical exercise-training studies suggest that increases in insulin sensitivity and reductions in HbA1c reliably occur after exercise at intensities of 60% to 80% of $\dot{V}O_2$max. In contrast, some studies have reported increased insulin sensitivity and decreased HbA1c levels after exercise training at low to moderate intensities of 50% to 60% $\dot{V}O_2$max (e.g., Trovati et al. 1984), but increases in maximal oxygen uptake after aerobic exercise performed near that intensity appear unrelated to changes in blood glucose and insulin levels measured at rest or after an oral glucose toler-

ance test (e.g., Wilmore et al. 2001). The normal HbA1c levels at the beginning of the Trovati study suggested that the participants had impaired glucose tolerance but had not yet developed type 2 diabetes. Hence, different levels of disease (e.g., IGT or type 2 diabetes) could moderate the intensity or amount of physical activity required to induce a meaningful change in glucose control.

Nonetheless, a multicultural cross-sectional study of nearly 1,500 men and women ages 40 to 69 of African American (29%), Hispanic (34%), and non-Hispanic white (38%) ethnicities found that insulin resistance measured by oral glucose tolerance test was inversely related to the usual weekly frequency of self-reported vigorous physical activity and to quintiles of weekly total energy expenditure estimated by a recall interview about physical activity during the past year (Mayer-Davis et al. 1998). Figure 9.6 shows that after adjustment for age, sex, ethnicity, dietary fat, alcohol intake, and smoking, insulin sensitivity among people who reported vigorous physical activity five or more times a week was significantly higher (1.59, 95% CI: 1.39–1.79) than that of people who reported that they rarely or never participated in vigorous physical activity (0.90, 95% CI: 0.83–0.97). The effect of physical activity was reduced but not removed after adjustment for BMI.

Biological Plausibility

The hallmark features of type 2 diabetes are impaired insulin sensitivity and insufficient insulin secretion. The sequence of the pathophysiology of type 2 diabetes still is not fully understood, but five events are key: a decrease in insulin receptor number, impaired chemical signaling for insulin,

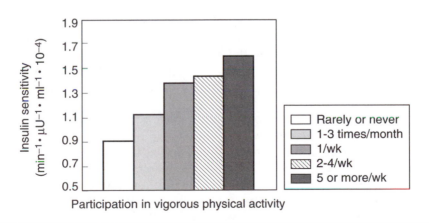

Figure 9.6 Insulin sensitivity according to frequency of self-reported participation in vigorous physical activity. Adjusted for ethnicity, clinic, age, sex, alcohol intake, smoking, dietary fat, and hypertension.

Data from Mayer-Davis et al. 1998.

impaired transport of glucose transporters to the cell membrane, impaired glucose transporter function, and impaired enzyme action. These features provide the framework for examining the biological plausibility that regular physical activity can prevent or normalize type 2 diabetes. Because high fat mass decreases insulin sensitivity, it is understandable that studies suggest that about half the effects of lowered risk of type 2 diabetes and improved insulin sensitivity can be explained by lowered fat mass among physically active people. However, physical activity also appears to exert an effect on insulin sensitivity and glucose control beyond its indirect effect of contributing to fat weight loss.

Insulin Resistance

More than 20 clinical studies have indicated that exercise training improves glucose tolerance by increasing sensitivity to insulin. Improvements in insulin sensitivity, inferred from lowered blood glucose levels, have been observed 12 h after a single exercise session. However, blood glucose levels typically return to preexercise levels 72 h after exercise. Long-term improvements, averaging about 10%, are most consistently seen after high-intensity exercise training five or more days a week.

Though exercise may improve glucose use and insulin action in fat cells, most of its effects occur in skeletal muscle. The uptake of glucose by a cell requires the function of a glucose transporter. Normally, glucose transporters lie inside the cell membrane and can help with the uptake of glucose into the cell only if they are situated on the cell membrane. There is evidence that glucose transport systems are altered in people with type 2 diabetes because of decreased movement of glucose transporters to the cell membrane. Muscle contraction has an insulin-like effect of promoting the transport of glucose from the blood through the muscle cell membrane (Holloszy and Hansen 1996).

Insulin increases the number of glucose transporters in plasma membranes. At least six glucose transporters have been discovered, two of which (GLUT1 and GLUT4) are found in skeletal muscle. Because glucose transporters, GLUT4 in particular, appear to be essential for insulin-mediated glucose transport in muscle, it appears plausible that an increase in the number or function of these transporters could help explain decreased insulin resistance after exercise training (Henriksen 2001).

Chronic Effects of Exercise on Diabetes

- Lowers circulating insulin
- Improves glucose tolerance
- Reduces insulin resistance
- Increases number of insulin receptors in skeletal muscle in people with type 2 diabetes
- Increases insulin-like effect of muscle contraction; increases GLUT4 transporter
- Increases insulin sensitivity in people with type 2 diabetes

---

Glucose Use During Exercise

It is plausible that changes in the metabolism of glucose after exercise training could alter the sensitivity of muscle cells to insulin. At the beginning of an exercise session, the energy for muscular contraction is provided by adenosine triphosphate (ATP). The body's natural response to compensate for ATP depletion is the recruitment of glycogen and triglycerides. The preferential recruitment of these two fuels depends on the intensity and duration of the exercise. During long sessions of low- to moderate-intensity exercise, the lipolysis of triglycerides is most important because more ATP can be derived from its oxidation than from the oxidation of glycogen. However, during high-intensity exercise, ATP can be generated faster from the metabolism of glycogen than of triglycerides. Thus, glycogen is the preferred fuel during high-intensity exercise. Physiological evidence suggests that insulin efficiency is most likely to be increased during the metabolism of glycogen. Therefore, the preferred fuel metabolized during high-intensity exercise, glycogen, could provide a potential mechanism for increased insulin efficiency.

Weight Loss

Regular physical activity also might prevent or retard the development of type 2 diabetes indirectly, by helping to reduce body fat, including intraabdominal fat, which is associated with insulin resistance. About 80% of patients with type 2 diabetes are also obese, which contributes to the development of the disease. Although exercise may promote metabolic improvements in obese individuals, severe obesity can limit the types and intensities of physical activity that can be performed safely. However, lower-intensity physical activity, possibly insufficient to make big changes in glucose metabolism, may lead to weight loss and thus indirectly improve insulin resistance.

Acute Effects of Exercise

Increased hepatic glucose

Increased glucose uptake in muscle

Increased lipolysis of free fatty acids from adipose cells

Decreased insulin secretion due to

- increased epinephrine secretion from adrenal medulla
- increased glucagon (secreted by alpha cells of pancreas, it activates glycogenolysis in the liver and yields 75% of the glucose from the liver)
- increased growth hormone
- increased cortisol from the **adrenal cortex**

Summary

Population-based studies and a few controlled clinical studies indicate that moderate physical activity is associated with a dose-dependent reduction in the risk of developing type 2 diabetes. That apparent protective effect is temporally correct; consistent among sexes, ages, and ethnic groups; and biologically plausible. The U.S. Diabetes Prevention Program, a multicultural randomized controlled trial of 3,234 obese adults ages 25 to 85 years with IGT confirmed that a three-year program combining 150 min per week of exercise and a low-fat diet led to a 5% weight loss and reduced the risk of developing diabetes by nearly 60% compared to placebo, superior to the approximately 30% reduction in risk after treatment with an oral hypoglycemic drug. It is not yet clear whether the effect of physical activity is wholly independent of BMI, fat loss, and diet. Though physical activity can indirectly help lower diabetes risk by contributing to weight loss, physical activity improves glucose tolerance and insulin sensitivity, and muscle contraction has an insulin-like effect on the transport of glucose from the blood. The effect of lowered glucose after acute exercise lasts about 72 h, so

exercising every two to three days each week may be sufficient to help maintain normalized blood glucose levels. The University of Pennsylvania alumni study indicated a dose-dependent reduction in the risk of developing NIDDM, with a 6% reduction in risk for each additional 500 kcal of weekly leisure-time physical activity. On balance, though, most studies suggest that vigorous physical activity two to three times a week provides most of the independent benefits of glucose control. Additional benefits of improved insulin sensitivity with daily moderate physical activity can occur through fat weight loss.

Bibliography

American College of Sports Medicine. 2000. Exercise and type 2 diabetes. *Medicine and Science in Sports and Exercise* 32: 1345–1360.

American Diabetes Association. 1998. Economic consequences of diabetes mellitus in the U.S. in 1997. *Diabetes Care* 21: 296–309.

Barnard, R.J., E.J. Ugianskis, D.A. Martin, and S.B. Inkeles. 1992. Role of diet and exercise in the management of hyperinsulinemia and associated atherosclerotic risk factors. *American Journal of Cardiology* 69: 440–444.

Bliss, M. 1982. *The discovery of insulin.* Chicago: University of Chicago Press.

Burstein, R., Y. Epstein, Y. Shapiro, I. Charuzi, and E. Karnieli. 1990. Effect of an acute bout of exercise on glucose disposal in human obesity. *Journal of Applied Physiology* 69 (1): 299–304.

Burstein, R., C. Polychronakos, C.J. Toews, H.J. MacDougall, and B.I. Posner. 1985. Acute reversal of the enhanced insulin action in trained athletes. *Diabetes* 34: 756–760.

Caro, J.J., A.J. Ward, and J.A. O'Brien. 2002. Lifetime costs of complication resulting from type 2 diabetes in the U.S. *Diabetes Care* 25: 476–481.

Centers for Disease Control and Prevention. 2002. *National diabetes fact sheet: General information and national estimates on diabetes in the United States, 2000.* Atlanta: U.S. Department of Health and Human Services, Centers for Disease Control and Prevention.

Centers for Disease Control and Prevention. 2003. Deaths: Preliminary data for 2001. *National Vital Statistics Reports* 51(5): 1–48.

Devlin, J.T., M. Hirshman, E.D. Horton, and E.S. Horton. 1987. Enhanced peripheral and splanchnic insulin sensitivity in NIDDM men after single bout of exercise. *Diabetes* 36: 444–449.

Douen, A.G., T. Ramlal, S. Rastogi, P.J. Bilan, G.D. Cartee, M. Vranic, J.O. Holloszy, and A. Klip. 1990. Exercise induces recruitment of the insulin-responsive glucose transporter. *Journal of Biological Chemistry* 265 (23): 13427–13430.

Durak, E.P., L. Jovanovic-Peterson, and C.M. Peterson. 1990. Randomized crossover study of effect of resistance training on glycemic control, muscular strength, and cholesterol in type I diabetic men. *Diabetes Care* 13: 1039–1043.

Eriksson, K.F., and F. Lindgarde. 1991. Prevention of type 2 (non-insulin-dependent) diabetes mellitus by diet and physical exercise: The 6-year Malmo feasibility study. *Diabetologia* 34: 891–898.

———. 1996. Poor physical fitness, and impaired early insulin response but late hyperinsulinaemia, as predictors of NIDDM in middle-aged Swedish men. *Diabetologia* 39: 573–579.

Goodyear, L.J., and B.B. Kahn. 1998. Exercise, glucose transport, and insulin sensitivity. *Annual Reviews in Medicine* 49: 235–261.

Gordon, B.L. 1960. *Medieval and Renaissance medicine.* New York: Philosophical Library.

Gudat, U., M. Berger, and P.J. Lefebvre. 1993. Physical activity, fitness, and non-insulin-dependent (type II) diabetes mellitus. In *Exercise fitness and health,* 2nd edition, edited by C. Bouchard, R.J. Shephard, T. Stephens, J.R. Sutton, and B.D. McPherson. Champaign, IL: Human Kinetics.

Harris, M.I., W.C. Hadden, W.C. Knowler, and P.H. Bennett. 1987. Prevalence of diabetes and impaired glucose tolerance and plasma glucose levels in US population aged 20 to 74 years. *Diabetes* 36: 523–534.

Heath, G.W., J.R. Gavin III, J.M. Hinderliter, J.M. Hagberg, S.A. Bloomfield, and J.O. Holloszy. 1983. Effects of exercise and lack of exercise on glucose tolerance and insulin sensitivity. *Journal of Applied Physiology* 55 (2): 512–517.

Heath, G.W., R.H. Wilson, J. Smith, and B.E. Leonard. 1991. Community-based exercise and weight control: Diabetes risk reduction and glycemic control in Zuni Indians. *American Journal of Clinical Nutrition* 53 (6 Suppl.): 1642S–1646S.

Helmrich, S.P., D.R. Ragland, R.W. Leung, and R.S. Paffenbarger. 1991. Physical activity and reduced occurrence of non-insulin-dependent diabetes mellitus. *New England Journal of Medicine* 325: 147–152.

Henriksen, E.J. 2001. Invited review: Effects of acute exercise and exercise training on insulin resistance. *Journal of Applied Physiology* 93: 788–796.

Hollander, P.A., and J. Nordstrom. 1991. Exercise and diabetes: Great for type II, good for type I. *Your Patient and Fitness* 5 (3): 6–13.

Holloszy, J.O., and P.A. Hansen. 1996. Regulation of glucose transport into skeletal muscle. *Reviews of Physiology, Biochemistry, and Pharmacology* 128: 99–193.

Hu, F.B., R.J. Sigal, J.W. Rich-Edwards, G.A. Colditz, C.G. Solomon, W.C. Willett, F.E. Speizer, and J.E. Manson. 1999. Walking compared with vigorous physical activity and risk of type 2 diabetes in women: A prospective study. *Journal of the American Medical Association* 282 (15): 1433–1439.

Kawate, R., M. Yamakido, Y. Nishimoto, P.H. Bennett, R.F. Garnman, and W.C. Knowler. 1979. Diabetes and its vascular complications in Japanese migrants on the island of Hawaii. *Diabetes Care* 2: 161–170.

Kelley, D.E., and B.H. Goodpaster. 2001. Effects of exercise on glucose homeostasis in type 2 diabetes mellitus. *Medicine and Science in Sports and Exercise* 33 (Suppl. 6): S495–S501.

King, H., and A.M. Kriska. 1992. Prevention of type II diabetes by physical training: Epidemiological considerations and study methods. *Diabetes Care* 15: 1794–1799.

King, H., R. Taylor, P. Zimmet, K. Pargeter, L.R. Raper, T. Beriki, and J. Tekanene. 1984. Non-insulin-dependent diabetes (NIDDM) in a newly independent Pacific nation: The Republic of Kiribati. *Diabetes Care* 7: 409–415.

Knowler, W.C., E. Barrett-Connor, S.E. Fowler, R.F. Hamman, J.M. Lachin, E.A. Walker, and D. Nathan. 2002. Reduction in the incidence of type 2 diabetes with lifestyle intervention or metformin. *New England Journal of Medicine* 346 (6): 393–403.

Kohl, H.W., N.F. Gordon, J.A. Villegas, and S.N. Blair. 1992. Cardiorespiratory fitness, glycemic status, and mortality risk in men. *Diabetes Care* 15 (2): 184–192.

Kriska, A. 1997. Physical activity and the prevention of type II (non-insulin-dependent) diabetes. *President's Council on Physical Fitness and Sports Research Digest* 2 (10): 1–7.

Kriska, A.M., S.N. Blair, and M.A. Pereira. 1994. The potential role of physical activity in the prevention of non-insulin-dependent diabetes mellitus: The epidemiological evidence. *Exercise and Sport Sciences Reviews* 22: 121–143.

Kriska, A.M., R.E. LaPorte, S.L. Patrick, L.H. Kuller, and T.J. Orchard. 1991. The association of physical activity and diabetic complications in individuals with insulin-dependent diabetes mellitus: The Epidemiology of Diabetes Complications Study VII. *Journal of Clinical Epidemiology* 44: 1207–1214.

Kriska, A.M., R.E. LaPorte, D.J. Pettitt, M.A. Charles, R.G. Nelson, L.H. Kuller, P.H. Bennett, and W.C. Knowler. 1993. The association of physical activity with obesity, fat distribution and glucose intolerance in Pima Indians. *Diabetologia* 36: 863–869.

Manson, J.E., D.M. Nathan, A.S. Krolewski, M.J. Stampfer, W.C. Willett, and C.H. Hennekens. 1992. A prospective study of exercise and incidence of diabetes among US male physicians. *Journal of the American Medical Association* 268: 63–67.

Manson, J.E., E.B. Rimm, M.J. Stampfer, G.A. Colditz, W.C. Willett, A.S. Krolewski, B. Rosner, C.H. Hennekens, and F.E. Speizer. 1991. Physical activity and incidence of non-insulin-dependent diabetes mellitus in women. *Lancet* 338: 774–778.

Manson, J.E., and A. Spelsberg. 1994. Primary prevention of non-insulin-dependent diabetes mellitus. *American Journal of Preventive Medicine* 10 (3): 172–184.

Mayer-Davis, E.J., R. D'Agostino, A.J. Karter, S.M. Haffner, M.J. Rewers, M. Saad, and R.N. Bergman. 1998. Intensity and amount of physical activity in relation to insulin sensitivity: The Insulin Resistance Atherosclerosis Study. *Journal of the American Medical Association* 279: 669–674.

Mokdad, A.H., E.S. Ford, B.A. Bowman, W.H. Dietz, F. Vinicor, V.S. Bales, and J.S. Marks. 2003. Prevalence of obesity, diabetes, and obesity-related health risk factors, 2001. *Journal of the American Medical Association* 289: 76–79.

Mokdad, A.H., E.S. Ford, B.A. Bowman, D.E. Nelson, M.M. Engelgau, F. Vinicor, and J.S. Marks. 2001. The continuing increase of diabetes in the US. *Diabetes Care* 24: 412.

Moy, C.S., T.J. Songer, R.E. LaPorte, J.S. Dorman, A.M. Kriska, T.J. Orchard, D.J. Becker, and A.L. Drash. 1993. Insulin-dependent diabetes mellitus, physical activity, and death. *American Journal of Epidemiology* 137: 74–81.

Olefsky, J.M., O.G. Kolterman, and J.A. Scarlett. 1982. Insulin action and resistance in obesity and noninsulin-dependent type II diabetes mellitus. *American Journal of Physiology, Endocrinology and Metabolism* 6: E15–E30.

Pan, X.R., G.W. Li, Y.H. Hu, J.X. Wang, W.Y. Yang, Z.X. An, Z.X. Hu, J. Lin, J.Z. Xiao, H.B. Cao, et al. 1997. Effects of diet and exercise in preventing NIDDM in people with impaired glucose tolerance: The Da Qing IGT and Diabetes Study. *Diabetes Care* 20 (4): 537–544.

Paternostro-Bayles, M., R.R. Wing, and R.J. Robertson. 1989. Effect of lifestyle activity of varying duration on glycemic control in type II diabetic women. *Diabetes Care* 12: 34–37.

Pedersen, O., J.F. Bak, P.H. Andersen, S. Lund, D.E. Moller, J.S. Flier, and B.B. Kahn. 1990. Evidence against altered expression of GLUT1 or GLUT4 in skeletal muscle of patients with obesity or NIDDM. *Diabetes* 39: 865–870.

Pereira, M.A., A.M. Kriska, M.L. Joswiak, G.K. Dowse, V.R. Collins, P.Z. Zimmet, H. Gareeboo, P. Chitson, F. Hemraj,

A. Purran, et al. 1995. Physical inactivity and glucose intolerance in the multiethnic island of Mauritius. *Medicine and Science in Sports and Exercise* 27 (12): 1626–1634.

Reitman, J.S., B. Vasquez, I. Klimes, and M. Nagulesparan. 1984. Improvement of glucose homeostasis after exercise training in noninsulin-dependent diabetes. *Diabetes Care* 7: 434–441.

Richter, E.A., L. Turcotte, P. Hespel, and B. Kiens. 1992. Metabolic responses to exercise. *Diabetes Care* 15 (Suppl. 4): 1767–1776.

Rogers, M.A., C. Yamamoto, D.S. King, J.M. Hagberg, A.A. Ehsani, and J.O. Holloszy. 1988. Improvement in glucose tolerance after one week of exercise in patients with mild NIDDM. *Diabetes Care* 11 (8): 613–618.

Schneider, S.H., L.F. Amorosa, A.K. Khachadurian, and N.B. Ruderman. 1984. Studies on the mechanism of improved glucose control during regular exercise in type 2 (non-insulin-dependent) diabetes. *Diabetologia* 26: 355–360.

Schneider, S.H., A.K. Khachadurian, L.F. Amorosa, L. Clemow, and N.B. Ruderman. 1992. Ten-year experience with an exercise-based outpatient life-style modification program in the treatment of diabetes mellitus. *Diabetes Care* 15 (4): 1800–1810.

Segal, K.R., A. Edano, A. Abalos, J. Albu, L. Blando, M.B. Tomas, and F.X. Pi-Sunyer. 1991. Effects of exercise training on insulin sensitivity and glucose metabolism in lean, obese and diabetic men. *Journal of Applied Physiology* 71 (6): 2402–2411.

Taylor, R., J. Badcock, H. King, K. Pargeter, P. Zimmet, T. Fred, M. Lund, H. Ringrose, F. Bach, R.L. Wang, et al. 1992. Dietary intake, exercise, obesity and noncommunicable disease in rural and urban populations of three Pacific Island countries. *Journal of the American College of Nutrition* 11 (3): 283–293.

Trovati, M., Q. Carta, F. Cavalot, S. Vitali, C. Banaudi, P.G. Luchhina, F. Fiocchi, G. Emanuelli, and G. Lenti. 1984. Influence of physical training on blood glucose control, glucose tolerance, insulin secretion, and insulin action in non-insulin-dependent diabetic patients. *Diabetes Care* 7 (5): 416–420.

Vanninen, E., M. Uusitupa, O. Siitonen, J. Laitinen, and E. Lansimies. 1992. Habitual physical activity, aerobic capacity, and metabolic control in patients with newly diagnosed type 2 (non-insulin-dependent) diabetes mellitus: Effect of a 1-year diet and exercise intervention. *Diabetologia* 4: 340–346.

Wallberg-Henriksson, H. 1992. Interaction of exercise and insulin in type II diabetes mellitus. *Diabetes Care* 15 (4): 1777–1782.

Wannamethee, S.G., A.G. Shaper, and G.M.M. Alberti. 2000. Physical activity, metabolic factors, and the incidence of coronary heart disease and type 2 diabetes. *Archives of Internal Medicine* 160 (14): 2108–2116.

Wilmore, J.H., J.S. Green, P.R. Stanforth, J. Gagnon, T. Rankinen, A.S. Leon, D.C. Rao, J.S. Skinner, and C. Bouchard. 2001. Relationship of changes in maximal and submaximal aerobic fitness to changes in cardiovascular disease and non-insulin-dependent diabetes mellitus risk factors with endurance training: The HERITAGE Family Study. *Metabolism* 50 (11): 1255–1263.

World Health Organization. 1998. *The World Health Report 1998. Life in the 21st century—a vision for all.* Geneva: World Health Organization.

Zimmet, P.Z., V.R. Collins, G.K. Dowse, K.G. Alberti, J. Tuomilehto, H. Gareeboo, and P. Chitson. 1991. The relation of physical activity to cardiovascular disease risk factors in Mauritians: Mauritius Noncommunicable Disease Study Group. *American Journal of Epidemiology* 134: 862–875.

Zimmet, P., G. Dowse, C. Finch, S. Serjeantson, and H. King. 1990. The epidemiology and natural history of NIDDM: Lessons from the South Pacific. *Diabetes Metabolic Review* 6: 91–124.

Web Site

www.diabetes.org. Site of the American Diabetes Association.

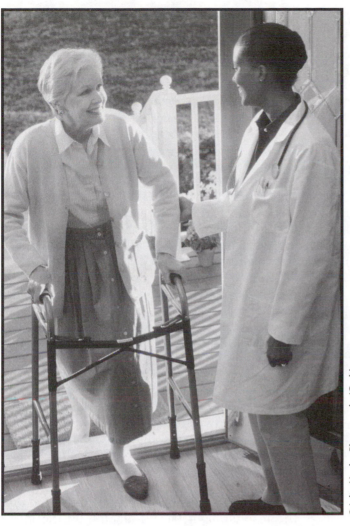

Chapter 10

© John Henley Photography/Corbis

Physical Activity and Osteoporosis

My strength faileth because of mine iniquity and my bones are consumed.

—*Psalms 31:10*

Osteoporosis, or "porous bone," is a disease characterized by abnormally low bone mass and microstructural deterioration of bone tissue that leads to brittle bones and increased risk of fractures. The World Health Organization (WHO) has defined osteoporosis as a bone mineral density (BMD) measurement more than 2.5 standard deviations below the average in young adults (WHO Study Group 1994; table 10.1). Based on this definition, bone is considered osteoporotic if it is unable to withstand the stress of normal physical activities or if a person has a history of spontaneous, nontraumatic fractures such as compression or crush fractures of the vertebrae. For each standard-deviation decrease in bone mass, there is a 50% to 100%

increase in the risk of fracture (Hui, Slemenda, and Johnston 1989). A standard-deviation loss of bone mass in the neck of the femur at the hip joint increases the risk of hip fracture by 300%. Bone mineral density between 1 and 2.5 standard deviations below that of young adults indicates **osteopenia** (i.e., low bone mass), which is a direct risk factor for osteoporosis (WHO Study Group 1994). According to the WHO, physical inactivity is also a risk factor for osteoporosis. After describing osteoporosis and its public health impact, this chapter presents the evidence that physical activity contributes to peak bone mass during youth and young adulthood, retards bone loss with aging, and can help reduce the risks of osteoporotic fractures.

TABLE 10.1	WORLD HEALTH ORGANIZATION DIAGNOSTIC CRITERIA FOR OSTEOPOROSIS
Normal	BMD within 1 SD of the mean of a young adult reference population
Osteopenia or low bone mass	BMD between 1.0 and 2.5 SD below the mean of a young adult reference population
Osteoporosis	BMD of 2.5 or more SD below the mean of a young adult reference population
Severe osteoporosis	Osteoporosis with one or more fragility fractures

••• *For each standard-deviation decline in bone mass in the hip, the risk of fracture increases threefold. A woman's lifetime risk of hip fracture is equal to her combined risk of breast, uterine, and ovarian cancer.*

Like the other chronic diseases discussed in this book, osteoporosis has existed since antiquity. As recorded in the Bible, King David, the ruler of Israel from about 990 to 970 B.C., probably suffered from osteoporosis in his later years (Ben-Noun 2002), and judging by the quotation that opened this chapter, he linked his bone loss to bad habits and failing strength. Bone archaeologists found a case of severe osteoporosis in the remains of a sixth-century female discovered in the Negev desert of southern Israel, who had compression fractures in two thoracic vertebrae and bone mineral densities at various sites that

were 5 to 8 standard deviations below the values expected for young adults (Foldes and Popovtzer 1996). Even in ancient times, it appears that women had lower bone mineral density and greater risk of osteoporosis than men, even though both men and women would have been physically active because of their nomadic or agrarian lifestyles. In a group of skeletons excavated in Unterhautzental, Austria, dated to the Bronze Age (i.e., 2200 to 1600 B.C.), the average (mean ± SD) bone mineral density in the neck of the femur of 14 women about 45 years old was $0.98 ± 0.15$ g/cm^2, significantly lower than the average of 5 men ($1.2 ± 0.26$ g/cm^2) found at the site (Frigo and Lang 1995).

Other archaeological evidence suggests that osteoporosis has become a more prevalent health problem in the 21st century as the incidence rate of osteoporotic hip fractures has become higher in the United States and Europe than would be expected merely from increased numbers of people living longer. During restoration of Christ Church at Spitalfields, London, skeletons of 87 white women ages 15 to 89 years who died between 1729 to 1852 were exhumed (Lees et al. 1993). The rate of bone mineral loss in their femoral necks was significantly less than found in a comparative sample of 294 modern-day women between 42 and 48 years old, before or after menopause. The authors suggested that the results might be explainable by the lower prevalence of daily physical activity in modern-day women compared with the Spitalfields sample, who were known to have worked typically 14 to 16 h a day operating weaving looms and walking for transportation. Other changes during the past 200 years that could contribute to greater loss of bone mass include lower consumption of dairy products, which contain calcium, and more tobacco smoking. All these factors are modifiable risks for the development of osteoporosis.

••• *About one in five patients who fracture a hip, most after age 75, dies in the year following the fracture, and 50% of the survivors become dependent on others for care.*

Magnitude of the Problem

The annual prevalence of diagnosed osteoporosis in the United States is about 10 million people; 80% are women. It is estimated that 44 million Americans ages 50 or older have either osteoporosis or osteopenia (National Osteoporosis Foundation 2002). Bone mass is generally lowest among women who are white or Asian, thin framed, and sedentary. Twenty percent of U.S. women ages 50 years or older who are non-Hispanic white or of Asian descent have osteoporosis. Black women and overweight or obese women have higher bone mass and thus are at comparatively lower risk of developing osteoporosis. Five percent of African American women ages 50 years or older have osteoporosis, and another 35% have osteopenia. Ten percent of Latina women 50 years or older have osteoporosis, and another 49% have osteopenia. The prevalence of osteoporosis is expected to continue to increase in nations that have increasing life expectancies and hence an increasing number of older people. Based on recent trends of increasing incidence, it is predicted that more than 52 million women and men 50 years old or older in the United States will have low bone mass or osteoporosis by the year 2010. By 2020 the prevalence is expected to be 61 million (National Osteoporosis Foundation 2002). Figure 10.1 illustrates the projected trends for osteoporosis and osteopenia among U.S. women and men.

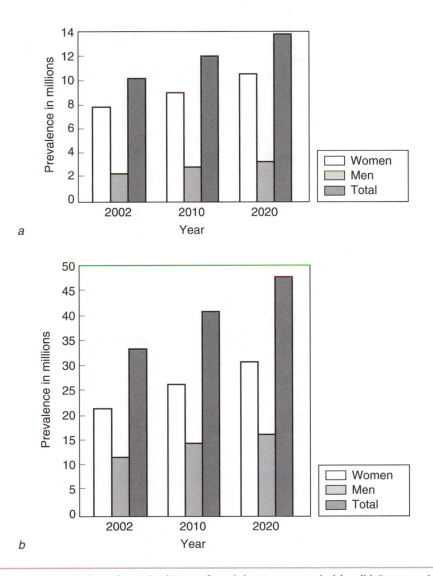

Figure 10.1   (a) Osteoporosis trends in the United States for adults 50 years and older. (b) Osteopenia trends in the United States for adults 50 years and older.

Data from the National Osteoporosis Foundation 2002.

Fractures and Mortality

Osteoporosis is responsible for more than 1.5 million fractures in the United States each year, including approximately 300,000 hip fractures, 700,000 vertebral fractures, 250,000 wrist fractures, and 300,000 fractures at other sites (National Osteoporosis Foundation 2002). Currently, about half of hip fractures worldwide occur in Europe and North America, but it has been estimated that by the year 2050 those regions will contribute only one fourth of total fractures, as incidence rates are predicted to increase markedly in Asia and Latin America (Riggs and Melton 1995). In the United States one in two women and one in eight men over age 50 will have an osteoporosis-related fracture in their lifetimes. A woman's risk of hip fracture is equal to her combined risk of breast, uterine, and ovarian cancer. Osteoporotic fractures are an important cause of disability and mortality in the elderly. About 20% of patients who fracture a hip die in the year following the fracture, and 50% of the survivors become dependent on others for care. Though men have fewer incidents of hip fracture, they have twice the risk of mortality after a fracture.

The lifetime risk for hip fracture has been estimated at 17.5% in white women and 6.0% in white men. Lower risks have been estimated for black women and men: 5.6% and 2.8%, respectively. White women have about a 16% lifetime risk for developing either vertebral or distal radius fractures. The lifetime risk for white females for fracture of the proximal femur, radius, or vertebrae is 40%. Vertebral fractures, including microcompression or crush fractures, account for half of all fractures. One in four people older than 70 years has some compression fractures of the vertebrae that can lead to **kyphosis** of the thoracic spine ("dowager's hump"). White women lose an average of 6.4 cm (2.5 in.) of height after menopause if they do not receive medical treatment. Complications of osteoporosis represent an economic burden to public health. The direct cost of treating osteoporotic fractures of the proximal femur, radius, and vertebrae is about $17 billion each year (National Osteoporosis Foundation 2002).

Sex Differences

The rate of bone loss differs between men and women as they age. At all ages, men have more bone mass than women, and men's natural bone loss is more gradual. Bone loss in men is thought to begin at age 40 to 45 years, proceeds at a rate of about 0.5% per year, then accelerates substantially after age 60 to a rate of up to 4% per decade until age 90 (Menkes et al. 1993). Women lose bone at a rate of about 1% to 2% beginning around age 35 (Whitfield and Morley 1998). During lactation, there is a slight, transient increase in bone loss to 7% in the first six months after childbirth, which returns to the normal rate of loss at the resumption of menses (Sowers, Corton, and Shapiro 1993). In addition, women can lose up to 20% of their bone mass in the five to seven years after menopause (Riggs and Melton 1986). The larger and faster decreases in bone mass in women explain most of the difference in prevalence of osteoporotic fractures between women and men.

It is believed that the marked decline in levels of estrogen after menopause accounts for the greater bone loss experienced by women; 75% or more of the bone loss that occurs in women during the first 15 years after menopause is attributable to estrogen deficiency. Men lose bone mass at an accelerated rate after about age 60; bone loss can be associated with a decline in gonadal function in some men (WHO Study Group 1994).

> ··· *Most of the higher prevalence of osteoporotic fractures among women than among men occurs after menopause. Without hormone replacement therapy, women can lose up to 20% of their bone mass within five to seven years after menopause.*

Etiology of Osteopenia and Osteoporosis

There are two main categories of osteoporosis. **Primary osteoporosis** includes age-related (type I, or senile) bone loss and postmenopausal (type II) bone loss (Garnero and Delmas 1997). **Secondary osteoporosis** is caused by another disease but may not be independent of age or menopause. This chapter deals mainly with primary osteoporosis because it can be positively affected by physical activity, especially by increasing peak bone mass during adolescence and young adulthood or by retarding bone loss during aging. Osteoporosis results mainly from loss of trabecular bone mass (i.e., trabeculae and their interconnections) and microdamage within the bone (Johnston and Slemenda 1995). Twin studies have demonstrated that several genes appear to regulate the fragility of bone, but the specific genes have not yet been identified fully (Slemenda et al. 1996). Dietary calcium and vitamin D, as well as regular physical activity, contribute to peak bone mass, particularly before age 20. Bone loss among women is related to estrogen levels and, to a lesser extent, androgen levels, and bone loss accelerates after menopause. Though men lose bone at about half the rate of women, the mechanisms for primary bone loss in men are poorly understood.

Generalized Secondary Osteoporosis Causes

- Hypogonadism
- Thyrotoxicosis
- Hyperprolactinemia
- Pregnancy
- Chronic liver disease
- Chronic heparin use
- Osteogenesis
- Rheumatoid arthritis
- Hyperadrenocorticism
- Anorexia nervosa
- Diabetes mellitus
- Vitamin D deficiency
- Alcoholism
- Anticonvulsants
- Homocystinuria
- Myeloma

Bone Renewal and Involution

To understand how **bone involution** might be retarded by physical activity, it is necessary to understand the basics of bone renewal. The **endosteum** is the layer of cells lining the inner surface of bone in the central medullary cavity. The **exosteum** refers to bone cells that are outside the central medullary cavity. After about age 30 to 40, endosteal bone is lost at a faster rate than exosteal bone is deposited. This is called bone involution, which results in osteopenia and is a risk factor for osteoporosis. One third of women who have bone involution develop osteoporosis.

There are two types of bone: **cortical bone** and **trabecular bone.** Cortical, or compact, bone is found mainly in the shaft of long bones and accounts for about 80% of all bone. Trabecular bone is spongy tissue found in the vertebrae, pelvis, flat bones, and ends of the long bones. Trabecular bone has a lattice or honeycomb design. It has more surface area per volume and is more metabolically active (e.g., a higher flux of minerals between bone and blood) than cortical bone; the formation and resorption of trabecular bone occur about six times faster than in cortical bone. Thus, trabecular bone is more susceptible to osteoporotic disease (figure 10.2).

White women lose an average of 50% of trabecular bone and 30% of cortical bone over their lifetimes (mainly after menopause), while men lose about 15% of trabecular and 12% of cortical bone mass (Sowers 1997). The loss of vertebral bone in the spine begins in the 20s but is usually negligible until after menopause. Bone density in

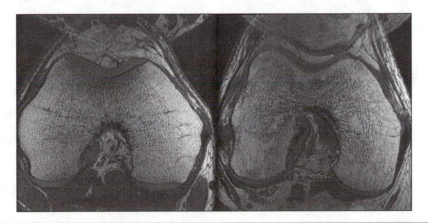

Figure 10.2   High-resolution cross-sectional images of osteoporotic distal femur bone of a spinal cord–injured subject on the right and an able-bodied control on the left. Notice the fewer black lines (bone) and more white (marrow) in the image of the spinal cord–injured subject.

Courtesy of Dr. Christopher Modlesky.

the neck of the femur peaks in the mid- to late 20s and starts to decline around age 30. Without intervention, about 5% of trabecular bone and 1% to 1.5% of total bone mass are lost each year during the 10 to 15 years after menopause. The rate of loss is slower among black women.

Bone remodeling is a continuous process involving hormonal and local regulation of three types of cells: **osteoclasts, osteoblasts,** and **osteocytes.** Osteoclasts are phagocytes that digest old bone cells and thus are involved in bone resorption (i.e., breakdown). Osteoblasts rebuild by forming new bone cells (i.e., osteocytes) from collagen to make an **osteoid matrix.** The osteoid matrix provides the infrastructure for the mineralization of bone (e.g., by calcium and phosphorus) and, along with trabecular bone, gives bone its mechanical, elastic, and tensile strength.

Increases (during growth) and decreases (with age) in bone mineral density depend on the balance of activity of osteoclasts and osteoblasts. During growth and maturation of skeletal bone in youth and young adulthood, osteoblastic activity exceeds osteoclastic activity, so bones grow and increase their mineral density. After peak bone mass is attained, the activity of osteoclasts gradually outpaces that of osteoblasts, leading to an accumulation of cavities in the bone's osteoid matrix (figure 10.3).

Hormonal Influences

Parathyroid hormone contributes to bone remodeling by stimulating resorption of calcium from the bone, while **calcitonin** inhibits resorption. It is not yet fully understood how reproductive hormones such as estrogen and testosterone help protect against bone loss. There is general consensus that the biologically active metabolite of **vitamin D** (1,25-dihydroxyvitamin D) enhances the absorption of dietary calcium by bone. Also, the presence of receptors for estrogen on osteoblasts indicates that estrogen can have a direct effect on osteogenesis. Estrogen stimulates several bone growth factors (e.g., insulin-like growth factors I and II) and inhibits the **lymphokines** interleukin-1 and interleukin-6 (cells that regulate the immune response during inflammation), which promote osteopenia. Estrogen also stimulates the synthesis of calcitonin, which inhibits bone resorption and increases vitamin D receptors in osteoblasts, thus influencing the activity of 1,25-dihydroxyvitamin D in bone (Speroff, Glass, and Case 1994).

Risk Factors

Several medical conditions that mainly occur in later life (e.g., Cushing's disease, Paget's disease, hypogonadism, acromegaly, thyroid or parathy-

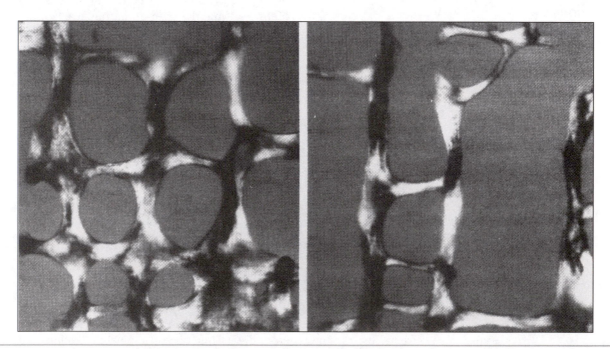

Figure 10.3   Stages of osteoporotic bone.

Reprinted, by permission, from Li Mosekilde, 1988, "Age-related changes in vertebral trabecular bone architecture assessed by a new method," *Bone* 9: 247-250.

roid disease, rheumatoid arthritis, and cancer) can lead to osteoporosis. Also, several drugs have been associated with decreased bone mass and increased risk of osteoporotic fractures. These drugs include glucocorticosteroids, anticonvulsants, excessive doses of thyroxin, and some antitumor drugs used to treat cancer.

The development of osteoporosis is inversely related to the maximum amount of bone accumulated during growth and positively related to the rate and duration of bone loss that occurs with aging, which accelerates after menopause among women. The lower the peak bone mass or the greater the rate of bone loss, the greater the risk of osteoporosis. Key unmodifiable and modifiable risk factors, including physical inactivity, are listed in table 10.2.

TABLE 10.2 RISK FACTORS FOR OSTEOPOROSIS

Modifiable	Unmodifiable
Cigarette smoking	Heredity
Excessive alcohol intake	Small body frame
Low testosterone levels	Female sex
Vitamin D intake	Race (European or Asian)
Physical inactivity	Age
Calcium intake	Postmenopause
Anorexia or bulimia	Amenorrhea
Amenorrhea	Premature menopause
Medications (e.g., benzodiazopenes)	

Steps to Prevent Osteoporosis

A comprehensive program that can help prevent osteoporosis includes

1. a balanced diet rich in calcium and vitamin D,
2. weight-bearing aerobic and resistance exercise,
3. a healthy lifestyle with limited alcohol intake and no smoking, and
4. bone density testing and prescribed medication when appropriate.

Dietary Calcium and Vitamin D

A diet containing an adequate amount of calcium, vitamin D, and protein is recommended to promote bone health and reduce the risks of osteopenia and osteoporosis. Calcium is the main component of bone, which stores 99.5% of the body's calcium and supplies calcium to meet the body's metabolic needs (e.g., nerve conductance and muscle contraction) via the blood. Inadequate calcium is a risk factor for osteopenia and osteoporosis. The recommended calcium intake during adolescence and adulthood, depending on age, is between 1,000 to 1,300 mg per day. This is not a problem for some populations. The Hunza, for example, live in a high mountain pass between China and Pakistan and have notoriety for being among the longest-living people in the world. Much of their longevity has been attributed to their water, called "Glacial Milk," which comes from the nearby Ultar Glacier and contains mineral-rich rock ground by the glacier, including 11,500 mg of calcium per liter (Wallach and Lan 1994). An 8-oz (237-ml) glass of cow's milk contains about 300 mg of calcium. However, most Americans do not have a calcium-rich water source, so their calcium intake is determined by dietary choice, which often leads to insufficient intake, especially by adolescent girls and women, who commonly consume less than half (mean of about 700 mg per day) of their recommended daily allowances (Alaimo et al. 1994).

Recommended Daily Allowance of Calcium

Children and adolescents (ages 9–18)	1,300 mg
Women (ages 19–50)	1,000 mg
Men (ages 19–50)	1,000 mg
Women and men older than 50	1,200 mg
Institute of Medicine 2003.	

Vitamin D is necessary for the body to absorb calcium from food. Its synthesis depends on sun exposure. Though sufficient amounts of vitamin D can be synthesized in the skin by 10 to 15 min of direct exposure of the face and extremities to sunlight two to three days each week, the biosynthesis of vitamin D is less in dark-skinned people and lessens as people age. Thus, vitamin D deficiency is common without dietary supplementation and results in resorption of stored calcium from bone. The recommended daily dietary intake of vitamin D is between 400 and 800 international units (IU). Dietary supplementation with calcium (500 mg a day) and vitamin D (700 IU a day) has been shown to reduce by 50% the three-year risk of developing osteoporosis among men and women over age 65 years (Dawson-Hughes et al. 1997).

FDA Approved Drugs for Treating Osteoporosis

- Estrogens (brand names include Premarin®, Ogen®, Estrace®, Estraderm®, Estratab®, and Prempro™)
- Alendronate (brand name Fosamax®)
- Calcitonin (brand name Miacalcin®)
- Raloxifene (brand name Evista®)
- Risedronate (brand name Actonel®)

Hormone Replacement Therapy

Hormone replacement therapy (HRT; i.e., estrogen alone or estrogen combined with progestin) is generally viewed as the most important intervention for both the prevention and treatment of osteoporosis in postmenopausal women. HRT can protect bone from rapid demineralization, typical of the early postmenopausal period, and thus decrease fracture rates in postmenopausal women. Women who take estrogen for at least seven years between the onset of menopause and the age of 75 have a 50% reduction in risk of fractures (Levinson and Altkorn 1998). A quantitative review of the evidence from 22 randomized controlled trials of HRT lasting at least 12 months found a cumulative 27% reduction in nonvertebral fractures after HRT (RR = 0.73, 95% CI: 0.56–0.94). The effect was greater (33% reduction in fractures) among women under age 60 (RR = 0.67, 95% CI: 0.46–0.98) than over age 60 (RR = 0.88, 95% CI: 0.71–1.08) (Torgerson and Bell-Syer 2001).

A recent report from the NIH Women's Health Initiative on a randomized, clinical trial of 16,608 postmenopausal women ages 50 to 79 recruited by 40 U.S. clinical centers in 1993 to 1998 found that HRT combining estrogen and progestin reduced the risk of hip fracture (RR = 0.66, 95% CI: 0.45–0.98) and all fractures (RR = 0.76, 0.69–0.85) (Rossouw et al. 2002). Notwithstanding the favorable effect of HRT on postmenopausal bone health, the trial was stopped by the National Heart, Lung, and Blood Institute because of the number of adverse events during the study. The investigators concluded that the overall health risks exceeded benefits across an average 5.2-year follow-up and that the regimen of estrogen plus progestin should not be initiated or continued for primary prevention of CHD, in contrast with many epidemiological studies that consistently showed reduced incidence of CHD and all-cause mortality among postmenopausal women using HRT (Mosca 2000). In the Women's Health Initiative study, increased risks (95% CI) after HRT were observed for total CVD, 1.22 (1.09–1.36); CHD, 1.29 (1.02–1.63); stroke, 1.41 (1.07–1.85); and breast cancer, 1.26 (1.00–1.59). A decreased risk after HRT was observed for colorectal cancer, 0.63 (0.43–0.92). Though all-cause mortality was not affected by HRT, absolute excess risks per 10,000 person-years attributable to estrogen plus progestin were seven more CHD events, eight more strokes, and eight more invasive breast cancers, while absolute risk reductions per 10,000 person-years were six fewer colorectal cancers and five fewer hip fractures.

••• The World Health Organization concluded about a decade ago that women who take estrogen for at least seven years between the onset of menopause and the age of 75 have a 50% reduction in risk of fractures as well as coronary heart disease (WHO Study Group 1994). However, some studies have shown increased risk of breast cancer and cardiovascular disease after estrogen or estrogen plus progestin replacement therapy.

Bone Measurement Techniques

No symptoms accompany bone loss, so it is difficult to diagnose. Bone mass is usually expressed as either bone mass density (BMD) or bone mass content (BMC). The two most common measurement techniques used are dual-energy X-ray absorptiometry (DXA), which provides area density (in grams per centimeter squared), and computed tomography (CT), which measures volumetric density (in milligrams per centimeter cubed). The DXA method is the most popular technique as it provides precise, fast measurement of BMD with minimal radiation exposure (less than one tenth of the amount used on a standard chest X-ray) and can scan virtually all skeletal sites (Garnero and Delmas 1997).

The anatomic sites most commonly measured by DXA or CT include the proximal femur (i.e., near the hip joint), the spine, and the proximal radius of the arm (near the wrist). The femoral neck and lumbar spine are usually considered optimal for BMD measurement because they are common fracture sites. There is no single site that predicts bone mineral density at other skeletal sites, but measurement of the femoral neck currently has the most general application (Sowers 1997).

Blood serum indexes of bone formation and resorption can help detect changes in BMD. Serum bone Gla protein (osteocalcin), the enzyme bone-specific alkaline phosphatase (BAP), and insulin-like growth factor I (IGF-I) are commonly used indicators of bone formation. Another enzyme, tartrate-resistant acid phosphatase (TRACP), and the protein C-terminal cross-linked telopeptide of type I collagen (ICTP) are indicators of bone resorption. Serum levels of 1,25-hydroxyvitamin D and urinary adenosine 3,5-cyclic monophosphate also have been used as indicators of bone turnover (Menkes et al. 1993). Measurement of bone turnover is a research tool rather than a clinical method for diagnosing or monitoring low bone mass (Sowers 1997).

Physical Activity and Osteoporosis: The Evidence

There is scientific consensus that physical inactivity is associated with decreased bone mass. Extreme losses of 2% to 10% have been found among young men after four months of bed rest (Buchner and Wagner 1992), but most of that loss is recovered soon after a return to upright posture and normal daily movement. The transience of this bone loss can be attributed to the reduced gravitational load, similar to the loss of bone mass that also occurs during microgravity (e.g., space travel). Nonetheless, there does seem to be a more insidious loss of bone mass among people who live sedentary lifestyles that compounds the natural history of bone loss with increasing age. A recent review of the research literature concluded that physical activity that involves high-intensity loading of bone promotes bone density and may help prevent osteoporosis, and that physical activity that involves static muscle contractions or slow movements has no effect or smaller effects on bone mass than activities that involve rapidly applied forces (Vuori 2001).

These are the conclusions from the current position statement on osteoporosis and exercise by the American College of Sports Medicine (ACSM 1995):

1. Weight-bearing physical activity is essential for the normal development and maintenance of a healthy skeleton. Activities that focus on increasing muscle strength may also be beneficial, particularly for non-weight-bearing bones.

2. Sedentary women might increase bone mass slightly by becoming more active, but the primary benefit of increased activity is avoiding further loss of bone from inactivity.

3. Exercise cannot be recommended as a substitute for hormone replacement therapy at the time of menopause.

4. "The optimal program for older women would include activities that improve strength, flexibility, and coordination that may indirectly, but effectively, decrease the incidence of osteoporotic fractures by lessening the likelihood of falling" (ACSM 1995).

Much of the evidence that formed the basis of that position statement by the ACSM came from cross-sectional studies that compared athletes or regular exercisers with sedentary people and from poorly controlled clinical studies of exercise training and bone mass. Cross-sectional studies are reviewed in the next section. Then we discuss population-based studies of whether physical activity boosts peak bone mass during adolescence and young adulthood. After that, we discuss clinical trials of the impact of endurance and resistance exercise training on bone mineral density during young adulthood, middle-age, and early old age, including comparisons of pre- and postmenopausal women. Finally, the evidence about whether exercise training retards bone loss as people grow older and whether it reduces the risk of osteoporotic fractures is summarized.

Cross-Sectional Studies

Though an early study reported that 41 recreational runners over the age of 50 years had 40% higher BMD than age-matched controls (N.E. Lane et al. 1986), bone mass among different types of athletes generally followed the peak weight-bearing activity or localized loading of bone, as in resistance exercise or strength training. For example, male tennis players 79 years old or older who played tennis for periods ranging from 25 to 72 years showed an increased BMD in their dominant forearms as compared with their age-matched controls (Huddleston et al. 1980). The following athletes are listed from highest to lowest bone mass: weightlifters, weight throwers, gymnasts, tennis players, runners, soccer players, swimmers, and nonathletes (Montoye 1984; Taaffe et al. 1995, 1997). This ranking does not indicate whether high BMD resulted from the particular sport or whether athletes excelled in these sports because of their optimal levels of bone mass. However, a study of college-aged gymnasts found that bone density at relevant sites responded dramatically to high-impact loading, independent of reproductive hormone status and despite high initial BMD values (Taaffe et al. 1997). This provides evidence that mechanical loading, rather than selection bias, underlies the high BMD values characteristic of female gymnasts. Swimming, which imposes smaller peak loads, did not increase BMD in another study (Emslander et al. 1998).

Greater muscle strength is positively associated with BMD; increased BMD possibly results from stimulation of bone modeling by the transfer of force from muscle to bone. For example, bone mass was positively associated with grip strength and peak torques at the hip and knee joints independently of body weight (Bauer et al. 1993). Among 709 men and 1,080 women over age 60 years in the Dubbo Osteoporosis Epidemiology cohort, quadriceps muscle strength predicted bone density at the proximal femur in the men but not the women. After adjustment for age and body weight, BMD at the femoral neck among men and women was about 5% higher in those who had high quadriceps strength and high calcium intake compared with those with

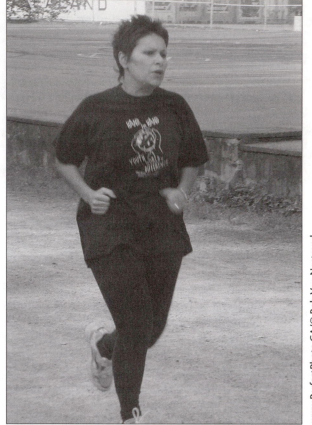

low quadriceps strength and low calcium intake (Nguyen et al. 1994).

Table 10.3 shows results from selected cross-sectional comparisons of bone mass in female athletes in sports that involve high peak forces and loading of bone (e.g., weightlifting and gymnastics) or repetitive weight-bearing activities (e.g., distance running and Nordic skiing). These comparisons generally show that, compared with nonathletes, bone mass in the lumbar spine, femoral neck, pelvis, and arm of athletes in high-load sports is 10% to 15% higher, but that of athletes who perform repetitive weight-bearing activities that don't involve a lot of peak loads is only about 3% to 8% higher. The differences in bone mass between nonathletes and female athletes in repetitive weight-bearing sports such as running or Nordic skiing were generally too small to be statistically significant in the small groups that were studied.

Prospective Cohort Studies

There have not been many prospective cohort studies of the effect of physical activity or fitness on bone mass or risk of osteoporosis. Most pro-

TABLE 10.3   CROSS-SECTIONAL COMPARISONS OF BONE MASS IN FEMALE ATHLETES WITH NONATHLETES

Study	Athletes	Difference in bone mass vs. nonathletes
HIGH-LOAD SPORTS		
Heinonen et al. 1993	18 weightlifters 25 ± 5 years old	Lumbar spine: 15% Femoral neck: 10% Distal radius: 29%
Nichols et al. 1995	14 basketball players 19 ± 1 year old	Lumbar spine: 10% Femoral neck: 14% Arm: 8%
Alfredson, Nordstrom, and Lorentzon 1997	13 volleyball players 21 ± 4 years old	Lumbar spine: 13% Femoral neck: 16% Humerus: 9%–10%
Courteix et al. 1998	18 gymnasts 10 ± 1 year old	Lumbar spine: 11% Femoral neck: 15% Radius: 16%
REPETITIVE WEIGHT BEARING		
Heinonen et al. 1995	30 orienteers 23 ± 3 years old	Lumbar spine: 8% Femoral neck: 3% Distal radius: –4%
	14 speed skaters 21 ± 9 years old	Lumbar spine: 6% Femoral neck: 4% Distal radius: –6%
	28 Nordic skiers 21 ± 3 years old	Lumbar spine: 3% Femoral neck: 5% Distal radius: –7%
Pettersson et al. 2000	16 Nordic skiers 16 years old	Spine: –1% Femoral neck: 9% Humerus: 7%–9%

spective studies included small samples of about 25 to 200 youths or young adults and lasted only 5 to 12 months. Despite the short time periods of the studies, most showed a 3% to 10% increase in BMD. Many of those studies did an incomplete job of controlling for diet and other potential confounders that influence bone mass. Nonetheless, the cumulative evidence is encouraging that vigorous physical activity, especially the types that involve high peak loads (e.g., resistance exercise or power sports), might promote higher peak bone mass (Modlesky and Lewis 2002). Some key studies are summarized next.

Nebraska Women

The effects of leisure-time physical activity, diet, and use of oral contraceptives on bone mass measured by DXA were observed for about 3.5 years among 156 healthy, college-aged (mean age 21 years at the beginning of the study), white women (Recker et al. 1992). Estimates of nutrient intake were obtained by repeated seven-day diet diaries. Physical activity was assessed using the Caltrac accelerometer for four days prior to each six-month visit to the clinic. The average gain in BMD in the lumbar spine was 6.8%, and the gain in bone density of the spine was related to both calcium intake and physical activity independently; the least-active women gained an average of 0.3%, and the most-active women gained 8.4%.

Finnish Youths

Bone mass was associated with exercise, smoking, and dietary calcium in a prospective cohort study of 153 females and 111 males ages 9 to 18, who were observed for 11 years; their BMD was assessed by DXA when they were 20 to 29 years old (Valimaki et al. 1994). After adjustment for age and body weight, femoral neck BMD was nearly 8% higher in the women and 10% higher in the men who were the most physically active compared with that of the least-active women and men. Similarly, BMD in the lumbar spine was 8% higher in the most-active men than in the least-active men. Exercise predicted BMD in the femoral neck and the lumbar spine of the men independently of smoking.

The University of Saskatchewan Bone Mineral Study

The influence of physical activity on gains in bone mass during adolescence was observed for six years among 53 girls and 60 boys who ranged from 8 to 14 years old at the start of the study (Bailey et al. 1999). Measures of physical activity, diet, height, weight, and bone mineral content (BMC) measured by DXA were taken every six months. Peak rates of gain in BMC were computed for the total body, lumbar spine, and proximal femur. After adjusting for height and weight gains, the peak rate of gain in BMC in the femoral neck, lumbar spine, and total body was higher for both males and females who were more physically active than in the less-active subjects. The BMC in the femoral neck measured one year after the peak rate of gain was 7% higher in boys and 9% in girls in the most-active quartile compared with the least-active quartile; total-body gains were 9% and 17% higher in the most-active boys and girls, respectively.

Amsterdam Growth and Health Longitudinal Study

Daily physical activity and fitness were monitored from age 13 to 29 years in a cohort of 182 males and females (Kemper et al. 2000). At a mean age of 28 years, BMD was measured by DXA at the lumbar spine, the femoral neck, and the distal radius. Physical activity during the previous three months was measured by interview when participants were between 13 and 16 years old and again between ages 21 and 27. Physical activity was expressed as energy expended (in MET-hours) per week or as peak intensity (in multiples of body mass), independently of the frequency and duration of activity. Physical fitness was measured with a neuromotor fitness test (a composite of six strength, flexibility, and speed tests) and as cardiopulmonary fitness (maximal oxygen uptake). After adjusting for sex, age, body composition, and dietary calcium, both measurements of physical activity and neuromotor fitness during adolescence and in young adulthood were positively related with the bone mass in the lumbar spine and femoral neck measured at a mean age of 28 years. Cardiorespiratory fitness was unrelated to bone mass.

Penn State Young Women's Health Study

The associations of cumulative teenage sports participation and calcium intake with gains in whole-body BMD measured using DXA between ages 12 and 18 years and with peak bone mass in the femoral neck at age 18 were studied in a small cohort of 81 females (Lloyd et al. 2000). Diets were assessed from 33 days of food records collected at regular intervals between ages 12 and 18 years. Calcium intake ranged from 500 to 1,500 mg per day and was unrelated to femoral bone mass and whole-body gains in bone mass at age 18. The cumulative amount of sports and exercise participation was correlated with peak femoral BMD at age 18 ($r = 0.42$) but not with gains in whole-body BMD.

Swedish Youth

A school-based intervention examined BMD measured by DXA in 40 boys and 40 girls who increased their physical education classes to four times each week for three to four years from age 12 to age 16, compared with a control group of 82 boys and 66 girls of the same age who had two days of physical education each week during the same time period (Sundberg et al. 2001). BMC, BMD, and volumetric BMD were 8% to 9% higher among the boys who increased the frequency of their physical education classes compared with the control boys. The differences remained after adjusting for possible confounders, including body weight and height, milk consumption, and physical activity after school.

Clinical Studies: Endurance Exercise Training

A quantitative review of 23 randomized and nonrandomized controlled trials of endurance exercise training conducted between 1966 and 1997 concluded that exercise training led to the prevention or reversal of about 1% of the annual loss of BMD or BMC in the lumbar spine and the femoral neck in both pre- and postmenopausal women in randomized controlled trials (I. Wolff et al. 1999). Effects were about twice that big in the nonrandomized controlled trials but were probably confounded by other factors that affect bone mass but were not controlled for because participants were not randomly assigned to the exercise intervention. Table 10.4 provides a summary of selected randomized controlled trials of endurance exercise training on bone mineral density.

••• *Cumulative evidence from 23 randomized and nonrandomized controlled trials indicates that endurance exercise training prevented or reversed about 1% of annual bone loss in the lumbar spine and the femoral neck.*

One of the earliest controlled studies of pre- and postmenopausal women conducted at the University of Wisconsin found that four years of endurance exercise retarded the loss of bone mass compared with the rate of loss in women who did not exercise (Smith et al. 1989). Similarly, 18 months of endurance training (walking, jogging, stationary cycling) at 55% to 75% of aerobic capacity was linearly related to increased BMD of the femoral neck among perimenopausal women (mean age = 52.5), while women who participated in light calisthenics or did not exercise had decreased BMD during the 18-month period of the study (Heinonen et al. 1998). No increases in BMD after exercise training were seen in the lumbar spine or distal radius. However, estrogen status may have been a confounder in the study because some women were premenopausal and some of the postmenopausal women were taking estrogen replacement therapy.

Though the effect of exercise observed in most studies averages to about a 1% to 2% decrease in annual bone loss, endurance exercise studies on postmenopausal women have shown mixed positive and null effects on bone mass. The interventions that have shown increases or maintenance of BMD with aging generally used intensities more vigorous than walking or extra weight in addition to the participants' body weight. The effect of long-distance running, between 33 and 37 miles (53–60 km) each week, on BMD was studied in pre- and postmenopausal women who were not receiving estrogen replacement therapy (Kirk et al. 1989). Computed tomography scans of vertebrae and the distal radius indicated increased

TABLE 10.4 SELECTED RANDOMIZED CONTROLLED TRIALS OF THE EFFECTS OF ENDURANCE EXERCISE TRAINING ON BONE MINERAL DENSITY

Study	Length of study	Participants	Type of exercise	Main findings
Snow-Harter et al. 1992	8 months	31 women 20 years old	Running 4–10 miles/wk (6.4–16.1 km/wk) 3 days/wk 70–80% HRmax	BMD gain: Lumbar spine: 1.2% Proximal femur: none
Friedlander et al. 1995	2 years	63 women 20–35 years old	Aerobic exercise plus weight training	BMD gain: Lumbar spine: 1.3% Proximal femur: 2.6%
Morris et al. 1997	10 months	71 girls 9–10 years old	30 min of high-impact aerobics 3 days/wk	BMD gain: Total body: 2.3% Lumbar spine: 3.6% Proximal femur: 10.3%
Bradney et al. 1998	8 months	40 boys 8–11 years old	Various weight-bearing activities	Increased BMD in total body and lumbar spine but not pelvis
Heinonen et al. 2000	9 months	58 premenarcheal and 68 postmenarcheal girls	Step aerobics 2 days/wk	Bone mineral content gain in premenarcheal girls: Lumbar spine: 3.3% Femoral neck: 4.0% No effects for postmenarcheal girls

vertebral bone density in the premenopausal but not the postmenopausal women when compared with nonrunning controls. Running had no effect on BMD of the radius. Similarly, a 12-month walking program at an intensity of 70% to 85% of maximal heart rate among postmenopausal women who did not smoke and were not taking estrogen replacement therapy had no impact on BMD (D. Martin and Notelovitz 1993). A running study found no changes in BMD among older women with an average age of 67 years (Blumenthal et al. 1991). Also, a combination of high- and low-impact aerobics for short periods (20 min each day) did not increase BMD in the lumbar spine of postmenopausal women, but nonexercising control participants who were not on estrogen replacement therapy lost an average of 6% of BMD, yielding a net benefit for the exercise group (Grove and Londeree 1992).

Small increases of about 0.5% to 1% in BMD of the lumbar spine of postmenopausal women after a year of high-intensity walking (either above ventilatory threshold or walking at an intensity of 70% to 85% of maximal heart rate while wearing a weighted belt) contrasted with 2% to 7% decreases in BMD among sedentary controls (Hatori et al. 1993; Nelson et al. 1991). Another study found that high-impact aerobic exercises (bench stepping and jumping) designed specifically to load the proximal femur and spine increased BMD by about 2% in the neck of the femur but had no effect on BMD in the lumbar spine (Welsh and Rutherford 1996).

Some training studies suggest that endurance exercise training can yield larger gains in BMD for postmenopausal women. Dalsky et al. (1988) used a multiple-mode aerobic intervention (50–60 min of walking, jogging, stair climbing, cycling, rowing, and bench press combined). Interventions lasted between 9 and 22 months, and results revealed a 5.2% to 6.1% increase in lumbar spine BMD. BMD subsequently declined to about 1% above the initial levels after 13 months of exercise detraining. However, the independent effect of exercise could not be determined because estrogen replacement was not controlled for and participants had calcium and vitamin D supplementation.

Kohrt, Ehsani, and Birge (1997) also demonstrated larger increases in BMD, especially in the femur, after a program of walking, jogging, and stair climbing up to 70% to 85% of maximal heart rate in women ages 60 to 74 years. BMD increases for the total body were 2.0% ± 0.8%; in the lumbar spine, 1.8% ± 0.8%; in the proximal femur, 6.1% ± 1.5%; and in the femoral neck, 3.5% ± 0.8%. Although the results by Dalsky et al. (1988) and by Kohrt, Ehsani, and Birge (1997) are encouraging, they probably overestimate the independent effect of aerobic training because some of the subjects were also receiving estrogen replacement therapy. On balance, it appears that vigorous, repetitive, weight-bearing aerobic training can result in a small net increase in bone mass of 1% to 2% per year among women regardless of age.

Clinical Studies: Resistance Exercise Training

Consensus is emerging that exercises that produce high peak forces that overload bone are effective for increasing and maintaining bone mass, regardless of age (Layne and Nelson 1999; Vuori 2001). Table 10.5 provides a summary of some of the randomized controlled trials that examined resistance exercise training (i.e., weight training) on bone mass in the lumbar spine and femoral neck.

TABLE 10.5   RANDOMIZED CONTROLLED TRIALS OF RESISTANCE EXERCISE AND BONE MASS IN PRE- AND POSTMENOPAUSAL FEMALES

Study	Length (months)	Participants	Training	Main findings
Sinaki et al. 1989	24	65 postmenopausal women, mean age 56 years	Back-strengthening exercises, lifting backpack 30%/max isometric back muscles strength, 5x/wk, 10x/day	Lumbar spine: Exercise: 1.4% loss Controls: 1.2% loss
Notelovitz et al. 1991	12	20 premenopausal women, mean age 45 years	5 stations, 8RM, 3x/wk, 15–20 min, plus estrogen in both groups	Lumbar spine: Exercise: 8.3% gain Controls: 1.5% gain

Study	Length (months)	Participants	Training	Main findings
Snow-Harter et al. 1992	8	20 premenopausal women 20 years old	14 exercises, 3 sets of 8–12 reps at 85% 1RM, 3x/wk	Lumbar spine: Exercise: 1.8% gain Controls: 1.2% loss
Nelson et al. 1994	12	39 postmenopausal women, mean age 60 years	High-intensity strength training: 3 sets of 8 reps at 80% 1RM, 2x/wk for 45 min	Lumbar spine: Exercise: 1.0% gain Controls: 1.8% loss Femoral neck: Exercise: 0.9% gain Controls: 2.5% loss
Pruitt, Taaffe, and Marcus 1995	12	26 postmenopausal women 65–79 years old	10 exercises 3x/wk for 60–70 min Low: 3 sets of 14 reps at 40% 1RM High: 1 set of 14 reps at 40% 1RM + 2 sets of 7 reps at 80% 1RM	Lumbar spine: Low exercise: 0.5% gain High exercise: 0.7% gain Controls: −0.1% loss Femoral neck: Low: 1.8% gain High: −0.2% loss Controls: 0.9% gain
Lohman et al. 1995	18	54 premenopausal women 28–39 years old	10 exercises 3 days/wk. Strength increased by 34% to 58%.	Lumbar spine: Exercise: 1.9%–2.8% gains compared with controls Femoral neck: Exercise: 1.8%–2.0% gains compared with controls
Blimkie et al. 1996	6	36 girls 14–18 years old	3x/wk	No effects on total-body or lumbar-spine BMD
Kerr et al. 1996	12	23 postmenopausal women, mean age 56 years	Unilateral upper- and lower-limb training, 3 sets, 20RM, 3x/wk, 20–30 min. Other side used as control.	Femoral neck: Exercise: no change Controls: 1% loss Radius: no change
Maddalozzo and Snow 2000	6	28 men, mean age 55 years 26 postmenopausal women, mean age 53 years	Moderate- or high-intensity free-weight training, 3x/wk. Participants were their own controls for 12 wk.	Spine: High-intensity: 1.9% gain in men No change in women No effects of moderate-intensity exercise
Hakkinen et al. 2001	24	62 men and women with rheumatoid arthritis	Strength training of major muscle groups at 50%–70% of 1RM, 2x/wk.	Spine: Exercise: 1.2% gain Controls: 0.9% loss Femoral neck: Exercise: 0.5% gain Controls: 0.7% loss
Nichols, Sanborn, and Love 2001	15	65 girls 14–17 years old	15 exercises, 30–45 min/day, 3x/wk.	Lumbar spine: Exercise: nonsignificant 2.6% Controls: nonsignificant 1% Femoral neck: Exercise: 3.6% gain Controls: nonsignificant 1%
Vincent and Braith 2002	6	62 men and women 60–83 years old	One set of 12 exercises, 3x/wk at low intensity (50% 1RM) or high intensity (80% 1RM)	Lumbar spine: No effect Femoral neck: Exercise: 2% gain in high intensity

RM = repetition maximum; x/wk = times per week

Postmenopausal Women

Several resistance-training studies have found that high-intensity (e.g., 80% of maximal strength) training can increase bone mass at specific sites among postmenopausal women without estrogen replacement. BMD in the lumbar spine was increased (mean ± SE) by 1.6% ± 1.2% after nine months of weight training among 17 postmenopausal women compared with a 3.6% ± 1.5% loss in BMD in a control group of 9 women who did not weight-train. Resistance exercise had no effect, though, on BMD at the femoral neck or distal radius at the wrist (Pruitt et al. 1992).

A randomized controlled trial examined whether a high-load, low-repetition program (three sets of 8RM) designed to maximize strength gains or a low-load, high-repetition program (three sets of 20RM) designed to maximize gains in muscular endurance would have the greatest effect on bone mass in 56 postmenopausal women (Kerr et al. 1996). BMD gains measured by DXA after a year of thrice weekly progressive resistance training of the forearms and hips on one side of the body were compared between the two types of training and with the other side of the body, which provided a nonexercise control. Strength (1RM) was increased for 10 exercises in both training groups, but with the exception of a single mid-radial site, the endurance program did not change bone mass. The high-load strength program led to increases of about 1.5% to 2% at the hip sites and 2.4% at the distal radius, whereas the control sites had reductions in BMD of 0.1% to 1.4%.

A subsequent randomized controlled trial conducted by the same investigators compared the effects of a two-year exercise intervention and calcium supplementation (600 mg) on BMD in 126 postmenopausal women (mean age, 60 ± 5 years), who were assigned to either progressive strength training or strength plus leg-cycling exercise at a minimal load (Kerr et al. 2001). The two exercise groups completed three sets of the same nine exercises three times a week. BMD was measured by DXA at the hip, lumbar spine, and forearm sites every six months. Both groups had a 0.9% increase in total-body BMD and a 1.1% increase in hip BMD.

Site-Specific Loading

Some studies have focused on the site-specific principles of mechanical loading. One study compared 12 men who engaged in strength training for at least one year with 50 age-matched controls (Colletti et al. 1989). The exercise group increased BMD compared with the control group in the weight-bearing sites of the lumbar spine, trochanter, and femoral neck, but no increase was seen in the non-weight-bearing site of the mid-radius. The effects of resistance training and bone density have been seen in older populations. A program of dynamic loading exercises of the distal forearm was done three times a week for five months by 14 postmenopausal osteoporotic women, and 26 osteoporotic women served as controls (Simkin, Ayalon, and Leichter 1987). After the five-month period, the exercise group had an increase in BMD of 3.8% in the radius, while the control group had a decrease of 1.9%.

Eccentric muscle training may be even more effective in bone formation than concentric training. Eccentric muscle contraction generates more force per muscle area. Twelve women ages 20 to 23 years at the University of Southern California participated in an 18-week strength-training program that involved training one leg using eccentric knee extension and flexion and the opposite leg using concentric extension and flexion (Hawkins et al. 1999). Eight similar women served as controls. There were no significant differences between exercise or control subjects in total BMD or hip BMD at the beginning or end of the study. The eccentric exercise significantly increased BMD in the mid-femur by 3.9%, concentric exercise produced a nonsignificant increase of 1.1%, and the control group had a 0.6% increase. These findings suggest that the greater force produced by eccentric exercise was responsible for the greater increase in bone mass.

Resistance exercise training also can be effective against glucocorticoid-induced bone loss, which can occur after antirejection drug therapy among heart transplant patients. In a prospective randomized controlled program, eight male transplant recipients participated in a resistance-training program and restored almost all of their preoperation total-body, femoral neck, and lumbar spine bone mass, while eight transplant patients in the control group lost bone mass (Braith et al. 1996).

Exercise Plus Hormone Replacement Therapy in Postmenopausal Women

Although estrogen-deficient women can benefit from weight-bearing exercise, exercise alone cannot substitute for HRT during the early postmenopausal phase of rapid bone loss. During the first five years after menopause, women who do not take estrogen can lose up to 35% of their bone mass. The combination of HRT and exercise may yield the greatest effect on bone because estrogen may enhance the osteogenic effect of mechanical loading. Several studies have examined whether estrogen plus weight training is more effective than just weight training or estrogen replacement alone. Notelovitz et al. (1991) showed that weight training enhanced the bone-conserving effect of estrogen in surgically postmenopausal women. After one year of weight training plus estrogen therapy, spine BMD significantly increased by 8.3% ± 5.3%, while an estrogen-only group merely maintained BMD, with a slight increase of only 1.5% ± 12.4%. Kohrt et al. (1995) described a one-year intervention trial that compared the combined and separate effects of HRT and weight-bearing exercises in 32 women with an average age of 66. The combination of HRT and high-intensity exercise had additive and synergistic effects on BMD, depending on the site measured. These findings suggest that each treatment acts via an independent mechanism; thus, exercise can have an additional beneficial effect on bone when used in conjunction with estrogen.

Prince et al. (1991) performed the first large prospective study. This two-year study compared four groups: sedentary controls, exercise subjects, an exercise plus calcium group, and an exercise plus HRT group. Each group consisted of 40 postmenopausal women, all with BMD at the distal radius one standard deviation below the fracture threshold, as determined by CT scan. The mean age of the subjects was 56. Calcium supplementation slowed bone loss, and HRT increased bone mass, but the rate of bone loss was similar for the exercise-only group and the sedentary controls. However, the exercise stimulus was inadequate in this study. It consisted of 1 h of supervised low-impact aerobics each week, and exercise compliance was less than 50%. Moreover, the wrist would not be expected to respond to low-impact weight-bearing exercise.

In contrast, a randomized controlled trial evaluated the effect of one month or three months of combination estrogen and progesterone therapy on menopausal symptoms, bone density, muscle strength, and lipid metabolism in 78 postmenopausal women ages 49 to 55 years (Heikkinen et al. 1997). HRT and placebo groups were further randomized to exercise or no-exercise subgroups. HRT was effective for slowing loss of BMD in the lumbar spine and proximal femur. In addition, exercise slowed bone loss in the placebo group, but exercise provided no additional benefit beyond the effects of HRT in the HRT-plus-exercise group.

Physical Activity and Risks of Falls or Fractures

A few studies have suggested that neuromuscular effects of resistance exercise training can aid in the prevention of falls and subsequent fractures in older people (Nelson et al. 1994). However, a recent review concluded that observational population-based studies and randomized controlled trials of the effectiveness of physical activity programs to prevent falls have been inconclusive, in part because many studies did not include enough people to show that the modest effects were statistically significant or didn't focus on types of exercise training most likely to reduce the risks of falling (Gregg, Pereira, and Caspersen 2000). The review concluded that recent clinical trials have suggested that exercise training that specifically used exercises designed to improve balance and leg strength can reduce the risk of falling, which could reduce the risk of hip and wrist fractures. Finally, the review concluded that there was consistent evidence from retrospective case–control and prospective cohort studies that leisure-time physical activity is associated with a 20% to 40% reduced risk of hip fracture but no association between physical activity and risks of wrist or spine fractures.

British Women and Men

The associations of low dietary calcium intake and physical inactivity measured by interview and medical exam in 1973 to 1974 with 15-year risk of hip fractures were evaluated in a case–control study of 441 women and 542 men 65 years old or older who lived in five areas in England, two areas in Scotland, and an area in Wales (Wickham et al. 1989). Incidence of hip fracture increased with age and was higher in women than men but was unrelated to a seven-day recall of calcium intake. After adjustment for smoking and BMI, the odds ratio of hip fractures in the lowest tertile for outdoor physical activity compared with the highest tertile was 4.3 (95% CI: 0.7–26.8) and 3.9 (95% CI: 0.7–23.0) in the lowest tertile for grip strength.

Finnish Men

The association between leisure physical activity measured in 1975 and future risk of osteoporotic hip fracture was studied prospectively for about

21 years in a cohort of 3,262 men 44 years old or older who did not have any diseases that limited their participation in physical activity (Kujala et al. 2000). After adjustment for the potential confounders height, BMI, baseline diseases, smoking, use of alcohol, work-related physical activity, and occupational group, the relative risk of osteoporotic hip fracture among men participating in vigorous physical activity was 0.38 (95% CI: 0.16–0.91) compared with sedentary men.

Strength of the Evidence

Randomized controlled studies provide the most valid evaluation of treatment effects by minimizing the effects of confounders that can influence bone outcomes, thus isolating the effects of physical activity. The cumulative, average effect in randomized trials of resistance training on BMD in the lumbar spine and the femoral neck in both pre- and postmenopausal women was about a 0.9% per year when compared with women who did not exercise (I. Wolff et al. 1999). In contrast, the effects of exercise reported by nonrandomized trials were nearly twice that size but probably overestimate the true effects as a result of poor control of confounders such as selection bias introduced by volunteers, who may be more likely to benefit than randomly selected subjects.

A few observational retrospective and prospective cohort studies and case–control studies have suggested that physical activity reduces the risk of falls and osteoporotic fractures. However, there is a virtual absence of controlled epidemiologic studies linking physical activity with risk of developing osteoporosis or fractures in a large population base. As we acknowledged in previous chapters on other chronic diseases, it is unlikely that a randomized, double-blind, placebo-controlled trial will ever be funded to demonstrate whether physical activity or vigorous exercise carried out during youth, adulthood, or old age reduces osteoporosis-related fractures in old age (Karlsson, Bass, and Seeman 2001). Nonetheless, a circumstantial body of evidence has accumulated that is encouraging. Namely, studies collectively suggest that resistance exercise is associated with (1) an increase in peak bone mass and (2) a slowing of osteopenia during middle age. A few studies also suggest that resistance exercise training has potential to promote (1) a reversal of bone mass loss in old age, (2) a reduc-

tion in risk factors for falls and the incidence of falls, and (3) a reduction in fractures resulting from falls among the elderly.

Modification and Confounders

Though increased bone mass after exercise training has been reported in both premenopausal and postmenopausal women, other age-related factors may modify the osteogenic effects of exercise. Several studies that failed to show a significant increase in bone density after strength training apparently did not impose the high strains, high strain rates, or strain distribution required to induce bone remodeling. Programs that fulfill all of these requirements may not be the most desirable ones for elderly people. For the frail elderly, they may even involve risks.

Beyond meeting the requirements of necessary strains on the bone, there are large differences among training programs in type, duration, frequency, and intensity. Comparing different programs' intensity may be the most difficult aspect because of insufficient and nonstandardized descriptions of intensity. Other important sources of heterogeneity among studies are the use of vitamin D, calcium supplementation, and HRT. All are known to have positive influence on BMD (Prince et al. 1991).

Bone mass differences at baseline can also explain various treatment effects. Individuals with low bone mass at the beginning of a training program are likely to show a greater increase in bone mass than those who start out with higher bone mass. Bone mass is positively related to body weight (Khosla et al. 1996; Alekel et al. 1995); therefore, weight loss in exercise groups can be a confounder in long-term interventions. Weight loss as a result of the training study might underestimate the effect of the programs (I. Wolff et al. 1999).

Temporal Sequence

Though more cross-sectional studies of physical activity and bone mass have been reported, several prospective cohort studies had follow-up periods ranging from about 3 months to 12 years, and randomized controlled trials typically lasted 5 to 12 months and as long as 2 years.

Strength of Association

The cumulative evidence from cross-sectional studies suggests that participants in repetitive weight-bearing activities have about 5% higher bone mass than sedentary controls and participants in resistance exercise training or sports that have high peak loads have 10% to 15% higher bone mass than sedentary controls. The few prospective cohort studies suggest a 3% to 10% increase in BMD and an average reduction in risk of fractures of the hip of 20% to 40% among physically active people. The aggregate effect of randomized controlled trials on middle-aged or older women is a reduction or reversal in the loss of bone mass with age of about 1% per year.

Consistency

Most prospective studies included small samples of about 25 to 200 youths or young adults. Though most randomized controlled trials have studied white women, who are at greatest risk of osteoporosis, the overall evidence for an osteogenic effect of physical activity is similar for men and women regardless of race, ethnicity, or age.

Dose Response

There is no evidence about whether the effects of physical activity on peak bone mass in youth and young adulthood depends on the type or intensity of physical activity. Similarly, there is no direct evidence to indicate whether the effect of physical activity on maintaining bone mass in premenopausal women and retarding or reversing bone loss in postmenopausal women is dose dependent. Nonetheless, it appears that site-specific effects on bone mineral content and density are greater for resistance exercise and sporting activities that place high peak loads on bone than for low-impact, repetitive, weight-bearing activities (Vuori 2001).

Biological Plausibility

The skeleton has two main extrinsic forces acting on it during exercise: (1) gravity and (2) the pull of the muscle–tendon unit during muscular contraction, locomotion, and maintenance of posture. These torsion, shearing, bending, and compression forces during exercise can provide the mechanical stress necessary to stimulate bone remodeling and increased bone mass (Khosla et al. 1996).

Research has indicated that the magnitude of loading stress on bone has a greater influence on bone density than the number of cycles of bone loading. Daily activities may provide several loading cycles but usually fail to provide sufficient loading magnitudes (Whalon, Carter, and Steele 1988). Generating the high inertial forces that increase bone mass requires greater muscular exertion and velocities than most people achieve during the physical activities of daily living, so most people consequently do not attain the bone densities observed among athletes whose sports require high ground reaction and joint reaction forces.

Although the geometric properties of bone are determined genetically, internal architecture, BMD, and internal and external bone diameter respond to environmental forces, which influence the balance of bone resorption and bone formation. Bone adapts to mechanical needs by atrophy and hypertrophy. The mechanical laws that regulate bone tissue's structural architecture are not fully understood (A.D. Martin and McCulloch 1987). However, several theories provide plausible ways that exercise could positively influence bone mass.

Proposed over 100 years ago, Wolff's law posits that mechanical loading applied to the bone causes change or remodeling of the bone's microstructural architecture (J. Wolff 1892). When bone is bent or under a mechanical load, it modifies its structure by building layers of new cells on the concave side of the bone and by resorption of old cells on the convex side of the bone. Long bones tend to align along the axis of force by hypertrophy in the areas that are compressed (Chamay and Tschantz 1972). The biochemical mechanisms that explain how mechanical strain is translated into an increase in BMD are still not fully understood. Several mechanisms have been proposed, including piezoelectric potentials; release of prostaglandins; increased bone blood flow and hormonal response; and a cascade of prostaglandins, nitric oxide, and growth factors in response to load imbalances communicated among bone cells. Most likely, a combination of the following proposed mechanisms is involved in bone formation.

Piezoelectric Effects

An early hypothesis of bone remodeling is that bone acts as a piezoelectric crystal (Bassett and Becker 1962; Brighton et al. 1985; Lanyon and Hartman 1977). Strains that are placed on the bone cause the bone to bend or vibrate. These strains are translated into biochemical

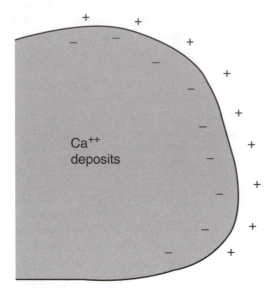

Figure 10.4   Mechanical osteogenesis. Bone acts as a piezoelectric crystal. When bone is bent or vibrated, Ca^{++} is deposited on the negatively charged side of the bone cell and Ca^{++} is reabsorbed from the positively charged side, thus balancing the osteoclast/osteoblast system.

Adapted from Bassett and Becker 1962.

signals that appear to be mediated by electric fields. As depicted in figure 10.4, loads cause transient electrical potential differences across the bone, which act as pulsed electric fields that stimulate deposits of positively charged calcium ions on the negatively charged side of the bone cell. Conversely, positively charged calcium ions are resorbed from the positively charged side of the bone cell. This is believed to result in an increased ratio of bone osteoblast activity to bone osteoclast activity at the points of stress, yielding formation of new bone. Early studies showed that application of electrical stimulation caused an increase in bone formation in animals (Bassett 1965), and applied electromagnetic fields have more recently been proposed as a clinically useful approach to the prevention of osteoporosis in people who are at high risk of developing osteoporosis (Bassett 1995; Tabrah et al. 1990).

Prostaglandins

Electrical stimulation of bone also increases the production of adenosine 3,5-cyclic monophosphate (cAMP) and prostaglandin E2 (PGE2) by osteoblasts. Prostaglandin is a necessary part of bone formation under loading conditions. The synthesis of PGE2 results from the stretch-

ing of bone cell membranes, which exposes cell membrane phospholipids to phospholipase A2 (Chamay and Tschantz 1972). The synthesis of PGE2 increases intracellular levels of cAMP, which acts to increase DNA and RNA synthesis of new bone proteins.

Blood Flow and Hormonal Response

Bone formation may also be stimulated by increased blood flow to the bones as a response to the metabolic demands of exercise, which can increase the diffusion surface area of bone cells and deliver more nutrients to osteocytes, perhaps increasing their production of bone growth factors (Chilibeck, Sale, and Webber 1995). Also, hormonal responses during exercise may stimulate the activity of osteoblasts. For example, osteoblasts have receptors for dihydrotestosterone, which can increase the gene expression of bone DNA by osteoblasts. Muscle contraction can result in spikes of increased testosterone in the blood, and weight training has reportedly led to increased production of endogenous testosterone (Kraemer, Marchitelli, and Gordon 1990). However, because it appears that bone formation is localized, as is seen in the dominant arm of tennis players or carpenters (Huddleston et al. 1980), the influence of general factors such as blood flow and hormonal action on bone changes after exercise seems very limited.

The Error-Strain Distribution Theory of Bone Remodeling

The error-strain distribution theory by Lanyon (1996) proposed that cells derived from osteoblasts and distributed on the surface of bone and in the bone matrix can sense mechanical strain, or load imbalances, and communicate with one another via gap junctions. The feedback about these load imbalances within bone tissue results in an influx of calcium ions, prostaglandins, nitric oxide, and growth hormones to the area of strain. This error-strain mechanism can explain bone remodeling, protection against fatigue cracks, mineral exchange, and repair of microdamage (Rawlinson, Pitsillides, and Lanyon 1996; Lanyon 1993).

These feedback responses are determined not only by the magnitude of the load placed on the bone but also by the frequency of the application of these loads (Rubin and Lanyon 1984). High loads and low frequencies, similar to typical resistance exercise, appear to be optimal for inducing bone hypertrophy.

> ### Error-Strain Distribution Hypothesis of Mechanical Osteogenesis
>
> 1. Bone cells sense mechanical strain from weight-bearing or resistance exercises.
>
> 2. Load imbalances are communicated among cells locally, leading to an influx of calcium ions.
>
> 3. The calcium ions are followed by prostaglandins, nitric oxide, and growth hormones, leading to bone remodeling.
>
> Adapted from Lanyon 1996.

Bone Turnover After Exercise

Cross-sectional studies have shown that strength training is associated with high BMD or with bone metabolism that favors a high BMD (Block et al. 1989). Bell et al. (1988) found higher levels of osteocalcin, serum 1,25-hydroxyvitamin D, and urinary cAMP, indicative of elevated bone turnover, among people who strength-trained than among inactive control subjects. In one longitudinal study, serum concentrations of osteocalcin, bone-specific alkaline phosphatase (BAP, an enzyme marker of bone formation), and tartrate-resistant acid phosphatase (TRACP, an enzyme marker of bone resorption) were measured before, during, and after a 16-week strength-training program (Menkes et al. 1993). Serum concentrations of osteocalcin increased by 19% ± 6% after 12 weeks of training and remained significantly elevated after 16 weeks of training compared with the control group. Blood levels of BAP increased by 26% ± 11% after 16 weeks of training. Blood levels of TRACP increased at each measured time point, but the differences were not statistically significant. When bone turnover was expressed as a ratio of bone formation to bone resorption (i.e., BAP/TRACP), the exercise-training group had a significant increase of 16% ± 9% in bone remodeling after four months.

A recent study suggests that increased bone density in older people after exercise training depends on bone turnover. Markers of bone turnover were assessed in 62 men and women ages 60 to 83 years after six months of progressive resistance exercise, either 13 repetitions at 50% of their one-repetition maximum (1RM) or 8 repetitions at 80% of 1RM, three times a week. Serum levels of BAP, osteocalcin, and pyridinoline cross-links were measured (Vincent and Braith 2002). The percentage increase in total strength was about 17% for both exercise intensities. BMD of the femoral neck increased by 2% in the high-intensity group only. The increase in osteocalcin was 25% after low-intensity training but 39% after high-intensity training. BAP increased by 7% only after high-intensity training.

The effects on bone mass and serum levels of insulin-like growth factor I (IGF-I) of six months of a moderate-intensity, seated, resistance-training program were compared with those of a high-intensity, standing, free-weight exercise program in healthy older men (mean age about 55 years) and postmenopausal women without estrogen replacement (Maddalozzo and Snow 2000). The high-intensity training resulted in a gain in BMD in the spine and hip in men but not in women, whereas moderate-intensity training produced no changes in either sex at these sites. Despite a nearly 38% increase in strength, the bone mass changes were unrelated to blood levels of IGF-I.

Another recent study examined the effects of four months of a progressive resistance-training program on blood markers of bone turnover, including osteocalcin, BAP, IGF-I, and C-terminal cross-linked telopeptide of type I collagen (ICTP; Sartorio et al. 2001). Thirty men ages 65 to 81 years were randomly assigned to a control group that sustained their usual physical activity or to a group that performed 10 repetitions each of six different sets of exercises using the major muscle groups (two for the lower limb and four for the upper limb) three times a week. The men warmed up each time with 15 min of cycling exercise at 50% of maximal oxygen uptake and 15 repetitions of each exercise at 20% of 1RM. Lower-limb training graduated from 50% to 80% of 1RM during the first month. Upper-limb exercises graduated from 40% to 65% of 1RM. Resistance exercise did not change osteocalcin or IGF-I levels, but BAP levels increased by 25%, and ICTP levels decreased by 5%. Bone turnover, expressed as the ratio of bone formation to bone resorption (i.e., BAP/ICTP), increased by 34% after the resistance exercise training, whereas no changes in the markers of bone turnover were seen in the control group.

Summary

The adaptation by bone to loads is apparently optimized when the load results in unusually high peak strain applied at a high rate for short intervals (Lanyon 1996). Hence, exercise sessions designed to promote increases in bone mass should hypothetically involve intermittent load-bearing cycles repeated daily or every other day. Resistance exercise training and endurance exercises that produce high ground reaction forces can increase peak bone mass in young adults by 5% to 10% and retard or reverse bone mass loss by about 1% per year in both pre- and postmenopausal women. Other studies show that estrogen and androgens help potentiate the osteogenic effects of bone loading and suggest that dietary intake of calcium needs to be within the range of 1,000 mg to 1,300 mg per day in order for the exercise stimulus to promote bone mass. Hence, the prevention and treatment of osteoporosis and osteoporotic fractures should be directed at maximizing peak bone mass by optimizing dietary calcium and vitamin D, normal menstruation, or sex-hormone replacement and using vigorous physical activity that involves high peak forces, such as resistance exercise (Layne and Nelson 1999). However, recent evidence from the Women's Health Initiative study that estrogen plus progestin HRT increases cardiovascular and breast cancer risks warrants careful consultation by women with their personal physician before the decision is made to use HRT to promote bone health after menopause. Though exercise with or without calcium supplementation is a potentially useful adjuvant for increasing or maintaining bone mass after menopause, maximal benefits for bone health may also require osteogenic drugs when medically indicated. Notwithstanding the encouraging results of clinical studies of exercise and bone mass, more population-based epidemiologic studies that do a better job of controlling for diet and adjusting for other potential confounders and more randomized controlled trials are needed to establish the generalizability of results to population segments at risk for developing osteoporosis and to establish the effect of physical activity on risk of osteoporotic fractures. Nonetheless, the cumulative evidence is encouraging that vigorous physical activity, especially the types that involve high peak loads (e.g., resistance exercise), might promote higher peak bone mass and might retard bone loss with aging.

Bibliography

Alaimo, K., M.A. McDowell, R.R. Briefel, A.M. Bischof, C.R. Caughman, C.M. Loria, and C.L. Johnson. 1994. Dietary intake of vitamins, minerals, and fiber of persons ages 2 months and over in the United States: Third National Health and Nutrition Examination Survey, phase 1, 1988–91. *Advance Data* 14 (258): 1–28.

Alekel, L., J.L. Clasey, P.C. Fehling, R.M. Weigel, R.A. Boileau, J.W. Erdman, and R. Stiliman. 1995. Contributions of exercise, body composition, and age to bone mineral density in premenopausal women. *Medicine and Science in Sports and Exercise* 27: 1477–1485.

Alfredson, H., P. Nordstrom, and R. Lorentzon. 1997. Bone mass in female volleyball players: A comparison of total and regional bone mass in female volleyball players and nonactive females. *Calcified Tissue International* 60: 338–342.

American College of Sports Medicine. 1995. American College of Sports Medicine position stand: Osteoporosis and exercise (review). *Medicine and Science in Sports and Exercise* 27 (4): I–VII.

Anderson, J.C., and C. Eriksson. 1970. Piezoelectric properties of dry and wet bone. *Nature* 227: 491–492.

Bailey, D.A., H.A. McKay, R.L. Mirwald, P.R. Crocker, and R.A. Faulkner. 1999. A six-year longitudinal study of the relationship of physical activity to bone mineral accrual in growing children: The University of Saskatchewan bone mineral accrual study. *Journal of Bone and Mineral Research* 14 (10): 1672–1679.

Bassett, C.A. 1965. Electrical effects in bone. *Scientific American* 213: 18–25.

———. 1995. Why are the principles of physics and anatomy important in treating osteoporosis? *Calcified Tissue International* 56 (6): 515–516.

Bassett, C.A., and R.O. Becker. 1962. Generation of electric potentials by bone in response to mechanical stress. *Science* 137: 1063–1064.

Bauer, D.C., W.S. Browner, J.A. Cauler, E.S. Orwoll, J.C. Scott, D.M. Black, J.L. Tao, and S.R. Cummings. 1993. Factors associated with appendicular bone mass in older women. *Annals of Internal Medicine* 18 (9): 657–665.

Bell, N.H., R.N. Godsen, D.P. Henry, J. Shary, and S. Epstein. 1988. The effects of muscle-building exercise on vitamin D and mineral metabolism. *Journal of Bone and Mineral Research* 3: 369–373.

Bemben, D.A. 1999. Exercise interventions for osteoporosis prevention in postmenopausal women. *Journal of the Oklahoma State Medical Association* 92 (2): 66–70.

Ben-Noun, L. 2002. What was the disease of the bones that affected King David? *Journal of Gerontology: Medical Sciences* 57A: M152–M154.

Blimkie, C.J.R., S. Rice, C.E. Wegger, J. Martin, D. Levy, and C.L. Gordon. 1996. Effects of resistance training on bone mineral content (BMC) and density in adolescent females. *Canadian Journal of Physiology and Pharmacology* 74: 1025–1033.

Block, J.E., A.L. Friedlander, J.S. Brooks, and P. Steiger. 1989. Determinants of bone density among athletes engaged in weight-bearing and non-weight-bearing activity. *Journal of Applied Physiology* 67: 1100–1105.

Blumenthal, J.A., C.F. Emery, D.J. Madden, R. Schniebok, M.W. Riddle, M. Cobb, M. Higginbotham, and R.W. Coleman. 1991. Effects of exercise training on bone density in older men and women. *Journal of the American Geriatric Society* 39 (11): 1065–1070.

Bradney, M., G. Pearce, G. Naughton, C. Sullivan, S. Bass, T. Beck, J. Carlson, and E. Seeman. 1998. Moderate exercise during growth in prepubertal boys: Changes in bone mass, size, volumetric density and bone strength: A controlled prospective study. *Journal of Bone and Mineral Research* 13: 1814–1821.

Braith, R.W., R.M. Mills, M.A. Welsch, J.W. Keller, and M.L. Pollock. 1996. Resistance exercise training restores bone mineral density in heart transplant recipients. *Journal of the American College of Cardiology* 28: 1471–1477.

Brighton, C.T., M.J. Katz, S.R. Goll, C.E. Nichols, and S.R. Pollack. 1985. Prevention and treatment of sciatic denervation disuse osteoporosis in the rat tibia with capacitatively coupled electric stimulation. *Bone* 6: 87–97.

Buchner, D.M., and E.H. Wagner. 1992. Preventing frail health. *Clinics in Geriatric Medicine* 8: 1–17.

Chamay, A., and P. Tschantz. 1972. Mechanical influences on bone remodeling: Experimental research on Wolff's law. *Journal of Biomechanics* 5: 173–180.

Chilibeck, P.D., D.G. Sale, and C.E. Webber. 1995. Exercise and bone mineral density. *Sports Medicine* 19 (2): 103–122.

Clinical practice guidelines for the diagnosis and management of osteoporosis [special supplement]. 1996. *Canadian Medical Association Journal* 155 (8): 1113–1129.

Colletti, L.A., J. Edwards, L. Gordon, J. Shary, and N.H. Bell. 1989. The effects of muscle-building exercise on bone mineral density of the radius, spine, and hip in young men. *Calcified Tissue International* 45: 12–14.

Courteix, D., E. Lespessailles, S.L. Peres, P. Obert, P. Germain, and C.L. Benhamou. 1998. Effect of physical training on BMD in prepubertal girls: A comparative study between impact-loading and non-impact-loading sports. *Osteoporosis International* 8: 152–159.

Dalsky, G.P., K.S. Stocke, A.A. Ehsani, E. Slatopolsky, W.C. Lee, and S.J. Birge. 1988. Weight-bearing exercise training and lumbar bone mineral content in postmenopausal women. *Annals of Internal Medicine* 108: 824–828.

Dawson-Hughes, B., S. Harris, E. Krall, and G. Dallal. 1997. Effect of calcium and vitamin D supplementation on bone density in men and women 65 years of age and older. *New England Journal of Medicine* 337: 670–676.

Emslander, H.C., M. Sinaki, J.M. Muhs, E.Y. Chao, H.W. Wahner, S.C. Bryant, B.L. Riggs, and R. Eastell. 1998. Bone mass and muscle strength in female college athletes (runners and swimmers). *Mayo Clinic Proceedings* 73: 1151–1160.

Fiatarone, M.A., E.F. O'Neill, N.D. Ryan, K.M. Clements, G.R. Solares, M.E. Nelson, S.B. Roberts, and W.J. Evans. 1994. Exercise training and nutritional supplementation for physical frailty in very elderly people. *New England Journal of Medicine* 330 (25): 1769–1775.

Foldes, A.J., and M.M. Popovtzer. 1996. Osteoporosis 4000 years ago. *New England Journal of Medicine* 334: 735.

Friedlander, A.L., H.K. Genant, S. Sadowsky, N.N. Byl, and C.-C. Gluer. 1995. A two-year program of aerobics and weight training enhances BMD of young women. *Journal of Bone and Mineral Research* 10: 574–585.

Frigo, P., and C. Lang. 1995. Osteoporosis in a woman of the early Bronze Age. *New England Journal of Medicine* 333: 1468.

Garnero, P., and P.D. Delmas. 1997. Osteoporosis. *Endocrinology and Metabolism Clinics of North America* 26: 913–936.

Gregg, E.W., M.A. Pereira, and C.J. Caspersen. 2000. Physical activity, falls, and fractures among older adults: A review of the epidemiologic evidence. *Journal of the American Geriatric Society* 48 (8): 883–893.

Gross, D., and W.S. Williams. 1982. Streaming potential and the electromechanical response of physiologically moist bone. *Journal of Biomechanics* 15: 277–295.

Grove, K.A., and B.R. Londeree. 1992. Bone density in post-menopausal women: High impact vs. low impact exercise. *Medicine and Science in Sports and Exercise* 24: 1190–1194.

Hakkinen, A., T. Sokka, A. Kotaniemi, and P. Hannonen. 2001. A randomized two-year study of the effects of dynamic strength training on muscle strength, disease activity, functional capacity, and bone mineral density in early rheumatoid arthritis. *Arthritis and Rheumatism* 44: 515–522.

Hatori, M., A. Hasegawa, H. Adachi, A. Shinozaki, R. Hayashi, H. Okano, H. Mizunuma, and K. Murata. 1993. The effects of walking at the anaerobic threshold level on vertebral bone loss in postmenopausal women. *Calcified Tissue International* 52: 411–414.

Hawkins, S.A., E.T. Schroader, R.A. Wiswell, S.V. Jaque, T.J. Marcell, and K. Costa. 1999. Eccentric muscle action increases site-specific osteogenic response. *Medicine and Science in Sports and Exercise* 31: 1287–1292.

Heikkinen, J., E. Kyllonen, E. Kurttila-Matero, G. Wilen-Rosenqvist, K.S. Lankinen, H. Rita, and H.K. Vaananen. 1997. HRT and exercise: Effects on bone density, muscle strength and lipid metabolism. A placebo controlled 2-year prospective trial on two estrogen-progestin regimens in healthy postmenopausal women. *Maturitas* 26 (2): 139–149.

Heinonen, A., P. Oja, P. Kannus, H. Sievanen, H. Haapasalo, A. Manttari, and I. Vuori. 1995. BMD in female athletes representing sports with different loading characteristics of the skeleton. *Bone* 17: 197–203.

Heinonen, A., P. Oja, P. Kannus, H. Sievanen, A. Manttari, and I. Vuori. 1993. BMD in female athletes of different sports. *Bone and Mineral* 23: 1–14.

Heinonen, A., P. Oja, H. Sievanen, M. Pasanen, and I. Vuori. 1998. Effect of two training regimens on bone mineral density in healthy perimenopausal women: A randomized control trial. *Journal of Bone and Mineral Research* 13: 483–490.

Heinonen, A., H. Sievanen, P. Kannus, P. Oja, M. Pasanen, and I. Vuori. 2000. High-impact exercise and bones of growing girls: A 9-month controlled trial. *Osteoporosis International* 11 (12): 1010–1017.

Huddleston, A.L., D. Rockwell, D.N. Kulund, and R.B. Harrison. 1980. Bone mass in lifetime tennis athletes. *Journal of the American Medical Association* 244: 1107–1109.

Hui, S.L., C.W. Slemenda, and C.C. Johnston Jr. 1989. Baseline measurement of bone mass predicts fracture in white women. *Annals of Internal Medicine* 111: 355–361.

Johnston, C.C. Jr., and C.W. Slemenda. 1995. Pathogenesis of osteoporosis. *Bone* 17 (Suppl. 2): 19S–22S.

Karlsson, M., S. Bass, and E. Seeman. 2001. The evidence that exercise during growth or adulthood reduces the risk of fragility fractures is weak. *Best Practice and Research: Clinical Rheumatology* 15 (3): 429–450.

Katz, W.A., and C. Sherman. 1998. Osteoporosis: The role of exercise in optimal management. *Physician and Sportsmedicine* 26 (2): 33–43.

Kemper, H.C., J.W. Twisk, W. van Mechelen, G.B. Post, J.C. Roos, and P. Lips. 2000. A fifteen-year longitudinal study in young adults on the relation of physical activity and fitness with the development of the bone mass: The Amsterdam Growth and Health Longitudinal Study. *Bone* 27 (6): 847–853.

Kerr, D., T. Ackland, B. Maslen, A. Morton, and R. Prince. 2001. Resistance training over 2 years increases bone mass in calcium-replete postmenopausal women. *Journal of Bone and Mineral Research* 16 (1): 175–181.

Kerr, D., A. Morton, I. Dick, and R. Prince. 1996. Exercise effects on bone mass in postmenopausal women are site-specific and load dependent. *Journal of Bone and Mineral Research* 11: 218–225.

Khosla, S., E.J. Atkinson, B.L. Riggs, and L.J. Melton. 1996. Relationship between body composition and bone mass in women. *Journal of Bone and Mineral Research* 11: 857–863.

Kirk, R., C.F. Sharp, N. Elbaum, D.B. Endres, S.M. Simons, J.G. Mohler, and R.K. Rude. 1989. Effect of long-distance running on bone mass in women. *Journal of Bone and Mineral Research* 4 (4): 515–522.

Kohrt, W.M., A.A. Ehsani, and S.J. Birge. 1997. Effects of exercise involving predominantly either joint reaction or ground reaction forces on bone mineral density in older women. *Journal of Bone and Mineral Research* 12: 1253–1261.

Kohrt, W.M., D.B. Snead, E. Slatopolsky, and S.J. Birge Jr. 1995. Additive effects of weight-bearing exercise and estrogen on BMD in older women. *Journal of Bone and Mineral Research* 10: 1303–1311.

Kohrt, W.M., K.E. Yarasheski, and J.O. Holloszy. 1998. Effects of exercise training on bone mass in elderly women and men with physical frailty. *Bone* 23: S499.

Kraemer, W.J., L. Marchitelli, and S. Gordon. 1990. Hormonal and growth factor responses to heavy resistance exercise protocols. *Journal of Applied Physiology* 69: 1442–1450.

Kujala, U.M., J. Kaprio, P. Kannus, S. Sarna, and M. Koskenvuo. 2000. Physical activity and osteoporotic hip fracture risk in men. *Archives of Internal Medicine* 160 (5): 705–708.

Lane, J.M., and M. Nydick. 1999. Osteoporosis: Current modes of prevention and treatment. *Journal of the American Academy of Orthodopaedic Surgeons* 7 (1): 19–31.

Lane, N.E., D.A. Bloch, H.H. Jones, W.H. Marshall Jr., P.D. Wood, and J.F. Fries. 1986. Long-distance running, bone density, and osteoarthritis. *Journal of the American Medical Association* 255: 1147–1151.

Lanyon, L.E. 1993. Osteocytes, strain detection, bone modeling and remodeling. *Calcified Tissue International* 53: 5102–5106.

———. 1996. Using functional loading to influence bone mass and architecture: Objectives, mechanisms, and relationship with estrogen of the mechanically adaptive process in bone. *Bone* 18 (Suppl. 1): 37S–43S.

Lanyon, L.E., and W. Hartman. 1977. Strain related electrical potentials recorded in vitro and in vivo. *Calcified Tissue International* 22: 315–327.

Layne, J.E., and M.E. Nelson. 1999. The effects of progressive resistance training on bone density: A review. *Medicine and Science in Sports and Exercise* 31 (1): 25–30.

Lees, B., T. Molleson, T.R. Arnett, and J.C. Stevenson. 1993. Differences in proximal femur bone density over two centuries. *Lancet* 341 (8846): 673–675.

Levinson, W., and D. Altkorn. 1998. Primary prevention of postmenopausal osteoporosis. *Journal of the American Medical Association* 280 (21): 1821–1822.

Lloyd, T., V.M. Chinchilli, N. Johnson-Rollings, K. Kieselhorst, D.F. Eggli, and R. Marcus. 2000. Adult female hip bone density reflects teenage sports-exercise patterns but not teenage calcium intake. *Pediatrics* 106 (1 Pt. 1): 40–44.

Lohman, T., S. Going, R. Pamenter, M. Hall, T. Boyden, L. Houtkooper, C. Ritenbaugh, L. Bare, A. Hill, and M. Aickin. 1995. Effects of resistance training on regional and total bone mineral density in premenopausal women: A randomized prospective study. *Journal of Bone and Mineral Research* 10 (7): 1015–1024.

Maddalozzo, G.F., and C.M. Snow. 2000. High intensity resistance training: Effects on bone in older men and women. *Calcified Tissue International* 66 (6): 399–404.

Martin, A.D., and R.G. McCulloch. 1987. Bone dynamics: Stress, strain, and fracture. *Journal of Sports Sciences* 5: 155–163.

Martin, D., and M. Notelovitz. 1993. Effects of aerobic training on bone mineral density of postmenopausal women. *Journal of Bone and Mineral Research* 8 (8): 931–936.

Menkes, A., S. Mazel, R.A. Redmond, K. Koffler, C.R. Libanati, C.M. Gundberg, T.M. Zizic, J.M. Hagberg, R.E. Pratley, and B.F. Hurley. 1993. Strength training increases regional bone mineral density and bone remodeling in middle-aged and older men. *Journal of Applied Physiology* 74: 2478–2484.

Modlesky, C.M., and R.D. Lewis. 2002. Does exercise during growth have a long-term effect on bone health? *Exercise and Sport Sciences Reviews* 30: 171–176.

Montoye, H.J. 1984. Exercise and osteoporosis. *American Academy of Physical Education Papers* 17: 59–75.

Morris, F.L., G.A. Naughton, J.L. Gibbs, J.S. Carlson, and J.D. Wark. 1997. Prospective ten-month exercise intervention in pre-menarcheal girls: Positive effects on bone and lean mass. *Journal of Bone and Mineral Research* 12: 1453–1462.

Mosca, L. 2000. The role of hormone replacement therapy in the prevention of postmenopausal heart disease. *Archives of Internal Medicine* 160: 2263–2272.

National Institutes of Health. 1994. NIH Consensus conference. Optimal calcium intake. NIH Consensus Development Panel on optimal calcium intake. *Journal of the American Medical Association* 272: 1942–1948.

National Osteoporosis Foundation. 2002. *America's bone health: The state of osteoporosis and low bone mass.* Washington, DC: National Osteoporosis Foundation.

Nelson, M.E., M.A. Fiatarone, C.M. Morganti, I. Trice, R.A. Greenberg, and W.J. Evans. 1994. Effects of high intensity strength training on multiple risk factors for osteoporotic fractures. *Journal of the American Medical Association* 272: 1909–1914.

Nelson, M.E., E.C. Fisher, F.A. Kilmanian, G.E. Dallal, and W.J. Evans. 1991. A 1-y walking program and increased dietary calcium in postmenopausal women: Effects on bone. *American Journal of Clinical Nutrition* 53: 1304–1311.

Nguyen, T.V., P.J. Kelly, P.N. Sambrook, C. Gilbert, N.A. Pocock, and J.A. Eisman. 1994. Lifestyle factors and bone density in elderly: Implications for osteoporosis prevention. *Journal of Bone and Mineral Research* 9 (9): 1339–1346.

Nichols, D.L., C.F. Sanborn, S.L. Bonnick, B. Gench, and N. DiMarco. 1995. Relationship of regional body composition to BMD in college females. *Medicine and Science in Sports and Exercise* 27: 178–182.

Nichols, D.L., C.F. Sanborn, and A.M. Love. 2001. Resistance training and bone mineral density in adolescent females. *Journal of Pediatrics* 139 (4): 494–500.

Notelovitz, M., D. Martin, R. Tesar, F.Y. Khan, C. Probart, C. Fields, L. McKenzie. 1991. Estrogen therapy and variable-resistance weight training increases bone mineral in surgically menopausal women. *Journal of Bone and Mineral Research* 6: 583–590.

Pettersson, U., H. Alfredson, P. Nordstrom, K. Henriksson-Larsen, and R. Lorentzon. 2000. Bone mass in female cross-country skiers: Relationship between muscle strength and different BMD sites. *Calcified Tissue International* 67: 199–206.

Prince, R.L., M. Smith, I.M. Dick, R.I. Price, P.G. Webb, N.K. Henderson, and M.M. Harris. 1991. Prevention of postmenopausal osteoporosis: A comparative study of exercise, calcium supplementation, and hormone-replacement therapy. *New England Journal of Medicine* 325: 1189–1195.

Pruitt, L.A., R.D. Jackson, R.L. Bartels, and H.J. Lehnard. 1992. Weight training effects on bone mineral density in early postmenopausal women. *Journal of Bone and Mineral Research* 7: 179–185.

Pruitt, L.A., D.R. Taaffe, and R. Marcus. 1995. Effects of a one-year high-intensity versus low-intensity resistance training program on BMD in older women. *Journal of Bone and Mineral Research* 10: 1788–1795.

Rawlinson, S.C., A.A. Pitsillides, and L.E. Lanyon. 1996. Involvement of different ion channels in osteoblasts' and osteocytes' early responses to mechanical strain. *Bone* 19: 609–614.

Recker, R.R., K.M. Davies, S.M. Hinders, R.P. Heaney, M.R. Stegman, and D.B. Kimmel. 1992. Bone gain in young adult women. *Journal of the American Medical Association* 268 (17): 2403–2408.

Riggs, B.L., and L.J. Melton. 1986. Involutional osteoporosis. *New England Journal of Medicine* 314: 1676–1686.

———. 1995. The worldwide problem of osteoporosis: Insights afforded by epidemiology. *Bone* 17 (5 Suppl.): 505S–511S.

Rossouw, J.E., G.L. Anderson, R.L. Prentice, A.Z. LaCroix, C. Kooperberg, M.L. Stefanick, R.D. Jackson, S.A. Beresford, B.V. Howard, K.C. Johnson, et al. 2002. Risks and benefits of estrogen plus progestin in healthy postmenopausal women: Principal results from the Women's Health Initiative randomized controlled trial. *Journal of the American Medical Association* 288: 321–333.

Rubin, C.T., and L.E. Lanyon. 1984. Regulation of bone formation by applied dynamic loads. *Journal of Bone and Mineral Research* 66: 397–402.

Sartorio, A., C. Lafortuna, P. Capodaglio, V. Vangeli, M.V. Narici, and G. Faglia. 2001. Effects of a 16-week progressive high-intensity strength training (HIST) on indexes of bone turnover in men over 65 years: A randomized controlled study. *Journal of Endocrinological Investigation* 24 (11): 882–886.

Shamos, M.H., and L.S. Lavine. 1964. Physical bases for bioelectric effects in mineralized tissues. *Clinical Orthopaedics and Related Research* 35: 177–188.

Sheth, P. 1999. Osteoporosis and exercise: A review. *Mount Sinai Journal of Medicine* 66 (3): 197–200.

Simkin, A., J. Ayalon, and I. Leichter. 1987. Increased trabecular bone density due to bone-loading exercises in postmenopausal osteoporotic women. *Calcified Tissue International* 40: 59–63.

Sinaki, M., L.A. Fitzpatrick, C.K. Richie, A. Montesano, and W. Wahner. 1998. Site-specificity of bone mineral density and muscle strength in women: Job related physical activity. *American Journal of Physical Medicine and Rehabilitation* 6: 470–476.

Sinaki, M., H.W. Wahner, K.P. Offord, and S.F. Hodgson. 1989. Efficacy of nonloading exercises in prevention of vertebral bone loss in postmenopausal women: A controlled trial. *Mayo Clinic Proceedings* 64: 762–769.

Slemenda, C.W., C.H. Turner, M. Peacock, J.C. Christian, J. Sorbel, S.L. Hui, and C.C. Johnston. 1996. The genetics of proximal femur geometry, distribution of bone mass and bone mineral density. *Osteoporosis International* 6 (2): 178–182.

Smith, E., C. Gilligan, M. McAdam, C.P. Ensign, and P.E. Smith. 1989. Deterring bone loss by exercise intervention in premenopausal and postmenopausal women. *Calcified Tissue International* 44: 312–321.

Snow-Harter, C., M.L. Bouxsein, B.T. Lewis, D.R. Carter, and R. Marcus. 1992. Effects of resistance and endurance exercise on bone mineral status of young women: A randomized exercise intervention trial. *Journal of Bone and Mineral Research* 7: 761–769.

Sowers, M.F. 1997. Clinical epidemiology and osteoporosis: Measures and their interpretation. *Endocrinology and Metabolism Clinics of North America* 26: 219–231.

Sowers, M.F., G. Corton, and B. Shapiro. 1993. Bone density and bone turnover with long-term lactation. *Journal of the American Medical Association* 269: 3130–3135.

Speroff, L., R.H. Glass, and N.G. Case. 1994. *Clinical gynecologic endocrinology and infertility.* Baltimore: Williams and Wilkins.

Steinberg, K.I.K., S.B. Thacker, S.J. Smith, S.F. Stroup, M. Sack, D. Flanders, and R.L. Berkelman. 1991. A meta-analysis of the effect of estrogen replacement therapy on the risk of breast cancer. *Journal of the American Medical Association* 265 (15): 1985–1990.

Sundberg, M., P. Gardsell, O. Johnell, M.K. Karlsson, E. Ornstein, B. Sandstedt, and I. Sernbo. 2001. Peripubertal moderate exercise increases bone mass in boys but not in girls: A population-based intervention study. *Osteoporosis International* 12 (3): 230–238.

Taaffe, D.R., T.L. Robinson, C.M. Snow, and R. Marcus. 1997. High-impact exercise promotes bone gain in well-trained female athletes. *Journal of Bone and Mineral Research* 12: 255–260.

Taaffe, D.R., C. Snow-Harter, D.A. Connolly, T.L. Robinson, M.D. Brown, and R. Marcus. 1995. Differential effects of swimming versus weight-bearing activity on bone mineral status of eumenorrheic athletes. *Journal of Bone Mineral Research* 10 (4): 586–593.

Tabrah, F., M. Hoffmeier, F. Gilbert Jr., S. Batkin, and C.A. Bassett. 1990. Bone density changes in osteoporosis-prone women exposed to pulsed electromagnetic fields (PEMFs). *Journal of Bone and Mineral Research* 5 (5): 437–442.

Torgerson, D.J., and S.E.M. Bell-Syer. 2001. Hormone replacement therapy and prevention of nonvertebral fractures: A meta-analysis of randomized trials. *Journal of the American Medical Association* 285: 2891–2897.

Valimaki, M.J., M. Karkkainen, C. Lamberg-Allardt, K. Laitinen, E. Alhava, J. Heikkinen, O. Impivaara, P. Makela, J. Palmgren, R. Seppanen, et al. 1994. Exercise, smoking, and calcium intake during adolescence and early adulthood as determinants of peak bone mass: Cardiovascular risk in young Finns study group. *British Medical Journal* 309 (6949): 230–235.

Vincent, K.R., and R.W. Braith. 2002. Resistance exercise and bone turnover in elderly men and women. *Medicine and Science in Sports and Exercise* 34 (1): 17–23.

Vuori, I.M. 2001. Dose-response of physical activity and low back pain, osteoarthritis, and osteoporosis. *Medicine and Science in Sports and Exercise* 33 (Suppl. 6): S551–S586.

Wallach, J., and M. Lan. 1994. *Rare earths forbidden cures.* California: Double Happiness Publications.

Welsh, L., and O.M. Rutherford. 1996. Hip bone mineral density is improved by high-impact aerobic exercise in postmenopausal women and men over 50 years. *European Journal of Applied Physiology* 74: 511–517.

Whalon, R.T., D.R. Carter, and C.R. Steele. 1988. Influence of physical activity on the regulation of bone density. *Journal of Biomechanics* 21: 825–837.

Whitfield, J.F., and P. Morley. 1998. *Anabolic treatments for osteoporosis.* Boca Raton, FL: CRC Press.

Wickham, C.A., K. Walsh, C. Cooper, D.J. Barker, B.M. Margetts, J. Morris, and S.A. Bruce. 1989. Dietary calcium, physical activity, and risk of hip fracture: A prospective study. *British Medical Journal* 299 (6704): 889–892.

Wolff, I., J.J. van Croonenborg, H.C.G. Kemper, P.J. Kostense, and J.W.R. Twisk. 1999. The effect of exercise training programs on bone mass: A meta-analysis of published controlled trials in pre- and postmenopausal women. *Osteoporosis International* 9: 1–12.

Wolff, J. 1892. *Das Gesetz der Transformation der Knochen* (The law of bone transformation). Berlin: Hirschwald.

World Health Organization Study Group. 1994. Assessment of fracture risk and its application to screening for postmenopausal osteoporosis. *WHO Technical Report Service* 843: 1–129.

Web Sites

www.nof.org. Site of the National Osteoporosis Foundation.

www.osteo.org. Home of the National Institutes of Health Osteoporosis and Related Bone Diseases National Research Center. Maintained by the National Osteoporosis Foundation, in collaboration with The Paget Foundation and the Osteogenesis Imperfecta Foundation.

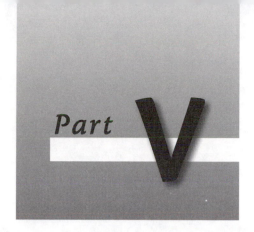

PHYSICAL ACTIVITY, CANCER, AND IMMUNITY

In the United States, cancer was predicted to kill about 556,000 people in 2003, second only to cardiovascular disease (CVD). Though groups such as the World Health Organization and the American Cancer Society have not formally recognized physical inactivity as a major risk factor for cancer, they do acknowledge that nearly a third of annual cancer deaths are attributable to lifestyle, including nutrition and physical inactivity. The chapters in this section describe the evidence that physical activity is associated with reduced risk of cancers of the colon, breast, and prostate, which, after lung cancer, are the most prevalent and deadly cancers in the United States.

Surgical treatment of breast cancer was documented as early as 1600 B.C. in Egyptian papyrus records, and in the fourth century B.C. Hippocrates coined the term *carcinoma*. However, he and Greco-Roman physicians such as Galen and Celsus believed that cancer was not curable. We now know that is not the case. We also have learned that behaviors, including physical activity, influence the risk of cancer. The first chapter in this part describes the contemporary epidemiologic evidence that physical activity indeed reduces the risk of developing cancers of the colon, breast, and prostate. The second chapter of this part focuses on the emerging evidence that moderate physical activity influences certain aspects of the immune system in ways that might help protect against some types of infection and tumor growth.

© David Sanders

Physical Activity and Cancer

Certain morbid affections come . . . from other causes, some particular posture of the limbs or unnatural movements of the body. We must advise men employed in standing trades to interrupt . . . that too prolonged posture by . . . walking about or exercising the body.

—*Benardino Ramazzini, The Diseases of Workers, 1713*

Cancer is a family of related diseases that result from uncontrolled growth and spread of abnormal cells, which usually become a tumor. Some of the oldest evidences of cancer are bone tumors **(osteosarcoma)** found in Egyptian mummies. Papyrus writings dated to about 1600 B.C. described the surgical treatment of eight cases of breast tumors, but the Greek physician Hippocrates is credited with coining a term for cancer in the fourth century B.C. He used the Greek word for crab, *carcinoma,* to describe ulcer-forming tumors, presumably because tumor projections resembled the shape of a crab's body and legs.

The epidemiologic study of cancer was catalyzed by the Italian physician Bernardino

Ramazzini (1633–1714) when he reported first in 1700 and later in 1713 that nuns seldom had uterine cervical cancer but had a high incidence rate of breast cancer. He speculated that the paradox might be explained somehow by their celibacy. Today, nulliparity (i.e., not giving birth) is recognized as a risk factor for breast cancer, and modern-day research on the hormonal effects of pregnancy on cancer risk can be traced in part to Ramazzini's views. He also believed that cancer risk was influenced by physical activity (Ramazzini 1983). Ramazzini is considered the father of occupational medicine (Franco 1999). He chronicled the risk factors associated with infectious diseases and cancer present in the workplace for 55 occupations, including runners and athletes, in his 1713 book *De Morbis Artificum Diatriba* (The Diseases of Workers, Ramazzini 1983). He observed that diseases, including cancer, among workers mainly were associated with the toxic materials that they handled and were exacerbated by "violent or irregular motions and unnatural postures of the body." He especially recommended exercise for sedentary workers such as cobblers and tailors (Ramazzini 1983). After a description of cancer and its public health impact, this chapter discusses whether the evidence supports Ramazzini's ideas about physical activity.

> ••• *Bernardino Ramazzini, the father of occupational medicine and early cancer epidemiologist, observed in the early 1700s that sedentary workers had elevated risks of chronic disease, including cancer.*

Magnitude of the Problem

Cancer is a leading cause of morbidity and mortality in developed nations. In the United States, cancer was predicted to kill about 556,000 people in 2003, second only to cardiovascular disease (CVD); nearly a third of annual cancer deaths are attributable to lifestyle, including nutrition and physical activity (American Cancer Society 2003). The financial burden of cancer is great: $170 billion in the year 2002 from medical services ($60 billion), lost productivity ($15 billion), and loss of life ($95 billion). Though the annual incidence of death from cancer is roughly half that of CVD in the United States, cancer deaths rose during the 1980s before leveling off during the 1990s. During that time, death rates from CVD steadily declined. Since the 1930s, the death rates from most cancers have stayed about the same or decreased. The exception is lung cancer deaths, which steadily increased until 1990 (figure 11.1, a and b).

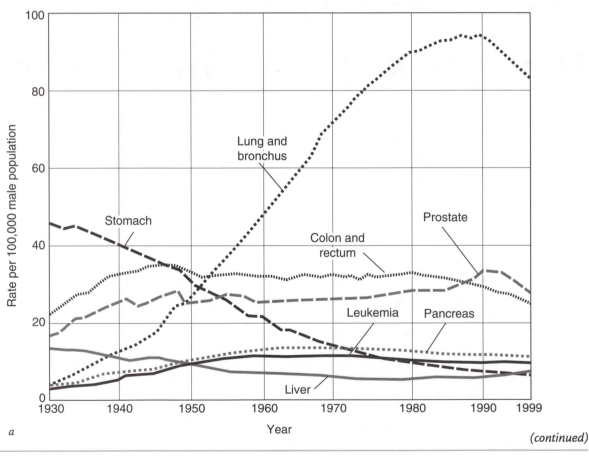

a

(continued)

Figure 11.1   *(a)* Age-adjusted cancer death rates for males by site. United States: 1930–1999.

U.S. Mortality Public Use Data Tapes 1960–1997, U.S. Mortality Volumes, 1930–1959. National Center for Health Statistics, Centers for Disease Control and Prevention 2000.

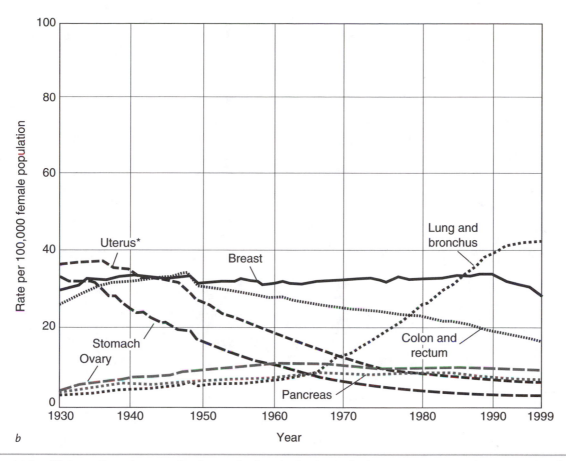

Figure 11.1 *(b)* Age-adjusted cancer death rates for females by site. United States: 1930–1999. *Uterus cancer death rates are for uterine cervix and uterine corpus combined.

U.S. Mortality Public Use Data Tapes 1960–1997, U.S. Mortality Volumes, 1930–1959. National Center for Health Statistics, Centers for Disease Control and Prevention 2000.

About 1.33 million new cases of cancer were expected in 2003. That represents nearly an 18% increase from the estimated incidence of 1.13 million new cases in 1992. About half of men and a third of women in the United States will develop some form of cancer during their lifetimes. Less than 15% of cancer is genetic, so the primary and secondary treatment of cancer are top priorities for public health.

> ••• *About half of men and a third of women in the United States will develop some form of cancer during their lifetimes. Less than 15% of cancer is genetic, so the primary and secondary treatment of cancer are top priorities for public health.*

Cancers differ in their numbers of new cases each year and annual death rates (figure 11.2). Though prostate cancer in men and breast can-cer in women are most prevalent in the United States, lung cancer is the most deadly in both men and women. Colorectal cancers rank third in both incidence and mortality, regardless of sex.

> ••• *Though prostate cancer in men and breast cancer in women are most prevalent in the United States, lung cancer is the most deadly in both men and women. Colorectal cancers rank third in both incidence and mortality, regardless of sex.*

Etiology of Cancer

Hippocrates believed that the body contained four humors (i.e., fluids), including blood, phlegm, yellow bile, and black bile. Health depended on maintaining a proper balance of these fluids. Hippocrates' idea that an excess of black bile in

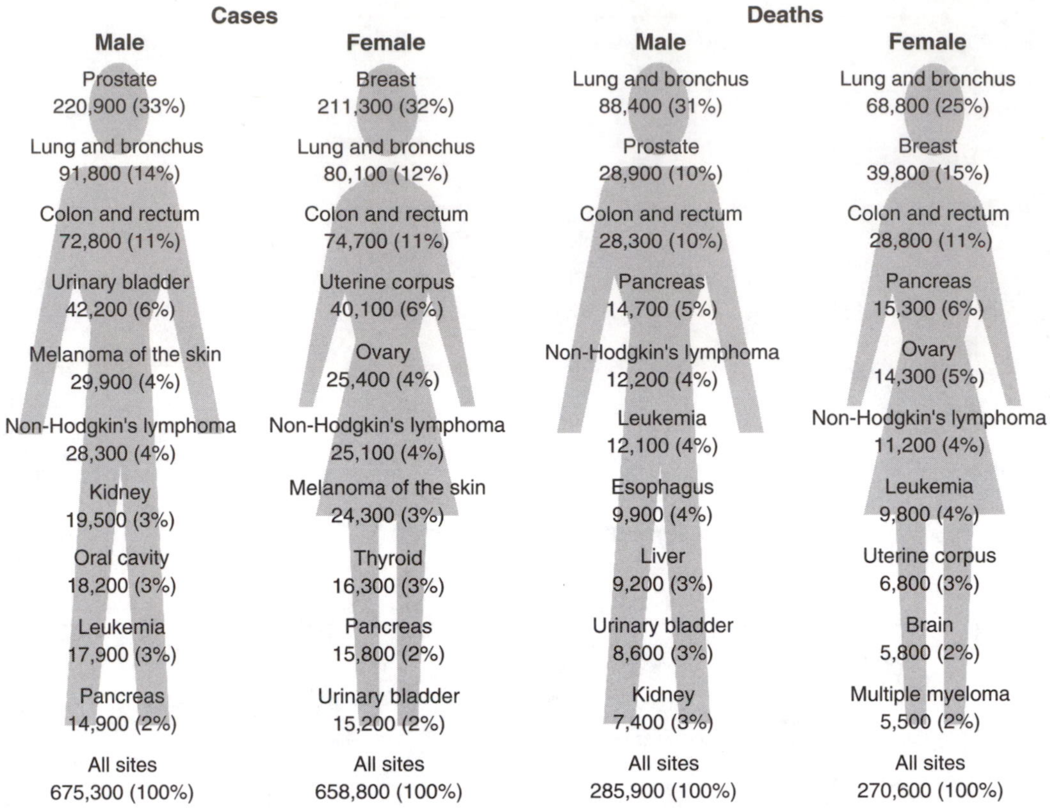

	Cases		Deaths	
	Male	**Female**	**Male**	**Female**
	Prostate 220,900 (33%)	Breast 211,300 (32%)	Lung and bronchus 88,400 (31%)	Lung and bronchus 68,800 (25%)
	Lung and bronchus 91,800 (14%)	Lung and bronchus 80,100 (12%)	Prostate 28,900 (10%)	Breast 39,800 (15%)
	Colon and rectum 72,800 (11%)	Colon and rectum 74,700 (11%)	Colon and rectum 28,300 (10%)	Colon and rectum 28,800 (11%)
	Urinary bladder 42,200 (6%)	Uterine corpus 40,100 (6%)	Pancreas 14,700 (5%)	Pancreas 15,300 (6%)
	Melanoma of the skin 29,900 (4%)	Ovary 25,400 (4%)	Non-Hodgkin's lymphoma 12,200 (4%)	Ovary 14,300 (5%)
	Non-Hodgkin's lymphoma 28,300 (4%)	Non-Hodgkin's lymphoma 25,100 (4%)	Leukemia 12,100 (4%)	Non-Hodgkin's lymphoma 11,200 (4%)
	Kidney 19,500 (3%)	Melanoma of the skin 24,300 (3%)	Esophagus 9,900 (4%)	Leukemia 9,800 (4%)
	Oral cavity 18,200 (3%)	Thyroid 16,300 (3%)	Liver 9,200 (3%)	Uterine corpus 6,800 (3%)
	Leukemia 17,900 (3%)	Pancreas 15,800 (2%)	Urinary bladder 8,600 (3%)	Brain 5,800 (2%)
	Pancreas 14,900 (2%)	Urinary bladder 15,200 (2%)	Kidney 7,400 (3%)	Multiple myeloma 5,500 (2%)
	All sites 675,300 (100%)	All sites 658,800 (100%)	All sites 285,900 (100%)	All sites 270,600 (100%)

Figure 11.2   Leading sites of new cancer cases and deaths—2003 estimates. Cancer cases by site and sex. New cancer cases exclude basal and squamous cell skin cancers and in situ carcinomas except urinary bladder.

Reprinted by the permission of the American Cancer Society, Inc.

organs was the cause of cancer was disseminated by the Roman physician Galen and remained the popular view in medicine until the European Renaissance, around the 14th century. The humoral theory of cancer was then supplanted by a theory that cancer was caused by the fermentation of lymph fluids. John Hunter, an 18th-century Scottish surgeon credited as the first modern physician to suggest that cancers could be cured by surgery, agreed that tumors grew from lymph filtered out of the blood. Around 1840, however, German pathologist Johannes Muller showed that cancer is composed of cells, not lymph. But he thought that cancer cells stemmed from buds (or blastema) extending between normal cells. Later, Muller's student Rudolph Virchow demonstrated that cancer cells, like all cells, result from the reproduction of existing cells (Gallucci 1985; Diamandopoulus 1996).

Cancer originates in two phases: initiation and promotion. In initiation, normal cells are changed into potentially harmful cells by damage from mutational factors. The second phase is promo-

tion, during which tumor growth is stimulated by other agents, including naturally circulating endogenous hormones. Genes located on chromosomes control the growth, division, and death of cells. Normally, body cells grow, divide, and die according to a systematic schedule. After a person reaches maturity, cell division occurs to replace injured or dying cells. In a normally aging cell, structures located at the end of chromosomes, called **telomeres,** shrink each time the cell divides until they reach a critical length that inhibits the cell from dividing further. Then the cell dies. Recent research has determined that 80% to 90% of cancer cells produce an enzyme called **telomerase,** which blocks the shrinking of telomeres, thus resulting in uncontrolled division of a cell into a tumor (Holland et al. 2000).

Certain genes that promote cell division are called **oncogenes.** Others that slow down cell division, or cause cells to die at the right time, are called **tumor suppressor genes.** Cancers can be caused by DNA mutations that activate oncogenes or inactivate tumor suppressor genes. Inherited DNA changes can cause certain cancers to occur very frequently and are responsible for the cancers that run in some families. Most cancer-causing agents (i.e., **carcinogens**) produce DNA mutations that lead to abnormal clones, which progressively become malignant clones that continue to reproduce (Holland and Frei 1993).

When cells break away from a tumor, they can **metastasize,** that is, migrate through the blood or lymph circulatory systems to other body tissues, where they build "colony" tumors at a new site and continue growing, a process first described by English surgeon Stephen Paget in 1889 after he had performed autopsies on 735 women who had died of breast cancer (Paget 1889). Cancers vary in their rates of growth, patterns of spread, and responses to different types of treatment. Benign (noncancerous) tumors do not metastasize and seldom kill people. Cancers are named by their site of origin, even if they spread to another part of the body. In general, those arising from epithelial cells are called **carcinoma.** Those arising from connective tissue are known as **sarcoma.** Cancers are generally categorized according to four stages or as recurrent. Stage I cancers are small, localized tumors that usually are curable. Stage II and III cancers are advanced, localized tumors or have spread to local lymph nodes. Stage IV cancers usually are inoperable or have metastasized. These stages are defined more precisely and differently for each type of cancer, and cannot be used to compare the progression of disease among different types of cancer. Other staging systems that are specific to the type of cancer are described later in this chapter for cancers of the colon, breast, and prostate.

> ••• *Cancers are named by their site of origin, even if they spread to another part of the body. In general, those arising from epithelial cells are called carcinoma. Those arising from connective tissue are known as sarcoma.*

Radiation and chemicals can alter a cell's DNA, causing mutations that result in cancer. One of the first practical uses of the X ray—discovered in 1896 by Wilhelm Conrad Roentgen, the first Nobel Prize winner for physics in 1901—was to treat cancer. It was subsequently determined that low daily doses of radiation can shrink tumors but that the wrong dose of radiation, including ultraviolet rays from the sun, also can cause cancer growth. The idea that chemicals can cause cancer probably had its origin in the writings of London physician John Hill, who popularized the idea that tobacco is a carcinogen. In 1761, he wrote a book titled *Cautions Against the Immoderate Use of Snuff.*

Viruses also are believed to contribute to cancer by injecting new DNA sequences into cells. For example, chronic hepatitis B infection can turn into liver cancer. A type of herpes virus, Epstein-Barr, which causes mononucleosis, is believed to contribute to non-Hodgkin's lymphoma and nose-and-throat cancer. Human immunodeficiency virus (HIV) increases the odds of developing non-Hodgkin's lymphoma, while human papilloma virus (HPV) appears to increase the risk of cervical cancer.

The discovery of two genes that cause some breast cancers, BRCA1 and BRCA2, permits genetic screening of people at exaggerated risk of developing breast cancer, thus permitting attempts at early primary and secondary prevention (Weber 1996). Other genes have been discovered that are associated with some cancers that run in families, such as cancers of the colon, rectum, kidney, ovary, esophagus, lymph nodes, skin, and pancreas.

Risk Factors

Different cancers have different risk factors, though some risk factors are associated with several cancers. For example, smoking is a risk factor for cancers of the lungs, mouth, throat, larynx, and bladder. In 2001, 172,000 cancer deaths (30% of all cancer deaths) were attributed to tobacco use; another 19,000 were attributed to alcohol abuse (American Cancer Society 2001). Though several factors like these are associated with higher rates of cancer, how they contribute to the pathophysiology that leads to specific-site cancers is less well understood than for some other chronic diseases such as cardiovascular disease and type 2 diabetes. For example, excessive sun exposure (especially in fair-skinned people and children and when the skin peels) increases the risk of basal cell and squamous cell carcinomas, which are diagnosed in about a million people each year. However, sun exposure has not been directly linked with the most serious form of skin cancer, melanoma, which had an incidence of about 51,000 new cases in 2001 and accounted for 7,800 (80%) of the estimated 9,800 deaths from all skin cancers (American Cancer Society 2001).

> ••• *The annual rate of cancer death among blacks in the United States is 15% to 30% higher than in whites and about twice as high as in Hispanics, American Indians, and Asian/Pacific Islanders. However, recent research suggests that the apparent discrepancy among races can mainly be explained by mortality from the higher prevalence of cardiovascular disease and diabetes among blacks (Bach et al. 2002). Cancer is not a different disease for different races.*

The American Cancer Society has not yet officially recognized physical inactivity as a major, independent risk factor of cancer to address in primary or secondary prevention. However, the number of studies that have examined the association of physical activity with the rates of some cancers has increased markedly in the past decade, yielding increasing evidence that leisure-time physical activity reduces the risk of breast cancer among women. In this chapter, we examine the evidence that physical inactivity is an independent, and plausibly causal, risk factor for some cancers.

Population Studies of Physical Activity: Specificity of Protection?

In 1996, the Surgeon General's report on physical activity and health concluded that sufficiently consistent epidemiologic evidence indicates that physical activity is associated with a reduction in the risk of colon cancer and that biologically plausible mechanisms for the reduced risk have been described, though not yet confirmed (U.S. Department of Health and Human Services 1996). In contrast, the report concluded that evidence linking physical activity with reduced risks for other cancers, such as breast, endometrial, ovarian, prostate, and testicular cancers, either was too sparse or inconsistent to permit firm judgments about the benefits of physical activity. Nonetheless, a scientific consensus panel convened in 1997 by the World Cancer Research Fund and American Institute for Cancer Research (1997) concluded that exercising regularly and controlling body weight can reduce incidence of cancer by 20%. A recent review used that scientific panel's definitions for the strength of

the evidence and evaluated nearly 170 epidemiological studies of physical activity and cancer risk according to cancer site (Friedenreich and Orenstein 2002). The review concluded that the evidence for decreased risk associated with higher levels of physical activity was convincing for colon and breast cancer, probable for prostate cancer, possible for lung and endometrial cancers, and insufficient for other cancer sites.

The following sections summarize the evidence about the relationship of physical activity and cancer and additional findings since the Surgeon General's report was released. Only cancers of the colon, breast, and prostate are discussed fully. They are prevalent and deadly cancers on which many physical activity studies have been conducted. Lung cancer, the deadliest and second most prevalent cancer in both men and women, is not discussed because too few studies of physical activity and lung cancer have been completed to permit any conclusions. It remains to be determined whether physical activity protects against all cancers or whether its benefits are site specific. Nonetheless, some well-done prospective studies of large cohorts have found that both physical activity and physical fitness are associated with reduced risk of all-site cancer deaths.

Harvard Alumni

Among 17,000 Harvard alumni who were observed for 12 to 16 years, a third of the deaths were attributed to cancer. After adjustment for age, smoking, and BMI, the men who said that they expended fewer than 500 kcal each week in physical activity had a 50% higher risk of cancer death than did men who expended 500 kcal or more each week (figure 11.3; Paffenbarger et al. 1987).

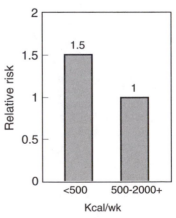

Figure 11.3 Harvard Alumni Study examining kilocalories burned per week with relative risk for cancer.

Aerobics Center Longitudinal Study (ACLS)

Among the ACLS cohort, over 10,000 men and 3,000 women were observed for about eight years after a clinic fitness test and health exam. The low-fit men and women were nearly three and two times, respectively, more likely to die of cancer than those who had an average level of fitness. Figure 11.4 illustrates that the lower risk associated with fitness was dose dependent. The low-fit men and women had relative risks of 4.3 and 16.3, respectively, compared with those who had a high fitness level. The high risk among low-fit women might not be accurate, though, because there were relatively few cancer deaths among women in the ACLS cohort.

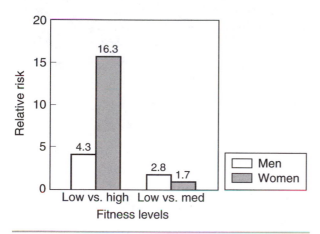

Figure 11.4 Aerobics Center Longitudinal Study comparing fitness levels to relative risk for cancer.
Data from Blair et al. 1989.

Colon and Rectal Cancer

According to the American Cancer Society (2003), about 105,500 new cases of colon cancer (49,000 men and 56,500 women) and 42,000 new cases of rectal cancer (23,800 men and 18,200 women) were predicted to occur in 2003. Colon and rectal cancers were expected to account for about 57,100 deaths (28,300 men and 28,800 women) during 2003. Colon cancer and rectal cancer have common features and often are referred to jointly as colorectal cancer. The death rate from colorectal cancers has been declining during the past 20 years, probably because of fewer new cases, early detection, and improved treatment. The five-year survival rate is 90% for people whose colorectal cancer is found and treated in an early stage, but only about 40% of colorectal cancers are detected before metastasis. After metastasis, the five-year survival rate goes down to 65%, and it is merely 8% after metastasis to the lungs or liver. The five-year survival rate in the United States is about 60% for whites and 50% for blacks (American Cancer Society 2001).

Types of Colon Cancer

The colon is a smooth-muscle vessel about 5 ft (1.5 m) long that absorbs water and minerals from fecal matter received from the small intestine. Fecal matter is then passed to the rectum for excretion from the body. The colon has four sections (figure 11.5): (1) The ascending colon (also known as the right colon) extends upward on the right side of the abdomen. (2) The transverse colon crosses the body to the left side, where it connects to (3) the descending colon (also known as the left colon), which continues downward on the left side. (4) The sigmoid colon, named for its S-like shape, connects to the

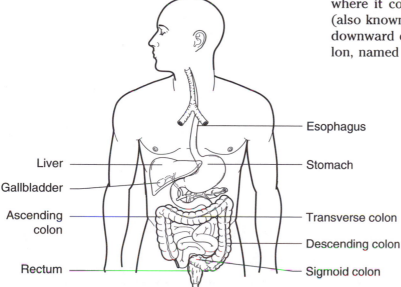

Figure 11.5 Diagram illustrating the four sections of the colon.
Adapted by the permission of the American Cancer Society, Inc.

rectum. Cancer can develop in any of the four sections of the colon or in the rectum and can cause different symptoms in each area (National Cancer Institute 1999).

Stages of Colon Cancer

Once cancer is detected, it is important that its severity be judged in order to plan treatment. Severity is graded in stages based on how far a tumor has spread within the rectum and colon, to nearby tissues, and to other organs as determined by palpation, sigmoidoscopy or colonoscopy, X rays, blood tests, and biopsy.

The most common staging systems are the TNM and the Dukes/Modified Astler-Coller equivalents systems, provided in tables 11.1 and 11.2 along with average survival rates. The TNM system is the one used most often. The T staging refers to the invasiveness of the tumor. N describes how far the cancer has spread to nearby lymph nodes. M indicates whether the cancer has me-

tastasized to other organs of the body. Stages 0 through IV also are used to describe increasing severity of the cancer.

Etiology of Colon Cancer

Like atherosclerosis and type 2 diabetes, colorectal cancers develop over a period of several decades. Before a true cancer develops, there usually are precancerous changes in the lining of the colon or rectum. These changes might be dysplasia (abnormal tissue formation) or adenomatous **polyps** (masses of tissue that bulge, usually on a stalk, from the interior lining of the colon). Polyps grow inward toward the center of the colon or rectum. In contrast, a cancer can grow either inward or outward through the walls of the colon or rectum and can metastasize if not treated. More than 95% of colorectal cancers are adenocarcinomas, glandlike cancers of epithelial cells in the lining of the colon and rectum. Most of this chapter deals with colon cancer because

TABLE 11.1   TNM STAGING TABLE

	T STAGE		N STAGE		M STAGE
T1	Invades submucosa	N0	No nodes involved	M0	No metastases
T2	Invades muscularis propria	N1	1 to 3 local lymph nodes involved	M1	Metastases present
T3	Invades through muscularis into subserosa	N2	4 or more pericolic lymph nodes involved		
T4	Invades other organs or perforates the visceral peritoneum	N3	Any lymph nodes along a named vascular trunk involved		

TABLE 11.2   TNM GROUP STAGING AND DUKES/MODIFIED ASTLER-COLLER EQUIVALENTS

TNM grouping	TNM stage	Dukes/MAC equivalent	5-year survival
T1 N0 M0	I	A	90%
T2 N0 M0		B1	75%
T3 N0 M0	II	B2	60%
T4 N0 M0		B3	50%
Any T N1 M0	III	C1	45%
Any T N2 M0		C2	40%
Any T N3 N0		C3	30%
Any T Any N M1	IV	D	10%

current evidence suggesting a protective effect of physical activity is much stronger for colon cancer than rectal cancer.

Risk Factors

Major risk factors of colorectal cancer include a personal or immediate family history of colorectal cancer or polyps, inflammatory bowel disease, age (about 90% of cases occur after age 50), a diet high in fat, and physical inactivity (American Cancer Society 2002; Shike 1996). About two thirds of colorectal cancers involve a missing allele in chromosome 18q (Laurent-Puig, Blons, and Cugnenc 1999), but it is not clear whether that causes the cancer or is an early result of cancer. Nonetheless, measures can be taken to reduce incidence and mortality rates. Three tests designed to detect colorectal cancer in its early stages are available. The stool blood test is recommended for men and women over 50 years of age. This test checks for hidden blood in the stool. The digital rectal exam can identify a tumor in the rectum and should be given to both men and women over age 40. A sigmoidoscopy, inspection of the rectum and lower colon by a camera attached to the end of a flexible tube, is more uncomfortable and complicated. This procedure is recommended every three to five years for everyone over 50 years of age (American Cancer Society 2001).

Any of these procedures can detect the presence of a polyp. An adenomatous polyp is one that is derived from glandular epithelial cells. The most common treatment for polyp removal is surgery. To prevent recurrence of polyps, most patients are given chemotherapy or radiation therapy. Fortunately, colorectal cancer has hallmark symptoms that are alarming enough to warn the patient before tumor surgery is needed. These symptoms include a change in usual bowel habits ranging from diarrhea to constipation; blood in the stool or narrower stool than usual; stomach discomfort such as gas pain, bloating, or cramps; a feeling that a bowel movement is not complete; weight loss without a reason; and persistent fatigue (National Cancer Institute 1999).

Physical Activity and Colon Cancer: The Evidence

Hard occupational work and leisure-time physical activity are associated with a reduction in the incidence of colon cancer (Arraiz, Wigle, and Mao 1992; Giovannucci et al. 1995; Markowitz et al. 1992; Shephard 1995, 1996; Sternfeld 1992; Thune and Furberg 2001). At the time of the Surgeon General's report on physical activity and health in 1996 (U.S. Department of Health and Human Services 1996), 29 population-based studies of physical activity and colon cancer had been reported. Of the 18 studies of occupational physical activity, 14 found lower rates of colon cancer incidence or mortality among people who were physically active on their jobs. The typical reduction in risk was between 25% and 50%. However, most of the studies had not controlled for other confounding factors such as social or economic status, diet, and other risk factors, so the independence of the reported effects usually was not determined. Eleven prospective cohort or case–control studies examined the association of leisure-time physical activity and colon cancer risk. Findings in eight of the studies generally were consistent between men and women and indicated that physical activity during middle age, but not early adulthood, was protective against colon cancer. There was a linear, dose-dependent decline in risk in 5 of 10 studies that permitted a test of a dose–response effect. Also, five of the studies controlled for diet and still found that leisure-time physical activity reduced the risk of colon cancer.

••• *A recent review of 48 epidemiological studies of 40,674 cases of colon or colorectal cancer showed a cumulative reduction in risk with increasing levels of physical activity. Results were clearest for colon cancer and when the intensity of physical activity was at least moderate (i.e., >4.5 METs; Thune and Furberg 2001). Another review reported that 43 of 51 studies found that physical activity was associated with an average reduction in colon cancer risk of 40% to 50% (Friedenreich and Orenstein 2002). Many studies did an incomplete job of adjusting for confounders, though, so the independent effect of physical activity remains unclear.*

Case–Control Studies

Sweden. Nearly 1,200 men and women were studied from 1986 to 1988 (352 cases of colon cancer, 217 cases of rectal cancer, and 624 controls; Gerhardsson et al. 1990). Both occupational and recreational physical activity levels were determined by self-reports. Sedentary men and women had a dose-dependent odds ratio of 3 for the rate cancer in the left colon, but not the right colon or rectum, compared with people who were classified as very active. Controlling for year of birth; sex; body mass; and intake of total energy, protein, total fat, and dietary fiber did not change the results.

Utah. A case–control study followed 119 women and 110 men with colon cancer and 204 female and 180 male controls (Slattery et al. 1988). Rectal cancer cases were not included. Physical activity quartiles were based on energy expended in both occupation and leisure-time physical activity. Self-reports, rather than occupational classification, were used. Odds ratios for the highest quartile of total physical activity compared with the lowest quartile were 0.70 for men and 0.48 for women. Intense physical activity by men was associated with a further reduction of 0.27 in the odds ratio. The benefit of physical activity was not influenced by dietary intake of calories, fat, or protein.

Seattle. Two hundred fifty men and 190 women ages 30 to 62 years who were diagnosed with colon cancer from 1985 to 1989 in three counties of the Seattle metropolitan area were matched by age, sex, and county of residence with about 230 male and 190 female controls (White, Jacobs, and Daling 1996). Physical activity was assessed by questions about the frequency and duration of various recreational and occupational activities performed at least twice a month during the 10-year period ending 2 years before diagnosis. Activities were classified as low intensity (<4.5 METs) or moderate to high intensity (>4.5 METs). Among men and women combined, participation in moderate- or high-intensity leisure-time physical activity two or more times each week was associated with a relative risk of 0.70 compared with people reporting no physical activity. The association was stronger for men than women. Paradoxically, the lowest risk was observed in people who said they exercised in their leisure time two to three times a week, rather than more often. Occupational activity was not associated with colon cancer, except a 70% reduction was found in men 55 years and younger who performed more than 14.5 h/wk of moderate activity compared with those who had sedentary jobs. Findings were independent of age, BMI, dietary factors, alcohol use, some other health behaviors, and region of the colon affected by cancer.

New York. Three hundred eight men with colon cancer were matched by age, race, hospital, and admission date with 1,164 male hospital patients to determine whether recreational activity was similarly protective among those engaging in high or low amounts of occupational activity (Markowitz et al. 1992). Occupational activity was determined by job title and was divided into three categories: involving physical activity more than 80% of the time, from 20% to 80%, and less than 20%. Recreational activity (20 min three times a week for at least one year) was assessed by questionnaire for three different periods of life (15–21 years, 22–44 years, and 45 years and older). The odds of colon cancer for moderate- and high-activity jobs were half those seen among sedentary workers, even after adjustment for age, race, geographical area, and leisure-time physical activity from ages 22 to 44. Thus, occupational physical activity was protective regardless of leisure physical activity during another period of life. Conversely, leisure-time physical activity performed from ages 22 to 44 was associated with a 10% to 25% lower rate of colon cancer regardless of the intensity of occupational work. However, men who exercised and had highly active jobs had the overall lowest cancer risk (OR = 0.3 to 0.6), indicating that the benefits of occupational and leisure-time physical activities were additive.

New England. The association of colorectal cancer with occupational and vigorous leisure-time physical activity was studied from 1986 to 1988 in 163 men with right ascending colon cancer, 242 men with rectal cancer, and 703 healthy men from the same community 31 years old or older (Longnecker et al. 1995). Subjects were categorized into four groups based on average time spent each week in vigorous (>4 METs) activity: none, 30 min, 1 h, and over 2 h. A physical activity score was assigned to each occupation reported 5 years previously and 20 years previously or for lifetime occupation. Vigorous physical activity during leisure time was associated with a decreased risk (OR = 0.6) of cancer of the right colon for men exercising about 2 h per week compared with those who did not exercise. Adjustment for diet, smoking, income, family history of colorectal cancer, BMI, and alcohol intake did not affect the association. Self-reported heavy occupational work was not associated with the odds of colon cancer.

Sweden. Nearly 100 colon and 79 rectal cancer cases were compared with two control groups of about 400, each sampled from a hospital and a population registry (Arbman et al. 1993). Subjects' jobs were classified as sedentary, intermediate, and physically active. Odds of left-sided colon cancer were lower by about 60% among people who had more than 20 years of physically active work compared with those who had never had a physically active job. Independence of the association was not tested, and no dose response was observed.

Taiwan. A hospital-based case–control study was conducted to determine the association between physical activity and histologically confirmed colorectal cancer risk in Taiwan (Tang et al. 1999). A total of 163 subjects ages 33 to 80 years with confirmed colorectal cancer and 163 hospital controls were enrolled during 1992. Dietary intake, physical activity, and other lifestyle activities were assessed using a food-frequency and lifestyle-activity questionnaire. The rate for colon cancer among men who engaged in leisure-time physical activity was 20% that of sedentary men, but physical activity was not associated with colon cancer risk among women.

Italy. A case–control study was conducted in Italy between 1992 and 1996 to estimate the odds ratios and population attributable risks (PARs) for colon cancer in relation to educational level, physical activity, energy and vegetable intake, eating frequency, and family history of colorectal cancer (Tavani et al. 1999; La Vecchia et al. 1999). Cases were 1,225 histologically confirmed colon cancer patients (688 men and 537 women) below the age of 75. Controls were 4,154 patients (2,073 men and 2,081 women) who had no history of cancer and were admitted to hospitals in the same areas for acute diseases other than cancer. Over 700 cases of rectal cancer also were analyzed. Compared with the lowest level of occupational physical activity at ages 30 to 39, the odds ratios for the highest level were 0.64 for men and 0.49 for women. This inverse association also was seen in both men and women at ages 15 to 19 and 50 to 59. Results were similar for the right ascending, transverse, left descending, and sigmoid regions of the colon. No association was found in either sex between colon cancer risk and leisure-time physical activity. PARs (i.e., the proportion of colon cancer that would have been avoided if all subjects were moved to the lowest exposure level) were 12% for high education, 14% for low physical activity, 14% for high energy intake, 22% for low vegetable consumption, 7% for high eating frequency, and 8% for a family history of colorectal cancer.

Hawaii. A population-based case–control study was conducted in the multiethnic population of Hawaii to examine whether colorectal cancer rates were associated with several characteristics of the Western lifestyle (high caloric intake, physical inactivity, obesity, smoking, and alcohol drinking) adopted by other ethnic groups that migrate to Western societies (Le Marchand et al. 1997). Interviews were conducted with 698 male and 494 female patients diagnosed from 1987 to 1991 with colorectal cancer who were of Japanese, European, Filipino, Hawaiian, or Chinese descent and were born in the United States or were immigrants. Nearly 1,200 population-based control participants were matched by age, sex, and ethnicity. Place of birth and duration of residence in the United States were unrelated to colorectal cancer risk. Energy intake and BMI were associated with increased risk, and lifetime recreational physical activity was associated with decreased risk. The associations were independent of each other, additive, and stronger in men; their additive odds ratios were 3.0 for men and 1.7 for women. The findings suggest that a positive energy imbalance, similar to the one involved in diabetes, may lead to colorectal cancer.

California, Utah, and Minnesota. A large population-based case–control study of colon cancer was conducted to determine whether leisure physical activity has a dose-dependent association with reduced risk of colon cancer (Slattery et al. 1997). Study participants came from Northern California, Utah, and the Minneapolis–Saint Paul metropolitan area in Minnesota. Long-term involvement (20 years) in high levels of physical activity, equivalent to 60 min or more of vigorous activity each session, was associated with a 30% reduction in risk of colon cancer. The amount of time involved in physical activity had a greater impact than the number of days per week that activities were performed. Those reporting the highest level of activity, as defined by both duration and intensity, had a 40% reduction in risk compared with those who were sedentary. Associations did not differ by age at diagnosis, site of the tumor within the colon, or sex. The protective effect of physical activity was slightly stronger among those without a family history of colorectal cancer. In the populations studied, 13% of colon cancers (4 cases out of 100,000) could be attributed to lack of vigorous leisure-time activity.

Prospective Cohort Studies

Over 20 prospective cohort studies have examined the association between occupational or leisure-time physical activity and risk of colon cancer.

Los Angeles. The protective effect of physical activity against the development of colon cancer was first suggested by an observational study of new colon cancer cases among men ages 20 to 64 years who lived in Los Angeles County from 1972 to 1981 (Garabrant et al. 1984). Physical activity levels were categorized as sedentary, moderately active, and highly active based on job titles. The age-adjusted incidence rates per 100,000 men declined linearly, from 24.6 to 21.6 to 13.4, with each increasing physical activity level. The relative risk for those in sedentary occupations was 1.8 times that in the highly active jobs, but the higher rate of cancer among the sedentary men might have been influenced by higher fat consumption, which was not controlled in the study.

Framingham, Massachusetts. The Framingham Heart Study also examined physical activity and the risk of colon cancer in a prospective cohort study of 1,900 men and 2,300 women ages 30 to 62 years who were observed for 28 years (Ballard-Barbash et al. 1990). Both men and women completed self-assessments of their leisure-time and occupational physical activity levels. One hundred fifty cases of colon cancer were observed. After adjustment for BMI, alcohol use, and serum total cholesterol, men in the lowest tertile of occupational activity had a relative risk of 1.8 and those in the middle tertile had a relative risk of 1.4 compared with men in the highest tertile. No association between activity levels and risk of colon cancer was seen among the women. A possible explanation is that the women's occupations required too little physical activity to exert a protective effect.

Sweden. Over 16,000 Swedish men and women born between 1886 and 1925 were observed for 14 years (Gerhardsson, Floderus, and Norell 1988). Occupational and leisure-time physical activity levels were assessed by self-reports. After adjustments for age, sex, and consumption of meat and coffee, those who had sedentary jobs had a relative risk 60% higher than those who performed heavy occupational work. The relative risk for men and women who were inactive during leisure time also was 60% higher than those engaging in vigorous physical activity during leisure time. The protective effects of occupational and leisure-time physical activity were additive. The relative risk of developing colon cancer was 3.6 among those who were physically inactive at

the workplace and during leisure time, but only when compared with those who did heavy work and vigorous leisure physical activity.

Another Swedish cohort study examined occupational work in more than a million men ages 20 to 64 years who were observed for 19 years (Gerhardsson et al. 1986). Sitting for 80% of the time at work was classified as a sedentary job, whereas sitting for less than 20% of the time was classified as a physically active job. More than 7,100 new cases of colon cancer and 5,290 new cases of rectal cancer were detected. After adjustments for age, socioeconomic class, and population density, those in sedentary occupations had a 30% higher risk of developing colon cancer. No associations were observed between occupational physical activity and rectal cancer.

Norway. The association between self-reported occupational and recreational physical activity and the risk of colorectal cancer was examined in a cohort from five areas in Norway (Thune and Lund 1996). More than 53,000 men and 28,000 women ages 20 to 69 years who entered the study between 1972 and 1978 were observed for an average of about 16 years. About 235 cases of colon cancer in men and 100 cases in women were detected. Participants were divided into four groups based on self-ratings of usual recreational activities: sedentary activities, physical activities for at least 4 h/wk, exercise to keep fit for at least 4 h/wk, and regular exercise training. Participants also were grouped according to occupational activity: sedentary work, work with walking, work with lifting and walking, and heavy manual work. Cancer rates were adjusted for age, BMI, serum cholesterol, and geographic region. Among men 45 years old or older and women of any age, physical activity (walking or bicycling) at least 4 h/wk was associated with a 25% reduction among men and a 40% reduction among women in risk of colon cancer compared with those who were sedentary. Diet was not controlled.

Male Health Professionals. Giovannucci et al. (1995) examined whether physical inactivity and obesity increase the risk for colon cancer and adenomas. A cohort of nearly 48,000 male health professionals 40 to 75 years of age responded in 1986 to a questionnaire about physical activity level and BMI. Participants were grouped into quintiles based on average energy expenditure from leisure-time activities. By 1992, 203 colon cancer cases and 586 adenoma cases were reported. The rate of left colon cancer was 50%

lower in the highest quintile compared with the lowest quintile after adjustment for age, history of colorectal polyps, previous endoscopy, parental history of colorectal cancer, smoking, BMI, use of aspirin, and intake of red meat, folate, dietary fiber, and alcohol. Modest levels of activity (11 MET-hours per week) substantially reduced the risk of colon cancer, with a dose–response relationship existing up to 46.8 MET-hours per week. The authors concluded that activities equivalent to about 1 h of running, 2 h of tennis, or 3 h of walking a week were sufficient to reduce the risk of colon cancer.

Nonetheless, the findings were limited to male health professionals, who might be more likely to engage in other healthful behaviors not controlled in the study. Also, only eight categories of common activities were assessed, which might lead to an underestimation of the amount of physical activity needed for protection against colon cancer. In addition, only six years were allowed for the cancer to develop.

Harvard Alumni Health Study. Previous investigations regarding the influence of physical activity on colon cancer risk generally used a single assessment of physical activity, thus failing to account for changes over time. In the Harvard Alumni Health Study, self-reported stair climbing, walking, and sports play were assessed between 1962 and 1966 and again in 1977 among 17,600 Harvard alumni ages 30 to 79 years who were followed prospectively for the occurrence of colon cancer (*n* = 280) and rectal cancer (*n* = 53) from 1965 through 1988 (Lee and Paffenbarger 1994). After adjusting for age, parental history of cancer, and BMI, the rate of colon cancer among inactive men was not different from that of the moderately and highly active men. Diet was not controlled.

Nurses' Health Study. None of the few prospective studies of women discussed so far showed a statistically significant reduction in colon cancer incidence or mortality associated with increased leisure-time physical activity. The Nurses' Health Study, which began in 1976, provides information about health and behavior updated every two years on about 90,000 women and thus permits an examination of whether leisure-time physical activity significantly influences the risk of colon cancer in women. Martinez et al. (1997) confirmed reported diagnoses of colon cancer by review of hospital records and pathology reports. After controlling for BMI, women who expended more than 21 MET-hours per week in various leisure-time physical activities had a relative risk of colon cancer of 0.54 compared with women who expended less than 2 MET-hours per week, consistent with observations in men. As in the male health professionals' study, only eight categories of physical activity were assessed, so the amount of activity needed for protection may have been underestimated.

Physicians' Health Study. Though most studies have indicated that physical activity is related inversely to colon cancer risk, whether a dose–response relationship exists, whether the relationship differs between nonobese and obese persons, and the effect of long-term physical activity remain unclear. Those issues were examined in the Physicians' Health Study (Lee et al. 1997). Physical activity among 21,807 men ages 40 to 84 years was assessed initially and again 36 months later. The men then were observed for an average of 11 years, during which 217 developed colon cancer. After adjusting for age, obesity, and alcohol intake, the relative risks of colon cancer for those who vigorously exercised either once, two to four times, or five or more times per week did not differ from men who did not exercise. Also, physical activity was not associated with colon cancer risk among obese or normal-weight men. Plausible explanations for the lack of association in this study include misclassification of physical activity and the possibility that the physically active men had increased surveillance for colon cancer (e.g., through more frequent screening).

Strength of the Evidence

In general, studies agree that physical activity appears to have a protective effect on the risk of colon cancer. That effect appears to be independent of other health factors (especially diet), but at this point there is not enough evidence to conclude whether it is fully consistent between men and women. Conclusions cannot be made about the type, frequency, intensity, and duration of physical activity that is most beneficial. Also, it is not clear whether leisure-time (Longnecker et al. 1995; Thune and Lund 1996; White, Jacobs, and Daling 1996) or occupational (Arbman et al. 1993; Markowitz et al. 1992) physical activity provides the greatest protection, in part because of the difficulty of measuring physical activity. Some evidence indicated that being physically active both in leisure time and at work confers the greatest protection (Markowitz et al. 1992).

One study found no difference by colon subsite in the protection provided by physical activity (White, Jacobs, and Daling 1996), while others found greater benefits for the right colon (e.g., Longnecker et al. 1995; Thune and Lund 1996), and still others found greater benefits for the left colon (e.g., Arbman et al. 1993; Giovannucci et al. 1995). The balance of the evidence has more consistently found reduced rates of left colon cancer among the physically active, but evidence for site-specific protection against colon cancer is not yet conclusive (Giovannucci et al. 1996; Lee and Paffenbarger 1994; Shephard 1996).

Lowered risk for colon cancer among physically active adults might be confounded by associations between physical activity and other health factors (e.g., diet, smoking, alcohol use, use of medications). For example, heavy drinkers tend to have low physical activity levels and high BMIs. Hence, low physical activity might be associated with more colon cancer in heavy drinkers because of their body fat, not directly because of their low physical activity. Chronic alcohol use can suppress the immune system, while excess adipose cells could provide a continuous source of carcinogens in the bloodstream (McTiernan et al. 1998). However, the protective effect of physical activity against colon cancer generally persists after controlling for relative weight or BMI (Shephard 1995, 1996) and diet (Lee 1995). The Nurses' Health Study and another large study that sampled U.S. women (Giovannucci et al. 1996) controlled for age, prior endoscopy, parental history of colorectal cancer, smoking, and intakes of aspirin, animal fat, dietary fiber, folate, methionine, and alcohol and still found an inverse association between physical activity and risk of large adenomas in the distal colon. On balance, the association between physical activity and lower incidence of colon cancer appears to be independent of other health factors.

Temporal Sequence

Many of the leisure-time physical activity studies and nearly all the occupational physical activity studies that showed lower rates of colon cancer used a cross-sectional design. However, a substantial number of prospective cohort studies lasting 5 to 20 years generally reported lowered risk for people who were more physically active.

Strength of Association

Most studies have reported a strong, inverse association between physical activity and risk

of colon cancer, but not rectal cancer, with the relative risk ranging from 1.2 to 3.9 for those who are most sedentary compared with those who are most active (Arraiz, Wigle, and Mao 1992; Lee 1995). On average, case–control and prospective cohort studies observed a reduction in colon cancer incidence of about 40% to 50% among people classified as most active either during leisure time or at work (Colditz, Cannuscio, and Frazier 1997; Friedenreich and Orenstein 2002). It has been estimated that colon cancer rates in the United States could be lowered by 7% if the roughly 25% of the U.S. adult population now sedentary were to increase energy expenditure by 10 MET-hours (about 3 h of moderate physical activity) each week (Colditz, Cannuscio, and Frazier 1997).

If the overall risk for colon cancer attributable to physical inactivity is 30%, about 15,000 deaths could be prevented if all sedentary Americans became vigorously active (Powell and Blair 1994). Based on those figures, had the national physical activity objectives for the year 2000 been met, mortality from colon cancer might have been reduced by as much as 5%, resulting in about 2,200 fewer deaths (Powell and Blair 1994).

> ••• *It has been estimated that colon cancer rates in the United States could be lowered by 7% if the 25% of the U.S. adult population now sedentary were to increase energy expenditure by 10 MET-hours (about 3 h of moderate physical activity) each week (Colditz, Cannuscio, and Frazier 1997).*

Consistency

Studies of leisure physical activity have shown significant protection against colon cancer in both men and women in different ethnic groups and nations, including the United States, Canada, China, Japan, Sweden, Denmark, Italy, New Zealand, Switzerland, Taiwan, and Turkey (Lee 1995; Markowitz et al. 1992; Thune and Furberg 2001). However, the findings have been less consistent among women, possibly because the surveys used to measure physical activity were developed mainly for men and are less precise in estimating household chores (Lee 1995).

Dose Response

A recent review of a dozen case–control and cohort studies of colon cancer published before August 2000 showed an overall dose–response reduction in risk with increasing level of physical activity (Thune and Furberg 2001). Results were clearest when the intensity of physical activity was at least moderate (i.e., >4.5 METs). Another review concluded that 25 of 29 observational studies found evidence of a dose–response reduction in risk (Frieden-reich and Orenstein 2002). At least five studies of occupational activity have shown a dose–response relationship between the amount of activity and the extent of protection against colon cancer (Shephard 1996). Among studies of leisure-time physical activity that included at least 100 cases of colon cancer, about two thirds of the case–control studies but only half of the prospective cohort studies showed a linear reduction in risk with higher levels of physical activity (figure 11.6; Thune and Furberg 2001). Despite several studies that showed a dose–response relationship between physical activity and risk of colon cancer, others have found no relationship (Longnecker et al. 1995; Shephard 1996). Some animal studies have even found lower doses of exercise to be more beneficial than high amounts (Shephard 1995, 1996).

Though studies have not yet indicated how much activity is needed, Lee (1995) proposed that a threshold of 1,000 kcal of weekly leisure physical activity is necessary, an amount

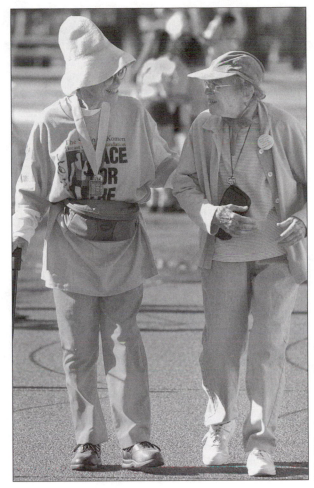

© David Sanders

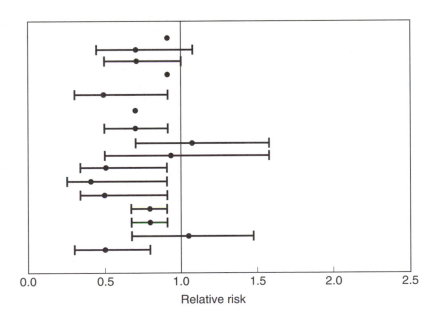

Relative risk

Figure 11.6   Summary of 16 prospective cohort studies—leisure-time physical activity and colon cancer risk (RR; 95% CI when available).

Data from Thune and Furberg 2001.

consistent with findings from the Nurses' Health Study and the male health professionals' study. Few data are available about the intensity of physical activity that is protective, but one study reported that incidence of colon cancer decreased in men who participated in highly intense exercise, while the reverse was true for women (Lee 1995). In contrast, other studies (e.g., Giovannucci et al. 1996) found that most of the benefit came from activities of moderate intensity, such as walking.

Biological Plausibility

Adenomatous polyps (adenomas) are precursors to most colorectal cancers, and some studies have reported lower risk of adenomas among physically active people. For example, in a colonoscopy study of 200 adenoma cases and 384 adenoma-free controls, women in the top three quartiles of leisure physical activity had half the incidence of colorectal adenomas of those in the least-active quartile (Sandler, Pritchard, and Bangdiwala 1995). There was no protective effect of occupational physical activity among men or women. Men who did not participate in sports had a 70% increase in risk for adenomas. In a recent prospective study of about 1,900 men and women, no associations between adenoma recurrence and moderate, vigorous, or total physical activity were found during a three-year follow-up period after colonoscopy (Colber et al. 2002).

The most popular explanation for reduced colon cancer among physically active people is that exercise results in a shortened gastrointestinal transit time (e.g., by increasing peristalsis and decreasing fecal segmentation), hence reducing the contact of potential carcinogens with the mucosal lining of the colon (Giovannucci et al. 1995; Lee 1995; Lee and Paffenbarger 1994; Markowitz et al. 1992; Shephard 1995, 1996; Thune and Lund 1996; White, Jacobs, and Daling 1996). Mechanisms might differ by colon site. Physical activity increases the tone of the vagus nerve to the heart. The vagus nerve also innervates the right colon and stimulates peristalsis, helping propel fecal contents along the colon. It is not established, though, whether physical activity affects the tone of the vagus nerve to the colon. In contrast, the left colon lacks parasympathetic innervation and serves as a storage site for fecal matter. By decreasing transit time, there is hypothetically less exposure to carcinogens from foods (Sternfeld 1992).

> ••• *The most popular explanation for reduced colon cancer among physically active people is that exercise results in a shortened gastrointestinal transit time, thereby reducing contact of potential carcinogens with the lining of the colon. But, like other plausible mechanisms, this idea has not yet been confirmed.*

Bowel transit time was decreased in one study after six weeks of running for 30 min at 70% to 80% of maximal heart rate three days a week (Cordain, Latin, and Behnke 1986). Untrained men ages 18 to 25 without previous irregularities of the gastrointestinal system were separated into an experimental group and a control group. Each subject ingested a dye capsule after performing a $\dot{V}O_2$max test and examined his fecal matter for the appearance of the dye. Transit time was recorded. There was a 22.8% decrease in bowel transit time in the experimental group but no change in the control group that did not run. Total bowel transit time also decreased in a small group of older men after a 13-week total-body strength training program (Koffler et al. 1992). However, other studies found that four weeks of exercise training had no effect on patients with idiopathic constipation (Meshkinpour et al. 1998) and no change in bowel transit time when sedentary men engaged in a few days of exercise (Coenen et al. 1992; Robertson et al. 1993). Also, some population-based studies found that cancer risk was not related to overall gastrointestinal transit time (Giovannucci et al. 1995; Shephard 1996).

Other studies argue that the protective effect of exercise is mediated by a reduction in body iron stores or by changes in prostaglandin levels (Markowitz et al. 1992; Shephard 1995, 1996; Thune and Lund 1996; White, Jacobs, and Daling 1996). Prostaglandin F increases gut motility and inhibits the division and spread of colon cancer cells. In contrast, prostaglandin E2, which is elevated in people with colorectal cancer or polyps, decreases gut motility and increases colonic cell proliferation. In a recent study, people who spent 28 MET-hours a week in physical activity had nearly 30% lower levels of prostaglandin E2 in mucosal cells of the rectum compared with those who spent 5 MET-hours each week in physical activity (Martinez et al. 1999).

People diagnosed with colon cancer have a higher-than-average rate of metabolic syndrome

X, characterized by hyperinsulinemia, hyper-glycemia, hypertriglyceridemia, and low HDL cholesterol levels. Physical inactivity is a strong determinant of hyperinsulinemia, which could mediate the effect of inactivity on colon cancer risk because insulin is an important growth factor for colon cancer cells (Giovannucci et al. 1995).

A single exercise session leads to increased secretion of gastroenteropancreatic hormones into the blood (Bartram and Wynder 1989), which can temporarily decrease bowel transit time, and an exercise session can temporarily elevate levels of some immune cells in the blood (e.g., natural killer cells, cytoxic T lymphocytes, monocytes, and interleukin-1), which might inhibit colon tumor growth (Lee 1995; Lee and Paffenbarger 1994; Shephard 1996; Thune and Lund 1996).

Most experimental studies used mice or rats that ran in an activity wheel or were forced to swim in order to examine whether physical activity affects tumor growth or survival after tumor implants (Shephard 1996). It is difficult to extrapolate age, duration of training, and rate of body fat accumulation from rats or mice to humans (Shephard 1996). Nevertheless, studies of rodents indicate that prior or concurrent exercise reduces the incidence of chemically induced tumors and produces a 25% to 100% slowing of tumor growth (Shephard 1995, 1996). This seems to hold true for both forced, strenuous activity that leads to weight loss and moderate, voluntary activity that does not lead to weight loss (White, Jacobs, and Daling 1996).

Summary and Conclusions

About 50 population-based studies of physical activity and colon cancer have been reported. Over 80% of the studies showed a protective effect of physical activity. This has been observed in different ethnic groups and nations, including the United States, Canada, China, Japan, Sweden, Denmark, Italy, New Zealand, Switzerland, Taiwan, and Turkey, indicating high consistency (Friedenreich and Orenstein 2002; Lee 1995; Markowitz et al. 1992; Thune and Furberg 2001). The reduction in rates of colon cancers among physically active people ranged from about 20% to 75%, with an average reduction of nearly 50% (Colditz, Cannuscio, and Frazier 1997; Friedenreich and Orenstein 2002). Occupational work is associated most clearly with reduced risks of tumors of the transverse and descending colon (Giovannucci et al. 1996;

Lee and Paffenbarger 1994; Shephard 1996). The benefits of leisure activity seem to be somewhat smaller, but occupational activity is usually classified more easily and may be sustained for longer periods (Shephard 1996). Some studies used subjects' participation in collegiate sport activities or a single question on a questionnaire to estimate leisure-time or total physical activity (Lee 1995). Studies of regular exercise (leisure activity) have shown that it significantly protects against colon cancer in both men and women (Shephard 1996), although the findings were less consistent for women, probably because questionnaires have been developed largely for men and are less precise in estimating household chores (Lee 1995). The protective effect of an active lifestyle is more clearly demonstrated when fitness rather than physical activity is assessed (Shephard 1996). Generally, study findings have satisfied the criteria of strength of association, consistency between sexes, temporal sequence, dose response, and biological plausibility. However, there have been no population-based studies of cancer risk in humans after experimental manipulations of physical activity. Also, there have been no studies showing that naturally occurring alterations in physical activity levels are associated with changes in colon cancer rates. The majority of human epidemiologic studies assessed physical activity only once, failing to allow for changes in activity over time (Lee and Paffenbarger 1994). Hence, randomized controlled trials are needed to confirm the protective effect of physical activity.

••• *About 50 population-based studies of physical activity and colon cancer have been reported worldwide. More than 80% of the studies showed a protective effect of physical activity. The reduction in rates of colon cancers among physically active people ranged from about 20% to 75%, with an average reduction of nearly 50% (Colditz, Cannuscio, and Frazier 1997; Friedenreich and Orenstein 2002).*

Breast Cancer

Next to skin cancers, breast cancer is the most prevalent cancer among women, accounting for one of every three cancer diagnoses in the United States. There were about 213,000 new cases of invasive breast cancer expected among women in 2003; only 1,300 cases were expected to be found among men (American Cancer Society 2003). In the United States, about 40,000 women were predicted to die from breast cancer in the year 2003; breast cancer mortality is second only to lung cancer mortality. About 1 in 8 women in the United States will develop breast cancer, and 1 in 28 women will die from it (Brinton and Devesa 1996). About 400 deaths from breast cancer were expected in men in 2001. Worldwide, the annual incidence of breast cancer is about one million cases. Incidence and mortality are highest in western Europe and North America and lowest in Asia and Africa (Brinton and Devesa 1996). Differences in incidence and mortality are greater among countries than within countries and are associated with variations in body weight, diet, reproductive hormone levels, and reproductive history, including menstrual cycle length, **parity,** and lactation (Kelsey and Horn-Ross 1993). Environmental factors, rather than genetic factors, are responsible for most of the variation in breast cancer rates among countries. Studies of migrants to the United States have shown that the incidence rate of migrants and their offspring approaches the level of the native-born population (Ewertz 1995).

> ••• *In the United States, about 40,000 women were predicted to die from breast cancer in the year 2003; breast cancer mortality is second only to lung cancer mortality.*

According to the American Cancer Society (2003), the five-year survival rate for localized breast cancer has increased from 72% in the 1940s to the present level of 97%; if the breast cancer is superficial, the survival rate approaches 100%. However, once the cancer has spread within the breast, the survival rate decreases to 77%. For people with distant metastases, the five-year survival rate is only 21%. In the United States, survival rates are higher for white women than black women (79.3% vs. 62.1% across all ages), and Asian American women have higher five-year survival rates than white American women (Kelsey and Horn-Ross 1993). Some cancer researchers have proposed that American blacks have poorer survival rates because of less aggressive treatment, lower incidence of estrogen receptor–positive tumors, a higher proportion of poorly differentiated tumors, poorer nutritional status, and higher BMI. In contrast, women of Asian descent have lower

body weight and fewer lymph node metastases than whites (Kelsey and Horn-Ross 1993). A recent cumulative review of studies involving 189,877 white and 32,004 black patients that controlled for deaths from causes other than cancer concluded that blacks were at a significantly higher risk of death from breast cancer but that the higher mortality rate among blacks was better explained by more advanced stages of cancer at the time of diagnosis rather than differences in cancer biology among racial groups (Bach et al. 2002).

Although the incidence rates have been increasing, possibly due to increased mammography utilization, mortality rates have remained virtually stable over the past 50 years, probably a result of earlier detection and better treatment. In the United States, the mortality rate in women less than 65 years old has fallen, but the rates have increased for older white women and black women of all ages.

Types of Breast Cancer

Most breast lumps are benign (not cancerous) and result from fibrocystic changes in breast tissue. Fibrosis refers to excessive scarlike connective tissue. Cysts are fluid-filled sacs. Fibrocystic lumps usually cause breast swelling and pain. The nipple might discharge a clear or cloudy liquid. Benign breast lumps such as fibroadenomas or papillomas are common growths. They cannot spread outside of the breast to other organs.

Mammographic abnormalities indicative of breast cancer include pointed, starlike lesions; small, asymmetric lumps; microcalcifications; and any distortion or asymmetry of the breast's shape (I.C. Henderson 1995). The most important physical sign of breast cancer is a painless lump in the breast. However, about 10% of patients have breast pain and no mass. Less common symptoms include persistent changes to the breast, such as thickening, swelling, skin irritation, or distortion, and nipple symptoms, including spontaneous discharge, erosion, inversion, or tenderness.

Carcinoma in Situ

When a cancer is confined to lobules (milk glands) or ducts (milk passages) and has not spread to surrounding fat cells in the breast or to other organs, it is called **breast carcinoma in situ** (figure 11.7). There are two types of in situ breast cancer: Lobular carcinoma in situ (LCIS) originates in the lobules and does not penetrate through the lobule walls. It usually does not become an invasive cancer, but it is a risk factor for developing

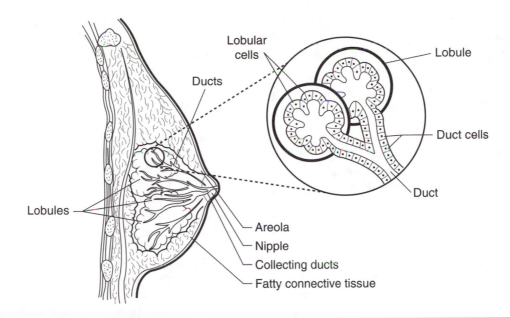

Figure 11.7   Diagram of breast structure.

Reprinted by the permission of the American Cancer Society, Inc.

invasive cancer. Ductal carcinoma in situ (DCIS) involves cancer cells inside the milk ducts that do not infiltrate the surrounding fat cells in the breast. It is the most common noninvasive breast cancer (National Cancer Institute 2000a).

Invasive Carcinoma

Invasive, or infiltrating, **carcinoma** spreads in the breast and to other parts of the body. Invasive ductal carcinoma (IDC) originates in a milk duct but breaks through the wall of the duct and invades the fatty tissue of the breast. It can pass into the lymph and blood circulatory systems and spread to other organs. About 80% of breast cancers are IDC. Another 10% to 15% of invasive breast cancers are infiltrating lobular carcinomas (ILC), which originate in the milk-producing glands. About 5% of breast cancers are medullary carcinomas, which have a distinct border between the tumor cells and normal breast tissue. Other rare forms of invasive breast cancer include colloid carcinoma, which produces mucus; tubular carcinoma; and adenoid cystic carcinoma, which usually develops in the salivary glands, not the breast. Each of these rare types of invasive cancer has a better prognosis than invasive lobular cancer, invasive ductal cancer, or inflammatory breast cancer (IBC), in which the skin is red, feels warm, and may thicken like an orange peel. Though called inflammatory, IBC results from the spread of cancer cells within the lymph circuits in the skin, not from inflammation.

It is classified as stage IIIB (breast cancers of any size that have spread to the skin, chest wall, or internal mammary lymph nodes) until it metastasizes (National Cancer Institute 2000a).

Stages of Breast Cancer

Stages indicate whether or how far a breast cancer has spread within the breast, to nearby tissues, and to other organs as determined by palpation, diagnostic blood tests, and X rays (National Cancer Institute 2000a).

Breast Cancer Stages

STAGE 0 (NONINVASIVE OR IN SITU BREAST CANCER)

Includes lobular carcinoma in situ and ductal carcinoma in situ.

STAGE I

Tumor is smaller than 2 cm (0.8 in.) in diameter and does not appear to have spread beyond the breast.

STAGE II

Tumor is larger than 2 cm (0.8 in.) in diameter and/or has spread to lymph nodes under the arm on the same side as the affected breast. Lymph nodes have not yet adhered to one

(continued)

another or to the surrounding tissues, a sign that the cancer has not yet advanced to stage III.

STAGE III

Stage IIIA: Tumor or tumors either are larger than 5 cm (2 in.) in diameter and/or have spread to lymph nodes that adhere to one another or surrounding tissue.

Stage IIIB: Breast cancer of any size has spread to the skin, chest wall, or internal mammary lymph nodes (located beneath the breast and inside the chest).

STAGE IV

The cancer, regardless of its size, has metastasized to distant sites, such as bones, lungs, or lymph nodes not near the breast.

Etiology of Breast Cancer

The etiology of breast cancer is not well understood. About 10% of breast cancer cases are hereditary; most hereditary cases are believed to result from mutations of the BRCA1 and BRCA2 genes, which normally express proteins that inhibit abnormal cell reproduction (Weber 1996). About 50% to 60% of women with inherited BRCA1 or BRCA2 mutations will develop breast cancer by the age of 70, and they also are at elevated risk for ovarian cancer. Inherited mutations of the p53 tumor suppressor gene can also increase a woman's risk of developing breast cancer, as well as leukemia, brain tumors, and sarcomas of bone or connective tissue. Most DNA mutations related to breast cancer, however, occur during a woman's life rather than being inherited. Acquired mutations of oncogenes or tumor suppressor genes may result from radiation or cancer-causing chemicals. So far, however, studies have not been able to identify any chemical in the environment or in our diets that is likely to cause these mutations or a subsequent breast cancer. The cause of most acquired mutations remains unknown.

> ••• *Only about 10% of breast cancer cases are hereditary; most hereditary cases are believed to result from mutations of the BRCA1 and BRCA2 genes, which normally express proteins that inhibit abnormal cell reproduction. About 50% to 60% of women with inherited BRCA1 or BRCA2 mutations will develop breast cancer by the age of 70.*

Tests to identify other acquired changes in oncogenes or tumor suppressor genes (such as p53) may help doctors more accurately predict the prognosis of some women with breast cancer. But, with the exception of the HER2 oncogene, these tests have not yet been shown to be useful in making decisions about treatment and are used only for research purposes. A monoclonal antibody therapy called trastuzumab (Herceptin®) has been developed that specifically interrupts the growth-promoting action of the HER2 oncogene.

Estrogen has been implicated in breast tumor growth since a Scot named Thomas Beatson discovered in 1878 that rabbits stopped producing milk after he removed the ovaries. He then tested whether breast cancer could be treated by oophorectomy (removal of the ovaries) and concluded from his sometimes successful results that the ovaries might be the cause of breast cancer. The incidence rate of breast cancer in women increases rapidly with age during the childbearing years, until around age 50; the slope rises at a slower pace after **menopause.** This changing rate is not apparent in men, for whom breast cancer incidence continues to increase linearly with age. This has been interpreted as evidence for the involvement of reproductive hormones in the etiology of breast cancer (Ewertz 1995). During menopause, the exposure to estrogen and progesterone decreases. Although these hormones are not carcinogenic themselves, they may act to promote the growth of cells that have already undergone malignant transformation.

Some women with genetic risk choose to take the medication tamoxifen in an attempt to reduce the likelihood of developing breast cancer. Results from the Breast Cancer Prevention Trial showed that women at high risk for breast cancer are less likely to develop the disease if they take tamoxifen, which blocks the effects of estrogen on breast cells. After an average of four years of tamoxifen, these women had 45% fewer breast cancers than women with the same risk factors who did not take tamoxifen. Whether tamoxifen prevents new breast cancer from developing or retards small, initially undetectable cancers has not been determined.

A woman's age increases her exposure to initiators and promoters of cancer. A woman's breast age differs according to the rate of cell divisions in breast tissue. Breast epithelial cell division begins at **menarche** and continues until menopause. The last menstrual cycle ends the division of breast epithelial cells. Physical activity has been proposed as a way to alter this exposure to estrogen and therefore may have a drastic affect on reducing risk by decreasing breast aging.

Estradiol is an endogenous estrogenic hormone that is not toxic to breast epithelial cells but stimulates cell proliferation in the body. Sometimes this proliferation can be excessively rapid and cause a mutation in the DNA. A DNA mutation could cause the production of defective repair enzymes or defective tumor suppressor genes. The defective enzymes might not allow the body to protect itself against excessively rapid proliferation of cells in the tissue, leading to cancer. Breast cancer has been hypothesized to form from excessive exposure to estradiol. Women have a higher risk of DNA mutations and breast cancer because of their increased lifetime exposure to estrogens. Factors such as age, age at menarche, age at menopause, obesity, hormone replacement therapy, and menstrual cycle length can increase hormone exposure in various ways.

••• *Estradiol can speed the rate of breast cell division. Coupled with gene mutations that inhibit tumor suppressor factors and enzymes that repair cells, this can promote tumor growth. Factors such as age, age at menarche, age at menopause, obesity, hormone replacement therapy, and menstrual cycle length increase lifetime estradiol exposure.*

Higher estradiol levels are associated with a doubling of breast cancer risk and have been found in girls whose menarche occurred before the age of 12. These girls were also found to be at higher risk for adiposity and fluctuating testosterone levels during their menstrual cycles, both of which also contribute to breast cancer risk. A delayed menarche may induce irregular menstrual cycles for up to 30 years and thus also lower lifetime estradiol exposure. Irregular cycles alone are associated with a reduction in risk around 50%.

The risk of breast cancer increases more slowly after menopause as female reproductive hormone levels decline. Nonetheless, postmenopausal women remain at greater risk because after menopause their levels of sex hormone–binding globulin (SHBG) decreases.

SHBG regulates the amount of active sex hormones circulating throughout the body. When it decreases, the body loses some of its ability to maintain a balance of sex hormones. Physical activity may help control this problem, mostly by preventing it from getting worse. Obesity in postmenopausal women further decreases the amount and function of SHBG; physical activity can fight obesity and thus counter further decreases in SHBG.

Risk Factors

Risk factors of breast cancer include being over the age of 40 years, high socioeconomic class, having family members with the disease, starting menstruation at an early age or menopause at a late age, and late first pregnancy or **nulliparity.** High fat intake or high overall calorie consumption is also associated with higher risk of breast cancer.

- *Age.* The incidence and mortality of breast cancer increases with age (table 11.3). Each year more than 75% of women newly diagnosed with breast cancer are over the age of 50. Breast cancer is rare in younger women, with an incidence rate of only 1 case per 100,000 for women ages 20 to 24. However, the rate climbs to about 25 cases per 100,000 for ages 30 to 34, 122 cases for ages 40 to 44, and 245 cases for ages 50 to 54. Breast cancer is the leading cause of cancer death in women between the ages of 15 and 54.

TABLE 11.3 LIKELIHOOD OF DEVELOPING INVASIVE BREAST CANCER AMONG WOMEN ACCORDING TO AGE, 1997–1999

Age interval	Percentage of age group	Likelihood
Birth to age 39 years	0.44%	1 in 228
Age 40 to 59 years	4.17%	1 in 24
Age 60 to 79 years	7.14%	1 in 14
Birth to death	13.3%	1 in 8

Data from American Cancer Society, 2003.

- *Race.* For all ages combined, white American women are more likely to develop breast cancer than African American women. In 1994, the incidence rate for white women in the United States was 113 cases per 100,000, and 100 per 100,000 for African American women. Among women younger than 50, African American women are more likely to develop breast cancer than white women. In 1994, African American women were more likely to die of breast cancer (31 per 100,000) than white women (25 per 100,000). Between 1988 and 1992, white, African American, and Hawaiian women had the highest rates of breast cancer incidence and mortality. Among different Asian American populations, incidence rates ranged from 29 per 100,000 for Korean American women to 106 per 100,000 for Hawaiian women, and mortality rates ranged from 11 per 100,000 for Chinese American women to 25 per 100,000 for Hawaiian women.

• *Sex.* Although breast cancer is a disease that affects primarily women, about 1,500 cases of breast cancer and 400 deaths occur in men each year. Male breast cancer accounts for less than 1% of the overall incidence and mortality of this disease. Even though men are at low risk of developing breast cancer, they should be aware of risk factors, especially family history, and report any change in their breasts to a physician.

• *Family history of breast cancer.* Having one first-degree relative (mother, sister, or daughter) with breast cancer doubles a woman's risk, and having two first-degree relatives increases her risk fivefold. A breast cancer susceptibility gene, BRCA1, has been identified on chromosome 17; it is implicated in approximately 5% of all breast cancers (Pleotis Howell 1995). Most of the inherited breast and ovarian cancer combinations are associated with BRCA1. Yet, only 45% of families with breast cancer have the BRCA1 gene.

• *Previous proliferative breast disease.* Women who have been diagnosed with proliferative breast disease with usual hyperplasia from an earlier breast biopsy have 1.5 to 2 times higher risk of breast cancer than other women. A previous biopsy result of atypical hyperplasia increases a woman's breast cancer risk four to five times. A woman with cancer in one breast has a three- to fourfold risk of developing a new cancer in the other breast. A biopsy diagnosed as fibrocystic changes without proliferative breast disease carries no risk of breast cancer.

• *Previous breast irradiation.* Women who have had chest-area radiation therapy as children or young women to treat another cancer (such as Hodgkin's disease or non-Hodgkin's lymphoma) are at significantly increased risk for breast cancer.

• *Menstrual history.* Women who started menstruating before age 12 have a 50% greater breast cancer risk than those who started at age 15 or later. Also, women who reached natural menopause at or after age 55 have twice the risk of women who experience menopause before age 45 (Brinton and Devesa 1996). Long-term, repetitive proliferation of breast endothelial cells during the childbearing years can promote the development of malignant cells.

• *High socioeconomic status.* Social class can be regarded as an indicator of a high-risk lifestyle, not necessarily as a direct risk factor of breast cancer. Women of higher socioeconomic status are more likely to have their first child at a later age, to have fewer children, and to use hormone replacement therapy during menopause, all of which may increase the risk of breast cancer (Ewertz 1995).

• *Oral contraceptive use.* It is still not clear what part oral contraceptives (birth control pills) might play in breast cancer risk. A recent analysis using data from most of the large, well-designed, published studies found that women now using oral contraceptives have a slightly greater risk of breast cancer than those women not using them. Women who stopped using oral contraceptives more than 10 years ago do not appear to have any increased breast cancer risk.

• *Nulliparity.* As first reported in 1713 by Bernardo Ramazzini, women who have had no children or who had their first child after age 30 have a slightly higher breast cancer risk. Protection against cancer-inducing factors may be one of the benefits of an early pregnancy. During pregnancy, a differentiation of breast tissue occurs that changes a woman's sensitivity to endogenous steroid hormones. Some evidence indicates that women who give birth before age 20 have about half the risk of developing breast cancer of nulliparous women (Stoll 1995). The increased risk with late pregnancy may be associated with the aging process, or involution, of the breasts.

• *Hormone replacement therapy.* Most studies suggest that long-term use (10 years or more) of estrogen replacement therapy (ERT) after menopause may increase the risk of breast cancer. Recent results of the Women's Health Initiative Study showed increased risk of breast cancer after about five years of hormone replacement therapy that combined estrogen plus progestin treatment. Another recent study found that the risk of ERT applies only to current and recent users and that a woman's breast cancer risk returns to that of the general population within five years of stopping ERT.

• *Alcohol consumption.* Compared with nondrinkers, women who consume one alcoholic drink a day have a very small increase in risk, and those who have two to five drinks daily have about 1.5 times the risk of women who drink no alcohol. Alcohol is also known to increase the risk of developing cancers of the mouth, throat, and esophagus.

• *Obesity and high-fat diets.* Risk appears to increase for women who gain weight as adults but not for those who have been overweight since childhood. Also, the effect of obesity on risk is more prominent among women taking estrogen replacement therapy than among those who do not. Most studies have found that breast cancer is less common in countries where the typical diet is low in total fat, low in polyunsaturated fat, and low in saturated fat. On the other hand, many studies of women in the United States have not found breast cancer risk to be related to dietary fat intake after controlling for other risk factors for breast cancer such as physical activity level and intake of other nutrients that might also alter breast cancer risk. The American Cancer Society recommends maintaining a healthy weight and limiting the intake of high-fat foods, particularly those from animal sources.

• *Environmental toxins.* Currently, research does not clearly show a link between breast cancer risk and exposure to environmental pollutants, such as the pesticide DDE (chemically related to DDT) or polychlorinated biphenyls (PCBs). Studies on other environmental toxins are under way.

• *Physical inactivity.* Physical activity has been hypothesized to reduce breast cancer, and it is one of the few modifiable behaviors that affect breast cancer risk. Unlike its protective effect against many of the diseases discussed in this book, the health benefits of physical activity in reducing breast cancer risk may depend on when activity occurs in a woman's life because of the role of menstruation and reproductive hormones in breast cancer risk. Plausible explanations for a protective effect of physical activity include reducing the number of lifetime ovulatory cycles or indirectly by association with lower body fat and reduced dietary fat or total caloric intake.

> ••• *Unlike its protective effect against many of the diseases discussed in this book, the health benefits of physical activity in reducing breast cancer risk may depend on when activity occurs in a woman's life because of the role of menstruation and reproductive hormones in breast cancer risk.*

Physical Activity and Breast Cancer: The Evidence

A recent review of the results of observational, epidemiological studies of physical activity and breast cancer reported that 32 of 44 studies found that physical activity was associated with an average reduction in breast cancer risk of 30% to 40% (Friedenreich and Orenstein 2002). The following sections discuss some of these studies, concluding with studies that examined the moderating effect of menopausal status.

Retrospective and Case–Control Studies

More than 40 population-based studies of physical activity and breast cancer risk involving nearly 110,000 cases of breast cancer have been reported (Thune and Furberg 2001). Eighteen of the 22 studies showed a lower rate of breast cancer among physically active women, but the reduced rates were big enough to be statistically significant in only about half the studies, as indicated by 95% confidence intervals that encompass an RR of 1.0.

College Alumnae Study. Frisch et al. (1985) conducted one of the first major studies of the protective effects of exercise against breast cancer. This study used a retrospective design to evaluate the prevalence of 10 breast cancers in a cohort of 5,398 living alumnae from the classes of 1925 to 1981 from 10 U.S. colleges. Women who had participated in intercollegiate or intramural athletics were compared with nonathletes to assess the effect of physical activity on risk for breast cancer. An athlete was defined as any woman who had been on at least one varsity team, house team, or other intramural team for one or more years. Figure 11.8 shows that after adjusting for potential confounding factors such as age, family history of cancer, age of menarche, number of pregnancies, use of oral contraceptives, use of hormones during menopause, smoking, and leanness, the relative risk of breast cancer for the nonathletes was 1.86 (95% CI: 1.00–3.47).

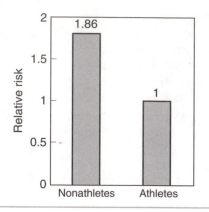

Figure 11.8 The relative risk for breast cancer in athletes versus nonathletes.

Data from R.E. Frisch et al., 1985.

The athletes were leaner and less likely to have used oral contraceptives and estrogens during menopause than the nonathletes. Athletes also had a later age of menarche (13.0 vs. 12.7 years) and an earlier age of natural menopause (51.3 vs. 52.0 years). Of the college athletes, 82% had been on precollege teams, compared with only 25% of the college nonathletes. As assessed by current physical activity, a larger percentage of the athletes than of the nonathletes were physically active after college (74% vs. 57%). Based on these findings, the authors concluded that long-term athletic training establishes a lifestyle that lowers the risk of breast cancer.

A limitation of the College Alumnae Study is that, although it shows physical inactivity's independence of known risk factors of breast cancer, only physical activity in college was studied. Given that nearly 60% of the college non-athletes were currently active at the time of the study, persistence of the results was not shown. In addition, by including only women who were alive in 1981, a selection bias may have occurred; mortality from breast cancer was not evaluated. Differences in the mortality rate might explain the lower prevalence rate of breast cancer in the athletes.

Washington State. In a retrospective study of occupational mortality in the state of Washington, Vena et al. (1987) examined the cause of death in 25,000 white females from 1974 to 1979. Occupation titles were taken from the death certificates in response to the question "usual occupation during most of working life, even if retired." Standardized proportionate mortality ratios of specific cause of death were determined for each of the 49 occupational categories. The observed number of deaths by cause was compared with expected mortality based on sex, cause-specific mortality, and calendar-year proportionate mortality across all occupations in the state of Washington. Physical activity was rated based on job categories. Women who held sedentary jobs were more likely to have died of breast cancer. In addition, occupations that were not sedentary were associated with significantly reduced breast cancer mortality. Women in the second quintile of occupational activity had reduced breast cancer mortality. These results indicate a threshold response to occupational activity level by reduced risk of breast cancer.

The Washington State study had several limitations. Independence was not determined. No adjustments were made for known risk factors of breast cancer. In addition, occupational physical activity was based only on the job title listed on the death certificate; lifetime occupational history was not considered. Vena et al. (1987) also noted that it was likely that the more sedentary jobs were related to a higher socioeconomic status and to a history of late first pregnancy, which are both associated with increased risk for breast cancer (Kelsey and Horn-Ross 1993).

Shanghai, China. A study of the incidence of breast cancer in Shanghai also used occupational information to assess physical activity (Zheng et al. 1993). In all 2,736 incidents of breast cancer, employment information for patients ages 30 years or older whose disease was diagnosed between 1980 and 1984 was compared with the 1982 census data on employment in Shanghai urban areas. Occupational physical activity was classified as low, moderate, or high based on time spent sitting and energy expenditure. Cancer incidence rates were based on the data collected by the Shanghai Cancer Registry. The expected number of breast cancer cases in a particular occupational group was determined using the incidence rates estimated for 1980 to 1984.

The observed number of cases was divided by the expected number of cases to obtain standardized incidence ratios for each occupational group. Risk of breast cancer was nearly 60% higher than average among white-collar professionals and about 15% lower than average among blue-collar service workers. Women with jobs that involved a lot of sitting had an incidence of breast cancer about 30% greater than average. Those with jobs that required relatively high energy expenditure had a 20% reduction in risk.

The Shanghai study did not demonstrate independence of physical activity from confounders. Other risk factors may have contributed to the association between cancer risk and occupational activity. The higher incidence of breast cancer in the white-collar workers may reflect socioeconomic status. Late age at first pregnancy is also common among professionals, and the analysis was not adjusted using parity data. Zheng et al. (1993) also commented that white-collar workers are usually better educated and are more likely to adopt Western lifestyles, including a high intake of dietary fat, which may be a risk factor for breast cancer (American Cancer Society 2003; Kritchevsky 1990). Lifetime occupational activity was not measured. Because of government policy, workers in Shanghai rarely change jobs, yet because of the study design, it is impossible to determine whether career choice or a change in careers resulted from the presence of the disease. Temporal sequence was not established.

Los Angeles County. Using a case–control design, Bernstein et al. (1994) matched 545 women (ages 40 and younger at diagnosis) who had been newly diagnosed with in situ or invasive breast cancer between 1983 and 1989 with 545 control subjects by date of birth (within 36 months), race (white), parity (nulliparous versus parous), and neighborhood of residence. Lifetime histories of participation in regular exercise activities were obtained during an interview. Figure 11.9 shows

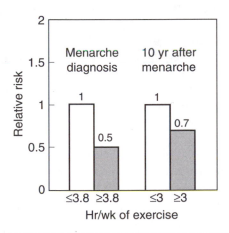

Figure 11.9 Using a case-controlled study of breast cancer incidence showed that the average number of hours spent in physical exercise activities per week from menarche to one year prior to the case patient's diagnosis was independently associated with reduced breast cancer risk.

Adapted from Bernstein et al. 1994.

that after adjustment for age at first pregnancy, age at menarche, birth date, family history, months of lactation, number of full-term pregnancies, parity, race, and oral contraceptive use, the average number of hours spent in exercise activities per week from menarche to one year prior to diagnosis was independently associated with reduced breast cancer risk.

The odds ratio of breast cancer among parous women who participated 3.8 h or more per week in exercise activities was 70% lower than inactive parous women, but the risk reduction from physical activity was not statistically significant among nulliparous women.

Seattle. A population-based case–control study examined the association between leisure-time physical activity and risk of breast cancer among women ages 21 to 45 years (Chen et al. 1997). Cases were 747 women diagnosed with invasive breast cancer between 1983 and 1990 in three counties of western Washington State in the Seattle–Puget Sound area. Controls were 961 women selected randomly from the same area. Physical activity was assessed by interview, with questions on the frequency and duration of various types of leisure physical activity during adolescence (between ages 12 and 21) and during the two-year period immediately prior to diagnosis. For the two-year time period before diagnosis, neither frequency of activity (four times or more per week), time spent in activity (4 h or more per week), nor energy expenditure (18 METs or more per week) was associated with the rate of cancer occurrence. Similarly, there was no association between leisure activity during adolescence and breast cancer risk. The lack of association between physical activity and risk was independent of BMI, age at menarche, age at first full-term pregnancy, parity, family history of breast cancer, or several health behaviors. Thus, this study did not find a protective effect of leisure-time physical activity either in adolescence or adulthood against breast cancer in premenopausal women.

A subsequent case–control analysis was conducted on postmenopausal women ages 50 to 64 years in the same western Washington area (McTiernan et al. 1996). The study included 537 patients with breast cancer diagnosed during 1988 to 1990 and 492 randomly selected women from the regional population who served as controls. Compared with women who reported no exercise, there was a 30% reduction in risk of breast cancer for women who exercised more than 1.5

h per week in the two years before diagnosis or who engaged in at least some high-intensity exercise, but there was no clear decline in risk at the highest categories of duration or intensity. There was no association between exercise of any intensity at ages 12 to 21 and risk of breast cancer. The findings indicated a weak inverse association between physical activity and risk of breast cancer in middle-aged women.

Premenopausal Women. In a population-based case–control study, 1,668 women under 45 years of age who had been recently diagnosed with breast cancer between 1990 and 1992 in Atlanta, central New Jersey, and Seattle were compared with 1,505 controls matched by age (within five years) and area of residence (Gammon, John, and Britton 1998). After adjustment for BMI, menopausal status, and caloric intake during the past year, breast cancer was not associated with recreational activity at ages 12 to 13, at age 20, or during the past year.

Italy. In a case–control study of 2,569 subjects with breast cancer and 2,588 controls conducted in Italy from 1991 to 1994, the population attributable risk of breast cancer in postmenopausal women was about 12% for low levels of physical activity (Mezzetti et al. 1998). That risk was similar to, but independent of, being overweight (10%).

Japan. Nearly 150 women ages 26 to 69 diagnosed with breast cancer by a physician between January 1990 and March 1997 were matched from hospital records with two controls by age (within one year) and city of residence (Ueji et al. 1998). After adjustment for BMI, family history of breast cancer, education, age at menarche, age at first birth, parity, and menopausal status, the odds ratio for breast cancer was 0.35 among women who reported that they regularly engaged in sports or exercise of more than 15.3 METs each week compared with women who reported no participation in sport or exercise. Occupational physical activity was unrelated to the risk of breast cancer.

A separate hospital-based case–control study examined whether risks of female breast cancer differed according to menopausal status (Hirose et al. 1995). Among 36,944 outpatients between 1988 and 1992, breast cancer was detected by histological exam in about 600 premenopausal and 450 postmenopausal women. More than 23,000 women without cancer were controls. Both pre- and postmenopausal women who reported two or more days a week of exercise had a 25% reduction in risk of breast cancer compared

with sedentary women, independently of diet, smoking, and BMI.

New England and Wisconsin. Nearly 6,900 women ages 17 to 74 years with breast cancer were interviewed between 1988 and 1991 in Maine, Massachusetts, New Hampshire, and Wisconsin and compared with about 9,500 controls (Mittendorf et al. 1995). Women who said that they had participated in any strenuous physical activity from ages 14 to 22 years had the same rate of breast cancer as their sedentary peers. However, those who exercised vigorously at least once a day (a small portion of the group) had a 50% reduction in risk of breast cancer, independently of diet and family history.

Switzerland. Almost 250 cases of breast cancer confirmed by histological exam between 1993 and 1998 in women younger than 75 were compared with about 375 controls who had been admitted to the same hospitals for acute illnesses that did not involve cancer or hormone-related diseases (Levi et al. 1999). High occupational physical activity was associated with about 50% less risk of breast cancer among women ages 30 to 39 years but not among those younger or older. In contrast, women who reported the highest leisure-time physical activity had 50% to 60% less risk of breast cancer among all women ages 15 to 59.

Carolina Breast Cancer Study. In a population-based case–control study, about 525 white women and 335 African American women with breast cancer were compared with nearly 800 controls matched by age and race (Marcus et al. 1999). Participants were asked about their participation in four physical activities at age 12: walking to school, biking to school, competitive sport training, and performing vigorous household chores. The women who reported participation in any of the four activities had a 20% reduction in the odds of breast cancer compared with women who said they had not been active.

Holland. Few studies have assessed the risk of breast cancer in relation to lifetime physical activity. In a population-based, case–control study in the Netherlands, self-rated physical activity was assessed among 918 case subjects (ages 20–54 years) and 918 age-matched controls (Verloop et al. 2000). Women who were more active at ages 10 to 12 or who had ever participated in leisure-time physical activity as an adult had a 30% reduction in breast cancer risk. Neither very early recreational activity (before age 20) nor recent activity (in the last five years) was associated with a greater reduction in risk than recreational activity in the intervening period. The protective effect of physical activity was not independent of body mass. Among the women who were active in their leisure time, those with a BMI less than 21.8 kg/m² had 40% fewer cancers than those with a BMI greater than 24.5 kg/m².

Canada. A population-based case–control study of 1,233 incident breast cancer cases and 1,237 controls conducted in Alberta, Canada, reported that total occupational and household physical activity accumulated across the lifetime reduced risk of postmenopausal breast cancer by 30% when the highest quartile of physical activity was compared with the lowest quartile of physical activity (Friedenreich, Bryant, and Courneya 2001; Friedenreich, Courneya, and Bryant 2001). Risk reduction was stronger among nonsmokers, non-alcohol-drinkers, and nulliparous postmenopausal women. Leisure-time physical activ-

ity was not associated with reduced risk of breast cancer, and no associations between physical activity and breast cancer were found for premenopausal women. A limitation of this study is the reliance on the women's recall of physical activity across their lifetimes and the resulting uncertainty about possible misclassification of the women according to activity levels.

Prospective Cohort Studies

A review of prospective cohort studies of both occupational and leisure-time physical activity and breast cancer is depicted in figure 11.10. About 50% of those studies found a significant reduction in breast cancer risk.

University of Pennsylvania Alumnae. A prospective study by Paffenbarger, Hyde, and Wing (1987) began following 4,706 female students who matriculated at the University of Pennsylvania in the period from 1916 to 1950 and followed them up through 1978. Physical activity was based on

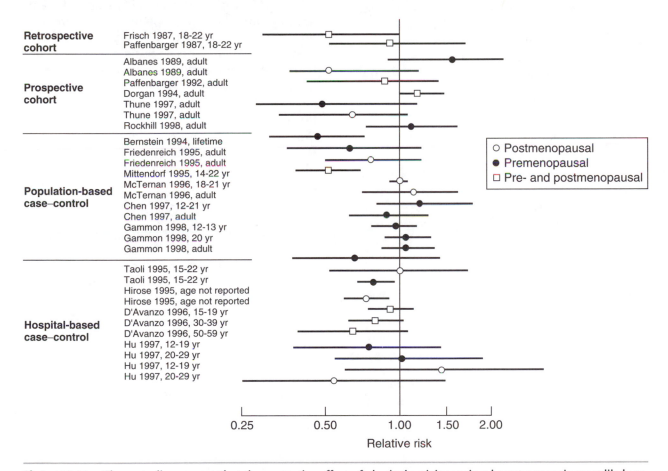

Figure 11.10 These studies suggest that the protective effect of physical activity against breast cancer is most likely to appear in later life.

Adapted, by permission, from M. Gammon, E. John, and J. Britton, 1998, "Recreational and occupational physical activities and risk of breast cancer," *Journal of the National Cancer Institute* 90: 100-117.

participation in college athletics. Age-adjusted incidence rates of both fatal and nonfatal breast cancers were determined by comparing those who engaged in sports 5 h or more a week during college against those who participated less than 5 h a week. No association was found between level of physical activity during the early years of college and incidence of breast cancer. The analysis did not control for key potential confounding factors.

NHANES I. The association between self-reported physical activity and breast cancer was studied in the first National Health and Nutrition Examination Survey (NHANES I) between 1971 and 1975 and followed up in the Epidemiologic Follow-Up Study in the years 1982 to 1984 (Albanes, Blair, and Taylor 1989). Among the 7,413 women, 84% were white and had a median age of 48 at the beginning of the study. Incidence rates for both fatal and nonfatal breast cancer were examined. There was a tendency for postmenopausal women who reported no participation in either recreational or nonrecreational physical activity to have more breast cancer risk than active women, but the difference was not large enough to be statistically significant, mainly because of the relatively small number of cancer cases. Adjustment for potential risk factors, including age at menarche and menopause, parity, age at first birth, family history of breast cancer, BMI, and dietary fat intake, did not change the results.

Cooper Clinic Cohort. To determine the association among three categories of physical fitness and nonfatal breast cancer, Brill, Barlow, and Blair (1992) examined 5,285 apparently healthy women who were free of cancer at baseline. The women received a preventive medical examination between 1972 and 1989 and completed a questionnaire in 1982 or 1990. The women were followed for an average of 4.5 years. The age-adjusted rates for incidence of breast cancer were calculated. Relative risk was determined by comparing the low and moderate fitness levels with the high fitness level. The analysis found no trends or significant decrease in risk, which suggests that fitness is not associated with incidence of nonfatal breast cancer.

Norway. Between 1974 and 1978 and again between 1977 and 1983, a total of 25,624 women, 20 to 54 years of age, answered questionnaires about leisure-time and occupational physical activity (Thune et al. 1997). Over nearly 14 years, 351 cases of invasive breast cancer were detected. Leisure-time physical activity was as-

sociated with a one third reduction in the risk of breast cancer after adjustment for age, BMI, parity, and county of residence. Among women who exercised regularly, the reduction in risk was greater in premenopausal women than in postmenopausal women, and greater in younger women (<45 years at study entry) than in older women (≥45 years). The risk of breast cancer was lowest (RR = 0.30) among women with a BMI under 23 who exercised at least 4 h each week. The risk was also reduced among women who had higher levels of occupational physical activity on the job, and that effect also was stronger among premenopausal women.

Framingham, Massachusetts. Physical activity of 2,300 women was determined by a physician-administered questionnaire from 1954 to 1956 at the fourth biennial examination of the Framingham Heart Study (Dorgan et al. 1994). Breast cancers were detected by self-report, surveillance of admissions to Framingham Union Hospital, and histological confirmation. During 28 years of follow-up, 117 breast cancer cases were diagnosed. After adjusting for age at physical activity assessment, menopausal status, age at first pregnancy, parity, education, occupation, and alcohol ingestion, there was a statistically weak trend of increasing risk of breast cancer with increasing physical activity.

Sweden. Three cohorts of women whose occupational titles permitted a classification of physical activity at work were sampled from the Swedish national censuses in 1960 (n = 704,904), in 1970 (n = 982,270), or in both 1960 and 1970 (n = 253,336; Moradi et al. 1999). Breast cancer incidence between 1971 and 1989 was determined from the Swedish Cancer Register. A total of 20,419, 22,840, and 8,261 breast cancers, respectively, were detected in the three cohorts. In all three cohorts, the risk for breast cancer increased linearly with decreasing level of occupational physical activity. Women who were sedentary on the job in both 1960 and 1970 had 30% more breast cancer than women who had jobs classified as high in physical activity. Except for women who were 50 to 59 years of age in 1970, the apparently protective effect depended on socioeconomic status.

Menopausal Status

University of Pennsylvania Alumnae. To determine whether the association between leisure-time physical activity and breast cancer differs according to postmenopausal status and body mass, nearly 1,600 University of Pennsylvania alumnae (average age 45.5 years) who were initially free of breast cancer in 1962 were observed until 1993 (Sesso, Paffenbarger, and Lee 1998). Women were classified by weekly energy expenditure from leisure physical activity into three levels (<500 kcal/wk, 500–999 kcal/wk, or ≥1,000 kcal/wk) based on questions about stairs climbed, blocks walked, and sports played in 1962. During 35,365 person-years of observation, 109 cases of breast cancer cases were detected. After adjustment for age and BMI, postmenopausal women who said they expended 1,000 kcal or more each week had 50% less risk of developing breast cancer than women who expended less than 500 kcal per week. Increased physical activity did not protect against breast cancer among premenopausal women.

Nurses' Health Study II. The associations between physical activity at two different times in life and breast cancer risk were examined in the Nurses' Health Study II, a prospective study of women who were 25 to 42 years old in 1989 (Rockhill et al. 1998). At the baseline survey, women were asked, "While in high school and between the ages 18 and 22 years, how often did you participate in strenuous physical activity at least twice a week?" Responses to the two time periods were averaged to estimate physical activity in late adolescence. Women were also asked how many hours each week they currently spent in several leisure physical activities. During six years of observation, 372 cases of invasive breast cancer were detected. Neither physical activity in adolescence nor contemporary leisure activity was associated with the risk of breast cancer.

In contrast, the average amount of physical activity that the nurses accumulated over the 16 years of observation was protective against breast cancer. From 1980 to 1996, 3,137 cases of invasive breast cancer (1,036 premenopausal and 2,101 postmenopausal women) were detected (Rockhill et al. 1999). In 1980 and on subsequent surveys, women were asked about the average number of hours per week they spent in various moderate and vigorous recreational physical activities during the past year. Women who said that they participated in moderate or vigorous physical activity for 7 h or more per week averaged across the 16 years of the study had nearly 20% less breast cancer than those who averaged less than 1 h per week.

Epidemiological Follow-Up Study (NHEFS) of NHANES I, 1971–1975. The association of long-term recreational physical activity with breast cancer risk was examined in a prospective cohort study of 6,160 women who were free of breast cancer at the first NHEFS follow-up in 1982 to 1984 (Breslow et al. 2001). Women were categorized as low, moderate, or high participants in leisure-time physical activity during the period between 1971 and 1975 and 10 years later in 1982 to 1984. One hundred thirty-eight women developed breast cancer between 1982 and 1992. Among women 50 years or older in 1982 to 1984, high physical activity was associated with a 67% reduction in breast cancer risk compared to low physical activity (RR = 0.33; 95% CI: 0.14–0.82) regardless of BMI or weight gain during adulthood.

Strength of the Evidence

Physical activity has been hypothesized to reduce breast cancer risk, but an inverse association has not been uniformly reported. An early review critically evaluated the epidemiologic studies examining breast cancer risk and leisure-time or occupational physical activity (Gammon, John, and Britton 1998). Results from seven of nine studies suggested that higher levels of occupational physical activity may be associated with a reduction in risk, at least among a subgroup of women. Eleven of 16 investigations on leisure-time physical activity reported a 12% to 60% decrease in risk among premenopausal and postmenopausal women.

Temporal Sequence

Prospective cohort studies have found a smaller risk reduction than case–control studies, which do not demonstrate temporal sequence. The temporal association between exercise and breast cancer development still needs to be addressed. When must exercise begin and for how long? Does exercise in adolescence provide protection for premenopausal and postmenopausal risk of breast cancer? Is there a protective benefit from beginning an exercise program after menopause? It is unclear when in the tumor development process exercise may have a protective effect.

Strength of Association

The mean relative risk from the studies shown in figure 11.10 indicates that physical activity reduced the risk of breast cancer by about 20% among all women, but this mainly occurred among women who were postmenopausal. This suggests that the protective effect of physical activity against breast cancer is most likely to appear in later life.

Figure 11.10 also shows that while most studies found a decreased risk, a few found increased risk. In addition, many of the results depicted had 95% confidence intervals (the horizontal lines through the group symbols) that included an RR of 1.0. Those results were too weak to be considered statistically reproducible, either because not enough women were studied to ensure a representative sample or because the rates varied a lot within the active and inactive groups.

Imprecise breast cancer estimates or physical activity measures can add to such variation. Indeed, most investigations did a poor job of assessing physical activity. This undoubtedly led to conflicting results about the duration, frequency, or intensity of activity necessary to minimize risk and whether the age when physical activity occurred influenced risk reduction. Also, most studies did not adequately control other risk factors for breast cancer, so the independent effect of physical activity was not clearly shown. Gammon, John, and Britton (1998) concluded that future studies should use a prospective cohort design to rule out bias from participants' recall of past physical activity and to improve the assessment of lifetime physical activity from all sources to clarify whether there is a dose–response relationship or an optimal time period or age to incur benefits from activity.

Consistency

The association between physical activity and breast cancer risk among women appears consistent across races and ethnicities but may differ with age, menopausal status, and body mass index. There is insufficient evidence to determine whether physical activity is associated with reduced risk of breast cancer among men.

> ••• *Most studies of physical activity and breast cancer risk used imprecise measures of physical activity and its timing, making it hard to determine the true dose response or whether the age when physical activity occurred influenced risk reduction. Many studies did not adequately control other risk factors for breast cancer, so the independent effect of physical activity was not clearly shown. More prospective cohort studies that control for confounders and use better measures of physical activity are needed.*

Dose Response

Recent reviews of more than 40 cross-sectional and prospective cohort studies that investigated physical activity and breast cancer risk concluded that the majority of the studies showed a linear reduction in risk of breast cancer with increasing level of physical activity (Friedenreich and Orenstein 2002; Thune and Furberg 2001). This was especially true when physical activity was at least moderate in intensity (>4.5 METs) (Thune and Furberg 2001). The measures of exercise in studies of physical activity and breast cancer risk have varied, from college athletic status to job classification to adult recreational activities and fitness levels. The type, intensity, or duration of exercise involved in the dose response is difficult to assess.

Biological Plausibility

A workshop sponsored by the National Cancer Institute of the United States summarized the most plausible, but as yet unproven, biological mechanisms that might explain the association between physical activity and reduced risk for breast cancer (Brinton, Bernstein, and Colditz 1998; Hoffman-Goetz et al. 1998). In addition to enhancing the immune system, which is discussed in chapter 12, the key possible mechanisms for the protective effect of physical activity generally include reducing the number of lifetime ovulatory cycles, reducing blood levels of insulin-like growth factor as a result of negative energy balance, or indirect associations with lower body weight or reducing dietary fat or total caloric intake.

Potential Mechanisms

- Reduction in endogenous estrogen exposure
- Alteration of menstrual cycles
- Delay of menarche and earlier menopause
- Increased energy expenditure and reduction in body weight

Hormones. A popular hypothesis for explaining how physical activity might protect against breast cancer is that it reduces the cumulative lifetime exposure to circulating ovarian hormones, especially estrogen. Physical activity has been found to decrease risk by delaying the age of menarche, decreasing adiposity, and helping maintain hormonal balance in the body. Thus, physical activity during early adolescence could have protective benefits on a woman's risk later in life. Physical activity also has an effect on post-menopausal breast cancer risk, but the main risk factors are obesity and decreased progesterone levels.

Menarche. Strenuous physical activity during adolescence may increase the age at menarche (Frisch et al. 1985; Gammon and John 1993) and is also associated with longer menstrual cycles (Hoffman-Goetz et al. 1998). In general, a 20% reduction in breast cancer risk is observed for every year that menarche is delayed (B.E. Henderson and Bernstein 1996). Conversely, women with relatively frequent, short, and regular ovulatory cycles are at increased risk for breast cancer. These women spend more of their time in the luteal phase of the menstrual cycle, when both estrogen and progesterone are high. Susceptibility to breast cancer increases because peak mitotic activity in breast epithelium occurs during the luteal phase (B.E. Henderson and Bernstein 1996). Therefore, if exercise delays menarche and lengthens regular menstrual cycles, cumulative exposure to estrogen and progesterone would be reduced, thus decreasing the risk of breast cancer. For menarche to occur, a girl must attain a critical ratio of body mass relative to height. Height is determined genetically, while weight is determined mostly by caloric intake. Once the critical mass-to-height ratio has been met, the critical mass must be maintained to maintain menstruation. Those who lose weight from vigorous activity and cease menstruating might gain protection against breast cancer. Irregular menstrual cycles and amenorrhea, with associated low levels of estrogen, have been reported among some competitive female athletes who train at very high levels of exertion.

Vigorous training in sports such as swimming, running, gymnastics, and dance has been associated with delayed menarche in young girls. Whether the delayed menarche is caused by the exercise or results from the smaller body mass of girls who naturally select such sports has not been established (Malina 1983). Nonetheless, one study found that even moderate physical activity of 600 kcal/wk increased the odds of irregular menstrual cycles when compared with those who engaged in less activity (Cooper et al. 1996). Thus, even moderate physical activity might have a protective effect against breast can-

cer by reducing lifetime exposure to endogenous steroid hormones.

Onset of Menopause. It is also plausible that physical activity could be associated with an earlier age at menopause. Women who experience natural menopause before age 45 are estimated to have half the risk of breast cancer of women whose natural menopause occurs after age 55 (Brinton and Devesa 1996). Physically active women tend to be leaner than inactive women, and obesity is associated with a late age at menopause (Friedenreich and Rohan 1995). Frisch et al. (1985) observed that athletes had an earlier age of natural menopause than nonathletes.

Energy Balance and Body Weight. Obesity also independently influences breast cancer risk. Abdominal obesity is related to higher circulatory estrogen levels and increased conversion of androgens to estrogen (Frisch et al. 1985). Exercise influences body composition by increasing energy expenditure, retarding loss of muscle mass, and increasing metabolic rate. Caloric availability is reduced by physical activity, and caloric restriction is proposed to be of benefit in reducing breast cancer risk. Exercise may also promote other health behaviors, including dietary changes in the type and amount of fat consumed. At present, the national per capita fat consumption estimates are correlated with breast cancer mortality rates (Hunter and Willet 1996). Thus, it is difficult to assess whether the relationships among exercise, estrogen, and breast cancer risk are related to activity's direct effect on ovulatory cycles; an indirect effect through diet, body composition, and caloric expenditure; or some combination of these.

Experimental studies have used chemically induced mammary tumors in rodents as the model for human breast cancer, though it remains unclear whether the carcinogens used and the dose and duration of exposure used in the animal studies would induce malignant tumor growth in humans. Despite those concerns, a summary of those studies indicates that mammary tumor incidence was decreased by exercise performed during the time of tumor initiation and promotion (Friedenreich and Rohan 1995). However, the effects of diet and energy balance were not well controlled in those studies, so the independent effect of exercise was not clearly shown (Hoffman-Goetz et al. 1998). Additionally, no dose–response relationship has been established for exercise and mammary tumors. Thus, the experimental studies also proved to be inconclusive regarding the protective effects of exercise on breast tumor growth.

Endogenous Steroid Exposure, Obesity, and Energy Balance.

Obese, postmenopausal women have been found to be at greater risk of breast cancer than obese, premenopausal women. Obese, premenopausal women under age 50 have little or no increased risk of breast cancer, but after age 60, 10 kg of excess body weight nearly doubles the risk of breast cancer. After menopause, estrogen is produced from other sources to compensate for lost production by shrinking ovaries. Adipose cells aid the conversion of androgens to estrogen. Maintenance of low body fat by energy expenditure during physical activity can help offset estrogen production by fat cells after menopause among obese women.

Low body fat has also been associated with increased metabolism of estradiol to its safer metabolite, 2-hydroxyestrone. Former female college athletes have been found to have lower body mass, higher 2-hydroxyestrone levels, and lower risk for breast cancer than nonathletes Thus, physical activity could protect both pre- and postmenopausal women by converting excess estradiol to 2-hydroxyestrone.

The effects of energy imbalance on breast cancer risk have been studied in premenopausal women. Both animal and human studies support the hypothesis that increased energy intake and decreased energy expenditure increase the risk of breast cancer. In premenopausal women, increased energy intake, unaccompanied by increased energy expenditure, leading to fat gain, has been shown to lead to an earlier age of menarche, a later age of menopause, and an increase in estrogen levels. An energy imbalance may also lead to immunosuppression, which decreases the body's ability to fight cancer growth. Because exercise has been proposed as a way to increase energy expenditure, premenopausal women may reduce risk by exercising.

> ••• The cumulative evidence from 41 studies that included nearly 110,000 cases of breast cancer showed that physical activity is associated with reduced risk of breast cancer (Thune and Furberg 2001).

Summary and Conclusions

A review of 21 studies published before December 1997 that examined physical activity and breast cancer outcomes was conducted as part of the 1997 National Cancer Institute Workshop on Physical Activity and Breast Cancer (Friedenreich et al. 1998). Fifteen of the 21 studies suggested that physical activity reduces the risk of breast cancer, whereas 4 studies found no association, and 2 studies found an increased risk of breast cancer associated with physical activity. More recently, a review of 41 studies that included over 108,000 cases of breast cancer concluded that most of the studies showed a protective effect of physical activity (Thune and Furberg 2001). A subsequent review concluded that 32 of 44 studies found that physical activity was associated with reduced risk of breast cancer (Friedenreich and Orenstein 2002).

Specific subgroups of the population may experience a greater decrease in breast cancer with increased levels of physical activity. These include women who are lean, parous, or postmenopausal. Postmenopausal women have shown a higher risk for breast cancer, presumably from lifetime exposure to estradiol, increased BMI, and decreased physical activity. To reduce postmenopausal risk, it is necessary to determine when in life physical activity has the greatest impact on risk. Menopausal status has been shown to affect the risk for women. Estradiol exposure seems to be the strongest predictor of risk, and physical activity can reduce this exposure both before and after menopause. It is plausible that physical activity affects risk by decreasing menstrual cycles; if so, physical activity would be most beneficial during preadolescence, adolescence, and young adulthood. However, chronic lifetime exercise may be more influential on risk if physical activity affects risk by decreasing obesity or increasing energy expenditure. Moderate physical activity seems to exhibit the same protective benefits for all women with minimal risks. Therefore, lifetime moderate physical activity seems to be a modifiable and protective measure against breast cancer for all women.

The overall evidence supports a reduction in breast cancer risk with increased physical activity. However, numerous questions remain regarding that association, including the underlying biological mechanisms that explain it; the features of physical activity that affect the risk, such as the type (occupational, recreational, or household), frequency, intensity, and duration; the times of life associated with risk reduction; and the important confounders and effect modifiers. Investigations that examine the effect of physical activity at different stages of breast cancer are needed. As was also the case for colon cancer, there have been no population-based studies of breast cancer risk in humans after experimental manipulations of physical activity. Also, there have been no studies showing that naturally occurring alterations in physical activity levels are associated with a change in breast cancer rates, so randomized controlled trials are needed to confirm the protective effect of physical activity.

Prostate Cancer

Next to skin cancer, prostate cancer is the most common type of cancer among men in the United States. Approximately 1 of every 11 men will eventually be diagnosed with prostate cancer. The American Cancer Society (2003) predicted that there would be about 221,000 new cases of prostate cancer in the United States during the year 2003. It is about twice as common among African American men as it is among white American men. About 28,900 men were expected to die of prostate cancer during 2003. Although men of any age can get prostate cancer, it is found most often in men over 50. More than 70% of men diagnosed with prostate cancer are over the age of 65 years.

Prostate cancer is also most common in North America and northwestern Europe and less common in Asia, Africa, Central America, and South America. The highest rate is 100 in 100,000 among African American men. The lowest rate of 1 in 100,000 occurs in Asia and North Africa. Migrants tend to acquire the prostate cancer patterns of their new home (Haenszel and Kurihara 1968).

> ••• *Nearly 10% of men in the United States will be diagnosed with prostate cancer. If the cancer is detected before it metastasizes, the five-year survival rate is 100%.*

Ninety-seven percent of men with prostate cancer live at least 5 years after diagnosis, and about 65% survive at least 10 years. If the cancer is found before it has spread outside the prostate, the five-year survival rate is 100%. If the cancer has spread to tissues near the prostate, the survival rate is 94%. And if the cancer has spread to other parts of the body when it is found, about 30% live at least five years. Survival rates also vary by race. In one population-based study, African American men had a five-year survival rate of 49%, compared

with 61% for white American men (Mettlin et al. 1995), possibly because of later diagnosis, mortality from other causes, lower income, poorer access to proper health care, and poorer nutritional status (Bach et al. 2002; Boyle 1994).

The incidence rate of prostate cancer in North America increased during the 25-year period preceding the mid-1990s from 39 to 47 per 100,000, about a 5% increase every five years (Boyle, Maisonneuve, and Napalkov 1996). The mortality rate has also been increasing but at a slower rate. Between 1980 and 1988 the mortality rate rose by 2.5% for white Americans and by 5.7% for black Americans. The difference between the increases in incidence and mortality may be explained by improvements in screening procedures and treatments; also a greater number of the detected tumors are nonmalignant (Boyle 1994).

Etiology of Prostate Cancer

The walnut-sized prostate, which produces seminal fluid, is located below the bladder, in front of the rectum (figure 11.11). The urethra passes through the prostate, and nearby nerves regulate erection of the penis. That is why prostate enlargement can contribute to urinary problems or erectile dysfunction disorder. Prostate cancer usually grows slowly, often without detection even into old age. Like other cancers, however, if prostate tumors metastasize into the **lymph system,** they spread quickly to other organs.

Cancers found early by a digital rectal exam or a **prostate-specific antigen (PSA)** blood test usually are smaller and have spread less than cancers found because of the symptoms they cause. But prostate cancer is unlike many other cancers in that it often grows very slowly. The digital rectal exam requires that a doctor insert a gloved finger into the rectum to feel for lumps on the prostate. The PSA blood test measures a protein made by prostate cells. The amount of PSA secreted into blood depends on the volume of the prostate, whereas productivity of the prostate epithelium remains constant or increases slightly with age. Levels of PSA in the blood under 4 ng/ml are usually considered normal. Levels between 4 and 10 ng/ml are borderline, and levels over 10 ng/ml are associated with high risk of developing prostate cancer and indicate that rectal ultrasound imaging or a needle biopsy of the prostate gland should be done to determine whether cancer is present (National Cancer Institute 2000b).

Problems with urinating may be a sign of prostate cancer. But more often this problem is

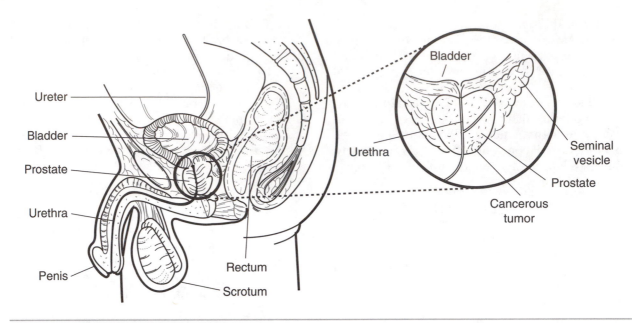

Figure 11.11   Diagram of the prostate gland.
Reprinted by the permission of the American Cancer Society, Inc.

caused by a less serious disease known as benign prostatic hyperplasia (BPH). Physical signs and symptoms of advanced prostate cancer include erectile dysfunction disorder, blood in the urine, swollen lymph nodes in the groin, and pain in the pelvis, spine, hips, or ribs, but those symptoms are not specific to prostate cancer.

If a prostate biopsy reveals a cancer, more tests are done to find out whether the cancer has spread and, if so, how far. The TNM system is most often used to stage prostate cancer. There are two T classifications for prostate cancer. The clinical stage is based on digital rectal exam, needle biopsy, and transrectal ultrasound findings. The pathologic stage is based on examination of the entire prostate gland; both seminal vesicles and nearby lymph nodes are removed and examined.

Grading is used to describe how fast a prostate tumor is growing. The Gleason system is used most often for grading. Under this system a lower number, such as 2 to 4, means a slower-growing tumor. A higher number, such as 8 to 10, means the cancer cells are aggressive and are likely to grow more quickly. Age, overall health, and the stage and grade of a prostate cancer influences decisions about treatment (National Cancer Institute 2000b).

Risk Factors

The causes of prostate cancer are not clearly known. Only about 10% of prostate cancers can be traced to genes. Two of the main biological risk factors, prolonged stimulation of androgen hormones (e.g., testosterone) and high intake of fat calories, have unclear associations with physical activity. These are some other risk factors:

• *Age.* The chance of getting prostate cancer goes up with age. Prostate cancer is found mostly among men over 50 years of age, and more than 70% of men diagnosed with prostate cancer are over the age of 65.

• *Race.* For unknown reasons, prostate cancer is more common among black American men than among white American men.

• *Diet.* A diet high in fat may play a part in causing prostate cancer. Tomatoes, grapefruit, and watermelon are rich in lycopenes, which help prevent damage to DNA and may help lower prostate cancer risk. The U.S. Health Professions Study followed 47,000 males ages 40 to 75 who were free of cancer (Boyle, Maisonneuve, and Napalkov 1996). Over four years, 300 prostate cancers were diagnosed. Total caloric intake and age were controlled for. The relative risk of a high fat intake was 1.8 times that of a low fat intake. Of at least 13 case–control studies, 10 showed positive evidence that a high-fat, high-calorie, and high-red-meat diet increases the risk of prostate cancer. The same as for other cancers, fat presumably exerts its effects on prostate cancer by modifying endogenous hormone levels and actions.

• *Family history.* Men with close family members who have had prostate cancer are more likely to get prostate cancer themselves. A Swedish study found that the incidence of prostate cancer in monozygotic twins was more than four times as great as in dizygotic twins (Boyle, Maisonneuve, and Napalkov 1996). Other studies have also reported a positive correlation with family history, yet it is difficult to exclude environmental influences on cancer that family members may be exposed to in common.

Physical Activity and Prostate Cancer: The Evidence

Results of a recent review of 28 studies that included 22,521 cases of prostate cancer in North America, Asia, and Europe concluded that half reported that leisure-time physical activity and/ or occupational physical activity significantly reduced the rate of cancer by 10% to 70% (Thune and Furberg 2001). A subsequent review similarly concluded that 17 of 30 studies found that physical activity was associated with an average reduction in breast cancer risk of 10% to 30% (Friedenreich and Orenstein 2002).

Case–Control and Retrospective Studies

U.S. Hospitals Study. In a case–control study of prostate cancer and socioeconomic factors, Yu, Harris, and Wynder (1988) studied 1,162 prostate cancer cases among white and black men and 3,124 controls matched by age. Adulthood physical activity was categorized into three groups by frequency: seldom (less than once per week), moderate (one to three times per week), and high (more than three times per week). Activity was defined as 20 min of exercise accompanied by sweating or shortness of breath. The study controlled for alcohol, smoking, BMI, marital status, education, and occupation. An age-adjusted elevation of 30% in the odds of prostate cancer was associated with low physical activity among white men, but there was no dose response to physical activity, and the effects were not independent of BMI, marital status, cigarette smoking, alcohol consumption, education, and occupation.

Washington State. In a study of occupational mortality, the causes of death for 430,000 men between 1950 and 1979 were examined (Vena et al. 1987). Specific occupations were taken from the death certificates, which indicated the individual's usual occupation during his lifetime.

These job titles were categorized into five levels of physical activity using codes from the Department of Labor. The number of deaths attributed to prostate cancer were compared with expected mortality based on sex, cause-specific mortality, and calendar-year proportionate mortality across all occupations in the state of Washington. Sedentary jobs had about a 10% higher age-adjusted odds ratio of prostate cancer than highly active jobs. That reduction was not persistent for each decade of study. The lower risk for high-activity jobs was observed only between 1960 and 1969, while the elevated risk for sedentary jobs was seen only in 1970 to 1979.

Missouri. Physical activity on the job and the incidence of cancer was examined in over 17,000 white male cancer patients in the Missouri Cancer Registry between 1984 and 1989 (Brownson et al. 1991). Patients' occupations were abstracted from hospital records and categorized by physical activity level. Occupations were classified as high activity if they required more than 80% of the time to be spent in physical activity, moderate for 20% to 80%, and low activity for less than 20%. Odds of prostate cancer increased by 10% in moderate-activity jobs and by 50% in low-activity jobs compared with high-activity jobs. Thus, a dose response was observed, but diet was not controlled.

Sweden. A population-based case–control study investigated whether physical activity during childhood and adolescence was associated with risk for prostate cancer (Andersson et al. 1995). Physical activity was assessed by interviews with 256 men with prostate cancer and 252 controls matched by age. Independent of diet and adult BMI, a weak reduction in odds for developing prostate cancer was not statistically significant.

Prospective Cohort Studies

Results of a recent review of prospective cohort studies of physical activity and prostate cancer risk (Thune and Furberg 2001) are shown in figure 11.12. About half the studies showed a reduction in risk of developing prostate cancer among physically active men.

San Francisco Longshoremen. About one third of the more than 60,000 San Francisco longshoremen ages 35 to 74 years were classified as having high-energy-expenditure jobs (>8,500 kcal expended per week), while the remaining two thirds were classified as having low-energy-expenditure jobs (Paffenbarger, Hyde, and Wing

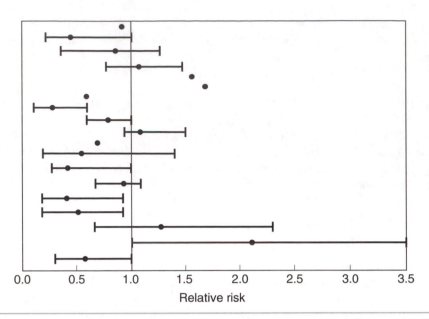

Figure 11.12   Relative risks of prostate cancer in prospective cohort studies comparing men according to their leisure-time physical activity.

Data from Thune and Furberg 2001.

1987). After 21 years of observation, from 1951 to 1972, the relative risk of developing prostate cancer for the men in the low-energy classification was 1.50 compared with men in the high-energy classification. There was no control for BMI, exposure to carcinogens on the job, or other potential confounders of the association between job activity and prostate cancer.

College Alumni Study.   Another study examined the physical activity of 51,977 male graduates of Harvard University and the University of Pennsylvania while they were in college between the years of 1916 and 1950 (Paffenbarger, Hyde, and Wing 1987). Participation in college sports was verified by school records for 1916 to 1950, and questionnaires were mailed to the men during the 1960s and 1970s. Age-adjusted incidence rates for both fatal and nonfatal prostate cancer were nearly 70% higher among those who said that they had played more than 5 h of sports a week compared to those who played less than 5 h a week. Those findings are difficult to interpret, though, because it is unlikely that exposure to college athletics would directly affect prostate disease in middle and old age (Kohl, LaPorte, and Blair 1988). Independence from confounders was not determined. There was no dose-dependent increase in risk, and a threshold of 5 h a week seems arbitrary.

Another analysis assessed leisure-time physical activity after college by nearly 17,000 Harvard alumni who had answered questionnaires about their health status in 1962 to 1966 and were observed for cause of death until 1978. Physical activity was classified into ordinal categories—less than 500 kcal/wk, 500 to 1,999 kcal/wk, and 2,000 or more kcal/wk—based on self-reports of city blocks walked, stairs climbed, and types of sports participation. After adjustment for age, smoking, and BMI, the relative risk was 0.60 for those who expended more than 2,000 kcal/wk compared with those who expended less than 500 kcal/wk, but this result was not statistically significant.

Harvard Alumni II.   In a later analysis of the Harvard alumni cohort (Lee, Paffenbarger, and Hsieh 1992), nearly 18,000 men ages 30 to 79 were observed from 1965 to 1977 and again from 1980 to 1988. Physical activity was based on self-reports of stair climbing, walking, and sports played. Physical activity tertiles were <1,000 kcal/wk, 1,000 to 4,000 kcal/wk, and >4,000 kcal/wk. The men who expended over 4,000 kcal/wk at both assessments had a 90% reduction in age-adjusted risk of prostate cancer compared with men who expended under 1,000 kcal/wk. Men ages 70 years and older who expended over 4,000 kcal/wk at either assessment had a risk about half that of all inactive men. Diet was not controlled, but adjustments were made for age, smoking, and family history. There was also no evidence of a dose–response relationship.

Harvard Alumni III.   Previous investigations regarding the influence of physical activity on the risk of developing prostate cancer used a single assessment of physical activity, thus failing to determine the persistence of lowered risk over time. In the Harvard Alumni III study, self-reported stair climbing, walking, and sports play were assessed between 1962 and 1966 and again in 1977 among 17,600 Harvard alumni ages 30 to 79 years who were followed prospectively for the occurrence of prostate cancer (n = 454) from 1965 through 1988 (Lee and Paffenbarger 1994). After classifying the men according to their reported physical activity between 1962 and 1966 and later in 1977 and after adjusting for age, parental history of cancer, and BMI, the rate of prostate cancer among inactive men was not different from that of the moderately and highly active men. Diet was not controlled.

NHANES I. The relationship between self-reported physical activity and prostate cancer was studied in the cohort of NHANES I, first examined between 1971 and 1975 and later observed in the Epidemiologic Follow-Up Study conducted between 1982 and 1984 (Albanes, Blair, and Taylor 1989). Among 5,138 men ages 25 to 74 years old, incidence rates for both fatal and nonfatal prostate cancer were examined using hospital records and death certificates. Physical activity was assessed by two questions about leisure-time and occupational activity at the beginning of the study. No association was observed between occupational physical activity and the risk of prostate cancer. However, men who reported little or no leisure-time physical activity had a relative risk of 1.8 compared with those who said they were very active.

NHANES I Follow-Up. The relationship between prostate cancer and self-reported physical activity was examined among 5,377 black and white participants in the NHANES I cohort (Clarke and Whittemore 2000). In this analysis, the cohort was first examined between 1971 and 1975 and then followed prospectively through 1992 in the Epidemiologic Follow-Up Study. Men who reported low levels of occupational physical activity had increased risk of prostate cancer compared with very active men. These findings were unchanged after adjustment for potential confounders and were stronger for blacks (RR = 3.7, 95% CI: 1.7–8.4) than whites (RR = 1.7, 0.8–2.3). Lower levels of recreational activity were weakly associated with increased prostate cancer risk among blacks but not among whites.

Norway. The association of leisure-time and occupational physical activity measured by questionnaire with the risk of prostate was examined in a population-based cohort study of over 53,000 Norwegian men ages 19 to 50 years (Thune and Lund 1994). During 16 years of observation, 220 prostate cancer cases were recorded in the Cancer Registry of Norway. When occupational and recreational physical activity were combined, after adjustment for age, BMI, serum cholesterol, and geographic region, a dose-dependent reduction in risk of prostate cancer was observed for men who walked during occupational hours and performed either moderate leisure-time physical activity (RR = 0.60) or regular exercise training (RR = 0.45) relative to sedentary men. That benefit occurred mainly among men older than 60 years but not among younger men.

A subsequent cohort of 22,895 Norwegian men ages 40 years or older was obtained from a health examination and two self-administered questionnaires. Information on incident cases of prostate cancer was obtained from the Cancer Registry of Norway (Lund Nilsen, Johnsen, and Vatten 2000). During a mean follow-up period of 9.3 years, 644 cases were diagnosed. Men who were the most physically active during their leisure time had a small, statistically nonsignificant reduction in risk of prostate cancer (RR = 0.80, 95% CI: 0.62–1.03) compared with the least active men.

U.S. Health Professionals Follow-Up Study. In a study begun in 1986, 47,542 men 40 to 75 years of age who were free of cancer responded to a mailed questionnaire that assessed physical activity (Giovannucci et al. 1998). From 1986 until 1994, 1,362 new cases of prostate cancer, 419 advanced (extraprostatic) cases, and 200 metastatic cases were detected. The weekly average MET-hours spent in leisure-time physical activities and in vigorous activities of 6 METs or more were not associated with total or advanced prostate cancer. However, after controlling for age, vasectomy, history of diabetes, height, smoking, and diet, the men in the highest category of vigorous activity (more than 25 MET-hours each week, or about 3 h of vigorous activity) had a 50% lower incidence of metastatic prostate cancer than men who reported no vigorous physical activity in their leisure time.

Finland. The association between physical activity and prostate cancer was evaluated among 29,133 participants in a clinical trial of the Alpha-Tocopherol, Beta-Carotene (ATBC) Cancer Prevention Study (Hartman et al. 1998). During up to nine years of observation, 317 men developed prostate cancer. The relationship between occupational, leisure-time, and total physical activity and prostate cancer was examined after adjustment for intervention group, benign prostatic hyperplasia, age, smoking, and urban residence. Compared with sedentary workers, risk of prostate cancer was lower for men who walked on the job (RR = 0.60) but not for men who walked and lifted or were heavy laborers. Participation in leisure-time physical activity reduced risk (RR = 0.70) among all working men except heavy laborers.

Iowa 65+ Rural Health Study. In 1982, 1,050 noninstitutionalized men ages 65 to 101 years who lived in two rural Iowa counties and had been cancer free for the past 10 years were interviewed about their health habits and physical activity (Cerhan et al. 1997). After nearly 8,500 person-years of observation, through 1993, 71 cases of prostate cancer were reported to the State Health Registry of Iowa. Paradoxically, a high level of physical activity was associated with increased risk of prostate cancer compared with inactive men (RR = 1.9), but there was no control for diet.

Aerobics Center Longitudinal Study. Nearly 13,000 men ages 20 to 80 years had a preventive medical exam, including a treadmill test of cardiorespiratory fitness, at the Cooper Aerobics Center in Dallas between 1970 and 1989 (figure 11.13; Oliveria et al. 1996). Ninety-four new cases of prostate cancer were reported on mail questionnaires sent to these men in 1982 and 1990. A dose-dependent reduction in the risk of developing prostate cancer was associated with higher fitness levels after controlling for age, BMI, and smoking habits, but only the most-fit quartile of men had a statistically significant reduction in relative risk,

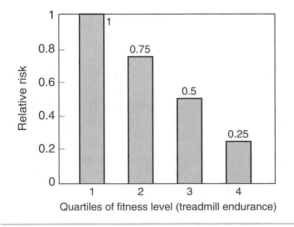

Figure 11.13 Aerobics Center Longitudinal Study prostate risk.

which was about 25% that of the least-fit quartile of men. Also, the protective effect was limited to participants younger than 60 years.

Physical activity also was associated with risk reduction. Men who said they expended between 1,000 and 2,000 kcal/wk or 3,000 or more kcal/wk had a two-thirds reduction in the risk of developing prostate cancer compared with those expending under 1,000 kcal/wk. Though men who expended 2,000 to 3,000 kcal/wk had a one third reduction in risk, it was not statistically significant. A limitation of the Cooper Clinic study was that less than half of the men originally tested were a part of the follow-up assessments, so results might have been biased in favor of finding a protective effect for physical activity and fitness.

Physicians' Health Study. The association between physical activity and prostate cancer risk was examined among 22,071 male participants ages 40 to 84 years in the Physicians' Health Study, a randomized trial of low-dose aspirin and beta-carotene (Liu et al. 2000). At baseline in 1982, the men reported that they had not had a myocardial infarction, stroke, or cancer. They also were asked about their frequency of exercise vigorous enough to work up a sweat in 1982 and again 36 months later. During 11.1 years of follow-up, 982 cases of prostate cancer were confirmed by medical records. After adjustment for the potential confounding factors of age, height, randomized treatment assignment, smoking status, alcohol intake, use of multivitamins, history of diabetes, history of hypertension or high cholesterol, and diagnosis of prostate cancer within the first 36 months of the study, there was no significant association between frequency of vigorous exercise and prostate cancer risk. The relative risks of prostate cancer associated with vigorous exercise, relative to those whose frequency was less than once per week, were 1.02 (95% CI: 0.82–1.26) for once per week, 1.07 (0.90–1.27) for two to four times per week, and 1.11 (0.90–1.36) for five or more times per week.

Britain. The relationship between physical activity and incidence of prostate cancer was examined in 7,588 British men ages 40 to 59 years who were cancer free at the outset of the study (Wannamethee, Shaper, and Walker 2001). The physical activity levels of the men at the beginning of the study were categorized as none/occasional, light, moderate, moderately vigorous, or vigorous. Cancer incidence data were obtained from death certificates, the national Cancer Registry, and self-reports of doctor-diagnosed cancer during an average follow-up of 18.8 years. After adjustments for age, smoking, BMI, alcohol intake, and social class, there was a linear dose–response reduction in prostate cancer risk only for time spent in vigorous activities.

Strength of the Evidence

At least five major review articles published during the past few years concluded that only half the published studies of physical activity and prostate cancer risk found a protective effect of physical activity (Colditz, Cannuscio, and Frazier 1997; Friedenreich and Orenstein 2002; Oliveria and Lee 1997; Thune and Furberg 2001; U.S. Department of Health and Human Services 1996). Other studies found no association between physical activity and prostate cancer risk, and a few reported a paradoxical increase in the risk of prostate cancer among physically active men. Despite the mixed results, the average of the studies' results was a reduction in risk between 10% and 30%. The weak agreement among the studies—coupled with weaknesses in the research designs (few prospective cohort studies adequately controlled for other risk factors, no randomized clinical trials), weaknesses in the measures of physical activity (many studies used invalidated self-reports, and only one study measured physical fitness), or weaknesses in the measures of prostate cancer incidence (many studies relied on self-reports rather than histological examinations) in most of the studies—prevents a strong conclusion that increased physical activity protects against prostate cancer. Nonetheless, there is sufficient evidence to recommend that more research be conducted to more accurately estimate the type, frequency, intensity, and duration of physical activity as well as the period during a man's lifetime when exercise might be beneficial.

Temporal Sequence

There have been nearly twice as many prospective cohort studies (about 20) as case–control studies, and the cohort studies typically lasted between 10 and 25 years; so, in general, a sufficient number of studies of physical activity and reduced prostate cancer risk demonstrated an appropriate temporal sequence that can suggest cause and effect.

Strength of Association

Recent reviews of about 30 studies concluded that about half the studies reported that leisure-time or occupational physical activity significantly reduced the rate of cancer by an average of 10% to 30% (Friedenreich and Orenstein 2002; Thune and Furberg 2001).

Consistency

Only about half the studies showed a significant reduction in prostate cancer risk among physically active men, but those studies included samples from the United States (including blacks, whites, and Japanese men from Hawaii), Canada, Britain, Norway, Finland, Sweden, Denmark, China, Turkey, and Serbia, so there has been reasonably good consistency of results across several nations, races, and ethnicities.

Dose Response

The evidence for a dose-dependent reduction in prostate cancer risk with increasing physical activity is not strong. Among studies that reported at least three levels of physical activity, a linear reduction in prostate cancer risk with increasing level of physical activity was observed in only 5 of 18 studies of leisure-time physical activity and in only 3 of 6 studies of occupational physical activity (Thune and Furberg 2001). Three studies reported increased risk among highly active men. However, many of the studies used imprecise or poorly validated self-report measures of physical activity or job classification.

Biological Plausibility

The etiology of prostate cancer remains unclear. Testosterone is believed to promote prostate cancer because testosterone and its metabolite, dihydrotestosterone, are the main hormones that regulate the growth and function of epithelial cells in the prostate. However, one case–control study showed no association between serum testosterone or dihydrotestosterone and prostate cancer risk (Vatten et al. 1997). Though muscle contraction is known to be accompanied by transient spikes in blood testosterone levels, heavy exercise training can reduce the level of circulating testosterone (Morville, Pesquies, and Guezennee 1979).

Obesity is another factor that is believed to influence the risk of prostate cancer, even though there is little evidence to support this. Physical activity can influence body composition by increasing energy expenditure, increasing lean body mass, and increasing resting metabolic rate. Changes in other health behaviors may also accompany physical activity, including dietary changes and changes in the amount and type of fat intake.

Benign prostatic hyperplasia leads to prostate enlargement and lower urinary tract symptoms and is highly prevalent among older men. Sympathetic nervous system activity, which can be decreased by physical activity, is associated with increased smooth-muscle tone of the prostate and symptoms that accompany prostate enlargement.

In a follow-up to the U.S. Health Professionals Study, men ages 40 to 75 years who were free of prostate cancer between 1986 and 1994 and had not had a radical prostatectomy but either had surgery for benign prostatic hyperplasia (*n* = 1,890) or scored 15 or more points out of 35 (*n* = 1,853) on seven questions about lower urinary tract symptoms were compared with controls who scored 7 points or less on symptoms (*n* = 21,745; Platz et al. 1998). After controlling for age, race or ethnicity, alcohol consumption, and smoking, the men in the highest quintile of physical activity (mainly walking 2–3 h each week) had a 25% reduction in the odds of having urinary tract symptoms indicative of benign prostatic hyperplasia and a 25% reduction in the odds of prostate surgery compared with the men in the lowest quintile of physical activity.

Measuring prostate-specific antigen (PSA) is an established tool in detecting prostate cancer. However, some evidence suggests that heavy exercise should be avoided before a diagnostic blood sampling of PSA. Serum concentrations of PSA were measured in 301 healthy outpatients before and after they performed standardized exercise (Oremek and Seiffert 1996). Immediately after 15 min of exercise on a cycle ergometer, PSA concentrations increased as much as threefold. The increase was age dependent and correlated with the PSA concentration before exercise.

Differences in endogenous androgen levels have been hypothesized to explain ethnic differences in prostate cancer risk. To examine this question, 1,127 men of African, European, Chinese, and Japanese descent, mostly ages 60 or older (mean age, 69.9 years), were selected from population bases in California, Hawaii, and Vancouver, Canada (Wu et al. 1995). Participants provided information on physical activity levels and donated an early morning fasting blood sample between March 1990 and March 1992. Serum concentrations of testosterone, dihydrotestosterone (DHT), and sex hormone–binding globulin (SHBG) and the ratio of DHT to total testosterone were measured. After adjustment for age and BMI, androgens and SHBG showed no clear and consistent relationships with physical activity.

Recently, the effects of a low-fat, high-fiber diet and exercise intervention on the growth of testosterone-dependent and testosterone-independent prostate cancer cells that were stimulated in culture by serum taken from the study's participants were studied. Fasting blood serum was obtained from 13 overweight men before and after they underwent an 11-day, low-fat, high-fiber diet and an exercise intervention and from another 8 men who had participated in the diet and exercise program for an average of 14 years (Tymchuk et al. 2001). The cell growth of the testosterone-dependent cancer cells was reduced by a mean of 30% after the 11-day intervention and another 15% after the 14-year intervention, suggesting that the exercise and dietary intervention blunted the growth of prostate cancer cells by mitigating testosterone's effect on growth. Levels of circulating testosterone were reduced after the 11-day intervention, but so were blood levels of glucose and lipids and body weight. Because the study was not otherwise controlled, changes in those factors could have confounded the associated drops in cancer cell growth and testosterone, precluding a clear conclusion of an independent effect of the intervention on testosterone-mediated cancer cell growth.

> ••• *To date, about half of 28 studies that included 22,521 cases of prostate cancer in North America, Asia, and Europe concluded that leisure-time or occupational physical activity significantly reduced the rate of cancer by 10% to 70% (Thune and Furberg 2001).*

Summary and Conclusions

Though it is encouraging that about half the available studies have shown lower rates of prostate cancer among physically active men, the existing evidence is inconclusive about the independent, protective effect of physical activity against prostate cancer. The majority of the studies failed to measure leisure-time or occupational physical activity precisely. This makes it impossible to unambiguously determine whether a true dose–response relationship between physical activity and prostate cancer risk exists. Other confounders that influence prostate cancer risk have generally been incompletely controlled, and none of the studies addressed the issue of when in life exercise should begin or for how long it should be done. Studies also have not addressed whether physical activity might affect the process of prostate tumor growth. Agreement among studies is modest, and evidence to confirm hypothesized plausible mechanisms of a protective effect of physical activity against prostate cancer is as yet uncompelling. Nonetheless, the evidence is sufficiently strong to justify better-controlled prospective cohort studies and possibly randomized controlled trials in the near future.

Bibliography

Albanes, D., A. Blair, and P.R. Taylor. 1989. Physical activity and risk of cancer in the NHANES I population. *American Journal of Health Promotion* 79 (6): 744–750.

American Cancer Society. 1993. *Cancer facts and figures.* Atlanta: American Cancer Society.

———. 2001. *Cancer facts and figures.* Atlanta: American Cancer Society.

———. 2003. *Cancer facts and figures.* Atlanta: American Cancer Society.

Andersson, S.O., J. Baron, A. Wolk, C. Lindgren, R. Bergstrom, and H.O. Adami. 1995. Early life risk factors for prostate cancer: A population-based case–control study in Sweden. *Cancer Epidemiology, Biomarkers and Prevention* 4 (3): 187–192.

Apter, D., and R. Vinko. 1975. Early menarche, a risk factor for breast cancer, indicates early onset of menses. *Journal of Clinical Endocrinology and Metabolism* 15: 617–631.

Arbman, G., O. Axelson, M. Fredriksson, E. Nilsson, and R. Sjödahl. 1993. Do occupational factors influence the risk of colon and rectal cancer in different ways? *Cancer* 72 (9): 2543–2549.

Arraiz, G.A., D.T. Wigle, and Y. Mao. 1992. Risk assessment of physical-activity and physical fitness in the Canada health survey mortality follow-up-study. *Journal of Clinical Epidemiology* 45 (4): 419–428.

Bach, P.B., D. Schrag, O.W. Brawley, A. Galaznik, S. Yakren, and C.B. Begg. 2002. Survival of blacks and whites after a cancer diagnosis. *Journal of the American Medical Association* 287 (16): 2106–2113.

Ballard-Barbash, R., A. Schatzkin, D. Albanes, M.H. Schiffman, B.E. Kreger, W.B. Kannel, K.M. Anderson, and W.E. Helsel. 1990. Physical activity and the risk of large bowel cancer in the Framingham study. *Cancer Research* 50: 3610–3613.

Bartram, H.P., and E.L. Wynder. 1989. Physical activity and colon cancer risk? Physiological considerations. *American Journal of Gastroenterology* 84: 109–111.

Bernstein, L., B.E. Henderson, R. Hanisch, J. Sullivan-Halley, and R.K. Ross. 1994. Physical exercise and reduced risk of breast cancer in young women. *Journal of the National Cancer Institute* 86: 1403–1408.

Boyle, P. 1994. Evolution of an epidemic of unknown origin. In *Prostate cancer 2000,* edited by L. Denis, pp. 5–11. Heidelberg: Springer-Verlag.

Boyle, P., P. Maisonneuve, and P. Napalkov. 1996. Prostate cancer: The threat to health and strategies for control. In *Questions and uncertainties about prostate cancer,* edited by W.B. Peeling, pp. 3–29. London: Blackwell Science.

Breslow, R.A., R. Ballard-Barbash, K. Munoz, and B.I. Graubard. 2001. Long-term recreational physical activity and breast cancer in the National Health and Nutrition Examination Survey I epidemiologic follow-up study. *Cancer Epidemiology, Biomarkers, and Prevention* 10 (7): 805–808.

Brill, P., C. Barlow, and S.N. Blair. 1992. Physical fitness and non-fatal site-specific cancer: Is there an association in women? (abstract). *Medicine and Science in Sports and Exercise* 24: S62.

Brinton, L.A., L. Bernstein, and G.A. Colditz. 1998. Summary of the workshop: Workshop on physical activity and breast cancer, November 13–14, 1997. *Cancer* 83 (Suppl. 3): 595–599.

Brinton, L.A., and S.S. Devesa. 1996. Etiology and pathogenesis of breast cancer: Incidence, demographics, and environmental factors. In *Diseases of the breast,* edited by J.R. Harris, M.E. Lippman, M. Morrow, and S. Hellman, pp. 159–168. Philadelphia: Lippincott-Raven.

Brownson, R.C., J.C. Chang, J.R. Davis, and C.A. Smith. 1991. Physical activity on the job and cancer in Missouri. *American Journal of Public Health* 81 (5): 639–642.

Centers for Disease Control and Prevention. 2002. Deaths: Preliminary data for 2001. *National Vital Statistics Reports* 51 (5): 1–45.

Cerhan, J.R., J.C. Torner, C.F. Lynch, L.M. Rubenstein, J.H. Lemke, M.B. Cohen, D.M. Lubaroff, and R.B. Wallace. 1997. Association of smoking, body mass, and physical activity with risk of prostate cancer in the Iowa 65+ Rural Health Study (United States). *Cancer Causes and Control* 8 (2): 229–238.

Chen, C.L., E. White, K.E. Malone, and J.R. Daling. 1997. Leisure-time physical activity in relation to breast cancer among young women. *Cancer Causes and Control* 8 (1): 77–84.

Clarke, G., and A.S. Whittemore. 2000. Prostate cancer risk in relation to anthropometry and physical activity: The National Health and Nutrition Examination Survey I Epidemiological Follow-Up Study. *Cancer Epidemiology, Biomarkers and Prevention* 9: 875–881.

Coenen, C., M. Wegener, B. Wedmann, G. Schmidt, and S. Hoffmann. 1992. Does physical exercise influence bowel transit time in healthy young men? *American Journal of Gastroenterology* 87 (3): 292–295.

Colber, L.H., E. Lanza, R. Ballard-Barbash, M.L. Slattery, J.A. Tangrea, B. Caan, E.D. Paskett, F. Iber, W. Kikendall, P. Lance, et al. 2002. Adenomatous polyp recurrence and physical activity in the Polyp Prevention Trial (United States). *Cancer Causes Control 2002* 13 (5): 445–453.

Colditz, G.A., C.C. Cannuscio, and A.L. Frazier. 1997. Physical activity and reduced risk of colon cancer: Implications for prevention. *Cancer Causes and Control* 8: 649–667.

Coogan, P.F., P.A. Newcomb, R.W. Clapp, A. Trentham-Dietz, J.A. Baron, and M.P. Longnecker. 1997. Physical activity in usual occupation and risk of breast cancer (United States). *Cancer Causes and Control* 8: 626–631.

Cooper, G.S., D.P. Sandler, E.A. Whelan, and K.R. Smith. 1996. Association of physical and behavioral characteristics with menstrual cycle patterns in women age 29–31 years. *Epidemiology* 7: 624–684.

Cordain, L., R.W. Latin, and J.J. Behnke. 1986. The effects of an aerobic running program on bowel transit time. *Journal of Sports Medicine and Physical Fitness* 26: 101–104.

DeWaard, F.J., J.P. Cornelis, K. Aoki, and M. Yoshida. 1977. Breast cancer incidence according to weight and height in two cities of the Netherlands and in Aichi prefecture, Japan. *Cancer* 40: 1269–1275.

Diamandopoulus, G.T. 1996. Cancer: An historical perspective. *Anticancer Research* 16: 1595–1602.

Dorgan, J.F., C. Brown, M. Barrett, G.L. Splansky, B.E. Kreger, R.B. D'Agostino, D. Albanes, and A. Schatzkin. 1994. Physical activity and risk of breast cancer in the Framingham Heart Study. *American Journal of Epidemiology* 139: 662–669.

Ewertz, M. 1995. Risk from age, race, and social class. In *Reducing breast cancer risk in women,* edited by B.A. Stoll, pp. 41–45. Dordrecht, The Netherlands: Kluwer Academic.

Ewertz, M., and S.W. Duffy. 1988. Risk of breast cancer in relation to reproductive factors in Denmark. *British Journal of Cancer* 38: 99–104.

Fentiman, I. 1993. *Prevention of breast cancer.* Austin, TX: R.G. Landes.

Franco, G. 1999. Ramazzini and worker's health. *Lancet* 354: 858–861.

Friedenreich, C.M., H.E. Bryant, and K.S. Courneya. 2001. Case-control study of lifetime physical activity and breast cancer risk. *American Journal of Epidemiology* 154: 336–347.

Friedenreich, C.M., K.S. Courneya, and H.E. Bryant. 2001. Influence of physical activity in different age and life periods on the risk of breast cancer. *Epidemiology* 12 (6): 604–612.

Friedenreich, C.M., and M.R. Orenstein. 2002. Physical activity and cancer prevention: Etiologic evidence and biological mechanisms. *Journal of Nutrition* 132 (11 Suppl.): 3456S–3464S.

Friedenreich, C.M., and T.E. Rohan. 1995. A review of physical activity and breast cancer. *Epidemiology* 6 (3): 311–317.

Friedenreich, C.M., I. Thune, L.A. Brinton, and D. Albanes. 1998. Epidemiologic issues related to the association between physical activity and breast cancer. *Cancer* 83 (Suppl. 3): 600–610.

Frisch, R.E., A.V. Gotz-Welbergen, J.W. McArthur, T. Albright, J. Witschi, B. Bullen, J. Birnholz, R.B. Reed, and H. Hermann. 1981. Delayed menarche and amenorrhea of college athletes in relation to age of onset of training. *Journal of the American Medical Association* 246: 1559–1563.

Frisch, R.E., G. Wyshak, N.L. Albright, I. Schiff, K.P. Jones, J. Witschi, E. Shiang, E. Koff, and M. Marguglio. 1985. Lower prevalence of breast cancer and cancers of the reproductive system among former college athletes compared to non-athletes. *British Journal of Cancer* 52: 885–891.

Gallucci, B.B. 1985. Selected concepts of cancer as a disease: From the Greeks to 1900. *Oncology Nursing Forum* 12: 67–71.

Gammon, M.D., and E.M. John. 1993. Recent etiologic hypotheses concerning breast cancer. *Epidemiologic Reviews* 15 (1): 163–168.

Gammon, M., E. John, and J. Britton. 1998. Recreational and occupational physical activities and risk of breast cancer. *Journal of the National Cancer Institute* 90: 100–117.

Garabrant, D.H., J.M. Peters, T.M. Mack, and L. Bernstein. 1984. Job activity and colon cancer risk. *American Journal of Epidemiology* 119: 1005–1014.

Garfinkel, L., C.C. Boring, and C.W. Heath. 1994. Changing trends: An overview of breast cancer incidence and mortality. *Cancer* 74: 222–227.

Gerhardsson, M., B. Floderus, and S.E. Norell. 1988. Physical activity and colon cancer risk. *International Journal of Epidemiology* 17: 743–746.

Gerhardsson, M., S.E. Norell, H. Kiviranta, N.L. Pedersen, and A. Ahlbom. 1986. Sedentary jobs and colon cancers. *American Journal of Epidemiology* 123: 775–780.

Gerhardsson, M., G. Steineck, U. Hagman, A. Reiger, and S.E. Norell. 1990. Physical activity and colon cancer: A case referent study in Stockholm. *International Journal of Cancer* 46: 985–989.

Giovannucci, E., A. Ascherio, E.B. Rimm, G.A. Colditz, M.J. Stampfer, and W.C. Willett. 1995. Physical activity, obesity, and risk for colon cancer and adenoma in men. *Annals of Internal Medicine* 122 (5): 327–334.

Giovannucci, E., G.A. Colditz, M.J. Stampfer, and W.C. Willett. 1996. Physical-activity obesity and risk of colorectal adenoma in women (United States) (abstract). *Cancer Causes and Control* 7: 253–263.

Giovannucci, E., M. Leitzmann, D. Spiegelman, E.B. Rimm, G.A. Colditz, M.J. Stampfer, and W.C. Willett. 1998. A prospective study of physical activity and prostate cancer in male health professionals. *Cancer Research* 58 (22): 5117–5122.

Haenszel, W., and M. Kurihara. 1968. Studies of Japanese migrants: Mortality from cancer and other diseases among Japanese in the United States. *Journal of the National Cancer Institute* 40: 43–68.

Hartman, T.J., D. Albanes, M. Rautalahti, J.A. Tangrea, J. Virtamo, R. Stolzenberg, and P.R. Taylor. 1998. Physical activity and prostate cancer in the Alpha-Tocopherol, Beta-Carotene (ATBC) Cancer Prevention Study (Finland). *Cancer Causes and Control* 9 (1): 11–18.

Henderson, B.E., and L. Bernstein. 1996. Etiology and pathogenesis of breast cancer: Endogenous and exogenous hormonal factors. In *Diseases of the breast,* edited by J.R. Harris, M.E. Lippman, M. Morrow, and S. Hellman, pp. 185–200. Philadelphia: Lippincott-Raven.

Henderson, B.E., M.C. Pike, and J.T. Casagrande. 1981. Breast cancer and the oestrogen window hypothesis (letter). *Lancet* 2 (8242): 363–364.

Henderson, I.C. 1995. Breast cancer. In *Clinical oncology,* edited by G.P. Murphy, W.L. Lawrence, and R.E. Lenhard. Atlanta: American Cancer Society.

Hirose, K., K. Tajima, N. Hamajima, M. Inoue, T. Takezaki, T. Kuroishi, M. Yoshida, and S. Tokudome. 1995. A large-scale, hospital-based case–control study of risk factors of breast cancer according to menopausal status. *Japanese Journal of Cancer Research* 86: 146–154.

Hoffman-Goetz, D. Apter, W. Demark-Wahnefried, M.I. Goran, A. McTiernan, M.E. Reichman. 1998. Possible mechanisms mediating an association between physical activity and breast cancer. *Cancer* 83 (3 Suppl.): 621–628.

Holland, J.F., and E. Frei (editors). 1993. *Cancer medicine.* 3rd ed. Philadelphia: Lea and Febiger.

Holland, J.F., D.W. Kufe, R.E. Pollock, R.R. Weichselbaum, E.I. Frei, and R.C. Bast Jr. (editors). 2000. *Holland-Frei Cancer Medicine.* 5th ed. Hamilton, ON: BC Decker.

Hunter, D.J., and W.C. Willet. 1996. Etiology and pathogenesis of breast cancer: Dietary factors. In *Diseases of the breast,* edited by J.R. Harris, M.E. Lippman, M. Morrow, and S. Hellman, pp. 201–212. Philadelphia: Lippincott-Raven.

Kelsey, J., and P.L. Horn-Ross. 1993. Breast cancer: Magnitude of the problem and descriptive epidemiology. *Epidemiologic Reviews* 15 (1): 7–15.

Koffler, K.H., A. Menkes, R.A. Redmond, W.E. Whitehead, R.E. Pratley, and B.F. Hurley. 1992. Strength training accelerates gastrointestinal transit in middle-aged and older men. *Medicine and Science in Sports and Exercise* 24 (4): 415–419.

Kohl, H.W., R.E. LaPorte, and S.N. Blair. 1988. Physical activity and cancer: An epidemiological perspective. *Sports Medicine* 6: 222–237.

Korenman, S.G. 1980. Oestrogen window hypothesis of the aetiology of breast cancer. *Lancet* 1: 700–701.

Kritchevsky, D. 1990. Nutrition and breast cancer. *Cancer* 66: 1321–1325.

Laurent-Puig, P., H. Blons, and P.H. Cugnenc. 1999. Sequence of molecular genetic events in colorectal tumorigenesis. *European Journal of Cancer Prevention* 8 (Suppl. 1): S39–S47.

La Vecchia, C., C. Braga, S. Franceschi, L. Dal Maso, and E. Negri. 1999. Population-attributable risk for colon cancer in Italy. *Nutrition and Cancer* 33 (2): 196–200.

Lee, I.-M. 1995. Exercise and physical health: Cancer and immune function. *Research Quarterly for Exercise and Sport* 66 (4): 286–291.

Lee, I.M., J.E. Manson, U. Ajani, R.S. Paffenbarger Jr., C.H. Hennekens, and J.E. Buring. 1997. Physical activity and risk of colon cancer: The Physicians' Health Study (United States). *Cancer Causes and Control* 8: 568–574.

Lee, I.M., and R.S. Paffenbarger Jr. 1994. Physical activity and its relation to cancer risk: A prospective study of college alumni. *Medicine and Science in Sports and Exercise* 26 (7): 831–837.

Lee, I.-M., R.S. Paffenbarger Jr., and C. Hsieh. 1992. Physical activity and risk of prostate cancer among college alumni. *American Journal of Epidemiology* 135 (2): 169–178.

Le Marchand, L., L.R. Wilkens, L.N. Kolonel, J.H. Hankin, and L.C. Lyu. 1997. Associations of sedentary lifestyle, obesity, smoking, alcohol use, and diabetes with the risk of colorectal cancer. *Cancer Research* 57: 4787–4794.

Levi, F., C. Pasche, F. Lucchini, and C. La Vecchia. 1999. Occupational and leisure time physical activity and the risk of breast cancer. *European Journal of Cancer* 35: 775–778.

Liu, S., I.M. Lee, P. Linson, U. Ajani, J.E. Buring, and C.H. Hennekens. 2000. A prospective study of physical activity and risk of prostate cancer in U.S. physicians. *International Journal of Epidemiology* 29: 29–35.

Longnecker, M.P., M. Gerhardsson de Verdier, H. Frumkin, and C. Carpenter. 1995. A case–control study of physical activity in relation to risk of cancer of the right colon and rectum in men. *International Journal of Epidemiology* 24 (1): 42–50.

Lund Nilsen, T.I., R. Johnsen, and L.J. Vatten. 2000. Socio-economic and lifestyle factors associated with the risk of prostate cancer. *British Journal of Cancer* 82 (7): 1358–1363.

Malina, R.M. 1983. Menarche in athletes: A synthesis and hypothesis. *Annals of Human Biology* 10 (1): 1–24.

Marcus, P.M., B. Newman, P.G. Moorman, R.C. Millikan, D.D. Baird, B. Qaqish, and B. Sternfeld. 1999. Physical activity at age 12 and adult breast cancer risk (United States). *Cancer Causes and Control* 10: 293–302.

Markowitz, S., A. Morabia, K. Garibaldi, and E. Wynder. 1992. Effect of occupational and recreational activity on the risk of colorectal cancer among males: A case–control study. *International Journal of Epidemiology* 21 (6): 1057–1062.

Martinez, M.E., E. Giovannucci, D. Spiegelman, D.J. Hunter, W.C. Willett, and G.A. Colditz. 1997. Leisure-time physical activity, body size, and colon cancer in women: Nurses' Health Study research group. *Journal of the National Cancer Institute* 89: 948–955.

Martinez, M.E., D. Heddens, D.L. Earnest, C.L. Bogert, D. Roe, J. Einspahr, J.R. Marshall, and D.S. Alberts. 1999. Physical activity, body mass index, and prostaglandin E2 levels in rectal mucosa. *Journal of the National Cancer Institute* 91: 950–953.

McTiernan, A., J.L. Stanford, N.S. Weiss, J.R. Daling, and L.F. Voigt. 1996. Occurrence of breast cancer in relation to recreational exercise in women age 50–64 years. *Epidemiology* 7: 598–604.

McTiernan, A., C. Ulrich, S. Slate, and J. Potter. 1998. Physical activity and cancer etiology: Associations and mechanisms. *Cancer Causes and Control* 9: 487–509.

Meshkinpour, H., S. Selod, H. Movahedi, N. Nami, N. James, and A. Wilson. 1998. Effects of regular exercise in management of chronic idiopathic constipation. *Digestive Diseases and Sciences* 43 (11): 2379–2383.

Mettlin, C.J., G.P. Murphy, L.S. McGinnis, and H.R. Menek. 1995. The National Cancer Data Base report on prostate cancer. *Cancer* 76 (6): 1104–1113.

Mezzetti, M., C. La Vecchia, A. Decarli, P. Boyle, R. Talamini, and S. Franceschi. 1998. Population attributable risk for breast cancer: Diet, nutrition, and physical exercise. *Journal of the National Cancer Institute* 90: 389–394.

Miller, A.B., and R.D. Bulbrook. 1986. UICC multidisciplinary project on breast cancer: The epidemiology, aetiology, and prevention of breast cancer. *International Journal of Cancer* 37: 173–177.

Miller, B.A., L.N. Kolonel, L. Bernstein, J.L. Young Jr., G.M. Swanson, D.W. West, C.R. Key, J.M Liff, C.S. Glover, and G.A. Alexander. 1996. *Racial/ethnic patterns of cancer in the United States, 1988–1992.* NIH Publication No. 96-4104. Bethesda, MD: National Cancer Institute.

Mittendorf, R., M.P. Longnecker, P.A. Newcomb, A.T. Dietz, E.R. Greenberg, G.F. Bogdan, R.W. Clapp, and W.C. Willett. 1995. Strenuous physical activity in young adulthood and risk of breast cancer. *Cancer Causes and Control* 6: 347–353.

Moradi, T., H.O. Adami, R. Bergstrom, G. Gridley, A. Wolk, M. Gerhardsson, M. Dosemeci, and O. Nyren. 1999. Occupational physical activity and risk for breast cancer in a nationwide cohort study in Sweden. *Cancer Causes and Control* 10: 423–430.

Morville, R., P.C. Pesquies, and C.Y. Guezennee. 1979. Plasma variations in testicular and adrenal androgens during prolonged physical exercise in man. *Annals in Endocrinology* 40: 501–515.

National Cancer Institute. 1999. *Information about detection, symptoms, diagnosis, and treatment of colon and rectal cancer.* Bethesda, MD: National Institutes of Health Publication No. 99-1552.

National Cancer Institute. 2000a. *Information about detection, symptoms, diagnosis, and treatment of breast cancer.* Bethesda, MD: National Institutes of Health Publication No. 00-1556.

National Cancer Institute. 2000b. *Information about detection, symptoms, diagnosis, and treatment of prostate cancer.* Bethesda, MD: National Institutes of Health Publication No. 00-1576.

Oliveria, S.A., H.W. Kohl III, D. Trichopoulos, and S.N. Blair. 1996. The association between cardiorespiratory fitness and prostate cancer. *Medicine and Science in Sports and Exercise* 28 (1): 97–104.

Oliveria, S.A., and I.M. Lee. 1997. Is exercise beneficial in the prevention of prostate cancer? *Sports Medicine* 23 (5): 271–278.

Oremek, G.M., and U.B. Seiffert. 1996. Physical activity releases prostate-specific antigen (PSA) from the prostate gland into blood and increases serum PSA concentrations. *Clinical Chemistry* 42: 691–695.

Paffenbarger, R.S., R.T. Hyde, and A.L. Wing. 1987. Physical activity and incidence of cancer in diverse populations: A preliminary report. *American Journal of Clinical Nutrition* 45: 312–317.

Paget, S. 1889. The distribution of secondary growths in cancer of the breast. *Lancet* 1: 571–573.

Parker, S.L., T. Tong, S. Bolden, and P.W. Wingo. 1997. Cancer statistics. *CA: A Cancer Journal for Clinicians* 47: 5–27.

Parkin, D.M., J. Stjernsward, and C.S. Muir. 1984. Estimates of worldwide frequency of twelve major cancers. *Bulletin of the World Health Organization* 62: 163–182.

Pike, M.C., M.D. Krailo, B.E. Henderson, J.T. Casagrande, and D.G. Hoel. 1983. 'Hormonal' risk factors, 'breast tissue age' and the age-incidence of breast cancer. *Nature* 303: 767–770.

Platz, E.A., I. Kawachi, E.B. Rimm, G.A. Colditz, M.J. Stampfer, W.C. Willett, and E. Giovannucci. 1998. Physical activity and benign prostatic hyperplasia. *Archives of Internal Medicine* 158 (21): 2349–2356.

Pleotis Howell, L. 1995. The pathway to cancer. In *A practical approach to breast disease,* edited by L.F. O'Grady, K.K. Lindfors, L. Pleotis Howell, and M.B. Rippon, pp. 23–39. Boston: Little, Brown.

Powell, K.E., and S.N. Blair. 1994. The public-health burdens of sedentary living habits: Theoretical but realistic estimates. *Medicine and Science in Sports and Exercise* 26 (7): 851–856.

Ramazzini, B. 1983. *Diseases of workers: Latin text of 1713 revised with translation and notes by Wilmer Cave Wright.* New York: Classics of Medicine Library, Division of Gryphon Editions.

Ries, L.A.G., C.L. Kosary, B.F. Hankey, and B.A. Miller. 1997. *SEER cancer statistics review, 1973–1994: Tables and graphs.* NIH Publication No. 97-2789. Bethesda, MD: National Cancer Institute.

Robertson, G., H. Meshkinpour, K. Vandenberg, N. James, A. Cohen, and A.J. Wilson. 1993. Effects of exercise on total and segmental colon transit. *Journal of Clinical Gastroenterology* 16 (4): 300–303.

Rockhill, B., W.C. Willett, D.J. Hunter, J.E. Manson, S.E. Hankinson, and G.A. Colditz. 1999. A prospective study of recreational physical activity and breast cancer risk. *Archives of Internal Medicine* 159 (19): 2290–2296.

Rockhill, B., W.C. Willett, D.J. Hunter, J.E. Manson, S.E. Hankinson, D. Spiegelman, and G.A. Colditz. 1998. Physical activity and breast cancer risk in a cohort of young women. *Journal of the National Cancer Institute* 90: 1155–1160.

Sandler, R.S., M.L. Pritchard, and S.I. Bangdiwala. 1995. Physical activity and the risk of colorectal adenomas. *Epidemiology* 6: 602–606.

Seeley, R., T. Stephens, and P. Tate. 1998. *Anatomy and physiology.* New York: McGraw-Hill.

Sesso, H.D., R.S. Paffenbarger Jr., and I.M. Lee. 1998. Physical activity and breast cancer risk in the College Alumni Health Study (United States). *Cancer Causes and Control* 9 (4): 433–439.

Shephard, R.J. 1995. Exercise and cancer: Linkages with obesity? *International Journal of Obesity* 19 (4): S62–S68.

———. 1996. Exercise and cancer: Linkages with obesity. *Critical Reviews in Food Science and Nutrition* 36 (4): 321–339.

Shike, M. 1996. Body weight and colon cancer. *American Journal of Clinical Nutrition* 63 (3S): 442S–444S.

Slattery, M., M.C. Schumacher, K.R. Smith, D.W. West, and N. Abd-Elghany. 1988. Physical activity, diet, and risk of colon cancer in Utah. *American Journal of Epidemiology* 128: 989–999.

Slattery, M.L., S.L. Edwards, K.N. Ma, G.D. Friedman, and J.D. Potter. 1997. Physical activity and colon cancer: A public health perspective. *Annals of Epidemiology* 7: 137–145.

Stallone, D.D. 1993. The influence of obesity and its treatment on the immune system. *Annals of Internal Medicine* 52: 37–50.

Sternfeld, B. 1992. Cancer and the protective effect of physical activity. *Medicine and Science in Sports and Exercise* 24: 1195–1207.

Stoll, B.A. 1995. Childbearing and related risk factors. In *Reducing breast cancer risk in women,* edited by B.A. Stoll, pp. 19–28. Dordrecht, The Netherlands: Kluwer Academic.

Tang, R., J.Y. Wang, S.K. Lo, and L.L. Hsieh. 1999. Physical activity, water intake and risk of colorectal cancer in Taiwan: A hospital-based case–control study. *International Journal of Cancer* 82 (4): 484–489.

Tavani, A., C. Braga, C. La Vecchia, E. Conti, R. Filiberti, M. Montella, D. Amadori, A. Russo, and S. Franceschi. 1999. Physical activity and risk of cancers of the colon and rectum: An Italian case–control study. *British Journal of Cancer* 79: 1912–1916.

Thune, I., T. Brenn, E. Lund, and M. Gaard. 1997. Physical activity and the risk of breast cancer. *New England Journal of Medicine* 336 (18): 1269–1275.

Thune, I., and A. Furberg. 2001. Physical activity and cancer risk: Dose-response and cancer, all sites and site-specific.

Medicine and Science in Sports and Exercise 33 (Suppl. 6): S530–S550.

Thune, I., and E. Lund. 1994. Physical activity and the risk of prostate and testicular cancer: A cohort study of 53,000 Norwegian men. *Cancer Causes and Control* 5 (6): 549–556.

———. 1996. Physical activity and risk of colorectal cancer in men and women. *British Journal of Cancer* 73 (9): 1134–1140.

Tymchuk, C.N., R.J. Barnard, D. Heber, and W.J. Aronson. 2001. Evidence of an inhibitory effect of diet and exercise on prostate cancer cell growth. *Journal of Urology* 166: 1185–1189.

Ueji, M., E. Ueno, D. Osei-Hyiaman, H. Takahashi, and K. Kano. 1998. Physical activity and the risk of breast cancer: A case–control study of Japanese women. *Journal of Epidemiology* 8: 116–122.

U.S. Department of Health and Human Services. 1996. *Physical activity and health: A report of the Surgeon General.* Atlanta: U.S. Department of Health and Human Services, Centers for Disease Control and Prevention, National Center for Chronic Disease Prevention and Health Promotion.

Vatten, L.J., G. Ursin, R.K. Ross, F.Z. Stanczyk, R.A. Lobo, S. Harvei, and E. Jellum. 1997. Androgens in serum and the risk of prostate cancer: A nested case–control study from the Janus serum bank in Norway. *Cancer Epidemiology, Biomarkers and Prevention* 6 (11): 967–969.

Vena, J.E., S. Graham, M. Zielenzy, J. Brasure, and M.K. Swanson. 1987. Occupational exercise and risk of cancer. *American Journal of Clinical Nutrition* 45: 318–327.

Verloop, J., M.A. Rookus, K. van Der Kooy, and F.E. van Leeuwen. 2000. Physical activity and breast cancer risk in women aged 20–54 years. *Journal of the National Cancer Institute* 92 (2): 128–135.

Wannamethee, S.G., A.G. Shaper, and M. Walker. 2001. Physical activity and risk of cancer in middle-aged men. *British Journal of Cancer* 85 (9): 1311–1316.

Weber, B.L. 1996. Genetic testing for breast cancer. *Scientific American Science and Medicine* 3 (1): 12–21.

White, E., E.J. Jacobs, and J.R. Daling. 1996. Physical activity in relation to colon cancer in middle-aged men and women. *American Journal of Epidemiology* 144 (1): 42–50.

World Cancer Research Fund and American Institute for Cancer Research. 1997. *Food, nutrition and the prevention of cancer: A global perspective.* Washington, DC: American Institute for Cancer Research.

Wu, A.H., A.S. Whittemore, L.N. Kolonel, E.M. John, R.P. Gallagher, D.W. West, J. Hankin, C.Z. Teh, D.M. Dreon, and R.S. Paffenbarger Jr. 1995. Serum androgens and sex hormone–binding globulins in relation to lifestyle factors in older African-American, white, and Asian men in the United States and Canada. *Cancer Epidemiology, Biomarkers and Prevention* 4 (7): 735–741.

Yu, H., R.E. Harris, and E.L. Wynder. 1988. Case–control study of prostate cancer and socioeconomic factors. *Prostate* 13: 317–325.

Zheng, W., X.O. Shu, J. McLaughlin, W. Chow, Y.T. Gao, and W.J. Blot. 1993. Occupational physical activity and the incidence of cancer of the breast, corpus uteri, and ovary in Shanghai. *Cancer* 71 (11): 3620–3624.

Ziegler, R.G. 1997. Anthropometry and breast cancer. *Journal of Nutrition* 127 (Suppl. 5): 924S–928S.

Web Sites

www.cancer.org. Site of the American Cancer Society.

www.nci.nih.gov. Site of the National Cancer Institute.

Chapter 12

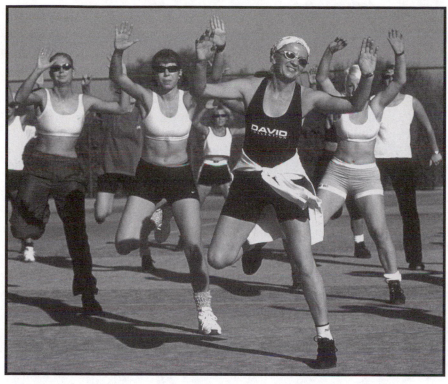
© SportsChrome

Physical Activity and the Immune System

Violent, prolonged, exhausting work produces a leucocytosis . . . made up principally by an increase in the polymorphonuclear . . . neutrophiles. . . . More than one cause acts to produce the leucocytosis—probably a temporary, mechanical cause, and a toxic cause, more slow to develop, but lasting as long as the exercise continues.

—Ralph C. Larrabee, "Leucocytosis After Violent Exercise," 1902

Though the site-specific mechanisms that explain the reduced risks for colon, breast, and prostate cancers are not yet understood clearly, the possibility that moderate levels of physical activity may have a positive influence on the immune system remains a likely explanation for general benefits that might extend to several different types of cancers. The acute effects of exercise on the immune system were first reported over 100 years ago, when German physiologist G. Schulz (1893) reported that muscle contractions produced an increase in the number of leukocytes circulating in the blood. Physical activity may also influence the risk of infections. A modern-day belief among athletes and coaches is that intense, strenuous exercise temporarily increases susceptibility to infection, especially upper-respiratory infection (URI). A few studies seem to confirm that view for some sports such as marathon running and training for cross-country skiing. In contrast, an equally common belief among the public is that regular physical activity of a moderate intensity and duration increases resistance to URI and may explain reduced risk for some cancers. None of these views is well documented by experimental evidence, but each remains plausible. Whether physical activity affects the immune system in a way that meaningfully reduces the risk of developing cancer is even less well established. No studies have shown such benefits among humans. However, experimental studies using rats and mice have shown that moderate physical activity seems to slow the growth of experimentally induced tumors (Cohen et al. 1992, 1993). Thus, there remains good reason to continue to study the effects of physical activity on the immune system. This chapter describes the immune system and its function and then discusses the scientific evidence about the effects of physical activity on the immune system.

An Abridged History of Immunology

The Greek historian Thucydides is credited with the first description of the concept of acquired immunity (from the Greek word *immunus,* meaning exemption) in his 430 B.C. account of the plague of smallpox that swept Greece after the Peloponnesian War: "It was with those who had recovered from the disease that the sick and the dying found most compassion. These knew what it was from experience, and had now no fear for themselves; for the same man was never attacked twice—never at least fatally" (Sprat 1667). Later, Chinese physicians around A.D. 1000 and the Circassians in Turkey during the 1600s practiced variolation, whereby people were inoculated by scratching the skin with smallpox taken from pustules of infected people.

> ••• *Immunology in Western medicine has its roots in the 1796 finding by British physician Edward Jenner that injection of cowpox virus into humans resulted in protection against human smallpox.*

However, **immunology** as a field of study in Western medicine has its roots in the 1796 observation by British physician Edward Jenner that injection of cowpox virus into humans resulted in inoculation against human smallpox, hence the term *vaccination,* from the Latin root *vaccinnus,* meaning "relating to a cow." Jenner reportedly got the idea when, while serving as an apprentice

to an apothecary, he overheard a farm girl tell her doctor that she could not contract smallpox because she had once had cowpox. That actually was a common observation among English milkmaids, who had reduced risk of contracting smallpox because of their exposure to cowpox. After 1770, Jenner was inspired to continue experiments with cowpox by his mentor, famous London surgeon and anatomist John Hunter. Jenner found that there were two forms of cowpox, but only one provided immunity against smallpox. On May 14, 1796, Jenner tested his hypothesis by inoculating a healthy eight-year-old boy, James Phipps, with cowpox. Two months later, he exposed the boy to smallpox virus from the dairymaid Sarah Nelmes, but the boy did not get the disease. Jenner submitted a manuscript describing his findings to the Royal Society of Medicine, but it was rejected. He then published a book about his studies in 1798 (figure 12.1), but it was largely ignored by physicians at the time. Later, an influential physician named William Woodville, who was director of London Smallpox and Inoculation Hospital, conducted extensive trials of successful vaccination

Early Discoveries

Milestones in the history of immunology include the discovery in the mid- to late 1800s by the French biochemist Louis Pasteur that most infectious diseases are caused by germs, including the discoveries of staphylococcus, streptococcus, and pneumococcus bacteria. He also discovered that weakened forms of a microbe could be used as an immunization against more virulent forms of the microbe and that rabies was transmitted by submicroscopic agents, thus discovering viruses and contributing to the development of vaccination against viruses. Around the same time, German physician Emil Adolph von Behring discovered antibodies through his pioneering research on immunization against diphtheria and tetanus by injecting what he termed "antitoxins." For that work, he received the first Nobel Prize in physiology and medicine in 1901. During the same era, the Russian biologist Ilya Mechnikov introduced the theory of **phagocytosis,** that is, that certain white blood cells can engulf bacteria. He won the 1908 Nobel Prize in physiology and medicine for using the concept of antibodies to treat diphtheria.

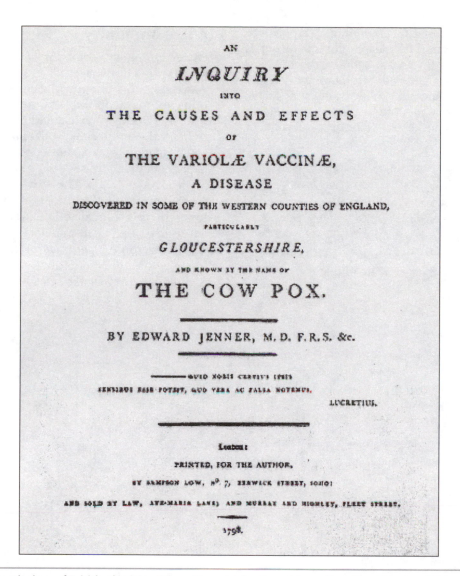

Figure 12.1   Frontispiece of British physician Edward Jenner's book on his studies of smallpox, published in 1798.

Cowpox

A farmer named Benjamin Jesty can be credited with the first cowpox inoculation after noticing that his milkmaid was seemingly protected from smallpox. However, when Jesty's children and wife became violently ill after a botched attempt at variolation (probably because of unsterile procedures in a barnyard), he was scorned by neighbors who felt his attempts were immoral.

on several thousand patients. Those studies led to the acceptance of Jenner's ideas by the Royal Society and set the stage for the modern study of immunology.

The Immune System

The **immune system** is an integrated network of molecules, cells, tissues, and organs that defends an organism against infection by foreign substances (e.g., bacteria and viruses) and against mutated native cells (i.e., tumors). It also helps to repair damaged tissues and to clean up the debris of dead cells (e.g., after muscle injury). Historically, the immune system has been regarded as self-regulating, independent of other regulatory mechanisms. However, it is now known that, in mammals at least, it interacts with the nervous and endocrine systems in ways that could plausibly be altered by exercise. There are two main types of immunities: innate (i.e., natural) and adaptive (i.e., acquired) immunity. They differ mainly in whether prior exposure is required for an immune response to occur. **Innate immunity** means that immune cells can recognize a foreign substance (an antigen) without prior exposure; **adaptive immunity** refers to immune cells' memory that recognizes a pathogen from a prior encounter, permitting a quicker and larger immune response upon a subsequent exposure (figure 12.2).

> ••• *The immune system is a network of molecules, cells, tissues, and organs that defend an organism against infection by foreign substances and against mutated native cells. It also helps repair damaged tissues by cleaning up the debris of dead cells.*

Innate Immunity

Innate immunity provides a defense against various infectious agents and cancer. It is accomplished by **phagocytic cells** such as macrophages, **neutrophils,** and **natural killer (NK) cells.** It includes physical and chemical barriers, such as the epidermis and epithelia. Even human sweat contains an antibacterial peptide that helps regulate microbes on the surface of the skin (Schittek et al. 2001). The innate immune system also is composed of factors that cause **inflammation,** which is a localized response of increased blood flow, increased capillary permeability, influx of neutrophils and macrophages, and secretion of **cytokines** (nonantibody proteins secreted by inflammatory leukocytes, and some other

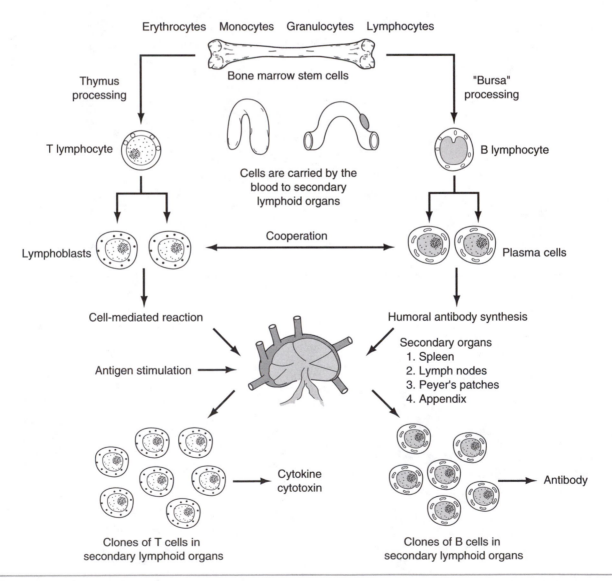

Figure 12.2　The immune system.

cells, that act as intercellular mediators). Innate immunity also involves blood proteins that are components of the **complement system**, which is capable of lysing bacteria and viruses coated with antibodies. The complement system is composed of about 25 proteins produced mainly by macrophages, the liver, and the intestine, which function in a cascade leading to cell lysis. Innate immunity is not very able to recognize specific antigens but provides general response against most infectious agents.

Adaptive Immunity

Adaptive immunity is able to recognize highly specific antigens as a result of previous exposure and offers different responses to different types of microbes. Memory enables a rapid and strong response to the same microbes when an organism is exposed to them again. Lymphocytes, such as T and B cells, and the products of plasma cells, **antibodies,** provide adaptive immunity. The molecules of the innate and adaptive immune systems function cooperatively as an integrated defense mechanism.

Cells of the Immune System

The immune system consists of different cell populations and molecules that migrate into and out of the blood and **lymph** circulations and are distributed in lymph organs and other tissues except the central nervous system. **Leukocytes** (white blood cells) include lymphocytes, monocytes, and granulocytes.

Lymphocytes are the major cells of adaptive immunity. **B lymphocytes** mature in bone marrow in mammals and differentiate into plasma cells, which produce antibodies after exposure to an antigen. B lymphocytes provide humoral (i.e., of the blood) immunity. They do not require mediating cell-to-cell contact in order to kill foreign cells during a primary (i.e., initial) infection by an antigen, but they require activation by helper T cells during a secondary (i.e., recurrent) infection by an antigen. Each B cell displays an antibody that has binding sites specific to a particular antigen. Antibodies are classified by five main types of **immunoglobulin (Ig)** that differ in their relative amounts in the blood: IgG, 80%; IgA, 10% to 15%; IgM, 5% to 10%; IgE, 1%; and IgE, 0.1%. Antibodies can coat antigens with opsonin (a process termed **opsonization**), a substance that makes it easier for antigens to be engulfed by a phagocyte. Binding of a B lymphocyte to an antigen presented by an **antigen-presenting cell** (APC) (cells that engulf antigens and present them to B or T lymphocytes in a recognizable form [e.g., in an MHC class II molecule], such as a macrophage or a dendritic cell, results in activation and **clonal expansion** of the B lymphocyte (figure 12.3). Other B lymphocytes are memory B cells, which mainly reside in the lymph nodes and spleen. Some memory B cells circulate in the blood as sentinels, ready to respond quickly and forcefully if they encounter the same antigen again. B cells can also serve as APCs for T lymphocytes. Macrophages and dendritic cells are

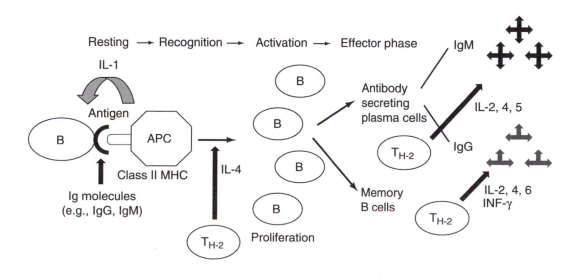

Figure 12.3 Activation of B cells and antibody secretion after presentation of an antigen.

termed "professional" APCs because they are effective at inducing a second-messenger signal needed for T and B cell activation.

T lymphocytes are derived from bone marrow and differentiate in the thymus. T lymphocytes are classified by the surface molecules, called the cluster of differentiation (CD), as CD4$^+$ or CD8$^+$ cells, which are also known by their functional names, helper T (T_H) cells and suppressor/cytotoxic T ($T_{S/C}$) cells, respectively. T cells participate in cell-mediated immunity, which means that they require cell-to-cell contact in order to generate cytotoxic cells and to activate macrophages. T_{H-1} cells activate macrophages. T_{H-2} cells activate cytotoxic T cells (figures 12.4 and 12.5). The specificity of T cells against antigens results from their ability to recognize peptide structures associated with the major histocompatibility complex (MHC) expressed on the surface of an APC. Cytotoxic T cells recognize MHC I proteins, while helper T cells recognize MHC II proteins. For example, when an APC first internalizes the antigen, it decomposes it into smaller peptides (epitopes) by digestion with lysosyme and then displays a fragment of the antigen on the APC's MHC class II molecule so that the helper T cell recognizes the antigen and is activated. The main function of cytotoxic T cells is **lysis** of tumor cells and virus-infected cells. When activated, helper T cells secrete cytokines that promote the growth and differentiation of T cells and other lymphocytes and activate inflammatory cells such as mononuclear phagocytes, neutrophils, and **eosinophils.**

Natural killer (NK) cells represent a distinct class of lymphocytes found in blood and **lymphoid** organs, especially the spleen. They have a similar shape as other lymphocytes but are granular, so they are also called large granular lymphocytes (LGL). NK cells are an important part of innate immunity that do not require prior exposure to recognize an antigen. Thus, NK cells play an important role in early defense against microbes by producing cell membrane damage (e.g., osmotically lysing) or inducing apoptosis (the process of genetically programmed cell death characterized by cell shrinkage and DNA fragmentation) in virus-infected cells and tumor cells. NK cells can also secrete cytotoxic cytokines, including TNF-α and IFN-γ.

> ••• *Natural killer (NK) cells are a class of large, granular lymphocytes found in blood and lymphoid organs, especially the spleen. They do not require prior exposure to recognize an antigen and thus play an important role in innate immunity. Acute exercise increases the numbers and possibly the activity of NK cells in the blood.*

Monocytes are produced in bone marrow and are released into the bloodstream, where they act as phagocytes, cytokine producers, regulators of blood clotting, and APCs for about a week while they travel to fixed sites in body tissues or special vessels. There they mature to become fully functioning macrophages, which are major phagocytes and APCs that produce cytokines during localized tissue infections. IL-1 secreted by macrophages is the key activator of helper T cells and stimulates the cascade of defense during an adaptive immune response to infection.

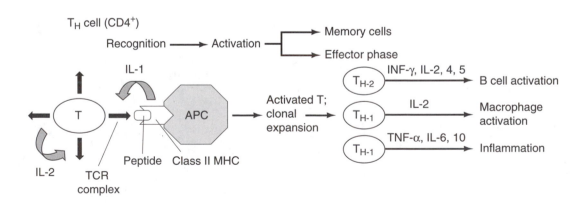

Figure 12.4   The presentation of an antigen to a helper T cell and the cascade of immune responses, including cloning of the activated helper T and subsequent activation of B cells, macrophages, granulocytes, and cytotoxic T cells, assisted by secretion of cytokines from other helper T cells.

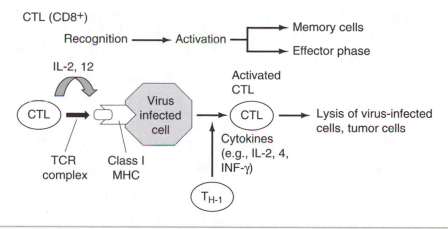

CTL (CD8+)

Recognition ⟶ Activation ⟶ Memory cells

⟶ Effector phase

IL-2, 12

Activated
CTL

CTL ➜ Virus
infected
cell ⟶ CTL ⟶ Lysis of virus-infected
cells, tumor cells

TCR   Class I
complex   MHC

Cytokines
(e.g., IL-2, 4,
INF-γ)

T_{H-1}

Figure 12.5   T cell activation. The presentation of an antigen directly to a cytotoxic T cell.

Dendritic cells are the most efficient APCs, but they are present in low numbers in the body.

Granulocytes, which originate in bone marrow, include neutrophils, eosinophils, **basophils,** and **mast cells.** Neutrophils make up about 80% to 90% of granulocytes and are major phagocytes of bacteria. They are abundant in the blood circulation but not in tissues. Neutrophils are chemically attracted and rapidly migrate from the blood to the site of an inflammation (a process called chemotaxis), especially a bacterial infection, where they ingest the bacteria. Neutrophils kill ingested bacteria by releasing lysosomal enzymes (e.g., proteases) or by an oxidative burst, using oxygen free radicals, nitric oxide, and hydrogen peroxide, which are toxic to microbes. Dead neutrophils comprise part of the pus that forms at the site of infection.

> ••• *Neutrophils are the main type of granulocytes that digest bacteria at the site of infection. They increase in number during and immediately after acute exercise.*

Cytokines differ from classical hormones because they are produced by several types of cells rather than by specialized glands. There are more than 60 cytokines, which are usually named according to their function or the cells that release them. Some cytokines that communicate between leukocytes are called **interleukins (IL).** Cytokines produced by lymphocytes are often termed lymphokines. Monocytes and macrophages secrete monokines.

Chemokines are a class of pro-inflammatory cytokines that are released by phagocytes, endo-thelial cells, fibroblasts, and smooth muscle cells in response to bacteria, viruses, and cell damage at the site of infection. Chemokines chemically attract and activate leukocytes in infected tissue by (1) binding with leukocytes and stabilizing the binding of integrin molecules with the endothelium, (2) providing a chemokine gradient across the endothelium that chemically attracts leukocytes across the vessel wall, and (3) activating phagocytic lysis. Chemokines are classified into two main types according to variations in shared cysteine molecules: C-X-C or α chemokines (e.g., IL-8) have paired cysteines separated by a different amino acid; they act as chemoattractants for neutrophils and fibroblasts involved with healing wounds. C-C or β chemokines (e.g., monocyte chemoattractant protein-1 [MCP-1]) have paired cysteines; they act as chemoattractants for monocytes, lymphocytes, eosinophils, and basophils.

Interferons boost resistance against viruses, inhibit proliferation of normal and malignant cells, impede multiplication of intracellular parasites, enhance macrophage and granulocyte phagocytosis, and augment natural killer cell activity. Interferon-gamma (IFN-γ) is the main interferon produced by stimulated lymphocytes. Cytokines mediate both innate (e.g., tumor necrosis factor-alpha [TNF-α], IL-1, IL-6, IL-10, IL-12, and IL-15) and adaptive immune responses (e.g., IFN-γ, transforming growth factor-beta [TGF-β], IL-2, IL-4, and IL-5). Cytokines released by resident phagocytes at the site of infection have local effects, including leukocyte adhesion to the vascular endothelium, expression of class I MHC molecules, and augmenting activity of phagocytes.

Cytokines also have general effects when they are released into the blood circulation. For example, pro-inflammatory cytokines such as IL-1β and TNF-α contribute to increased body temperature, which can inhibit the growth of some bacteria and enhance some immune reactions. They also induce the **acute-phase response,** which can result in fever, fatigue, loss of appetite, and nausea, as well as output by the liver of proteins that function like antibodies and boost innate immunity. A key acute phase protein is C-reactive protein (discussed in chapter 4 regarding inflammation and coronary heart disease), which binds to some bacteria and fungi, serving as both an opsonin and a complement catalyst. Another general effect of pro-inflammatory cytokines during initial infection is **leukocytosis,** which is an increase in the number of leukocytes circulating in the blood coming from bone marrow and, to a much lesser extent, the marginal pool.

Key Cytokines of the Immune System

Interleukin-1 (IL-1) is produced mainly by macrophages and activates acute-phase responses during the first few hours of infection or tissue damage. Such responses include fever, redistribution of amino acids, and increased liver production of antimicrobial plasma proteins. IL-1 also activates the cascade of humoral and cellular immune responses against infection by activating helper T cells and the clonal expansion of B cells, and by inducing the expression of adhesion molecules to aid emigration of leukocytes from the blood to infected tissue (Cannon et al. 1986).

Interleukin-2 (IL-2) is produced mainly by activated T_H lymphocytes. Its main functions are self-priming (i.e., it up-regulates its own activity), activation of cytotoxic T cells and natural killer cells, increased expression of IL-2 receptors on other lymphocytes, and stimulation for the release of other cytokines such as IFN.

Interleukin-6 (IL-6) is produced primarily by activated T_{H-2} lymphocytes, monocytes, and macrophages (Mackinnon 1999). Its main functions are to stimulate B cells to form plasma cells and secrete antibodies and to induce acute-phase protein synthesis by the liver in response to inflammation (Sprenger et al. 1992). Hence, it is an anti-inflammatory cytokine. IL-6 is secreted by skeletal muscle during violent exercise that induces muscle injury and also during moderate exercise. The IL-6 response to moderate exercise is a putative regulator of fuel metabolism during exercise (Febbraio and Pedersen 2002), but it also has potentially positive immunological effects. It promotes an anti-inflammatory cascade characterized by increased levels of cytokine inhibitors, IL-1 receptor antagonist (IL-1ra), TNF receptors (TNF-R), and the anti-inflammatory cytokine IL-10.

Interleukin-8 (IL-8) is a chemokine released mainly by resident macrophages and epithelial cells in damaged tissue. It acts as a chemoattractant for neutrophils and fibroblasts involved with healing wounds.

Interleukin-10 (IL-10) is an anti-inflammatory cytokine produced by T_{H-2} lymphocytes. It was initially termed cytokine synthesis inhibitory factor because it inhibits cytokine production by macrophages in order to down-regulate T_{H-1} cells. IL-10 also down-regulates MHC II expression on antigen-presenting cells and acts in concert with IL-4 to decrease macrophage inflammatory activity.

Interleukin-12 (IL-12) is secreted by macrophages and B cells. It activates T_{H-1} lymphocytes and natural killer cells. In combination with IL-2, IL-12 also activates cytotoxic T cells.

Tumor necrosis factor-alpha (TNF-α) is primarily produced by macrophages. It activates the killing of tumor cells and plays a role in antiviral activity (Mackinnon 1999). It also is an anti-inflammatory mediator of the acute-phase response (Rivier et al. 1994). Paradoxically, high levels of TNF-α have harmful effects, including inflammation and muscle wasting (Mackinnon 1999).

Tumor necrosis factor-beta (TNF-β) is produced by T lymphocytes. It activates tumor lysis, enhances phagocytic activity by macrophages, and is involved with mediating inflammation.

Interferon-gamma (IFN-γ) is produced by activated T_{H-1} and cytotoxic lymphocytes and natural killer cells. It plays a major role in antimicrobial and antitumor responses as well as antiviral effects and inhibition of antigen proliferation and differentiation (Sprenger et al. 1992). IFN-γ activates macrophages so that they are more phagocytic and increases their expression of class II MHC so that they have increased capacity as an APC.

Transforming growth factor-beta (TGF-β) is released by platelets, macrophages, and lymphocytes. It increases IL-1 production by activated macrophages, converts proliferating B cells to IgA, and is a chemoattractant for monocytes and macrophages. It also inhibits lymphocyte proliferation during inflammation, thus facilitating wound healing by restraining inflammation after cell injury.

Colony Stimulating Factors

Leukocytosis from bone marrow is regulated by colony stimulating factors (CSF), which are glycoproteins (conjugated protein–carbohydrate compounds) found in the blood that stimulate the proliferation of bone marrow cells and the formation of colonies of granulocytes or macrophages. They include granuloctye–macrophage colony stimulating factor (GM-CSF), granulocyte colony stimulating factor (G-CSF), macrophage colony stimulating factor (M-CSF), and IL-3. GM-CSF is produced in response to several inflammatory factors in blood and at the site of infection. It stimulates the production of neutrophils, macrophages, and mixed granulocyte–macrophage colonies from bone marrow cells. It can also stimulate the formation of eosinophil colonies and stimulate activities in mature granulocytes and macrophages. G-CSF induces the survival, proliferation, and differentiation of neutrophilic granulocyte precursor cells and functionally activates mature blood neutrophils. M-CSF stimulates the survival, proliferation, and differentiation of monocyte–macrophages. IL-3, also termed multi-CSF because it is secreted by lymphocytes, epithelial cells, and astrocytes, stimulates clonal proliferation and differentiation of various types of blood and tissue cells.

Organs of the Immune System

Immune cells migrate to and are concentrated in the primary and secondary lymphoid organs. The primary lymphoid organs include bone marrow, where hematopoiesis (generation of blood cells) occurs, and the thymus, where thymocytes mature to become T lymphocytes. The secondary lymphoid organs, where the contact between lymphocytes and antigens occurs, consist of lymph nodes, the spleen, the mucosal associated lymphoid tissue (MALT) (e.g., **Peyer's patches** in the small intestine and the tonsils), and the cutaneous immune system (e.g., epidermic or dermic lymphocytes). Foreign antigens in the lymph are collected and transported to lymph nodes, which are located throughout the lymphatic vessels, and other lymphoid tissues, where they can be recognized by lymphocytes. The spleen removes foreign substances from the blood, stores immune cells, and provides another site for immune responses to blood-borne antigens. Migration and recirculation of monocytes, neutrophils, and lymphocytes to the different sites in the body where antigens can be localized are critical in immune responses.

Responses to Infection

Host responses to an infection have three main phases: (1) innate, nonadaptive defense involving epithelial cell surfaces, resident phagocytes, and complement activation; (2) early induced responses, including inflammation, activation of phagocytes, natural killer cells, and cytokine release; and (3) the adaptive immune response involving the clonal expansion of cytoxic T cells and B cells (Abbas, Lightman, and Pober 1997).

The first phase occurs within a few hours after infection. If the complement system and resident phagocytes do not sufficiently limit the infection, the second phase of early nonadaptive responses is induced. Key aspects of this phase are inflammation and the migration of leukocytes (e.g., monocytes and granulocytes) to the site of infection. Inflammation and migration are regulated by cytokines (e.g., IL-6 and IL-8) and other inflammatory factors such as prostaglandins and leukotrienes released by phagocytes during the initial, innate response, as well as by complement proteins C5a, C3a, and C4a. Localized actions of these inflammatory factors culminate in local dilation of postcapillary venules, a reduced rate of blood flow, and increased permeability of vessel walls leading to edema (i.e., swelling), heat, and pain. The vascular changes also result in **margination** of leukocytes to the slower, peripheral area of the bloodstream, thereby increasing contact between circulating leukocytes and the endothelial cells that line the vessels and facilitating the transmigration of leukocytes circulating in the blood across the vessel walls into infected tissues. This margination and emigration from the blood of leukocytes is a three-step process termed **extravasation,** which is regulated by **adhesion molecules** expressed by both the leukocyte and the endothelium (Collins 1995) (figure 12.6). Expression of adhesion molecules by endothelial cells is regulated by inflammatory cytokines including IL-1 and TNF-α.

The first step of extravasation is mediated by **selectin molecules** (e.g., L-selectin, P-selectin, E-selectin) expressed by the endothelium of venules, which bind with glycoproteins on leukocytes and cause leukocytes to roll along a "sticky" endothelial surface of the blood vessel. This is a rapid process. For example, E-selectin is activated by TNA-α in about one hour. The second step involves binding of **integrin molecules** (e.g., lymphocyte function associated antigen-1 [LFA-1], leukocyte adhesion receptor [Mac-1], very late antigen-4 [VLA-4], and murine mucosal homing receptor-1 [LPAM-1]) on leukocytes with

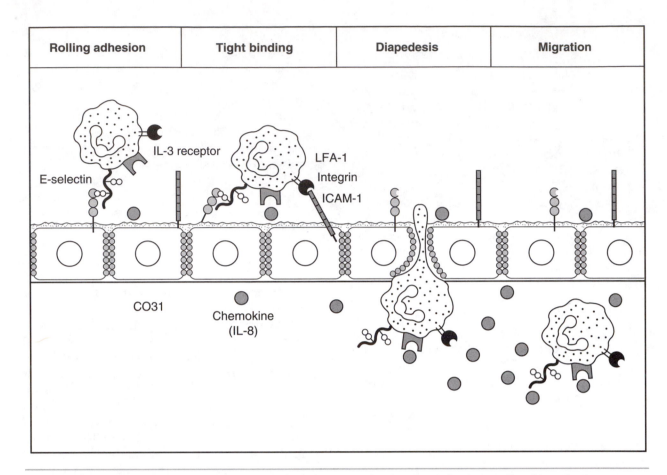

Figure 12.6   Extravasation and transmigration of a leukocyte to the site of an infection regulated by adhesion molecules and chemokines.

adhesion molecules on the endothelial surface (e.g., intercellular adhesion molecule-1 [ICAM-1] binds with LFA-1 integrin, vascular cell adhesion molecule-1 [VCAM-1] binds with integrin VLA-4 and LPAM-1, and mucosal addressin cell adhesion molecule-1 [MAdCAM-1] assists homing of lymphocytes to specific lymphoid sites) so that leukocytes stop rolling and become loosely attached to the endothelium, where they form the **marginal pool.** This is a slower process. For example, activation of VCAM-1 by IL-4 and other pro-inflammatory cytokines and ICAM-1 by IFN-γ takes five or more hours. The last step is transmigration of the leukocyte through the vascular wall into the infected tissue. This step is termed **diapedesis** and depends on the binding of leukocyte integrins with platelet endothelial cell adhesion molecule-1 (PECAM-1), an adhesion molecule expressed by platelets and on the junctions between endothelial cells, and erosion of the endothelial basement membrane by proteas-

es (enzymes that decompose proteins) released by the leukocyte. After an infection is contained, lymphocytes return to the bloodstream via the thoracic duct, and some recirculate in the lymph and blood through the same tissue acting as antigen sentinels based on memory of past antigen exposure (this is called "homing"). Monocytes and granulocytes do not reenter the lymph and blood circulation from infected tissue.

Immunomodulation by the Nervous and Endocrine Systems

Activation of the sympathetic nervous system (SNS) and the **hypothalamic-pituitary-adrenocortical axis (HPA axis)** helps regulate the immune response during heavy exercise and other types of stress (figure 12.7).

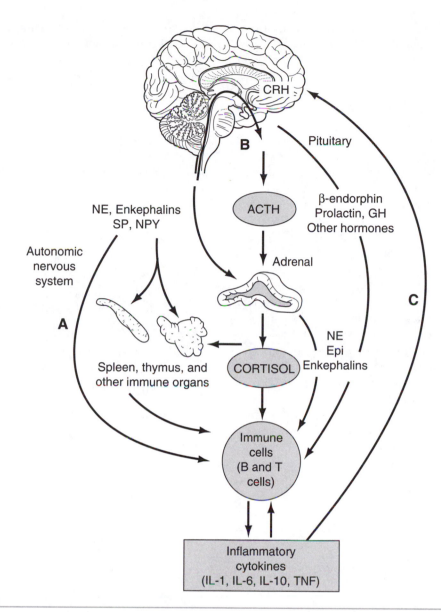

Figure 12.7 Schematic of the interaction between the autonomic nervous and hypothalamic-pituitary-adrenal cortical systems and the immune system.

Adapted from S.F. Maier and L.R. Watkins, 1998, "Cytokines for psychologists: Implications of bi-directional immune-to-brain communication for understanding behavior, mood, and cognition," *Psychological Review* 105(1): 83-107. © 1998 by the American Psychological Association. Adapted with permission.

Sympathetic Innervation and Immunomodulation

The autonomic nervous system (ANS) includes the parasympathetic nervous system (PNS) and the sympathetic nervous system (SNS), which regulate the organism's internal environment. The SNS controls the flight-or-fight reaction to **stressors,** whereas the PNS governs rest and, along with the **enteric nervous system,** digestion. In a stressful situation, the SNS is activated by the **hypothalamus,** resulting in increased sympathetic nerve traffic to target organs such as the heart and immune tissues. Immune organs are stimulated by catecholamines (norepinephrine and epinephrine) released from the sympathetic nerve terminals and are modulated by the hormonal effects of these catecholamines after they are secreted into the blood from the adrenal medulla (Maier and Watkins 1998).

Figure 12.8 illustrates the influence of catecholamines on leukocytosis, the migration of leukocytes from lymphoid organs into the blood. Noradrenergic nerves to the spleen and noradrenergic nerve ends in the spleen have been found in rats. In humans, β-adrenergic receptors have been identified on lymphocytes, including NK cells. Infusion of epinephrine results in increased numbers of NK cells activated by lymphokines such as IL-2 (Kappel et al. 1998) and an immediate but short-lived increase in the **cytolytic** (i.e., cell killing) activity of NK cells (Tonnesen, Christensen, and Brinklov 1987).

It is now known that epinephrine increases the number of lymphocytes, especially NK cells, that leave the spleen or other lymphoid organs by activating β_2-adrenoreceptors. The influence of catecholamines on the trafficking of granulocytes from the spleen to the blood is regulated by α-adrenoreceptors (Ernstrom and Sandberg 1973). Prior to those findings, it was thought that epinephrine caused the spleen to contract, spilling its store of lymphocytes by mechanical action. This view was abandoned, though, when other studies showed that epinephrine still induced lymphocytosis in animals after the spleen had been removed. In the 1990s it was found that emotional stress or an injection of norepinephrine increased blood levels of NK cells in people without a spleen as much as or more than in people with spleens. The most likely explanation for this observation is that catecholamines cause

NK cells to leave the marginal pool, apparently by inhibiting adhesion molecules on NK cells. The shearing force of increased blood flow can also contribute to the exit of leukocytes from the marginal pool. The additional circulating granulocytes induced by catecholamines come both from the marginal pool and from bone marrow. In contrast, the increased NK cells appear to come mainly from the marginal pool rather than bone marrow. NK cells do not follow the same recirculation pathway between lymph and blood (i.e., via lymph nodes and the thoracic duct) as do other lymphocytes.

> ••• *Leukocytosis from the marginal pool is mainly explained by inhibition of adhesion molecules by catecholamines and by shearing forces of increased blood flow during exercise.*

Activation of the HPA Axis and Immunomodulation

Neuroendocrine responses to stressors include increased levels of **glucocorticoids,** such as **cortisol** and corticosterone, in circulating blood as a result of activation of the HPA axis. Synthesis and secretion of releasing factors such as **corticotropin-releasing hormone (CRH)** by the hypothalamus

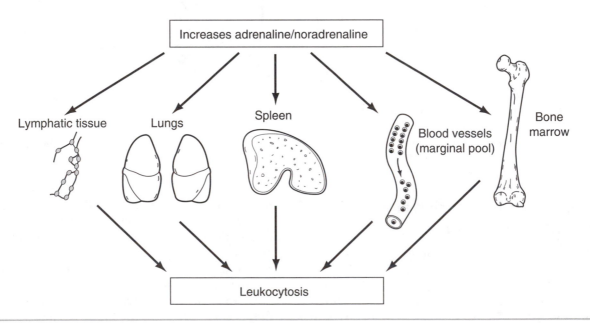

Figure 12.8 Effects of catecholamines on leukocyte circulation.

Adapted from *Brain, Behavior, and Immunity* 10, R.J. Benschop, M. Rodriguez-Feuerhahn, and M. Schedlowski, "Catecholamine-induced leukocytosis: Early observation, current research, and future directions," pgs. 77-91, Copyright 1996, with permission from Elsevier.

activate the pituitary gland to secrete hormones such as **adrenocorticotropic hormone (ACTH),** which in turn leads to the release of glucocorticoids from the adrenal cortex. Increased levels of circulating glucocorticoids regulate organs and cells of the immune system that possess receptors for these hormones (Maier and Watkins 1998). The effects of cortisol on immunity are inconsistent in humans, but many studies show that short-term increases in blood levels of cortisol contribute to the migration of granulocytes and lymphocytes from the blood circulation back to lymph organs as a stress response ends. However, long-term exposure of lymphocytes to cortisol, as during periods of repeated severe stress, can contribute to suppression of the immune system's ability to fight an infection.

> ••• *Short-term increases in blood levels of cortisol help regulate the migration of granulocytes and lymphocytes from the blood circulation back to lymph organs after a stress response ends. Long-term exposure of lymphocytes to cortisol during repeated stress can suppress the immune system's ability to fight an infection.*

Other Mechanisms

In addition to the SNS stimulation of immune tissues and increased level of adrenal hormones, opiates and **endogenous** opioid peptides appear to play a role in the regulation of immunity during stress. Opioid receptors have been found on large, granular lymphocytes, which include NK cells. Intermittent stress can activate the opioid system and suppress NK cell activity. That suppression is blunted by opioid antagonists.

Physical Activity and Immunity: The Evidence

After the German physiologist G. Schulz (1893) reported that muscle activity produced an increase in the number of leukocytes in the blood, several-fold increases in blood leukocytes were reported in four men after they ran the Boston Athletic Association's marathon of 1901 (Larrabee 1902) and in another group of men after a 400-m race (Garrey and Butler 1929). Lymphocytes increased in number within the first 10 min

of exercise, and this was followed by an increase in neutrophils—the same pattern seen after an injection of epinephrine. Hence, it was hypothesized that an increase in epinephrine levels during exercise was responsible for leukocytosis during exercise (Martin 1932). Modern studies have generally confirmed those early observations of leukocytosis in response to exercise (Pedersen and Hoffman-Goetz 2000; Woods, Ceddia et al. 1999; Woods, Lowder, and Keylock 2002).

Acute Exercise

Among normal, healthy people, the numbers of several types of immune cells, especially natural killer cells and neutrophils, are usually elevated during and immediately after a session of moderate- to high-intensity exercise (50%–85% $\dot{V}O_2$max; Fiatarone et al. 1988; Lewicki et al. 1988; Moyna et al. 1996; Murray et al. 1992; Palmo et al. 1995; Rhind et al. 1999). Neutrophils remain elevated for several hours, and lymphocytes return to normal levels within 2 h (Lewicki et al. 1988) to 24 h after the exercise (Espersen et al. 1996). However, after heavy, prolonged exercise, numbers of lymphocytes and NK cells can be depressed below normal levels for up to 6 h after exercise (Espersen et al. 1996). One view is that this period of immunosuppression after heavy exercise provides a window of susceptibility to infection if exposure to a pathogen occurs while the number of cytotoxic cells is below normal (Hoffman-Goetz and Pedersen 1994).

> ••• *A temporary suppression of the immune system after heavy exercise may provide a window of susceptibility to infection if exposure to a pathogen occurs while the number of cytotoxic cells is below normal.*

Macrophages

Acute exercise increases the number of monocytes circulating in the blood. This increase in monocytes (as for other leukocytes) is best explained by an influx of cells from the marginal pool. Exceptions to this increase are the migration of monocytes from the blood during prolonged exercise of several hours and a likely increase in the region of an infection after exhaustive exercise. The latter exception makes sense, as a localized infection would logically have higher biological priority than would circulatory adjustments during exercise. Exercise also has stimulatory effects on phagocytosis, antitumor activity, reactive oxygen and nitrogen metabolism, and chemotaxis of macrophages, but most of the studies that investigated these effects used mice rather than humans as subjects (Woods, Davis et al. 1999). Studies of mice also have shown that exercise training can increase macrophage antitumor activity, regardless of age. However, not all macrophage functions are enhanced by exercise. Reductions in the expression of MHC II by macrophages and in their antigen-presenting capacity have been reported. Hence, it has been suggested that exercise temporarily increases the phagocytic function of macrophages while inhibiting their accessory cell functions (Woods et al. 2000).

Lymphocytes

Many studies have suggested that the ability of T lymphocytes and B lymphocytes to proliferate (i.e., to grow and to reproduce by cloning) is increased when they are exposed to some mitogenic factors (factors that induce clonal expansion by lymphocytes, e.g., IL-2 and pokeweed) and inhibited when exposed to other mitogenic factors (e.g., phytohemagglutinin and concanavalin A). However, it appears that those changes merely reflect the number of lymphocytes circulating in the blood during and immediately after exercise, not a real change in the growth and division of individual lymphocytes (Pedersen and Hoffman-Goetz 2000) (table 12.1). Generally, acute exercise temporarily decreases the number of T lymphocytes and increases the number of natural killer cells circulating in the blood.

Natural Killer Cells

A recent quantitative review of 27 published studies conducted on a total of 390 people indicated that the cumulative effect of acute exercise was an increase in NK cytotoxicity (i.e., the killing of tumor cells **in vivo** by NK cells) of 1.2 standard deviations (95% CI: 0.37–2.1; Hong and Dishman 2004). Results changed distinctly over time, with a marked increase in cytotoxicity during and soon after exercise, a decrease below pre-exercise basal levels 1 to 3 h after exercise, and a return to the basal level within 24 h. Changes did not differ according to the mode or intensity of the exercise but were larger for exercise that lasted between 20 min and 2 h than for exercise longer than 2 h (e.g., Espersen et al. 1996; Nielsen et al. 1998; Rhind et al. 1999). Changes were

TABLE 12.1   EFFECT OF STRENUOUS EXERCISE ON THE IMMUNE SYSTEM

	During exercise	After exercise
Neutrophil count	↑	↑↑
Monocyte count		↑
Lymphocyte count	↑	↓
CD4+ T cell count	↑	↓
CD8+ T cell count	↑	↓
CD19+ B cell count	↑	↓
CD16+56+ NK cell count	↑	↓
Lymphocyte apoptosis	↑	↑
Proliferative response to mitogens	↓	↓
Antibody response in vitro	↓	↓
Saliva IgA	↓	↓
Delayed type hypersensitivity response (skin test)		↓
NK cell activity	↑	↓
Lymphokine activated killer cell activity	↑	↓
C-reactive protein		↑

↑, increase; ↓, decrease; ↑ ↑, marked increase; TNF-α, tumor necrosis factor-α; TNF-R, tumor necrosis factor receptors; IL, interleukin; MIP, macrophage inflammatory protein.

Reprinted, by permission, from B.K. Pedersen and L. Hoffman-Goetz, 2000, "Exercise and the immune system: Regulation, integration, and adaptation," *Physiological Reviews* 80: 1055-1081.

larger among people who were either sedentary or physically active in their leisure but had not undergone exercise training designed to increase their physical fitness. The changes in NK cytotoxicity after exercise are probably the result of changes in the number of NK cells in the blood more so than changes in the ability of individual NK cells to lyse tumor cells. For example, most studies have found that when cytolytic activity of NK cells in the blood is appropriately expressed relative to NK cell number, it is not changed by exercise (Moyna et al. 1996; Nieman et al. 1995; Palmo et al. 1995).

Levels of prostaglandins (e.g., PGE2), β-endorphin, and catecholamines have been investigated as possible mechanisms or mediators of altered NK cell activity after acute exercise (Fiatarone et al. 1988; Moyna et al. 1996; Murray et al. 1992; Rhind et al. 1999), but there are too few studies using uniform methods to draw conclusions. Some evidence indicates that the activity of neutrophils, including chemotaxis, phagocytosis, and the oxidative burst, is enhanced after moderate-intensity exercise, especially in the upper airways.

*** *The increased killing of tumor cells by NK cells after acute exercise is probably the result of an increased number of NK cells in the blood rather than an increase in the ability of individual NK cells to kill tumor cells.*

Eccentric Muscle Contraction

Eccentric resistance exercise involving smaller muscle groups has been found both to increase (Palmo et al. 1995) and decrease (Malm, Lenkei, and Sjodin 1999) NK cell numbers in the blood circulation during exercise. In addition, the number of NK cells increases after a heavy exercise bout (80% $\dot{V}O_2$max) but not after light exercise (40% $\dot{V}O_2$max; Strasner et al. 1997). Other studies have shown that prolonged endurance exercise (e.g., 2-3 h) and shorter-term, heavy eccentric exercise can induce an inflammation-like response resulting in increased secretion of inflammatory cytokines (e.g., IL-1, IL-6, and TNF-α) by stimulating the liver's biosynthesis of acute-phase proteins. Also, neutrophils and macrophages migrate to the area of muscle damage to remove the debris of dead cells.

Natural Killer Cells After Exercise Training

Too few studies of the effects of chronic exercise on macrophages, neutrophils, and T and B lymphocytes have been conducted to draw conclusions about the adaptations of these immune cells to repeated physical activity (Woods, Davis

et al. 1999). Results are somewhat clearer for NK cells. A half dozen exercise training studies and another handful of cross-sectional comparisons between exercise-trained and untrained people have shown cumulative mean increases in numbers of NK cells of 0.6 standard deviation (95% CI: 0.3–0.9) and 1.0 standard deviation (95% CI: 0.7–1.4), respectively (Hong and Dishman 2004).

Results of individual studies have not consistently shown significant changes in NK cell activity, however (Shephard and Shek 1999). No change in NK cell activity or in blood mononuclear cell numbers or proliferation was found in 18 rheumatoid arthritis patients after eight weeks of progressive cycle exercise training (Baslund et al. 1993). Neither 12 to 15 weeks of a walking exercise program (45 min at 60%–75% maximal HR, five days per week; Nieman, Nehlsen-Cannarella et al. 1990) nor 8 weeks of combination of aerobic and resistance training (Scanga et al. 1998) influenced NK cell activity or circulating levels. Six months of aerobic exercise by elderly men and women did not significantly affect NK cell activity or leukocyte counts (Woods, Davis et al. 1999). In contrast, a cross-sectional study by Rhind et al. (1994) found that physically trained individuals (with $\dot{V}O_2$max of 57 ml · kg^{-1} · min^{-1}) showed higher levels of circulating total leukocytes, granulocytes, and NK cells compared with previously untrained control individuals ($\dot{V}O_2$max of 39 ml · kg^{-1} · min^{-1}).

Compared with the evidence from human studies, the effect of exercise training on NK cell cytotoxicity in mice has been more consistent. An hour and a half of daily, moderate-intensity swimming for 20 days increased NK cell activity in mice (Ferrandez and De la Fuente 1996). Hoffman-Goetz, Arumugam, and Sweeny (1994) conducted a series of studies on NK cell activity and tumor metastasis following exercise training in mice. After nine weeks of wheel running and treadmill training exercise, male C3H mice were injected with tumor cells. After three weeks of tumor development and no exercise, the mice were killed. Trained mice demonstrated enhanced splenic NK cell activity and lower tumor cell retention in the lungs (MacNeil and Hoffman-Goetz 1993b). Treadmill training for 10 weeks enhanced NK cytotoxicity in mice measured **in vitro** (Simpson and Hoffman-Goetz 1990), and 9 weeks of both voluntary wheel running and treadmill training resulted in increased cytotoxicity both in vivo and in vitro (MacNeil and Hoffman-Goetz 1993a). A dissociation between NK cytotoxicity and tumor metastasis was found in female mice that received an injection of tumor cells; mice with previously elevated LAK cell (NK cells activated by lymphokines) activity measured in vitro showed higher tumor multiplicity after eight weeks of voluntary wheel running (Hoffman-Goetz, Arumugam, and Sweeny 1994).

In contrast to studies of mice, basal splenic NK cell activity in rats did not change after 6 weeks of voluntary wheel running (Dishman et al. 1995), 6 weeks of treadmill running (Dishman, Warren et al. 2000), or 15 weeks of treadmill running (Nasrullah and Mazzeo 1992). Conversely, reduced immune functions including NK cell activity in obese Zucker rats were restored after treadmill exercise five days per week for 40 weeks (Moriguchi et al. 1998).

The balance of the evidence in humans and in rodents is that chronic physical activity does not alter basal NK activity, despite a temporary enhancement of NK cytotoxicity right after an exercise session. However, other studies in rats indicate that chronic physical activity, independently of any fitness changes, protects against the suppression of NK cell activity after stress (Dishman et al. 1995; Dishman, Hong et al. 2000; Dishman, Warren et al. 2000).

> ••• *Despite strong evidence that acute exercise temporarily increases the number of NK cells in the blood, the effects of exercise training on basal NK activity have been inconsistent in studies of both humans and rodents.*

Investigators have not always clearly described the use of force in studies of swimming and treadmill running and have used different strains of rats and mice that differ in their inherent running behavior. Hence, it remains important to determine the effects of chronic exercise independently of the co-occurring stress of forced, rather than voluntary, exercise. Although exercise training has been found to augment NK cell activity in rats and mice, it has not been shown whether exercise training enhances peripheral blood NK cytotoxicity in humans. The insignificant effect of exercise training on resting NK cell activity observed in human studies raises questions regarding the nature of the exercise program (its

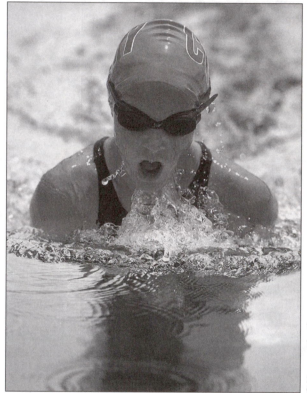

© Human Kinetics

Effects of Exercise

Acute exercise	Chronic exercise
Increases • Blood levels of granulocytes (mainly neutrophils) • Blood levels of monocytes • Phagocytic activity of macrophages • Blood levels of NK cells	Increases • NK cell cytotoxicity? • Risk of upper-respiratory infection (strenuous exercise)
Decreases • Blood levels of T lymphocytes • NK cell cytotoxicity (strenuous exercise)	Decreases • Risk of upper-respiratory infection (moderate exercise) • Tumor growth

Reprinted, by permission, from B.K. Pedersen and L. Hoffman-Goetz, 2000, "Exercise and the immune system: Regulation, integration, and adaptation," *Physiological Reviews* 80: 1055-1081.

intensity, duration, etc.) as it might affect different adaptations in NK cell activity.

Overtraining and Immune Suppression?

A few population-based surveys suggested that heavy, prolonged exercise can have a negative impact on immunity. Among 2,300 runners in the 1987 Los Angeles Marathon, the incidence of self-reported infection during the week after the race was six times higher (13%) than among similar runners who did not run the marathon (Nieman, Johannsen et al. 1990). In a cohort of over 500 runners, those who trained more than 17 miles (27 km) a week for a year had twice the rate of upper-respiratory infections (URI) as those who ran less than 10 miles (16 km) a week (Heath et al. 1991). Some small clinical studies have reported decreased levels of neutrophils and increased rates of URI among endurance athletes undergoing heavy training, but, to date, no clear association between those two responses has been shown (Davis and Colbert 1997).

In cross-country skiing, the chronic stress of strenuous training may combine with the drying effect of breathing cold, dry air to both suppress immunoglobulin responses in the airways and reduce the mucous barrier against bacteria and viruses. Also, some studies suggest that temporary immune suppression for 24 to 48 h after prolonged running (e.g., a marathon race) may lower resistance to URI (Nieman and Pedersen 1999). A common clinical recommendation by physicians is to avoid exercise when the symptoms of an infection extend below the neck, as is the case during a bout of flu or high fever. When symptoms are localized about the neck, exercise does not appear to worsen symptoms.

Men Infected With the Human Immunodeficiency Virus

Several studies have examined whether men diagnosed as positive for human immunodeficiency virus (HIV) respond favorably to chronic exercise. Though long-term morbidity and mortality studies with large numbers of men have not been conducted, small clinical studies generally have found that the prudent use of aerobic and resistance exercise training within professionally accepted guidelines for healthy adults (e.g., Pollock et al. 1998) leads to increased cardiorespiratory and muscular fitness without adverse effects on the numbers of blood lymphocytes or health (LaPerriere et al. 1990; Rigsby et al. 1992).

Cancer Survivors

There have been at least a half dozen studies of whether regular exercise can positively influence the immune system of cancer survivors. A comprehensive review of those studies published between 1994 and 2000 reported that four out of the six studies found statistically significant improvements in a number of cancer-related immune system components associated with exercise (Fairey et al. 2002). Nonetheless, methodological problems of small samples, weak research designs that incompletely controlled for confounders, poorly standardized prescriptions of the exercise dose, or limited measures of physical fitness and immune responses were noted by the authors of the review as limitations that prevent a clear interpretation of the results. Nonetheless, the preliminary findings are sufficiently encouraging to show the need for controlled clinical trials of whether exercise can independently reduce the risk of cancer recurrence and secondary malignancies and increase survival times among cancer survivors.

Mechanisms of Alterations in Monocytes, Granulocytes, and Natural Killer Cells After Acute Exercise

Acute exercise induces leukocytosis, but the mechanisms have yet to be clearly elucidated. The major catalysts to leukocytosis during infection are colony stimulating factors. If exercise induces an acute-phase-like response, as several researchers believe, it is plausible that increases in circulating granulocytes and monocytes in response to exercise are mainly the result of increases in colony-stimulating factors, independently of epinephrine. A recent study found that increases in blood levels of IL-6 and G-CSF after a maximal treadmill exercise test each were correlated with the increase in circulating neutrophils measured 1 to 2 hours after the exercise ended (Yamada et al. 2002). Another study of vigorous, prolonged exercise (running at 75% of $\dot{V}O_2max$ for 2.5 h) reported a nearly 30-fold increase in circulating IL-6 and a 3-fold increase in circulating neutrophils (Steensberg et al. 2001). Epinephrine infusion resulted in just a 6-fold increase in IL-6 and no increase in neutrophils. In contrast, both exercise and epinephrine infusion increased the numbers of circulating lymphocytes to a similar level (Steensberg et al. 2001).

Likewise, the mechanisms underlying the marked increase in NK cell percentage after exercise are not fully known. The role of the spleen in leukocyte redistribution during or after acute exercise was investigated in individuals who had undergone splenectomy (Baum, Geitner, and Liesen 1996). Marked leukocytosis was shown after exhaustive cycling exercise but did not differ between splenectomized and control individuals. Markedly increased blood pressure and cardiac output during acute exercise might contribute to leukocytosis by freeing cells that are loosely attached to the vessel walls. It has been hypothesized that acute exercise results in a shedding of adhesion molecules on lymphocytes, resulting in lymphocytes' detaching from the vascular endothelium and surging into the circulation.

Increased levels of neutrophils and lymphocytes have been observed after intense resistance exercise (six sets of 10RM leg squats) in women, but the percentages of T, B, and NK cells that expressed the adhesion molecule L-selectin decreased in peripheral blood (Miles et al. 1998). That finding suggests a shedding of L-selectin. Adrenergic mechanisms have been hypothesized to influence shedding of adhesion molecules on lymphocytes, including NK cells, which affects lymphocytes' migration and homing to circulation and lymphoid tissues (Benschop, Rodriguez-Feuerhahn, and Schedlowski 1996; Benschop, Schedlowski et al. 1997; Carlson, Fox, and Abell 1997). Treadmill running to exhaustion led to increased levels of circulating adhesion factors, which was diminished by administering a β-adrenoreceptor-blocking drug treatment (Rehman et al. 1997).

Whether these results indicate an exercise-induced decrease in the capacity of NK cells to adhere to adjacent tissues and cells or whether they indicate altered NK cell cytotoxicity during or after acute exercise is not established. However, it is possible that the molecular signaling that results in shedding of the adhesion molecules during exercise might also affect adhesion of NK cells to target cells, which could influence NK cell cytotoxicity.

Exercise and Cytokines

Only a few of the more than 60 known cytokines are likely to be influenced by exercise (Pedersen et al. 2001). Table 12.2 shows the effects of acute exercise on specific cytokines, such as IL-1, IL-2, IL-6, IL-7, interferons, and TNF as determined by experimental studies (Moldoveanu, Shephard, and Shek 2001). Those known as inflammatory cytokines (e.g., IL-1, IL-6, IL-8, IL-10, and TNF) are part of the acute-phase response to infection or injury. Some researchers believe that acute exercise produces an acute-phase-like response. It is also likely that very heavy exercise, especially novel eccentric exercise that damages muscle cells, evokes an inflammation-like response to clean up the debris of dead muscle cells.

TABLE 12.2 PLASMA LEVELS OF LYMPHOKINES DURING AND AFTER VIGOROUS EXERCISE	During exercise	After exercise
Interleukin-1	↑	↑
Interleukin-6	↑↑	↑
Interleukin-8	↑	↑
Interleukin-10	↑	↑
Tumor necrosis factor-α	↑	↑
Tumor necrosis factor-receptors	↑	↑
Interferon	↔	↔

↑, increase; ↑↑, marked increase; ↔, no change.

Adapted from data in Pedersen, B.K., and L. Hoffman-Goetz. 2000. Exercise and the immune system: Regulation, integration, and application. *Physiological Reviews* 80: 1055-1081.

Interleukin-1 (IL-1)

Blood levels of IL-1 are unchanged from resting levels immediately after exercise but are elevated 2 to 3 h after exercise (Cannon et al. 1986; Evans et al. 1986; Haahr et al. 1991; Lewicki et al. 1988). Most studies did not use a control group that did not exercise, however, so some of the increases in IL-1 after exercise might be explainable by natural circadian variations in IL-1 levels during the day (e.g., Smith et al. 1992). Other possible explanations include a delay in the synthesis of new cytokines that requires some time after exercise ends or altered migration of cytokines between lymph tissues and the blood.

IL-1 levels in muscles are elevated immediately after heavy eccentric resistance exercise of the type that damages muscle cells (Fielding et al. 1993). Levels remained elevated five days postexercise, in spite of decreasing muscle damage. This is consistent with the concept that IL-1 contributes to prolonged metabolic alterations following eccentric exercise.

Interleukin-2 (IL-2)

IL-2 levels in blood are lowered during exercise (Espersen et al. 1990; Lewicki et al. 1988; Tvede et al. 1993) and 2 h after exercise (Lewicki et al. 1988; Tvede et al. 1993). That decrease in IL-2 is followed by a compensatory increase in the numbers of IL-2 receptors observed after exercise (Espersen et al. 1990; Sprenger et al. 1992). The changes in IL-2 numbers after exercise probably reflect the initial exit and subsequent return to the blood circulation of T lymphocytes, which produce IL-2. An increase in IL-2 levels has been found 24 h after strenuous exercise sufficient to cause muscle damage and inflammation (Espersen et al. 1990).

Interleukin-6 (IL-6)

Blood levels of IL-6 are increased by as much as 100 times basal levels after acute exercise, depending upon the intensity, duration, and type of exercise (Febbraio and Pedersen 2002). The timing of peak levels of IL-6 in the blood also depends upon the type of muscle contraction. IL-6 levels increased during a graded cycling or treadmill test to exhaustion and remained elevated between about 20 min and 1 h after the tests ended (Rivier et al. 1994; Yamada et al. 2002). A 20-km run lasting about 2 h resulted in increased levels of IL-6 in both blood and urine during, 1 h after, and 5 h after the run (Sprenger et al. 1992). Treadmill running at 75% of VO_2max for 2.5 h led to a 29-fold increase in blood levels of IL-6 during exercise (Steensberg et al. 2001). Though the main sources of IL-6 are activated monocytes, macrophages, fibroblasts, and vascular endothelial cells, increased levels of IL-6 in the blood after exercise appear to come from contracting skeletal muscle. It is plausible that increases in IL-6 with exercise promote muscle energy metabolism (e.g., glycogenolysis and lipolysis) and enhance insulin sensitivity by inhibiting TNF-α (which has an insulin resistance effect). It also is likely that IL-6 is indicative of an inflammatory response to muscle damage, depending upon the nature of the muscle contraction. IL-6 increases resulting from muscle damage are smaller and occur later than increases resulting directly

from muscle contraction (Febbraio and Pedersen 2002); they seem to be independent of epinephrine and lactate responses to exercise but are blocked by indomethacin, a nonsteroidal anti-inflammatory drug (Rhind et al. 2002). Increases in IL-6 after prolonged, intense exercise are followed by smaller increases in the anti-inflammatory cytokine IL-10 (Febbraio and Pedersen 2002), suggesting a compensatory, homeostatic response.

Tumor Necrosis Factor-Alpha

Studies generally agree that plasma TNF-α levels are unchanged during exercise (Espersen et al. 1990; Haahr et al. 1991; Rivier et al. 1994; Smith et al. 1992), 20 min after exercise (Rivier et al. 1994), and 2 to 24 h after exercise (Haahr et al. 1991; Smith et al. 1992). One study reported increased levels of TNF-α in urine during and 1 h after exercise (Sprenger et al. 1992), suggesting that TNF-α is rapidly removed from circulation. Quick excretion of TNF-α is plausible as a protection against the toxic effects of the accumulation of high levels of TNF-α in blood and other tissues. The response by TNF-α to exercise may depend upon the duration or intensity of exercise, as strenuous, prolonged exercise such as marathon running is accompanied by a small increase in blood levels of TNF-α near the end of the run and afterward (Febbraio and Pedersen 2002).

Interferon-Gamma

Studies of IFN-γ in response to exercise have found no effects. Haahr et al. (1991) reported no change in plasma levels of IFN-γ during exercise and 2 and 24 h following exercise. Sprenger et al. (1992) reported elevated urine levels of IFN-γ during exercise but a return to baseline levels within 1 h. Responses of IFN to exercise are not well investigated.

Chronic Effects of Exercise in Trained Versus Untrained People

Though a single session of vigorous exercise appears to be accompanied by a temporary activation of the immune system that is similar to the acute phases of inflammation and response to infection, it is not clear that chronic exercise has a meaningful effect on cytokines. In one study, basal levels of IL-1 in the blood at rest were higher among exercise-trained men than in untrained men (Evans et al. 1986). Also, all the untrained men, but only one of the trained men, had an increase in IL-1 blood levels 3 h after exercise. That finding could be plausibly explained by more muscle cell damage in the untrained men than in the trained men. In another study (Smith et al. 1992), exercise-trained and untrained men had the same blood levels of IL-1, IL-6, and TNF-α measured at rest and after exercise. The discrepant findings might be explainable by the extent or type of exercise training.

Possible Mechanisms

One plausible mechanism to explain the effects of strenuous, intense exercise on cytokine levels is that it elicits a response similar to the acute-phase response of infection. However, the elevation in blood IL-1 levels induced by exercise is smaller than that found during infection (Cannon et al. 1986; Evans et al. 1986). A popular hypothesis is that cytokine release in response to exercise occurs most reliably in response to localized muscle damage, especially IL-1 increases after eccentric resistance exercise (Fielding et al. 1993), in order to activate phagocytic removal of dead or injured cells as part of the healing process.

Another plausible mechanism is a hormone-induced elevation of cytokine levels. Elevated blood levels of stress hormones, especially epinephrine and norepinephrine, during exercise cause changes in lymphocyte number, which suggests that increased IL-1 and IL-6 levels after exercise may be the result of increased blood levels of catecholamines (Cannon et al. 1986; Haahr et al. 1991) or other neuropeptides (Jonsdottir 2000). Another possible explanation is that increased blood flow during exercise results in synthesis and release of cytokines in order to regulate a greater flux and mixing of leukocytes caused by the increased blood flow. A recent study concluded that prolonged (3 h) cycling and inclined walking was accompanied by leukocytosis and elevated blood concentrations of IL-1, IL-6, and TNF-α but no changes in **messenger RNA** for those cytokines, suggesting that acute upregulation of gene expression does not explain the increased levels of cytokines (Moldoveanu, Shephard, and Shek 2000).

Problems With the Research

Several problems with the methods used limit conclusions about whether exercise has an independent effect on cytokines. Few studies of acute effects of a single session of exercise used an appropriate control group to show that the changes after exercise were not just normal fluctuations that would also have been seen at rest during the same amount of time. Also, the intensity, duration, and type of exercise were dissimilar among many studies, making it impossible to compare dose responses among studies. Studies of whether exercise training affects cytokines typically compare a group of people who are already trained with a group who are regarded as untrained. Randomized clinical trials have not been reported, and mostly men have been studied. Few of the cross-sectional studies controlled for medication intake, alcohol intake, diet, activity level prior to the experiment, or existing illnesses. The methods used to assay cytokines also differed widely among studies, introducing unknown sources of error in the measurements.

Nonetheless, exercise appears to enhance the release of cytokines in plasma, urine, and muscle. IL-1 and IL-6 levels appear to increase after exercise. IL-2 levels decrease, with a concomitant increase in IL-2 receptor expression. TNF and IFN remained constant during exercise in the few studies that examined these particular cytokines. Trained individuals have higher cytokine levels than untrained individuals. Extremely intense activity has been shown to reduce immune function, presumably by reducing the production of glutamine in skeletal muscles and increasing oxidative stress. Glutamine metabolism has been found to provide essential fuel to immune cells, and decreased production leads to slower immune response and recovery. The oxidative stress that physical activity may cause may also increase the body's vulnerability to cell and tissue damage by free radicals. Free radicals have been hypothesized to be initiators of cancer; therefore, overtraining should be avoided in order to experience the protective benefits of physical activity.

Summary

Acute exercise results in a temporary increase in the numbers of white blood cells circulating in the blood, mainly neutrophils, natural killer cells, and monocytes. This leukocytosis is plausibly explained by increases in pro-inflammatory cytokines that induce an inflammatory-like, acute-phase response that activates colony stimulating factors to induce the proliferation of neutrophils and monocytes from bone marrow. The influx of natural killer cells into the blood probably comes mainly from the marginal pool, resulting from shearing forces of increased blood flow and inhibition of adhesion molecules that help lymphocytes adhere briefly to the endothelial cells of blood vessels. The general pattern of the leukocytosis is a marked increase during and shortly after moderate-intensity to vigorous exercise of durations of 20 min up to 2 h, followed by a reduction below preexercise basal levels that lasts for 1 to 3 h but returns to basal levels within 24 h. The clinical meaning of this pattern of leukocytosis has not yet been confirmed in humans, but some experts have proposed that the transient reduction in leukocytes after heavy exercise might open a window of susceptibility to infections. A limited amount of epidemiologic evidence showing increased risk of upper-respiratory infections after marathon running has been interpreted by some researchers as being consistent with that idea. Acute exercise also results in elevations of several lymphokines in the blood, suggesting that acute exercise mimics an acute-phase response to infection. However, increases in many of these lymphokines (e.g., interleukins and interferons) can simply be explained by the fact that the numbers of the lymphocytes that secrete them have increased, so whether exercise simulates an infection-like response remains to be verified.

Adaptations by the immune system to chronic exercise have been harder to document, but the majority of exercise training studies and cross-sectional comparisons of exercise-trained men and women with sedentary people generally suggest an enhancement of innate immunity as evidenced by increased killing of tumor cells by NK cells. A very few studies found increased killing of bacteria by neutrophils and greater phagocytosis by macrophages.

To date, most studies of physical activity and the immune response among humans have understandably been limited to descriptions of cells in the blood. Animal studies using mice and rats have been able to examine the effects of exercise on immune responses in lymph tissues other than blood and have begun to clarify the potential mechanisms and health consequences of immune responses to exercise. Preliminary findings suggest that moderately intense exercise can have a positive influence on cancer survivors, increase fitness among men who have HIV disease without further impairing the immune system, and possibly reduce the risk of upper-respiratory infections. In contrast, exhausting exercise and heavy endurance training has been associated with increased risk of infection in a few studies. Though limited in quantity and scientific quality,

the available evidence is encouraging enough to justify more randomized controlled trials and prospective cohort studies to clarify the health implications of short- and long-term physical activity on overall immune function, resistance to infection, and cancer risk.

Bibliography

Abbas, A.K., A.H. Lightman, and J.S. Pober. 1997. *Cellular and molecular immunology.* 3rd ed. Philadelphia: Saunders.

Baslund, B., K. Lyngberg, V. Andersen, J. Halkjaer-Kristensen, M. Hansen, M. Klokker, and B.K. Pedersen. 1993. Effect of 8 wk of bicycle training on the immune system of patients with rheumatoid arthritis. *Journal of Applied Physiology* 75 (4): 1691–1695.

Baum, M., T. Geitner, and H. Liesen. 1996. The role of the spleen in the leukocytosis of exercise: Consequences for physiology and pathophysiology. *International Journal of Sports Medicine* 17: 604–607.

Benschop, R.J., R. Geenen, P.J. Mills, B.D. Naliboff, J.K. Kiecolt-Glaser, T.B. Herbert, G. van der Pompe, G.E. Miller, K.A. Matthews, G.L.R. Godaert, et al. 1997. Cardiovascular and immune responses to acute psychological stress in young and old women: A meta-analysis. *Psychosomatic Medicine* 60: 290–296.

Benschop, R.J., M. Rodriguez-Feuerhahn, and M. Schedlowski. 1996. Catecholamine-induced leukocytosis: Early observations, current research, and future directions. *Brain, Behavior, and Immunity* 10: 77–91.

Benschop, R.J., M. Schedlowski, H. Wienecke, R. Jacobs, and R.E. Schmidt. 1997. Adrenergic control of natural killer cell circulation and adhesion. *Brain, Behavior, and Immunity* 11: 321–332.

Brines, R., L. Hoffman-Goetz, and B.K. Pedersen. 1996. Can you exercise to make your immune system fitter? *Immunology Today* 17 (6): 252–254.

Cannon, J., W. Evans, V. Hughes, C. Meredith, and C. Dinarello. 1986. Physiological mechanisms contributing to increased interleukin-1 secretion. *Journal of Applied Physiology* 61 (5): 1869–1874.

Carlson, S.L., S. Fox, and K.M. Abell. 1997. Catecholamine modulation of lymphocyte homing to lymphoid tissues. *Brain, Behavior, and Immunity* 11: 307–320.

Cohen, L.A., E. Boylan, M. Epstein, and E. Zang. 1992. Voluntary exercise and experimental mammary cancer. *Advances in Experimental and Medical Biology* 322: 41–59.

Cohen, L.A., M.E. Kendall, C. Meschter, M.A. Epstein, J. Reinhardt, and E. Zang. 1993. Inhibition of rat mammary tumorigenesis by voluntary exercise. *In Vivo* 2: 151–158.

Collins, T. 1995. Adhesion molecules in leukocyte emigration. *Scientific American Science and Medicine* 2 (6): 29–37.

Davis, J.M., and L.H. Colbert. 1997. The athlete's immune system, intense exercise, and overtraining. In *Perspectives in exercise science and sports medicine,* edited by D.R. Lamb and R. Murray, vol. 10, *Optimizing sport performance,* pp. 269–311. Carmel, IN: Cooper.

Dishman, R.K., S. Hong, J. Soares, G.L. Edwards, B.N. Bunnell, L. Jaso-Friedmann, and D.L. Evans. 2000. Activity wheel running blunts suppression of natural killer cell cytotoxicity after sympathectomy and footshock. *Physiology and Behavior* 71: 297–304.

Dishman, R.K., J.M. Warren, S. Hong, B.N. Bunnell, E.H. Mougey, J.L. Meyerhoff, L. Jaso-Friedmann, and D.L. Evans. 2000. Treadmill exercise training blunts suppression of splenic natural killer cell cytolysis after footshock. *Journal of Applied Physiology* 88: 2176–2182.

Dishman, R.K., J.M. Warren, S.D. Youngstedt, H. Yoo, B.N. Bunnell, E.H. Mougey, J.L. Meyerhoff, L. Jaso-Friedmann, and D.L. Evans. 1995. Activity-wheel running attenuates suppression of natural killer cell activity after foot shock. *Journal of Applied Physiology* 78 (4): 1547–1554.

Ernstrom, U., and G. Sandberg. 1973. Effects of adrenergic alpha- and beta-receptor stimulation on the release of lymphocytes and granulocytes from the spleen. *Scandinavian Journal of Haematology* 11: 275–286.

Espersen, G., A. Elbaek, E. Ernst, E. Toft, S. Kaalund, C. Jersild, and N. Grunnet. 1990. Effect of physical exercise on cytokines and lymphocyte subpopulations in human peripheral blood. *APMIS: Acta Pathologica, Microbiologica, et Immunologica Scandinavica* 98: 395–400.

Espersen, G.T., A. Elbaek, S. Schmidt-Olsen, E. Ejlersen, K. Varming, and N. Grunnet. 1996. Short-term changes in the immune system of elite swimmers under competition conditions: Different immunomodulation induced by various types of sport. *Scandinavian Journal of Medicine and Science in Sports* 6 (3): 156–163.

Evans, W., C. Meredith, J. Cannon, C. Dinarello, W. Frontera, V. Hughes, B. Jones, and H. Knuttgen. 1986. Metabolic changes following eccentric exercise in trained and untrained men. *Journal of Applied Physiology* 61: 1864–1868.

Fairey, A.S., K.S. Courneya, C.J. Field, and J.R. Mackey. 2002. Physical exercise and immune system function in cancer survivors: A comprehensive review and future directions. *Cancer* 94 (2): 539–551.

Febbraio, M.A., and B.K. Pedersen. 2002. Muscle-derived interleukin-6: Mechanisms for activation and possible biological roles. *Journal of the Federation of American Societies for Experimental Biology* 16: 1335–1347.

Felten, D.L., S.Y. Felten, D.L. Bellinger, S.L. Carlson, K.D. Ackerman, K.S. Madden, J.A. Olschowka, and S. Livnat. 1987. Noradrenergic sympathetic neural interactions with the immune system: Structure and function. *Immunological Review* 100: 225–260.

Felten, D.L., and J. Olschowka. 1987. Noradrenergic sympathetic innervation of the spleen: II. Tyrosine hydroxylase (TH)–positive nerve terminals form synapticlike contacts on lymphocytes in the splenic white pulp. *Journal of Neuroscience Research* 18: 37–48.

Ferrandez, M.D., and M. De la Fuente. 1996. Changes with aging, sex and physical exercise in murine natural killer activity and antibody-dependent cellular cytotoxicity. *Mechanisms of Ageing and Development* 86 (2): 83–94.

Fiatarone, M.A., J.E. Morley, E.T. Bloom, D. Benton, T. Makinodan, and G.F. Solomon. 1988. Endogenous opioids and the exercise-induced augmentation of natural killer cell activity. *Journal of Laboratory Clinical Medicine* 112 (5): 544–552.

Fielding, R., T. Manfredi, W. Ding, M. Fiatarone, W. Evans, and J. Cannon. 1993. Acute phase response in exercise: III. Neutrophil and IL-1 beta accumulation in skeletal muscle. *American Journal of Physiology* 265: R166–R172.

Gahmberg, C.G., L. Valmu, S. Fagerholm, P. Kotovuori, E. Ihanus, L. Tian, and T. Pessa-Morikawa. 1998. Leukocyte integrins and inflammation. *Cellular and Molecular Life Sciences* 54: 549–555.

Garrey, W.E., and V. Butler. 1929. Physiological leucocytosis. *American Journal of Physiology* 90: 355–356.

Haahr, P., B. Pedersen, A. Fomsgaard, N. Tvede, M. Diamant, K. Karlund, J. Halkjaer-Kristensen, and K. Bendtzen. 1991. Effect of physical exercise on in vitro production of interleukin-1, interleukin-6, tumor necrosis factor-α, interleukin-2 and interferon-γ. *International Journal of Sports Medicine* 12: 223–227.

Heath, G.W., E.S. Ford, T.E. Craven, C.A. Macera, K.L. Jackson, and R.R. Pate. 1991. Exercise and the incidence of upper respiratory tract infections. *Medicine and Science in Sports and Exercise* 23: 152–157.

Hoffman-Goetz, L., ed. 1996. *Exercise and immune function*. Boca Raton, FL: CRC Press.

Hoffman-Goetz, L., D. Apter, W. Denmark-Wahnefried, M.I. Goran, A. McTiernan, and M.E. Reichman. 1998. Possible mechanisms mediating an association between physical activity and breast cancer. *Cancer* 83 (3 Suppl.): 621–628.

Hoffman-Goetz, L., Y. Arumugam, and L. Sweeny. 1994. Lymphokine activated killer cell activity following voluntary physical activity in mice. *Journal of Sports and Medicine in Physical Fitness* 34 (1): 83–90.

Hoffman-Goetz, L., and B.K. Pedersen. 1994. Exercise and the immune system: A model of the stress response? *Immunology Today* 15: 382–387.

Hong, S., and R.K. Dishman. 2004. The effect of exercise on natural killer cell activity: A quantitative synthesis. Unpublished manuscript, The University of Georgia, Athens.

Irwin, M., R.L. Hauger, and M. Brown. 1992. Central corticotropin releasing hormone activates the sympathetic nervous system and reduces immune function: Increased responsivity of the aged rat. *Endocrinology* 131: 1047–1053.

Irwin, M., R.L. Hauger, M. Brown, and L. Britton. 1988. CRF activates autonomic nervous system and reduces natural killer cytotoxicity. *American Journal of Physiology* 5 (2): R744–R747.

Irwin, M., R.L. Hauger, L. Jones, M. Provencio, and K.T. Britton. 1990. Sympathetic nervous system mediates central corticotropin-releasing factor induced suppression of natural killer cytotoxicity. *Journal of Pharmacology and Experimental Therapeutics* 255: 101–107.

Jonsdottir, I.H. 2000. Neuropeptides and their interaction with exercise and immune function. *Immunology and Cell Biology* 78: 562–570.

Kanter, M.M. 1994. Free radicals, exercise, and antioxidant supplementation. *International Journal of Sport Nutrition* 4: 451–455.

Kappel, M., T.D. Poulsen, H. Galbo, and B.K. Pedersen. 1998. Influence of minor increases in plasma catecholamines on natural killer cell activity. *Hormone Research* 49: 22–26.

Katafuchi, T., S. Take, and T. Hori. 1993. Roles of sympathetic nervous system in the suppression of cytotoxicity of splenic natural killer cells in the rat. *Journal of Physiology (London)* 465: 343–357.

LaPerriere, A.R., M.H. Antoni, N. Schneiderman, G. Ironson, N. Klimas, P. Caralis, and M.A. Fletcher. 1990. Exercise intervention attenuates emotional distress and natural killer cell decrements following notification of positive serologic status for HIV-1. *Biofeedback and Self-Regulation* 15: 229–242.

Larrabee, R.C. 1902. Leucocytosis after violent exercise. *Journal of Medical Research* 7: 76–82.

Lee, I.M. 1995. Exercise and physical health: Cancer and immune function. *Research Quarterly for Exercise and Sport* 66: 286–291.

Lewicki, R., H. Tchorzewski, E. Majewska, Z. Nowak, and Z. Baj. 1988. Effect of maximal physical exercise on T-lymphocyte subpopulations and on interleukin-1 (IL-1) and interleukin-2 (IL-2) production in vitro. *International Journal of Sports Medicine* 9 (2): 114–117.

Mackinnon, L. 1999. *Advances in exercise immunology*. Champaign, IL: Human Kinetics.

MacNeil, B., and L. Hoffman-Goetz. 1993a. Chronic exercise enhances in vivo and in vitro cytotoxic mechanisms of natural immunity in mice. *Journal of Applied Physiology* 74 (1): 388–395.

———. 1993b. Exercise training and tumour metastasis in mice: Influence of time of exercise onset. *Anticancer Research* 13 (6A): 2085–2088.

Madden, K.S., K.D. Ackerman, S. Livnat, S.Y. Felten, and D.L. Felten. 1993. Neonatal sympathetic denervation alters development of natural killer (NK) cell activity in F344 rats. *Brain, Behavior, and Immunity* 7: 344–351.

Maier, S.F., and L.R. Watkins. 1998. Cytokines for psychologists: Implications of bidirectional immune-to-brain communication for understanding behavior, mood, and cognition. *Psychological Review* 105 (1): 83–107.

Maisel, A.S., T. Harris, C.A. Rearden, and M.C. Michel. 1990. β-adrenergic receptors in lymphocyte subsets after exercise: Alterations in normal individuals and patients with congestive heart failure. *Circulation* 82 (6): 2003–2010.

Malm, C., R. Lenkei, and B. Sjodin. 1999. Effects of eccentric exercise on the immune system in men. *Journal of Applied Physiology* 86 (2): 461–468.

Mandler, R.N., W.E. Mandler, and S.A. Serrate. 1986. β-endorphin augment the cytolytic activity and interferon production of natural killer cells. *Journal of Immunology* 136: 934–939.

Martin, H.E. 1932. Physiological leucocytosis. *Journal of Physiology* 75: 113–129.

Miles, M.P., S.K. Leach, W.J. Kraemer, K. Dohi, J.A. Bush, and A.M. Mastro. 1998. Leukocyte adhesion molecule expression during intense resistance exercise. *Journal of Applied Physiology* 84 (5): 1604–1609.

Moldoveanu, A.I., R.J. Shephard, and P.N. Shek. 2000. Exercise elevates plasma levels but not gene expression of IL-1beta, IL-6, and TNF-alpha in blood mononuclear cells. *Journal of Applied Physiology* 89 (4):1499–1504.

———. 2001. The cytokine response to physical activity and training. *Sports Medicine* 31 (2): 115–144.

Moriguchi, S., M. Kato, K. Sakai, S. Yamamoto, and E. Shimizu. 1998. Exercise training restores decreased cellular immune functions in obese Zucker rats. *Journal of Applied Physiology* 84 (1): 311–317.

Morville, R., P.C. Pesquies, and C.Y. Guezennee. 1979. Plasma variations in testicular and adrenal androgens during prolonged physical exercise in man. *Annals in Endocrinology* 40: 501–515.

Moyna, N.M., G.R. Acker, K.M. Weber, J.R. Fulton, F.L. Goss, R.J. Robertson, and B.S. Rabin. 1996. The effects of incremental submaximal exercise on circulating leukocytes in physically active and sedentary males and females. *European Journal of Applied Physiology* 74 (3): 211–218.

Murray, D.R., M. Irwin, C.A. Rearden, M. Ziegler, H. Motulsky, and A.S. Maisel. 1992. Sympathetic and immune interactions during dynamic exercise: Mediation via a beta 2-adrenergic-dependent mechanism. *Circulation* 86 (1): 203–213.

Nasrullah, I., and R.S. Mazzeo. 1992. Age-related immunosenescence in Fischer 344 rats: Influence of exercise training. *Journal of Applied Physiology* 73: 1932–1938.

Newsholme, E.A., and M. Parry-Billings. 1994. Effects of exercise on the immune system. In *Physical activity, fitness, and health,* edited by C. Bouchard, R. Shepard, and T. Stephens, pp. 451–455. Champaign, IL: Human Kinetics.

Nielsen, H.B., N.H. Secher, M. Kappel, and B.K. Pedersen. 1998. N-acetylcysteine does not affect the lymphocyte proliferation and natural killer cell activity responses to exercise. *American Journal of Physiology* 275 (4 Pt. 2): R1227–R1231.

Nieman, D.C., D.A. Henson, G. Gusewitch, B.J. Warren, R.C. Dotson, D.E. Butterworth, and S.L. Nehlsen-Cannarella.

1993. Physical activity and immune function in elderly women. *Medicine and Science in Sports and Exercise* 25: 823–831.

Nieman, D.C., D.A. Henson, C.S. Sampson, J.L. Herring, J. Suttles, M. Conley, M.H. Stone, D.E. Butterworth, and J.M. Davis. 1995. The acute immune response to exhaustive resistance exercise. *International Journal of Sports Medicine* 16 (5): 322–328.

Nieman, D.C., L.M. Johannsen, J.W. Lee, and K. Arabatzis. 1990. Infectious episodes in runners before and after the Los Angeles Marathon. *Journal of Sports Medicine and Physical Fitness* 30: 316–328.

Nieman, D.C., S.L. Nehlsen-Cannarella, P.A. Markoff, A.J. Balk-Lamberton, H. Yang, D.B. Chritton, J.W. Lee, and K. Arabatzis. 1990. The effects of moderate exercise training on natural killer cells and acute upper respiratory tract infections. *International Journal of Sports Medicine* 11: 467–473.

Nieman, D.C., and B.K. Pedersen. 1999. Exercise and immune function. *Sports Medicine* 27: 73–80.

Palmo, J., S. Asp, J.R. Daugaard, E.A. Richter, M. Klokker, and B.K. Pedersen. 1995. Effect of eccentric exercise on natural killer cell activity. *Journal of Applied Physiology* 78 (4): 1442–1446.

Pedersen, B.K., and L. Hoffman-Goetz. 2000. Exercise and the immune system: Regulation, integration, and adaptation. *Physiological Reviews* 80: 1055–1081.

Pedersen, B.K., A. Steensberg, C. Fischer, C. Keller, K. Ostrowski, and P. Schjerling. 2001. Exercise and cytokines with particular focus on muscle-derived IL-6. *Exercise Immunology Review* 7: 18–31.

Pollock, M.L., G.A. Gaesser, J.D. Butcher, J.P. Despres, R.K. Dishman, B.A. Franklin, and C.E. Garber. 1998. Recommended quantity and quality of exercise for developing and maintaining cardiorespiratory and muscular fitness, and flexibility in healthy adults. *Medicine and Science in Sports and Exercise* 30: 975–991.

Rehman, J., P.J. Mills, S.M. Carter, J. Chou, J. Thomas, and A.S. Maisel. 1997. Dynamic exercise leads to an increase in circulating ICAM-1: Further evidence for adrenergic modulation of cell adhesion. *Brain, Behavior, and Immunity* 11: 343–351.

Rhind, S.G., G.A. Gannon, R.J. Shephard, and P.N. Shek. 2002. Indomethacin modulates circulating cytokine responses to strenuous exercise in humans. *Cytokine* 19: 153–158.

Rhind, S.G., G.A. Gannon, M. Suzui, R.J. Shephard, and P.N. Shek. 1999. Indomethacin inhibits circulating PGE2 and reverses postexercise suppression of natural killer cell activity. *American Journal of Physiology* 276 (5 Pt. 2): R1496–R1505.

Rhind, S.G., P.N. Shek, S. Shinkai, and R.J. Shephard. 1994. Differential expression of interleukin-2 receptor alpha and beta chains in relation to natural killer cell subsets and aerobic fitness. *International Journal of Sports Medicine* 15 (6): 311–318.

Rigsby, L.W., R.K. Dishman, A.W. Jackson, G.S. Maclean, and P.B. Raven. 1992. Effects of exercise training on men seropositive for the human immunodeficiency virus-1. *Medicine and Science in Sports and Exercise* 24: 6–12.

Rivier, A., J. Pene, P. Chanez, F. Anselme, C. Caillaud, C. Prefaut, P. Godard, and J. Bousquet. 1994. Release of cytokines by blood monocytes during strenuous exercise. *International Journal of Sports Medicine* 15 (4): 192–198.

Scanga, C.B., T.J. Verde, A.M. Paolone, R.E. Andersen, and T.A. Wadden. 1998. Effects of weight loss and exercise training on natural killer cell activity in obese women. *Medicine and Science in Sports and Exercise* 30 (12): 1666–1671.

Schittek, B., R. Hipfel, B. Sauer, J. Bauer, H. Kalbacher, S. Stevanovic, M. Schirle, K. Schroeder, N. Blin, F. Meier, G.

Rassner, and C. Garbe. 2001. Dermcidin: A novel human antibiotic peptide secreted by sweat glands. *Nature Immunology* 2: 1133–1137.

Schulz, G. 1893. Experimentelle Untersuchungen über das Vorkommen und die diagnostische Bedeutung der Leukozytose. *Deutsches Archiv für Klinische Medizin* 51: 234.

Shavit, Y., G.W. Terman, J.W. Lewis, et al. 1986. Effects of footshock stress and morphine on natural killer lymphocytes in rats: Studies of tolerance and cross-tolerance. *Brain Research* 372: 382–385.

Shephard, R.J. 2002. Cytokine responses to physical activity, with particular reference to IL-6: Sources, actions, and clinical implications. *Critical Reviews in Immunology* 22: 165–182.

Shephard, R.J., and P.N. Shek. 1995. Cancer, immune function, and physical activity. *Canadian Journal of Applied Physiology* 20: 1–25.

———. 1999. Effects of exercise and training on natural killer cell counts and cytolytic activity. *Sports Medicine* 28: 177–195.

Simpson, J.R., and L. Hoffman-Goetz. 1990. Exercise stress and murine natural killer cell function. *Proceedings of the Society for Experimental Biology and Medicine* 195 (1): 129–135.

Smith, J., R. Telford, R. Baker, A. Hapel, and M. Weidermann. 1992. Cytokine immunoreactivity in plasma does not change after moderate endurance exercise. *Journal of Applied Physiology* 73 (4): 1396–1401.

Sprat, T. 1667. *The plague of Athens which hapned in the second year of the Peloponnesian Warr / first described in Greek by Thucydides, then in Latin by Lucretius, now attempted in English by Tho. Sprat.* London: Printed by E.C. for Henry Brome.

Sprenger, H., C. Jacobs, M. Nain, M. Gressner, H. Prinz, W. Wesemann, and D. Gemsa. 1992. Enhanced release of cytokines, interleukin-2 receptors, and neopterin after long-distance running. *Clinical Immunology and Immunopathology* 63 (2): 188–195.

Steensberg, A., C. Keller, R.L. Starkie, T. Osada, M.A. Febbraio, and B.K. Pedersen. 2002. IL-6 and TNF-alpha expression in, and release from, contracting human skeletal muscle. *American Journal of Physiology Endocrinology and Metabolism* 283: E1272–E1278.

Steensberg, A., A.D. Toft, P. Schjerling, J. Halkjaer-Kristensin, and B.K. Pedersen. 2001. Plasma interleukin-6 during strenuous exercise: Role of epinephrine. *American Journal of Physiology Cell Physiology* 281: C1001–C1004.

Strasner, A., J.M. Davis, M.L. Kohut, R.R. Pate, A. Ghaffar, and E. Mayer. 1997. Effects of exercise intensity on natural killer cell activity in women. *International Journal of Sports Medicine* 18 (1): 56–61.

Tonnesen, E., N.J. Christensen, and M.M. Brinklov. 1987. Natural killer cell activity during cortisol and adrenaline infusion in healthy volunteers. *European Journal of Clinical Investigation* 17: 497–503.

Tvede, N., M. Kappel, J. Halkjaer-Kristensen, H. Galbo, and B. Pedersen. 1993. The effect of light, moderate and severe bicycle exercise on lymphocyte subsets, natural and lymphokine activated killer cells, lymphocyte proliferative response and interleukin 2 production. *International Journal of Sports Medicine* 14 (5): 275–282.

Woods, J.A., M.A. Ceddia, B.W. Wolters, J.K. Evans, Q. Lu, and E. McAuley. 1999. Effects of 6 months of moderate aerobic exercise training on immune function in the elderly. *Mechanisms of Ageing and Development* 109 (1): 1–19.

Woods, J.A., J.M. Davis, J.A. Smith, and D.C. Nieman. 1999. Exercise and cellular innate immune function. *Medicine and Science in Sports and Exercise* 31: 57–66.

Woods, J.A., T.W. Lowder, and K.T. Keylock. 2002. Can exercise training improve immune function in the aged? *Annals of the New York Academy of Sciences* 959: 117–127.

Woods, J.A., Q. Lu, M.A. Ceddia, and T. Lowder. 2000. Special feature for the Olympics: Effects of exercise on the immune system: Exercise-induced modulation of macrophage function. *Immunology and Cell Biology* 78: 545–553.

Wu, A.H., A.S. Whittemore, L.N. Kolonel, E.M. John, R.P. Gallagher, D.W. West, J. Hankin, C.Z. Teh, D.M. Dreon, and R.S. Paffenbarger Jr. 1995. Serum androgens and sex hormone–binding globulins in relation to lifestyle factors in older African-American, white, and Asian men in the United States and Canada. *Cancer Epidemiology, Biomarkers and Prevention* 4 (7): 735–741.

Yamada, M., K. Suzuki, S. Kudo, M. Totsuka, S. Nakaji, and K. Sugawara. 2002. Raised plasma G-CSF and IL-6 after exercise may play a role in neutrophil mobilization into the circulation. *Journal of Applied Physiology* 92: 1789–1794.

Web Sites

www.biology.arizona.edu/immunology/immunology.html. An introductory, interactive site developed and maintained by the biology department at the University of Arizona that contains problem sets and tutorials about the immune system.

http://www.med.sc.edu:85/book/welcome.htm. An award-winning online textbook developed and maintained by the Department of Pathology and Microbiology at the University of South Carolina School of Medicine. Includes in-depth, illustrated chapters on immunology, bacteriology, and virology.

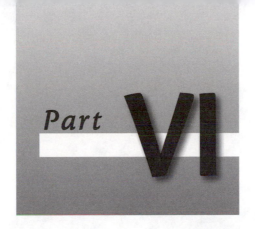

Part **VI**

PHYSICAL ACTIVITY AND SPECIAL CONCERNS

For the new millennium, the American Psychological Association has initiated the "Decade of Behavior," an interdisciplinary effort to promote behavioral and social science research. One of the themes of that effort is health. The preceding parts of this book have shown why the promotion of leisure-time physical activity has emerged as an important initiative for public health and quality of living in many economically developed nations and, more recently, in developing nations. The chapters in this part expand the view of public health beyond chronic diseases and premature death. The World Health Organization has already endorsed disability-adjusted life expectancy as an important way to judge healthy living beyond mere life expectancy in years. Moreover, the WHO has projected that depression will be second only to cardiovascular disease as the world's leading cause of death and disability by the year 2020. Nonetheless, it is important to acknowledge that participation in vigorous physical activity carries with it some risk. Chapter 15 discusses the hazards of physical activity. Leisure-time physical activity has remained below recommended levels in nations that keep population statistics about physical activity. The final chapter deals with the promotion of a safe, physically active lifestyle among all segments of the population.

Physical Activity and Mental Health

Opposite to Exercise is Idleness or want of exercise, the bane of body and minde . . . the chiefe author of all mischiefe, one of the seven deadly sinnes, and the sole cause of melancholy.

—*Robert Burton, Anatomy of Melancholy, 1632*

Our muscular vigor will . . . always be needed to furnish the background of sanity, serenity, and cheerfulness to life, to give moral elasticity to our disposition, to round off the wiry edge of fretfulness, and make us good-humored. . . .

—*William James, Talks to Teachers on Psychology:*
And to Students on Some of Life's Ideals, 1899

Mental health problems are a public health burden worldwide, decreasing the quality of life and adding substantially to health care costs. In the United States, about $150 billion are spent each year on mental health (Greenberg et al. 1993; Rice and Miller 1995). The most common disorders in the United States, **anxiety disorder** and depression, each cost about $45 billion a year and have annual prevalence rates of 17% and 11%, respectively, among people ages 15 to 54. Their lifetime prevalence rates are higher—25% for anxiety disorder and 20% for depression—and are nearly twice as high among women than men. The lifetime prevalence of depression is 21% among women and 13% among men. Anxiety disorders have a lifetime prevalence rate of 30% in women and 19% in men. The most common type of depression, major depressive episode, occurs at least once in a lifetime among 21% of adolescent girls and women through age 54; in contrast, the rate is about 12% in boys and men of those ages (Kessler et al. 1994). In contrast, men (35%) are almost twice as likely to have a substance abuse disorder during their lifetime as are women (18%).

The father of American psychology, William James, recognized the usefulness of exercise for decreasing worry and elevating **mood** at the turn of the 20th century. Nearly 600 years earlier, Hippocrates had prescribed exercise for his patients suffering from depression, which he called *melancholia,* a term still used today for severe, somatic depression. As noted by the 17th-century theologian Robert Burton (1632) in *The Anatomy of Melancholy,* sloth or physical inactivity has been regarded as a cause of depression since antiquity. The recent report of the U.S. Surgeon General on mental health included physical activity as an important part of mental hygiene (U.S. Department of Health and Human Services 1999). This chapter describes the evidence that supports the clinical observations of James and Hippocrates.

A protective effect of physical activity against the primary (i.e., initial incidence) and secondary (i.e., recurrence) risk of developing depression and anxiety disorders would have great potential importance for public health. Not only are anxiety disorders the most prevalent mental health problem in the United States, they are also risk factors for cardiovascular morbidity and mortality. Moreover, the World Health Organization (WHO) has projected that depression will be second only to cardiovascular disease as the world's leading cause of death and disability by the year 2020 (Murray and Lopez 1997).

Depression

The American Psychiatric Association recognizes four types of mood disorders: (1) depression, (2) bipolar or **manic-depressive disorder,** (3) mood disorders due to a medical condition, and (4) substance-induced mood disorders. The first category includes **major depression** and the milder chronic form, **dysthymia.** The two principal subtypes of major depression are melancholic and atypical depression, although 53% of patients who meet the criteria for major depression do not meet the criteria for either subtype. The second category, bipolar or manic-depressive disorder, is characterized by periods of depression alternating with periods of elevated, expansive, or irritable mood, exaggerated self-confidence, risky or asocial behavior, or even paranoia.

Manic-Depressive Disorders

Bipolar I: Major depression alternates with mania, or uncontrollable elation.

Bipolar II: Major depression alternates with hypomania, a milder form of elation.

Cyclothymia: Swings between hypomania and milder depression.

According to the *Diagnostic and Statistical Manual of Mental Disorders,* 4th ed. (DSM-IV) (American Psychiatric Association 2000a), people have a major depressive episode when they experience at least five of the following eight symptoms during the same two-week period and these symptoms represent a change from previous functioning. In addition, one of the symptoms must be depressed mood or marked loss of interest or pleasure. These are the eight diagnostic symptoms of major depression:

- Depressed mood most of the day, nearly every day
- Marked loss of interest or pleasure in almost all activities most of the day, nearly every day
- Significant weight loss or weight gain when not dieting (e.g., more than 5% of body weight in a month), decrease or increase in appetite nearly every day
- Insomnia or hypersomnia nearly every day
- Psychomotor agitation or retardation nearly every day, observable by others
- Fatigue or loss of energy nearly every day
- Feelings of worthlessness or of excessive and inappropriate guilt nearly every day
- Recurrent thoughts of death (not just fear of dying), recurrent ideas of suicide with or without a specific plan, or a suicide attempt

In Europe, the **International Classification of Diseases (ICD-10)** endorsed in 1992 by the WHO in Geneva, Switzerland, defines a depressive episode as depressed mood, loss of interest and enjoyment, and reduced energy leading to increased fatigability (often after only slight effort) and diminished activity (WHO 1992). The depressive episode is classed as mild, moderate, or severe.

Common Symptoms of a Depressive Episode According to the International Classification of Diseases (ICD-10)

- Reduced concentration and attention
- Reduced self-esteem and self-confidence
- Ideas of guilt and unworthiness (even in a mild type of episode)
- Bleak and pessimistic views of the future
- Ideas or acts of self-harm or suicide
- Disturbed sleep
- Diminished appetite

WHO 1992.

During a depressive episode, the lowered mood is usually persistent from day to day for at least two weeks, regardless of circumstances, yet tends to improve during the day. A depressive episode may be diagnosed when symptoms have not lasted for two weeks but are very severe and appeared very rapidly. In some cases, **anxiety** and motor agitation can be more prominent symptoms than depressed mood. Also, mood disturbance can be less apparent than other features such as irritability, abuse of alcohol, and worsening of existing comorbid phobias, obsessions, or preoccupation with physical symptoms.

Some symptoms included in the ICD-10 classification system have special clinical significance for defining typical somatic depression and are similar to the American DSM-IV system for the diagnosis of **melancholia.** At least four of the following are required for diagnosis of somatic depression:

- Loss of interest or pleasure in activities that are normally enjoyable
- Lack of emotional reactivity to normally pleasurable surroundings and events
- Waking in the morning two hours or more before the usual time
- Depression worse in the morning
- Objective evidence of definite psychomotor retardation or agitation (remarked on or reported by other people)

- Marked loss of appetite
- Weight loss (defined as 5% or more of body weight in the past month)
- Marked loss of libido

When a person experiences a major depressive episode, these symptoms cause significant distress and impairment in social and occupational settings as well as in other areas of the person's life. Depression is not considered a major depressive episode if it is caused by drug abuse or medication or a medical condition such as hyperthyroidism, heart disease, diabetes, multiple sclerosis, hepatitis, or rheumatoid arthritis. Also, many people have these symptoms within the first two months after a loved one has died, but it is not considered major depression unless the symptoms are associated with marked functional impairment, a preoccupation with worthlessness, ideas of suicide, psychotic symptoms, or psychomotor retardation.

••• *The WHO has projected that depression will be second only to cardiovascular disease as the world's leading cause of death and disability by the year 2020.*

Magnitude of the Problem

Estimates from epidemiologic research in England, Finland, Australia, and the United States suggest that 8% of women and 4% of men have some form of clinical depression at any point in time (Lehtinen and Joukamaa 1994). In the United States, 4.5% to 9.3% of all women and 2.3% to 3.2% of all men have a major depressive disorder. The annual prevalence of major depression in the United States has increased steadily during the past 50 years. African Americans tend to experience less depression than white Americans, while nonwhites of Hispanic ancestry have more depression than whites. As shown in figure 13.1, the National Comorbidity Survey found a lifetime rate of 17% for major depression (21% for women and 13% for men) and a rate of 5% when people were asked whether they had been depressed in the previous month (Kessler et al. 1994). The recently completed replication of that survey estimated that the lifetime prevalence of major depression among U.S. adults was 16% (Kessler et al. 2003). Except for manic episodes in bipolar disorder, women have about twice the rate of depression as men.

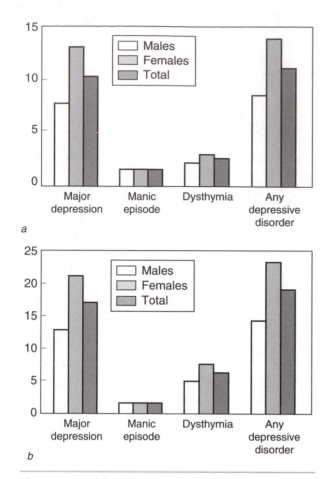

a

b

Figure 13.1 *(a)* Twelve-month and *(b)* lifetime prevalence of depression.

Date from Kessler et al., 1994. Reprinted, by permission, from J. Buckworth and R.K. Dishman, 2001, *Exercise psychology* (Champaign, IL: Human Kinetics), 132.

Half of suicide deaths, one of the nation's top 10 killers, can be attributed to depressive disorders, and about 15% of people who have ever been hospitalized for the treatment of depression commit suicide (Coryell, Noyes, and Clancy 1982). In 1990, an estimated 15,000 men and 3,400 women in the United States committed suicide as a result of depression (Greenberg et al. 1993). The onset of increased rates of depression occurs during early adolescence, affecting about 8% to 9% of boys and girls annually (Rushton, Forcier, and Schectman 2002). The annual rate of depression among teenagers and young adults is about twice that of adults 25 to 44 years of age and four times the rate among people over age 65 (Kessler et al. 1994). In addition, the rate of suicide attributable to depressive disorders increases dramatically from age 10 through young adulthood (Greenberg et al. 1993). Suicide is the third leading cause of death among teenagers and young adults. Depression is especially prevalent

among girls and women under age 25, who have twice the rate of depression as boys and men of the same age and six times the rate of women ages 25 to 54 (Regier et al. 1988).

Why Is the Rate of Depression Higher in Women?

Four possible reasons have been proposed:

- They ruminate more about their problems.
- They are more introspective and more likely to seek help.
- In many cultures they have less control over their lives than men, leading to helplessness and despair.
- Flux in reproductive hormones such as estrogen increases risk of depression during menstruation, menopause, while taking birth control pills, and after childbirth.

Etiology of Depression

There are many causes of depression, and at least 10 different theoretical models of the etiology of depressive disorders have been proposed, including existential models, based on loss of purpose; social models, based on loss of role status; cognitive models, based on irrational thought; learning modes, based on loss of control and helplessness; and biochemical models, based on malfunction of brain neurotransmission.

A modern biological framework, which encompasses social and psychological factors, for the etiology and treatment of depression and other mental disorders is based on the following five principles proposed by Nobel Prize–winning psychiatrist Eric Kandel (1998):

1. Actions at the brain level are responsible for all mental and psychological processes.
2. Brain functioning is controlled by genes.
3. Social, developmental, and environmental factors can produce alterations in gene expression.
4. Alterations in gene expression induce changes in brain functioning.
5. Treatments for mental illness exert their effect by producing alterations in gene

expression, resulting in beneficial changes in brain function.

Within this framework, depression is thought to result from disturbances in brain neuronal function, and effective treatments for depression, such as psychotherapy, medication, or exercise, are hypothesized to produce treatment responses in brain function at a genetic level that result in alleviation of depressive symptoms.

The etiology of depression can include catastrophic events such as major physical illness, loss of a loved one through death or separation, loss of **self-esteem** (e.g., feeling unworthy for not meeting academic goals), or chronic anxiety or stress (e.g., worry or a feeling that life is out of one's control). Depression, especially somatic or melancholic depressive episode, can also occur for no apparent reason. A direct genetic abnormality leading to depression has not been confirmed, but some people are more vulnerable to depression. Regardless of cause, depression is associated with imbalances in **neurotransmitters,** chemicals that influence the activity of brain cells that regulate mood, pleasure, and rational thought.

Studies of neurotransmitter systems involved in depression have focused primarily on **noradrenergic** and **serotonergic** systems primarily because most effective pharmacotherapies modulate either or both of these neurotransmitter systems. The norepinephrine system originates primarily in the **locus coeruleus,** a small region in the brain stem, and projects to numerous brain regions, including areas associated with the regulation of **emotion.** The **serotonin,** or 5-hydroxytryptamine (5-HT), system sends projections from the **raphe nuclei** in the brain stem to various brain regions, including those that control norepinephrine release (figure 13.2).

Brain Neurobiology in Depression

A neurobiological perspective on depression integrates cognitive and neurological theories. For example, neural circuits involved with depression must involve brain neural circuits that regulate mood, pleasure, pain, memories about reward for behavior, and abstract **cognitions** such as optimism. The effects of these different neural systems are dependent on several neurotransmitters, which have been targets for the pharmacologic treatment of depressive disorders.

The evidence accumulated from neuroscience studies that have used the techniques of brain lesioning, **electrophysiological measures,** and **neuroimaging** has so far identified six key brain regions that seem to be most involved in the expression of human emotion, including depression and anxiety (R.J. Davidson and Irwin 1999; Drevets 1998). These include (1) the **prefrontal cortex;** (2) the **amygdala,** especially the central portion; (3) the **hippocampus;** (4) the **ventral striatum,** especially the **nucleus**

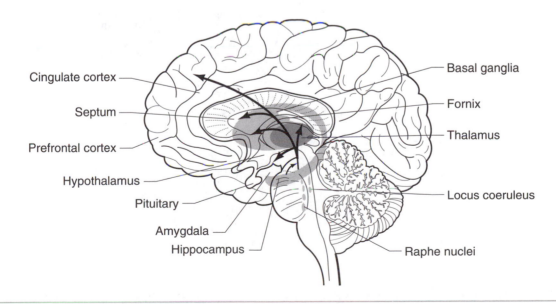

Figure 13.2 Cross section of the central nervous system showing limbic structures (hippocampus, amygdala, cingulate cortex, fornix). Arrows show the pathways from the raphe nuclei to the central structures.

Reprinted, by permission, from J. Buckworth and R.K. Dishman, 2001, *Exercise psychology* (Champaign, IL: Human Kinetics), 48.

accumbens located below the front of the caudate and putamen; (5) the **cingulate cortex,** a layer of gray matter lying between the cerebrum and the lateral ventricle; and (6) the **insular cortex,** an island of involuted cortex near the temporal lobe. These brain regions function synergistically, but they each appear to have some unique functions:

• The prefrontal cortex stores memories of the consequences of behaviors or experiences that were aversive or pleasurable; this permits an emotion to be sustained long enough to direct behavior toward the goal that is appropriate for that emotion.

• The amygdala plays a key role in integrating overt behavior, autonomic responses, and hormonal responses during stress and emotion. Also, its tonic level of activity is sensitive to negative mood. For example, activity in the amygdala is elevated among patients diagnosed with depression and anxiety disorders.

• The hippocampus processes memories of the environmental context in which an emotion occurs. People who have damage to the hippocampus still experience emotion but often at inappropriate times or places.

• The ventral striatum, especially the nucleus accumbens, is in the pathway of **dopamine** neurons in the midbrain that are key in what is known as reward-motivated behavior. It plays a role in regulating approach behaviors that accompany pleasure.

• The anterior cingulate cortex is part of the primitive cortex common to species other than humans. It helps regulate attention during the processing of pleasure or displeasure during an emotion.

• The insular cortex receives sensory inputs from the autonomic nervous system, especially cardiovascular responses, and sends signals to the central amygdala and the hypothalamus, which each regulate cardiac and endocrine responses during stress.

In addition to these brain regions, the dopaminergic neuronal circuit between the **ventral tegmental area (VTA)** (a group of neural cell bodies in the underside of an area at the top of the brainstem, between the pons and the fourth ventrical of the brain), the nucleus accumbens, and the prefrontal cortex is key in regulating motivation by its involvement in pleasure and the memory of pleasurable events (figure 13.3).

Many antidepressant drugs target the monoamines (i.e., serotonin, norepinephrine, and dopamine). The currently most popular drugs target serotonergic systems by blocking serotonin reuptake or acting on serotonergic receptors as agonists or antagonists. In addition, norepinephrine reuptake inhibitors have a long history of **efficacy** in the treatment of depression, and new dopamine agonists are also efficacious as antidepressants.

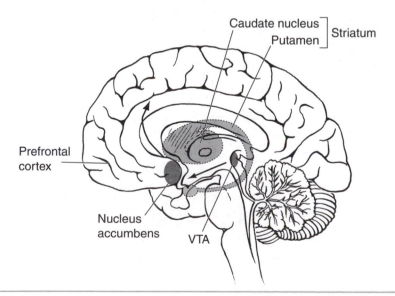

Figure 13.3   The VTA, a major site of brain DA, is shown in respect to the basal ganglia (caudate nucleus, putamen, and nucleus accumbens). Reward pathway from the ventral tegmental area (VTA) to the nucleus accumbens to the prefrontal cortex.

Reprinted, by permission, from J. Buckworth and R.K. Dishman, 2001, *Exercise psychology* (Champaign, IL: Human Kinetics), 55.

The roles of monoamines in the etiology of depression arose from observations in the 1950s that about 15% of patients with hypertension developed depression when they were treated with the drug reserpine, which is an alkali derived from Indian snakeroot *(Rauwolfia serpentina),* that depletes monoamines in neurons by damaging their storage vesicles, thus exposing them to degrading by the enzyme monoamine oxidase. At about the same time, about 15% of patients being treated for tuberculosis with the drug iproniazid, a monoamine oxidase inhibitor (MAOI), were observed to develop mania. Subsequently, studies conducted in the 1960s and 1970s found that depressed individuals often exhibit decreased levels of the main metabolite of norepinephrine (i.e., **3-methoxy-4-hydroxyphenylglycol,** or **MHPG**) or of serotonin (i.e., **5-hydroxyindoleacetic acid,** or **5-HIAA**) in cerebrospinal fluid and urine compared with nondepressed individuals (Bunney and Davis 1965; Prange 1964; Schildkraut 1965). Additional support for monoamine involvement in depression has come from pharmacologic studies that demonstrated alterations of these amines in brain synapses upon treatment with antidepressant agents. The primary action of several antidepressant medications is to increase the level of norepinephrine at the synapse. MAOIs exert their effect by preventing the breakdown of norepinephrine, while tricyclic antidepressants prevent reuptake of norepinephrine by blocking presynaptic receptors.

Subsequent research revealed that it is not the level of norepinephrine, serotonin, or their metabolites that accounts for depression or the therapeutic effects of drugs, but rather impairment of the neuronal function of the brain cells that synthesize, release, and respond to norepinephrine and serotonin. It is still not fully understood what aspect of impaired function occurs first to lead to depression. One early view, the permissive amine hypothesis (Prange 1964), proposed that low serotonin function was not sufficient to cause depression but made it possible for altered norepinephrine function to cause depression. More recent views suggest that altered balance between the serotonin and norepinephrine systems may be mainly responsible for symptoms related to appetite, sleep, and hyperarousal, while dopamine dysfunction may be involved with loss of pleasure and depressed mood, and acetylcholine abnormalities may alter sexual function, especially in men.

The synthesis and metabolic pathways for norepinephrine and its receptors in the brain are the same as for peripheral noradrenergic nerves to

---

Historical Models of Monoamines in Depressed Patients

Schildkraut and colleagues (1983) proposed three types:

- Low MHPG
  - Low synthesis
- Normal MHPG
  - Other systems involved
- High MHPG
  - Subsensitive norepinephrine receptors
  - Increased cholinergic activity

Maas (1979) proposed two types:

- Low urinary MHPG and normal 5-HIAA
- Normal MHPG and low 5-HIAA

---

the heart and blood vessels that were illustrated in figure 6.2 of chapter 6 on hypertension. Other commonly prescribed antidepressant medications specifically target the serotonin system. For example, selective serotonin reuptake, inhibitors (SSRIs) act to block serotonin reuptake, allowing the neurotransmitter to remain in the synapse. Serotonin's synthesis from the amino acid, tryptophan, its metabolic pathways, and its receptors are illustrated in figure 13.4.

Although research has focused primarily on the role of norepinephrine and serotonin in depression, recently more attention has been paid to understanding the role of dopamine in the etiology of depression and its symptoms. Because the dopamine system plays a critical role in reward, motivation, and motor functions, **dysregulation** of this system may contribute to the anhedonia (i.e., loss of pleasure) and psychomotor disturbances that are observed in depression. Also, prolonged elevations in cortisol during chronic stress have been accompanied by dysfunction of dopamine neurons (Chrousos 1998), and some antidepressant drugs influence the activity of dopamine neurons by targeting dopamine receptors or altering dopamine metabolism (Willner 1995). Dopamine is the precursor molecule for the synthesis of norepinephrine, so they share the same synthetic and metabolic pathways. Key receptors for dopamine in brain neurons are depicted in figure 13.5. Later in this chapter, evidence is presented that exercise could protect against depression by altering brain monoamines and the function of their neurons.

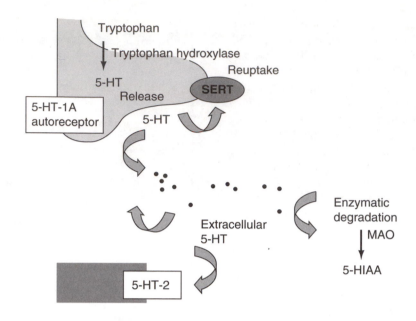

Figure 13.4 Serotonin synapse.

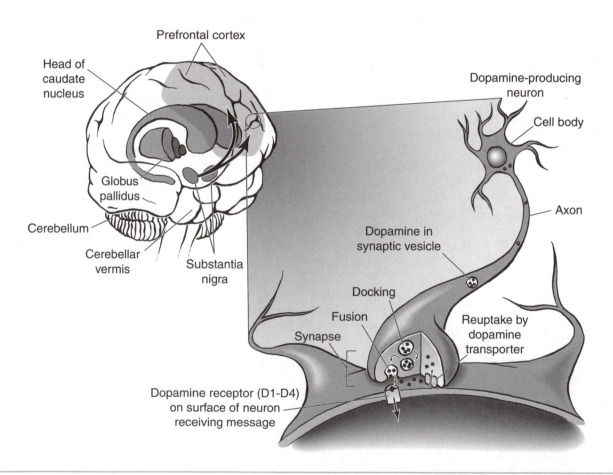

Figure 13.5 Structures of the basal ganglia and the actions of dopamine from production to postsynaptic activation.

Treatment of Depression

Despite their higher prevalence of depression, women respond to treatment as well as or better than men. About 80% to 90% of adults who suffer depression can be effectively treated as outpatients with antidepressant medications, psychotherapy, or a combination of the two treatments. People who do not respond to those treatments may be helped by electroconvulsive therapy (ECT), or electroshock treatment, in which small amounts of electric current are passed through the brain. The efficacy of psychotherapy is about 65% among adolescents, and the efficacy and safety rates of drug therapy among adolescents have not yet been established. Most depression is called unipolar, characterized only by depressed mood. A smaller percentage of people have manic-depressive disorder. They experience periods of depressed mood alternating with periods of elevated, expansive, or irritable mood, exaggerated self-confidence, risky or asocial behavior, or even paranoia. They are often treated with a drug called lithium carbonate.

The treatment of depression, either by drugs or psychotherapy, involves acute, continuation, and maintenance stages, as depicted in figure 13.6. Hospitalization is required for about 5% to 10% of major depressive episodes and for about half of manic episodes, mainly because of debilitating symptoms and risk of suicide or self-harm. Because of high costs, the average hospital stay is about a week for depression and 10 days to two weeks for mania, but depressive symptoms are seldom reduced within one to two weeks, and patients usually require follow-up outpatient care.

Acute Phase

Acute-phase treatment continues until a clinically meaningful treatment response is observed, which is defined as a reduction in symptoms of more than 50%, enough so that the patient no longer meets diagnostic criteria of a depressive episode. When pharmacotherapy is indicated, this commonly takes six to eight weeks, during which patients are observed each or every other week in order to monitor symptoms and side effects and to adjust medication dosage. Psychotherapy commonly consists of 6 to 20 weekly sessions during the acute phase of depression treatment. About 50% to 70% of depressed patients treated as outpatients respond favorably to drug treatment or psychotherapy. Drugs are typically changed if a patient does not respond within four to six weeks and are

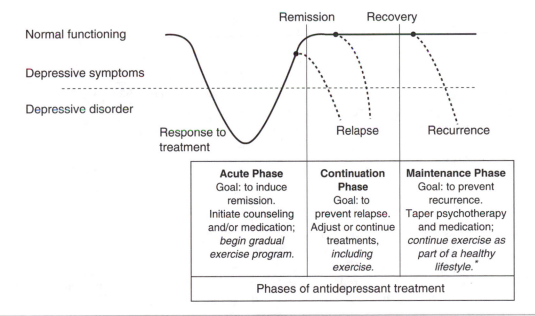

Figure 13.6 Phases of antidepressant treatment. * Because depressive episodes often recur, long-term maintenance of remission is an important clinical issue. While pharmacotherapy and psychotherapy are tapered and withdrawn following remission of depression, exercise may be continued and incorporated into the individual's lifestyle. Thus, unlike most other traditional treatments, potential antidepressant effects of exercise are not time-limited.

Adapted, by permission, from H.A. O'Neal, A.L. Dunn, and E.W. Martinsen, 2000, "Depression and exercise," *International Journal of Sports Psychology* 31: 113.

often added to psychotherapy if symptoms have not improved within three to four months.

It is acknowledged that acute response to treatment includes the combined effects of placebo expectancy, spontaneous remission, and active treatment. The magnitude of the active treatment effect can be estimated from randomized clinical trials by subtracting the placebo response rate from that of active medication. Overall, the active treatment effect for major depression typically ranges from 20% to 40%, after accounting for a placebo response rate of about 30% (American Psychiatric Association 2000b). The dropout rates from acute-phase therapy commonly range from 30% to 40%, and rates of nonadherence to the prescribed therapy among those who stay in treatment are higher, mainly because of side effects or unrealistic expectations about benefits.

Continuation Phase

Acute-phase antidepressant drug therapy or ECT is nearly always followed by at least six months of continuation-phase treatment during which patients are seen every two weeks or monthly in order to prevent relapse to clinical depression and to maintain remission at normal levels of functioning (American Psychiatric Association 2000b; Rudorfer, Henry, and Sackheim 1997). Continuation pharmacotherapy reduces the risk of relapse from between 40% and 60% to between 10% and 20%. Full recovery should be attained before the antidepressant drugs are ceased. Psychotherapy also is usually tapered by reducing sessions to once every two weeks or monthly, but some evidence has shown that relapse is less common after **cognitive-behavioral therapy** than after pharmacotherapy.

Maintenance Phase

Maintenance pharmacotherapy is intended to prevent a future recurrence of depression, which is defined as a new depressive episode rather than merely a relapse, which is the return of symptoms during the initial episode. Maintenance pharmacotherapy is especially indicated for people who have a history of three or more depressive episodes, chronic depressive state, or bipolar disorder. It commonly involves monthly or quarterly visits to a physician and may last for several years in some people.

Psychotherapy

The two most effective types of psychotherapy used to treat depression are behavioral therapy and cognitive-behavioral therapy. Behavioral therapy teaches patients how to control their environment in ways that reduce the risk of depression and how to minimize situations that compound symptoms. Cognitive-behavioral therapy builds upon the behavioral approach by helping patients to better understand faulty thinking that contributes to their feelings of helplessness, hopelessness, and despair.

Pharmacotherapy

More than 20 drugs are being used to treat depression (table 13.1). The most common drugs used to treat depression are tricyclics, introduced in the 1940s, which block the reuptake of monoamines released by brain neurons; monoamine oxidase inhibitors (MAOIs), introduced in the 1950s, which block the deamination (i.e., metabolism) of monoamines after neuronal release; and

TABLE 13.1 COMMON ANTIDEPRESSANT DRUGS

Tricyclics

Anafranil® (clomipramine)*
Asendin® (amoxapine)
Aventyl® (nortriptyline)
Elavil® (amitriptyline)
Norpramin® (desipramine)
Sinequan® (doxepin)
Tofranil® (imipramine)
Vivactil® (protriptyline)

Monoamine oxidase inhibitors

Marplan® (isocarboxazid)
Nardil® (phenelzine sulfate)
Parnate® (tranylcypromine sulfate)

Selective serotonin reuptake inhibitors

Desyrel® (trazodone)
Ludiomil® (maprotiline)
Paxil™ (paroxetine)
Prozac® (fluoxetine)
Zoloft® (sertraline)

Selective serotonin and noradrenaline reuptake inhibitor

Effexor® (venlafaxine)
Serzone® (nefazodone)

Dopamine agonist

Wellbutrin® (bupropion)

*The generic name of each drug appears in parentheses.

Side effects: low blood pressure, blurred vision, irregular heartbeat, stomach and gastrointestinal upsets, male sexual dysfunction, toxicity after extended use, especially with lithium.

selective serotonin reuptake inhibitors (SSRIs), introduced in the late 1980s, that block reentry of serotonin into the neuron after release. The SSRIs are currently the most popular, not because they are more effective, but because they have fewer side effects. In 2000, the SSRI Prozac was the most-prescribed antidepressant in the United States, with sales exceeding $2.7 billion; sales for another SSRI, Zoloft, reached $2 billion (a month's supply of either drug costs about $100).

During the 1990s, selective norepinephrine reuptake inhibitors (SNRIs; e.g., reboxetine), which selectively block the reuptake of norepinephrine, and drugs that simultaneously block the reuptake of both norepinephrine and serotonin (e.g., venlafaxine) or that block reuptake of dopamine (e.g., amineptine and bupropion) more than norepinephrine and serotonin became popular. Some other tetracyclic antidepressants, first introduced in the 1970s, have a different chemical structure from tricyclics and MAOIs. They do not affect the reuptake or metabolism of monoamines; rather, they block receptors (e.g., mianserin blocks 5-HT$_2$ [serotonin] receptors, and mirtazapine blocks α_2 [norepinephrine] autoreceptors).

Neuronal Effects of Antidepressant Drugs

FIRST LINE, ACUTE

- Blocked reuptake of norepinephrine or serotonin
- Reduced norepinephrine cell firing in brain stem
- Temporary reduction of norepinephrine synthesis and turnover
- Blocked α_1 and α_2 receptors for norepinephrine

SECOND LINE, CHRONIC (10–20 DAYS)

- Sustained blockade of norepinephrine or serotonin reuptake
- Transient **down-regulation** of α_2 receptors
- Normalization of norepinephrine cell firing rate and turnover; increased norepinephrine synthesis and release
- Down-regulation of β_1 and up-regulation of α_1 and serotonin receptors

Baldessarini 1989.

The overall effect of drugs that block monoamine reuptake is an average reduction of about three standard deviations in depression symptoms, regardless of whether they selectively block norepinephrine or serotonin or otherwise alter the function of monoamine neurons (Workman and Short 1993). However, when the treatment response to drug therapy or psychotherapy, or their combination, is not clinically effective or is too slow (e.g., in a person with delusional depression and intense thoughts of suicide), ECT is considered. ECT use, which began in the 1930s, was based on the faulty belief that epilepsy (seizure disorder) and schizophrenia could not coexist at the same time in an individual. Accumulated clinical experience and controlled clinical trials found that ECT is ineffective for treating dysthymia but has a 60% to 70% response rate for mania and severe depression, similar to drug therapy but faster, making it a treatment of choice when the risks of suicide and self-harm are high (Rudorfer, Henry, and Sackheim 1997). The most common adverse side effects of ECT are temporary confusion and short-term memory loss about events near the time of the ECT treatment. These usually end within an hour or so of awakening from the treatment, but some memory problems can persist in some people.

People suffering from bipolar disorder, or manic depression, are usually treated with lithium carbonate (Baldessarini et al. 2002). Lithium is an alkaline metal like sodium and potassium and forms a salt when combined with carbonate. The mechanism by which lithium controls manic episodes and reduces severe depression is not fully known, but lithium alters sodium transport and may interfere with ion exchange mechanisms and nerve conduction. Lithium enhances the reuptake of norepinephrine and serotonin by the brain neurons that release them, reduces the release of norepinephrine from brain neurons, and inhibits production of the neural second messenger cyclic AMP. Lithium can replace sodium in extracellular fluid and is not effectively removed from cells by the sodium pump during the cell depolarization. Hence, the reentry of potassium into brain neurons is prevented. Thus lithium interferes with electrolyte distribution across the neuronal membrane, leading to a fall in membrane potential and changes in conduction and neuronal excitability. This process is accompanied by clinical improvements in mania and to a lesser degree depression, but the precise therapeutic action is not yet known. Though lithium can disturb the regulation of body water and electrolytes, which can impair temperature regulation and cardiovascular function, studies have confirmed that exercise does not alter lithium metabolism (Jefferson et al. 1982).

Though many people with depression respond well to prescription drugs or psychological treatments, it is alarming that only 30% of those who report symptoms or signs of depression actually seek the help of a mental health professional. About half the people who have an episode of clinical depression go undiagnosed or misdiagnosed. Of people who are correctly diagnosed with depression and would be helped by antidepressant drugs, half have never taken them, and less than a third are prescribed the appropriate dose. The drugs usually have varying negative side effects for many people, including somnolence (sleepiness), dry mouth, stomach and intestinal distress, increased appetite, weight gain, dizziness, blurred vision, and sexual impairment, as well as more serious cardiovascular problems, such as low blood pressure and irregular heart rate. These facts indicate the potential importance of self-help behaviors, which can enhance mental hygiene. Many studies agree that regular physical activity can reduce symptoms after a person is depressed and can reduce the odds that a person will experience depression. As discussed later, exercise may have effects on the brain monoamine systems similar to the effects of antidepressant drugs, or the exercise setting may have cognitive effects that are beneficial, such as increasing physical self-esteem.

Physical Activity and Depression: The Evidence

The first reports by psychiatrists using exercise to treat depression in the United States appeared in 1905. The mood and reaction times of two depressed men were improved on days they exercised for about 2 h compared with days that they rested (Franz and Hamilton 1905). The use of exercise in psychiatry continued in the United States through the 1950s (Campbell and Davis 1939–1940; Layman 1960) without scientific evaluation. Morgan et al. (1970) conducted the first experimental study showing that self-ratings of depressive symptoms could be reduced in men after an exercise training program. That finding was extended in a small, randomized, clinical trial of psychiatric outpatients, which found that the reduction in depressive symptoms after 12 weeks of running therapy was equivalent to or greater than two forms of group psychotherapy (Greist et al. 1978). Moreover, 9 of the 10 patients treated with running therapy were still running and not depressed nine months later, while depressive symptoms had returned in the other patients.

In 1984, the National Institute of Mental Health Workshop on Exercise and Mental Health concluded that exercise is associated with a decreased level of mild to moderate depression (Morgan and Goldston 1987). That conclusion was upheld at the Second International Consensus Symposium on Physical Activity, Fitness, and Health held in Toronto in 1992 (Bouchard, Shephard, and Stephens 1994) and by the U.S. Surgeon General's report *Physical Activity and Health* (U.S. Department of Health and Human Services 1996). The documentation of an association between exercise and the reduction in symptoms of mild to moderate depression has come from population studies, narrative and quantitative (i.e., **meta-analyses**) research literature, and exercise training studies conducted with clinical and nonclinical populations. About 30 studies qualify as population-based, epidemiologic studies, and about 30 studies were randomized controlled trials of people diagnosed as having depression.

Physical Activity and Depression in Youth

No randomized controlled trials of children or adolescents diagnosed with depression have been reported. However, two quasi-experimental studies with small samples of adolescents reported small reductions in depressive symptoms after exercise training (Brown et al. 1992; Norris, Carroll, and Cochrane 1992). Whether that apparent effect is generalizable to a reduction in the primary risk of developing depression among adolescents is not yet established. About 10 observational studies using cross-sectional or prospective designs showed lower depressive symptoms associated with physical activity among adolescents, but those studies did not adjust for depression risk factors that might have been confounders. In contrast, a recent prospective, cohort study examined naturally occurring changes in physical activity, and changes in depressive symptoms were studied during early adolescence, when depression risk begins to increase markedly (Motl, O'Connor, and Dishman 2003). More than 2,000 boys and girls reported their frequency of physical activity outside of school and completed the Center for Epidemiological Studies Depression scale in the fall of 1998 (beginning of 7th grade; baseline data), spring of 1999 (end of 7th grade; interim data), and spring of 2000 (end of 8th grade; follow-up data). Results indicated that a one standard-deviation change in the frequency of leisure-time physical activity was inversely related to a one third standard-deviation change in depressive symptoms in both boys and girls. This effect was attenuated but remained statistically significant when the confounding effects of smoking and alcohol consumption were controlled (Motl, O'Connor, and Dishman 2003). Thus, physical activity was independently and inversely related to depressive symptoms, providing evidence that physical activity indeed represents a feasible target of population-based interventions designed to reduce depression risk among adolescent boys and girls.

Most studies of exercise and depression have been conducted on young to middle-aged adults. Among people over age 65, the evidence suggests that the benefits of exercise for *reducing* symptoms of depression may diminish as people age (Chambliss and Dishman 2003; O'Connor, Aenchbacher, and Dishman 1993); however, despite more age-related symptoms of depression

among older people (e.g., sleep and cognitive disorders), older people have a lower prevalence of clinically diagnosed depression than young and middle-aged adults. The benefits of physical activity for helping *prevent* depression usually occur regardless of people's age, sex, race, or socioeconomic status.

> ••• *The benefits of physical activity for helping prevent depression occur regardless of people's age, sex, race, or socioeconomic status.*

Preventing Depression: Population Studies

About 30 population-based studies of exercise and depression have been reported around the world since the first one in 1988. Nearly all of them reported an inverse relationship between physical activity and depression in at least one analysis (Chambliss and Dishman 2003; Dunn, Trivedi, and O'Neal 2001). Nearly all of them showed that symptoms of depression are more likely among people who report little or no leisure-time physical activity, but about half the results did not reach a high level of statistical significance, often because the sample sizes were too small given relatively small and variable reductions

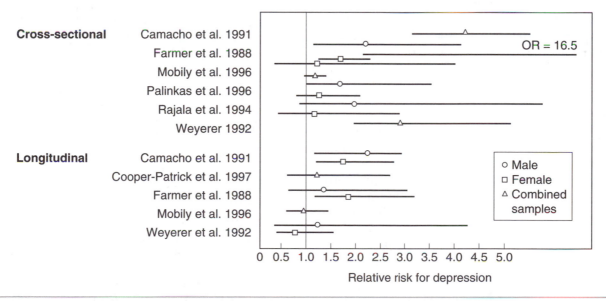

Figure 13.7   The relative risks and 95% confidence intervals (odds ratios in the cross-sectional studies) from selected studies.

Adapted from Chambliss and Dishman 2004.

in risk. Figure 13.7 illustrates relative risks (odds ratios in the cross-sectional studies) and 95% confidence intervals from selected studies.

These were three important early studies of physical activity and depression:

- The National Health and Nutrition Examination Survey I (NHANES I), a 1975 survey of nearly 7,000 Americans ages 25 to 74, found that people who said they got little or no exercise in their leisure time also reported more symptoms of depression (Stephens 1988).

- The Canada Fitness Survey of 22,000 Canadians ages 10 years and older yielded similar findings (Stephens 1988). In this 1981 survey, inactive people reported more symptoms related to negative moods than people who said they were moderately or very active in their leisure time.

- A study was conducted in Upper Bavaria, Germany, between 1975 and 1984 of 1,500 people ages 15 and older (Weyerer 1992). It found that the prevalence of several types of depressive disorders among those who stated that they currently did not exercise for sports was three times higher than those who stated that they did regularly exercise for sports.

In all three studies, higher rates of depression occurred among inactive people regardless of physical illness, sex, age, and social class. However, the studies reported only cross-sectional comparisons of active and inactive people and thus did not determine whether it was inactivity or depression that occurred first. It is very possible that people became less active after becoming depressed rather than becoming depressed due to inactivity. As shown in figure 13.8, physical inactivity did not predict higher depression five years later in the Upper Bavarian study.

More encouraging results were found in the NHANES study, depicted in figure 13.9. About 1,500 of the people originally interviewed in NHANES I were interviewed again eight years later (Farmer et al. 1988). That follow-up survey first measured physical activity and then looked for the later occurrence of the symptoms of depression. Among the findings of the NHANES I follow-up were these:

- The rate of depression among sedentary, white women who were not depressed in 1975 and who remained inactive was twice that of women who said they participated in a moderate

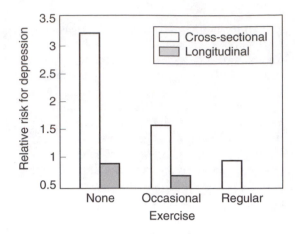

Figure 13.8 Upper Bavarian field study. N = 1,536 community residents. Depression assessed by clinical interview. OR = 3.15 for inactive. Physical inactivity did not significantly increase risk for depression at five-year follow-up.

Weyerer, *Int J Sports Med,* 1992.

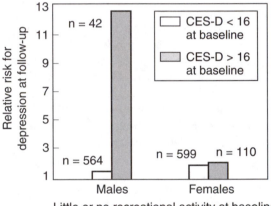

Figure 13.9 NHANES I: Longitudinal analysis. N = 1,497, ages 25 to 77 years. Examined relationship between self-reported physical activity and depressive symptoms (CES-D) in 1971 to 1975 and depressive symptoms in 1982 to 1984.

Data from Farmer et al., *Am J of Epidemiol,* 1988.

amount of physical activity and who remained active over the eight years.

- White men who were depressed and inactive in 1975 and remained inactive were 12 times more likely to be depressed after eight years than those who were initially depressed but had become physically active. Again, these findings were observed regardless of age, education level, and socioeconomic status.

In the NHANES cross-sectional study, inactive black men had a 16-fold increase in odds of depression, but inactive black women had no increased rate of depression symptoms, as shown in figure 13.10. Those effects were independent of age, socioeconomic status, and general health, but there was no dose response. Being inactive increased the odds of depression, but being highly active did not further reduce the odds beyond those of people who were moderately active. The results probably were not very representative of true risk among African Americans, though, as there were fewer than 100 each of black men and women in the study.

Two other important prospective studies followed depression over time and compared people's risk with their physical activity:

• In the Alameda County (California) Study, about 5,000 nondepressed adult men and women completed surveys on physical activity and depression in 1965 (Camacho et al. 1991). Those who were not depressed in 1965 were studied again in 1974 and 1983. Participants were classified as low active, medium active, or high active based on self-reported frequency (i.e., never, sometimes, often) and intensity of physical activity in the categories of active sports, swimming, walking, doing exercises, or gardening. Inactive people who were not depressed in 1965 had a 70% increase in risk of depression in 1974 compared with those who were initially highly active (figure 13.11). Associations between changes in activity between 1965 and 1983 and symptoms of depression in 1983 suggested that the risk of

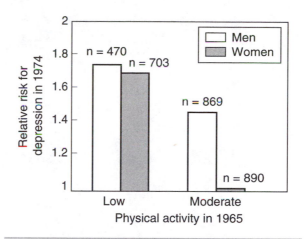

Figure 13.11   Alameda County study of longitudinal analysis. Individuals reporting low levels of physical activity in 1965 were at higher risk for depression in 1974. Data from Camacho et al., *Am J of Epidemiol*, 1991.

depression was alterable by increasing exercise, but this association was not independent of the other risk factors for depression.

• In a study of about 10,000 male Harvard University alumni from the mid-1960s through 1977, physical activity was shown to reduce the likelihood of developing physician-diagnosed depression (Paffenbarger, Lee, and Leung 1994). Figure 13.12 illustrates that those who expended 1,000 to 2,500 kcal per week by walking, climbing stairs, or playing sports had 17% less risk of developing depression compared with their less-active peers. Those who expended more than 2,500 kcal per week had a 28% lower risk.

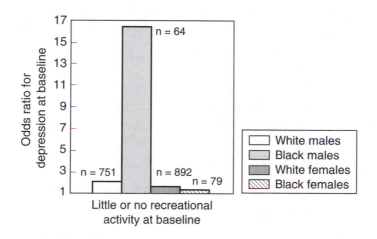

Figure 13.10   NHANES I: Cross-sectional analysis. N = 1,900, ages 25 to 77 years. Physical activity was assessed by self-report. Depression was assessed by self-report of symptoms (CES-D). Little or no recreational activity was associated with more depressive symptoms in cross-sectional analysis.
Data from Farmer et al., *Am J of Epidemiol*, 1988.

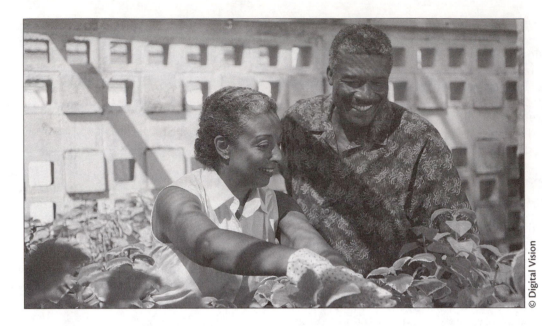

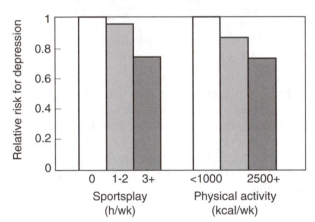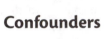

Figure 13.12　Harvard alumni study. N = 10,201 males. Measured activity habits in 1962 to 1966 and incidence of depression during 23- to 27-year follow-up.

Adapted, by permission, from R.S. Paffenbarger, I.M. Lee, and R. Leung, 1994, "Physical activity and personal characteristics associated with depression and suicide in American college men," *Acta Psychiatrica Scandinavica*, Suppl. 337: 16-22.

Other Risk Factors for Depression Often Controlled Statistically in Population Studies of Physical Activity

Age	Education
Chronic health conditions	Perceived health
Physical disability	Physical symptoms
Feelings of autonomy	Social isolation

Stressful life events: moving, job loss, separation or divorce, death of spouse, and financial difficulties

Confounders

To build a case that physical activity causes reduced risk of depression, it must be demonstrated that the effect of physical activity is independent of other factors, such as age, overall health, and psychosocial variables, that might be associated with physical activity levels and also influence depression. For example, cross-sectional analysis of baseline data from NHANES I revealed significant associations between little or no recreational exercise and depressive symptoms after adjusting for age, education, employment status, chronic conditions, and income (Farmer et al. 1988). While controlling for other risk factors or moderating variables may lessen the association between physical activity and depression in some studies, significant effects for physical activity are often observed even after adjusting for other potential influences on depression. Thus, there is limited evidence that physical inactivity is an independent risk factor for depression. However, stronger evidence for causality comes from randomized controlled trials.

Treating Depression: Experimental Studies

Most of the experimental research showing that exercise improves self-ratings of depressive mood has been done with people who had normal mental and physical health, but about 30 randomized controlled trials involving people diagnosed with mild to moderate unipolar depression have shown improvements in mood after several weeks of moderately intense exercise. When the exercise program lasted several months, the improvements in people's self-ratings of depression were as large as those usually seen after psychotherapy. The best results for fighting depression occurred when outpatients were in an exercise program and also received psychotherapy. A few studies of exercise programs lasting four to six months showed improvements comparable to those typically seen after drug treatment. Though exercise appears comparable to drug therapy for treating mild to moderate depression, its clinical effects on reducing symptoms occur later than those of drug therapy. The minimal or optimal type or amount of exercise for reducing depression is not yet known, but it appears that an increase in physical fitness is not required, and resistance exercise has been effective in a few studies.

Reviews and Meta-Analyses

Several subjective reviews and quantitative meta-analyses of exercise and depression research indicate that exercise reduces depression symptoms among people diagnosed with depression by three fourths to one standard deviation and among people without depression by about one half standard deviation (Chambliss and Dishman 2003; Craft and Landers 1998; Lawlor and Hopker 2001; Morgan 1994; North, McCullagh, and Zung 1990). Those changes represent reductions of about 5 to 10 points on standard self-rating scales of symptoms. Exercise also compares well with traditional forms of treatment.

Most studies of chronic exercise and depression have used an aerobic exercise intervention such as walking or jogging. However, the type of people studied, the severity of initial depression, the use of appropriate comparison groups, and the type and amount of exercise used varied among studies. Nonetheless, it appears that aerobic endurance exercise and resistance exercise each have potential to reduce depression symptoms.

> ••• *Both aerobic and resistance exercise training have a positive effect on patients diagnosed as having mild to moderate depression.*

Meta-Analysis of Randomized Controlled Trials

A meta-analysis of 14 trials of chronic exercise among people diagnosed with depression (Lawlor and Hopker 2001) showed that exercisers had a 1.1 SD (95% CI: −1.5 to −0.60) reduction in depression symptoms measured using the Beck Depression Inventory compared with people who were not treated. This was a seven-point reduction (95% CI: −10.0 to −4.6). The effects of exercise were similar to the effects of cognitive psychotherapy. Collectively, the studies had several scientific weaknesses that made it hard to conclude that the reduced depression symptoms were the independent result of exercise:

- Use of volunteers
- Use of symptom ratings rather than clinical diagnoses as the measure of treatment response
- Failure to conceal group assignment
- Exclusion of dropouts from the treatment response tally

Early studies of the effects of exercise training on symptoms among hospitalized psychiatric patients diagnosed with major depression were conducted by Norwegian psychiatrist Egil Martinsen and his colleagues at the Modum Bads Nervesanatorium (Martinsen, Hoffart, and Solberg 1989b; Martinsen, Medhus, and Sandvik 1985). In the first study, 43 patients were randomly assigned to either exercise or an occupational therapy control group in addition to their standard treatment, which included psychotherapy and medication. After nine weeks of training, patients in the exercise group had significantly larger reductions in self-reported symptoms of depression than the control group. In the second study, 99 patients diagnosed with unipolar depressive disorders (major depression, dysthymic disorder, and atypical depression) were randomly assigned to either aerobic or nonaerobic exercise. After eight weeks of training, both groups had significant reductions in depression scores. The change in depression scores did not differ between the two conditions, but the aerobic group had significant increases in fitness, defined as maximal oxygen uptake ($\dot{V}O_2$max), while the fitness of the nonaerobic group did not change.

The first experimental report comparing the effectiveness of resistance exercise with aerobic exercise for reducing depression symptoms was reported by Doyne et al. (1987). Forty women ages 18 to 35 years who were diagnosed with depression were assigned to an aerobic exercise (running) or a weightlifting group. After eight weeks of exercise training, both exercise groups exhibited significant reductions in depression scores, while no changes were found in a control group. The reduction in depression scores was similar for both forms of exercise. Singh, Clements, and Fiatarone (1997b) conducted a 10-week, progressive, resistance exercise training study among elderly subjects who met DSM-IV criteria for depression or dysthymia. Compared with a control group that received health education only, the resistance exercise group had larger reductions (about four to five standard deviations) in depressive symptoms on both Beck self-ratings and diagnostic interview ratings by clinicians. Results from these studies and those by Martinsen in Norway show that changes in aerobic capacity are not necessary for the antidepressant effects of physical activity.

The cumulative evidence shows that exercise can be as effective as psychotherapy (North, McCullagh, and Zung 1990). Whether the effects of exercise operate through a different mechanism from psychotherapy and thus are additive to the treatment response of psychotherapy alone is not yet known. For example, Fremont and Craighead (1987) compared aerobic exercise to traditional psychotherapy for depression in a sample of 49 men and women 19 to 62 years of age with self-reported symptoms of mild to moderate depression (figure 13.13). Participants were randomly assigned to supervised running, individual cognitive psychotherapy, or combined running and psychotherapy. After 10 weeks of treatment, all groups exhibited significant reductions in depression scores, but no differences were found among the groups. Thus, exercise was found to be as effective as a traditional psychotherapy, but there was no additional benefit when exercise was added to psychotherapy.

Recent research has shown that exercise can be generally as effective as drug therapy for reducing depression symptoms. Aerobic exercise was compared with standard medication in a training study of 156 older men and women who were clinically diagnosed with major depressive disorder (figure 13.14) (Blumenthal et al. 1999). Participants were randomly assigned to an aerobic exercise, antidepressant, or combined exercise and medication group. Figure 13.14 illustrates that after the 16-week program, all three groups demonstrated similar decreases in depression that were statistically and clinically significant. The medication-only group exhibited the fastest initial response, but by the end of the program, the exercise treatment was equally effective in reducing depression in this older sample. Also, the exercise group was more likely to have fully recovered and less likely to have relapsed into depression six months after treatment than the drug-treatment patients (Babyak et al. 2000).

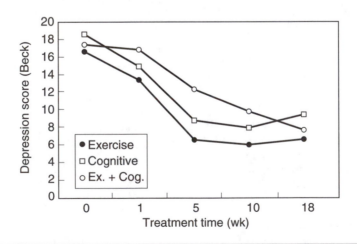

Figure 13.13   Early studies of the effects of exercise training on symptoms among hospitalized psychiatric patients diagnosed with major depression showed that after eight weeks of training, both groups exhibited significant reductions in depression scores.

Data from Fremont and Craighead, 1987, *Cog. Therapy & Res.* 11: 241–251.

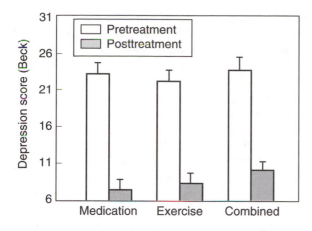

Figure 13.14 Changes in depression scores across treatment.

Adapted from Blumenthal et al., 1999, *Archives of Internal Medicine* 159: 2349–2356.

Experimental Evidence of Improved Depression Symptoms

About a dozen experiments have found that patients recovering from a heart attack report a moderate reduction in self-rated depression (about half a standard deviation) when they participate in a cardiac rehabilitation exercise program (Kugler, Seelbach, and Kruskemper 1994). Improvements in symptoms of depression have also been reported among breast cancer survivors who exercised (Segar et al. 1998).

Strength of the Evidence

The case for a protective effect of leisure-time physical activity on the primary and secondary prevention of depression is encouraging but as yet incomplete. Most of the population-based studies of physical activity and depression show lower risk of depression among people who say they are physically active in their leisure time, but only about half of the studies found big enough effects to be statistically significant, often because of relatively small population samples. Also, only about half the population studies used a prospective cohort design and covered a time period sufficient to show a benefit. Many did an incomplete job of controlling confounders, and they used imprecise measures of physical activity or depression.

Many clinical studies have found that both acute and chronic exercise are followed by lower scores on self-report questionnaires designed to measure depressed mood. This has been found in about 30 randomized controlled trials of depressed adults, but most of the studies did not report whether the reduction in symptoms was enough to result in a diagnosis of remission (i.e., over 50% reduction in symptoms). Also, exercising patients commonly received treatment by psychotherapy or drug therapy, so it wasn't possible to determine the sole, independent effect of exercise on their symptoms. Many exercise programs with depressed patients were conducted in groups outdoors during daylight, so it was hard to determine whether the benefits attributed to exercise could be explained by social effects or light exposure; each could have antidepressant effects regardless of the physical exertion. Reduced scores on depression scales have also been reported after exercise by people who have normal fluctuations in mood but have not been diagnosed with depression. However, it has not been determined whether this mood-elevating response reduces the risk of future development of depression.

Temporal Sequence

Examples of population studies that demonstrate temporal sequence include studies of Alameda County residents (Camacho et al. 1991) and Harvard alumni (Paffenbarger, Lee, and Leung 1994). Future exercise interventions in experimental studies should be of sufficient length to observe whether reductions in depression occur in a manner consistent with theoretical biological explanations and should incorporate follow-up assessments to evaluate whether antidepressant effects are maintained over time.

Strength of Association

Though the results from population-based studies have been mixed, usually because the cohorts studied were too small for the risk reduction among active people to reach statistical significance, the average rate of elevated depression symptoms was about double among people who were physically inactive in their leisure time. Several quantitative reviews of randomized controlled trials using people with normal mood and people diagnosed with mild to moderate depression have found a moderately large reduction in symptoms of depression, ranging from about one half to two thirds of a standard deviation. For comparison, symptoms are reduced by about one standard deviation after psychotherapy and about three standard deviations after drug therapy.

Exercise studies did not, however, determine whether the reduction in symptoms was large enough for a diagnosis of remission or maintenance of remission, though a recent study was encouraging that exercise might be more effective for maintenance than drug treatment is (Babyak et al. 2000).

Consistency

It is important to consider whether the effects of exercise are the same between the sexes and among races or ethnicities and ages to establish the scientific consistency of the effects and for the practical reason of implementing optimal physical activity interventions within segments of the population. In general, physical activity has been associated with decreased risk for depression in both males and females, across age groups, and in multiple cultures (Krause et al. 1993; Rajala et al. 1994; Weyerer 1992). However, the evidence for consistency is limited since most studies consist of homogeneous samples, and inconsistencies exist both within and among studies. Quantitative reviews have reported statistically similar reductions in depression for men and women (0.82 ± 1.09 vs. 0.45 ± 0.86 SD) that were inversely related to increasing age. In contrast, exercise was inversely associated with depression symptoms independently of age in two community-based studies and one national sample. Most studies were not designed to compare demographic groups on their depression responses to exercise and were limited to ages younger than 55 years or arbitrarily used middle age (e.g., 40–45 years) as a criterion for aging effects. There have been few observational or controlled studies of children and adolescents, and most studies of people over age 65 measured symptoms of depression but did not demonstrate clinically meaningful remission of symptoms among people diagnosed with a depressive disorder. Cross-sectional population studies in the United States and Canada showed that sedentary leisure time was associated with increased depression differently for men and women when they were grouped above or below 40 years of age, although both men and women who were sedentary had increased relative risk for developing depression symptoms during an eight-year follow-up of a U.S. study. In the NHANES I study, for example, among subjects who did not exhibit elevated depressive symptoms at baseline, little or no recreational physical activity was a significant predictor of self-reported depression in women at the follow-up assessment. Women who reported being inactive were twice as likely as active women to exhibit elevated symptoms of depression; however, this effect was found only for white women (Farmer et al. 1988). Inconsistent results were also obtained in the Upper Bavarian Field Study (Weyerer 1992), which used a psychiatrist-administered clinical interview to diagnose depression according to ICD criteria and classified subjects by level of self-reported physical activity. After adjusting for sex, age, social class, and physical disorders, cross-sectional analysis of baseline data revealed that nonexercisers were approximately three times as likely to exhibit depression as regular exercisers. However, upon analysis of longitudinal data, physical inactivity did not appear to increase the risk of developing depression five years later.

Dose Response

At present, there does not seem to be a clear dose–response relationship between the intensity or total amount of daily physical activity and depression (Dunn, Trivedi, and O'Neal 2001). On balance, it appears that being sedentary increases risk of depression, but high levels of exercise may not be more protective against depression than moderate levels. For example, in the NHANES I study of physical activity and depressive symptoms in 1,497 men and women ages 25 to 77 years, people who reported little or no physical activity in leisure or at work exhibited significantly greater depressive symptoms than individuals who reported being moderately active (Farmer et al. 1988). However, there was no difference in depression scores between moderately active and highly active groups. In the Canada Fitness Survey, people were seemingly protected from symptoms of depression if their daily leisure energy expenditure was at least 1 kcal per kilogram of body weight per day, which is a low level of activity (e.g., about 20 minutes of walking) (Stephens 1988). Risk of depression was not further reduced when the energy expenditure was raised to 2 to 5 kcal per kilogram of body weight per day.

Data from the Harvard alumni study did suggest a dose-dependent reduction in depression with increased exercise. Men who spent 3 h or more per week playing sports or expended about 2,500 kcal each week during their leisure time had about a 28% reduction in the risk of being diagnosed with depression by a physician compared with their less-active peers over a 12-year period. However, the significance of those findings is limited because fewer than 1 in 10 adults in America expends this much energy in leisure-time physical activity.

The effects of setting and exercise intensity on depressive mood were experimentally examined in a study of 357 healthy, older adults without clinical depression (King, Taylor, and Haskell 1993). Sedentary men and women between the ages of 50 and 65 were randomly assigned to one of three exercise training programs (high-intensity group exercise, high-intensity home exercise, and low-intensity home exercise). After 12 months, no significant differences among groups were observed. However, subsequent data analysis revealed an inverse relationship between level of exercise participation and depression scores independent of exercise format and intensity.

Few studies have appropriately manipulated intensity and duration of exercise to allow examination of the dose–response relationship between exercise and depression. Epidemiologic studies typically classify subjects into two or three activity groups. These grouping procedures have prevented or limited the evaluation of the dose–response relationship across the full range of reported physical activity and may have misclassified individuals who overestimate or underestimate their activity. For example, a reduction in risk of depression for active individuals was not found in the Precursors Study, a prospective study of 752 former medical students (Cooper-Patrick et al. 1997). However, level of physical activity was determined by self-report of the number of times per week a person exercised until sweating; thus, information regarding the duration, intensity, frequency, and mode of exercise is not available to adequately evaluate the dose.

Plausibility

The second-century Greek physician Galen recognized the importance of exercise for stimulating the four humors of Hippocrates, which Galen extended to help explain mood. In modern times, it was proposed that exercise was beneficial to people who were depressed because it stimulated nerves and increased glandular secretions (Vaux 1926). The following paragraphs discuss the evidence that supports a biological explanation of activity's effect on mood. However, unlike the other chronic diseases discussed in this book, biological mechanisms are not the only plausible explanations for the mental health effects of physical activity. Cognitive explanations, especially increased self-esteem, and social support are also popular hypotheses to explain physical activity's antidepressant effect. It is important to remember, though, that regardless of whether the pivotal mechanism whereby physical activity reduces depression is viewed as cognitive or social, it ultimately can be explained in biochemical and physiological terms as the regulation of neurons by genes (e.g., Kandel 1998).

Cognitive and Social Factors. Cognitive changes, such as enhancement of self-esteem, and social support have been proposed as explanations for the effects of physical activity on depression. However, there's little evidence to permit conclusions about their roles. Observational, population studies have not included measures of self-esteem and social support to determine whether they confound or mediate the lower rates of depressive symptoms found among physically active people. Also, most randomized controlled trials did not examine whether reduced depression after exercise training was mediated by enhanced self-esteem nor did they use the proper comparison groups to demonstrate that reduced depression after exercise was independent of social support. Nonetheless, such cognitive and social factors deserve further study, especially self-esteem.

Self-esteem is a cornerstone of mental health and behavior, and depression is often associated with low self-esteem. Because body image is related to general **self-concept,** an improvement in body image or physical skills can contribute to general self-esteem in people who place high value on physical attributes relative to the other aspects of self-concept (Sonstroem 1998) and might reduce the primary or secondary risk of depression.

• *Self-esteem.* Self-esteem is the value people place on their conception or view of themselves. It reflects a person's feelings about and evaluations of specific personal features, including physical attributes—such as appearance, endurance, strength, and sport skills—and social, academic or professional, emotional, and spiritual attributes (Sonstroem and Morgan 1989). Positive comments from others about one's fitness or physique, or merely expectations of increased fitness, can improve self-esteem even when actual fitness has not improved. A sense of achievement is the key. The Preventive Services Task Force of the U.S. Office of Disease Prevention and Health Promotion concluded in 1989 that regular exercise can improve self-esteem (Harris et al. 1989). Participants' self-esteem tends to improve more after fitness training than after participating in competitive sports, where success and feelings of accomplishment are less predictable (Fox 2000). The biggest gains in self-esteem usually occur for people who value physical fitness or appearance and are not satisfied with their current status in these areas. Believing that you are doing something positive for yourself may be enough to improve self-esteem. Supporting this idea is a study by Desharnais et al. (1993) in which college students' self-esteem improved after participating in an exercise program whose stated goal was to improve psychological well-being. Students in the same study who were not told of the goal did not report improvements in self-esteem, even though they showed similar fitness improvements. People who improve their fitness can gain an increased sense of mastery over physical tasks. Some evidence suggests that this confidence can extend beyond physical activity settings to enhance overall self-concept and life adjustment and therefore help reduce depression.

• *Social support.* In one randomized controlled trial of 30 depressed elderly men and women, participants either walked outdoors for 20 min twice weekly for six weeks with a young companion or spent the same amount of time with another young companion. Compared with a control group, both conditions resulted in reductions in self-ratings of depression but the condition that combined walking with social contact was not more effective than the condition of social contact alone (McNeil, LeBlanc, and Joyner 1991). Hence, walking added no benefit beyond social contact.

Although enhanced self-esteem remains a plausible explanation for the antidepressant effects of exercise, it has not been empirically tested as a mediator of depression reduction after exercise in well-designed studies. Moreover, if self-esteem was the only mechanism underlying the treatment responses observed in exercise programs, this mechanism would not be unique to exercise and would not support an independent, causal effect of exercise for reducing depression symptoms because self-esteem can exert its influence in many settings that do not involve physical ac-

tivity. Likewise, social influences that contribute to reductions in depression after exercise would be part of the setting in which exercise takes place, not exercise itself, that might be no different from other therapeutic settings.

Biological Plausibility. Several neurobiological mechanisms represent potential avenues by which exercise could potentially influence physiological mediators of depression. The following discussion provides an overview of the primary biological hypotheses regarding exercise and depression.

• ***Endorphin hypothesis.*** One proposed mechanism for the antidepressant effect of exercise is that elevations in **endorphin** levels following exercise produce improvements in mood. Endorphins and **enkephalins** are proteins with analgesic properties that occur naturally in the brain, spinal cord, adrenal gland, gut, and sympathetic nerves. They help modulate body temperature and the cardiovascular system during stress; they can elevate mood and reduce pain, with effects similar to those of the powerful drug morphine. Beta-endorphin, though found in the brain, is released from the pituitary into the blood during stress. Although blood levels of β-endorphin have been shown to be elevated following exercise, β-endorphin has not been shown to cross the blood–brain barrier during or after exercise. For β-endorphin to be a plausible mechanism for the antidepressant effects of exercise, it must induce changes in brain regions that regulate mood. Endorphins modulate the actions of monoamines throughout brain regions involved with emotions and increase in the brain after exercise in rats and mice (Hoffman 1997). However, that study was not designed to show changes in depression-like behaviors. In addition, most studies of humans that have used drugs to block the action of opioids have not prevented changes in depressive mood following exercise. Thus, the available experimental evidence in humans has failed to support the endorphin hypothesis of mood change after exercise (Dishman 1998). Nonetheless, one action of β-endorphin in the brain is to inhibit the tonic inhibition of dopamine, the key neurotransmitter involved in brain regions involved with pleasure (e.g., the ventral tegmental area) and motivation (e.g., the nucleus accumbens). So, it is plausible that β-endorphin could indirectly influence positive moods through its role in regulating dopamine. The dopaminergic effect of endorphins' response to exercise and its impact on symptoms of depression hve not yet been tested.

• *Brain blood flow hypothesis.* Research has demonstrated that blood flow to areas of the brain involved in the control of movement and cardiovascular responses increases during exercise. Because an increase in blood flow is associated with elevated cellular metabolism, enhanced blood flow to brain regions involved in the regulation of emotion could mediate changes in mood with exercise. However, alterations in blood flow to brain areas that are involved with the regulation of mood have not been reliably shown during exercise, so there is currently little evidence to support the role of brain blood flow in mediating the effects of exercise on depression (Dishman 1998).

• *HPA hypothesis.* Disruption of the hypothalamic-pituitary-adrenocortical (HPA) axis, the system that regulates much of the body's endocrine response to stress, has also been implicated in the etiology of depression. In response to a physical or psychological stressor, the hypothalamus produces corticotropin-releasing factor (CRH), which acts on the pituitary to signal the release of adrenocorticotropic hormone (ACTH). ACTH then exerts its effect on the adrenal gland to stimulate the release of cortisol. The integrated function of this system is to prepare the body for fight or flight in response to a real or perceived threat. Although activation of this system is critical for an appropriate stress response, excess activation of the HPA axis may play a role in the development of depression. Depressed individuals frequently exhibit a blunted ACTH response to CRH, and hyperactivation of the HPA axis and hypercortisolism are also commonly seen in patients with depression. Because CRH and glucocorticoids such as cortisol influence brain regions important in emotional responses, including the nucleus accumbens, amygdala, and hippocampus, elevated levels of CRH and cortisol under conditions of chronic stress may disrupt functioning in brain regions that regulate mood and lead to depression (Gold and Chrousos 1998).

Both acute and chronic exercise can influence functioning of the HPA axis. Acute bouts of exercise result in activation of this system, whereas exercise training attenuates the effect of acute exercise at a given absolute workload. However, the effect of exercise training on this system in relation to depression is unclear. For example, when rats with access to activity wheels were compared with sedentary animals following a foot-shock stressor, responses in plasma levels of ACTH and corticosterone did not differ between the groups (Dishman et al. 1995, 1997). In contrast, increased levels of ACTH have been observed in treadmill-trained rats after immobilization stress (White-Welkley et al. 1995). Further investigation is needed to clarify the effects of exercise on the HPA axis and to determine how these effects may influence depression.

• *Improved sleep.* Chronic insomnia increases mortality and psychiatric problems and decreases work productivity. About one third of all adults will experience insomnia sometime in their lives, and people suffering from depression or an anxiety disorder commonly have disturbed sleep. Exercise is frequently included as a component of good sleep hygiene and could plausibly reduce other depression symptoms by improving sleep (Youngstedt 2000). Sleep is measured by **polysomnography,** which measures changes in electrical potentials that come from the brain cortex, the chin muscles, and eye movements. Sleep is composed of periods of rapid eye movement (REM) sleep, when most dreaming occurs, and four stages of non-REM sleep with decreasing activation of brain and skeletal muscle. During sleep, activity of the brain cortex, estimated by electrical waves or cycles, fluctuates along a continuum from harmonious, low-frequency, high-amplitude waves to irregular, high-frequency, low-amplitude waves. This continuum includes periods of delta (0.5–3 cycles/s), theta (3.5–7.5 cycles/s), alpha (8–12 cycles/s), and beta (13–30 cycles/s) activity. **Alpha wave activity** is commonly described as relaxed wakefulness. Sleep progresses from drowsiness to stage 1, marked by theta activity. Stage 2 occurs later, denoted by theta activity, sleep spindles (short bursts of 12–14 cycles/s), and K complexes (sudden sharp spikes). Spindles occur several times a minute throughout stages 1 to 4, while K complexes occur only in stage 2. Stage 3, which follows, is characterized by delta activity. Increasing delta activity denotes stage 4, or deep sleep. REM sleep, when dreaming occurs, typically begins about 45 min after the onset of stage 4 sleep and is marked by beta activity, rapid eye movements, and little skeletal muscle activity. During the night, a normal sleeper (someone who sleeps 8 h) commonly has four or five sleep cycles, each lasting about 90 min and consisting of 20 to 30 min of REM sleep. Measures used to describe sleep include the time spent in stage 2, time spent in stages 3 and 4 (together called slow-wave sleep), time spent in REM, time before REM begins, wakefulness during sleep, time to fall asleep, and total sleep time.

About 40 studies of acute exercise and another dozen or so studies of chronic exercise have examined the effects of physical activity on polysomnographic measures of sleep among normal sleepers. They generally agree in showing small increases in slow-wave (deep) sleep and total sleep time, with decreases in the time needed to fall asleep and in wakefulness during sleep. Moderately large reductions (nearly half a standard deviation) in REM sleep (about 7–10 min) and increased **latency** for REM sleep (about 12–15 min) have been reported (Kubitz et al. 1996; Youngstedt, O'Connor, and Dishman 1997). The changes in REM sleep after exercise could help explain the antidepressant effects of exercise, as REM sleep deprivation has been shown to be an effective treatment for some depressed patients. How exercise facilitates sleep is unknown; possible but unconfirmed explanations include body restitution, energy conservation, anxiety reduction, body warming, and increased production of **melatonin** and adenosine, body chemicals that help regulate sleep.

Only a few studies have examined whether regular exercise promotes sleep for people with sleep problems. Stanford University researchers found that elderly patients with insomnia reported improvements in self-rated sleep after a 16-week exercise program of moderate intensity consisting of 30 to 40 min of aerobic exercise four times a week (King et al. 1997). Tufts University researchers reported that a 10-week, three-day-a-week, resistance training program improved self-ratings of sleep in depressed adults with sleep problems (Singh, Clements, and Fiatarone 1997a). A separate publication from that study also showed a reduction in depression symptoms (Singh, Clements, and Fiatarone 1997b).

• *Monoamine hypothesis.* Much of the physiological research on exercise and depression has focused on the brain monoaminergic systems, which include the neurotransmitters dopamine, norepinephrine, and serotonin (Chaouloff 1997a, 1997b; Dishman 1997b; Meeusen and De Meirleir 1995), primarily because most effective pharmacotherapies modulate one or more of these neurotransmitter systems. Animal research has provided evidence of a mediating effect of exercise on the monoaminergic systems implicated in depression. Studies using rats have demonstrated that acute exercise results in increased release of norepinephrine, dopamine, and serotonin in the brain (Meeusen, Piacentini, and De Meirleir 2001; Wilson and Marsden 1996) and that repeated treadmill training attenuates norepinephrine release during exercise (Pagliari and Peyrin 1995b).

Subsequent studies on rats conducted at the University of Georgia showed that brain noradrenergic adaptations to chronic exercise are related to antidepressant-like effects. First, Dunn and colleagues (1996) found that both treadmill exercise training and activity-wheel running led to increased levels of norepinephrine in regions of the brain stem that contain norepinephrine cell bodies. Next, it was shown that such increases in brain norepinephrine in the locus coeruleus and raphe nuclei were accompanied by protection against depletion of brain norepinephrine (Dishman et al. 1997). That was the first study to experimentally test a neurobiological mechanism for the antidepressant effects of exercise. Next, a pharmacologic model of depression was used to compare exercise and antidepressant treatment in animals treated neonatally with clomipramine, a serotonin reuptake inhibitor (Yoo, Tackett et al. 2000). Treadmill exercise training and activity-wheel running each increased brain levels of norepinephrine and decreased the number of β-adrenoreceptors in the brain frontal cortex, effects that are similar to those obtained by chronic administration of the antidepressant imipramine. Chronic activity-wheel runners also had attenuated release of norepinephrine in the frontal cortex during uncontrollable foot electric shock compared with sedentary animals but no change in gene expression for the synthetic enzyme tyrosine hydroxylase (Soares et al. 1999). Those findings suggest a downregulation in activity by the locus coeruleus that could preserve brain norepinephrine during stress. Subsequent research suggested that this attenuated stress response after wheel running can be partly explained by increased gene expression for **galanin,** a neuropeptide that appears to inhibit neuronal discharge by the locus coeruleus (O'Neal et al. 2001).

In addition, both acute and chronic exercise in animals have been shown to influence dopaminergic activity, and changes in the density and affinity of dopamine receptors have been observed following chronic training in animals (for reviews, see Chaouloff 1989; Mazzeo 1991;

Meeusen and De Meirleir 1995; Tantillo et al. 2002). Dishman et al. (1997) found that sedentary animals had 50% higher dopamine concentrations in the hypothalamus than animals with access to activity wheels following uncontrollable foot shock; this brain region is important in the regulation of hormone release from the pituitary. Moreover, sedentary animals exhibited 30% more serotonin in the amygdala following foot shock. Thus, exercise training appears to influence monoamine systems, and these adaptations may help explain the biological effects of exercise as a treatment for depression.

- *Depression-like behavior.* In rats, the escape-deficit model after uncontrollable stress, first reported by McCulloch and Bruner (1939), was the first animal model of depression. The hallmark response to uncontrollable, inescapable foot shock is increased latency to escape from controllable shock administered 24 to 72 h later, presumably resulting from depletion of norepinephrine in the locus coeruleus and a subsequent up-regulation of β-adrenoreceptors in the brain cortex. The escape-deficit model is an attempt to simulate the so-called learned helplessness or behavioral despair common in human depression. The escape-deficit model is mostly **isomorphic** with human depression, featuring weight loss, reduced sexual behavior, sleep disturbances (decreased REM sleep latency), and anhedonia. Though self-reward tasks such as feeding choices between water and water with sucrose added and intracranial self-stimulation are used as surrogate measures in the rat for the phenomenological **construct** of pleasure experienced by humans, it is not possible to determine whether a rat feels helpless or hopeless.

Some types of depression and anxiety in humans appear to be endogenous; they cannot be attributed to an uncontrollable stressor. One model of endogenous depression in the rat involves injecting neonatal pups with clomipramine, leading to decreased REM sleep latency and other key behavioral signs of depression upon reaching adulthood. Another endogenous model disturbs brain neurotransmitter systems, including norepinephrine and serotonin, by surgically removing the olfactory bulbs located below the brain frontal cortex (Kelly, Wrynn, and Leonard 1997). These models each are responsive to pharmacotherapy. Studies conducted at the University of Georgia showed that chronic activity-wheel running protects against depression-like behavioral abnormalities in all of the rat models mentioned. Female wheel runners were protected from learned helplessness when exposed to electrical shock (Dishman et al. 1997), and male wheel runners were protected against impaired sexual behavior after neonatal clomipramine injections (Yoo, Tackett et al. 2000) and after olfactory bulbectomy (Van Hoomissen et al. 2001). Not only were behavioral signs of depression reduced among wheel runners, but responses by the brain noradrenergic and serotonergic systems, as well as enhanced neuron growth factors, were comparable to antidepressant drug treatment (Dishman et al. 1997; O'Neal et al. 2001; Van Hoomissen et al. 2003; Yoo, Tackett et al. 2000).

Because the procedures used to study the monoaminergic systems directly are extremely invasive, much of the research has been limited to animal models of depression, with obviously limited application to human depression. However, refinement of neurobiological diagnostic procedures in humans, including brain-imaging techniques such as **functional magnetic resonance imaging (FMRI)** and **positron emission tomography (PET),** should allow researchers and clinicians to gain a better understanding of the effects of exercise on neuronal activity in brain systems and their role in the etiology of depression (Davidson et al. 2003; Kalin et al. 1997; Nemeroff 1998; Nemeroff, Kilts, and Berns 1999). It is likely that future studies of exercise and depression that include brain-imaging assessments will greatly enhance our understanding of the neurobiological adaptations associated with exercise. For the time being, however, although there is evidence that neurobiological mechanisms underlying depression may be responsive to exercise stimuli, current evidence is inadequate to conclusively determine a biologically plausible explanation for physical activity's effect on depression.

Summary and Conclusions

A limitation of the exercise and depression research literature has been the failure to fully characterize the mental status of subjects. There are several types of depressive disorders, and symptoms exhibited by individuals with depression can vary widely depending on the nature of their illness. Furthermore, depressed individuals often suffer from anxiety or other mental disorders (Kessler et al. 1994), yet most studies do not assess comorbidity or analyze data to investigate whether effects are dependent on the nature of the depressive disorder. Well-controlled studies that encompass a range of demographic groups and fully consider subject characteristics are needed to determine whether the relationship between exercise and depression is consistent across sexes, ages, races, ethnicities, levels of education, socioeconomic levels, and mental status. In addition, better descriptions of the exercise stimulus are needed to determine whether the effects are consistent for all modes, intensities, frequencies, and durations of physical activity.

Numerous studies have demonstrated the antidepressant effect of chronic exercise. However, most prospective studies had methodological limitations that may have obscured the actual effect of exercise training. For example, many studies used preexperimental or quasi-experimental designs. Studies have often failed to randomly assign subjects to experimental conditions, resulting in bias due to self-selection and nonequivalence of groups. Furthermore, few studies have been conducted using a blinded design to protect against experimenter bias, and it is difficult to protect against bias due to participant expectancies. The failure to use appropriate comparison groups is another common design limitation in this area of research. Studies that compare an exercise group to a no-treatment control group reveal little about the clinical meaningfulness of the results since the only conclusion that can be made is that exercise is better than no treatment and thus might merely be a placebo effect. Because standard therapies have been shown to be effective in treating depression, a placebo group or minimal-intervention control group is needed to adequately evaluate the effectiveness of exercise in alleviating depression. Medication is the best-documented treatment for depression, but only one published study has compared exercise and medication in the treatment of depression—with promising results, however (Blumenthal et al. 1999). Research design must also provide rigorous control of other factors that could potentially influence mood and depression, such as increased social contact and increased light exposure, so that the effect of the exercise stimulus can be established.

The use of valid measures of physical activity and depression is also an important experimental consideration. Physical activity should be adequately described, and physiological status before and after training should be measured using appropriate methods. Level of depression should be assessed with valid inventories with good psychometric properties. Therapist interviews as well as self-report questionnaires should be employed because both methods are needed to confirm that a clinically meaningful remission of symptoms occurs after exercise.

> ••• *Although moderate exercise during leisure time is associated with reduced risk of depression and with reduced depression symptoms, excessive exercise training (i.e., overtraining), especially in endurance sports, can result in depression in some athletes (Morgan et al. 1987). Most youths and adults are sedentary, though, so depression resulting from overtraining is not a concern for the general population.*

Few studies used resistance or flexibility exercise; most studies used jogging as the mode of activity, and a few used cycling. Exercise training usually was prescribed based on the guidelines of the American College of Sports Medicine for the types and amounts of exercise recommended for cardiorespiratory fitness in otherwise healthy people (Pollock et al. 1998). Because no adverse effects were reported in these studies, the following exercise guidelines should be appropriate for people with depression who are otherwise healthy:

- Three to five days a week
- 20 to 60 min each session
- 55% to 90% of maximal heart rate

Though beginners should always increase the intensity and length of their workouts gradually, gradual progress is especially important for someone who is depressed. Gradual progress helps to maximize feelings of success and control and to minimize potential feelings of failure if the person cannot sustain the exercise program due to overly rapid progression. It is important to remember that continued participation is more important for reducing depression than is increasing fitness.

> ••• *Being sedentary increases the risk for depression, but high levels of physical activity may not be any more protective than moderate levels.*

Anxiety Disorders

Anxiety is characterized by apprehension or worry and is typically accompanied by agitation, feelings of tension, and bodily arousal. Other signs and symptoms of anxiety disorders vary in number and severity. They include agitation, excessive alertness, confusion, muscle tension, tremors, high heart rates, palpitations, flushing, sweating, dry mouth, and urinary and gastrointestinal problems. Though anxiety often occurs with depression, and chronic anxiety can contribute to the risk of depression, people most often experience anxiety apart from depression. Anxiety is a common human experience during imagined or real threatening circumstances. **State anxiety** can be used to describe this condition if the feelings of anxiety are temporary and fluctuate from moment to moment ("How do I feel right now?"); the term **trait anxiety** is used if these feelings and symptoms are constant and persistent ("How have I been feeling generally?").

Anxiety disorders, however, are illnesses that cause people to feel frightened, distressed, and uneasy for extended periods of time for no apparent reason. Left untreated, these disorders can reduce productivity and diminish the quality of life.

Though apprehension, agitation, and activation of the autonomic nervous system are core signs and symptoms present to varying degrees in all anxiety states, there are several recognized types of anxiety disorders. According to the American Psychiatric Association (2000a), the major types include the following:

• *Phobias.* A **phobia** is an intense fear of an object, place, or situation. A person with a specific phobia experiences extreme fear of something that poses little or no actual danger; the fear causes people with phobias to avoid these objects or situations and most likely limits their lives unnecessarily.

• *Social phobia.* People with social phobia have an overwhelming fear of scrutiny and embarrassment in social situations, which causes them to avoid many potentially enjoyable activities. Social phobias are equally common in men and women. They may be discrete (e.g., restricted to eating in public, to public speaking, or to encounters with the opposite sex) or diffuse, involving almost all social situations outside the family circle. A fear of vomiting in public may be important. Direct eye-to-eye confrontation may be particularly stressful in some cultures. Social phobias are usually associated with low self-esteem and fear of criticism. Symptoms often involve flushing, hand tremor, nausea, or urgent need to urinate; a person with social phobia is sometimes sure that one of these secondary symptoms of anxiety is the primary problem. Symptoms may progress to panic attacks. Agoraphobia, which is fear of open spaces, and depressive disorders are often prominent, and both may contribute to the person's becoming housebound.

• *Panic disorder.* Panic disorder involves repeated episodes of intense fear that strike without warning and without an obvious source. Physical symptoms include chest pain, heart palpitations, choking sensations or shortness of breath, dizziness, abdominal distress, feelings of unreality, and fear of dying, losing control, or going crazy. A panic attack usually lasts for minutes, during which a crescendo of fear and autonomic symptoms builds and leads the person to flee and subsequently avoid the situation where the attack occurred, often producing fear of being alone or going into public places and persistent fear of another attack.

• *Obsessive-compulsive disorder (OCD).* Repeated, unwanted thoughts or compulsive behaviors that seem impossible to stop, typified by repetitive acts or rituals to relieve anxiety.

• *Post–traumatic stress disorder.* A delayed or prolonged response to a stressful event or situation (either short- or long-lasting) that was especially threatening or catastrophic (e.g., natural disaster, combat, serious accident, witnessing the violent death of others, or being the victim of torture, terrorism, rape, or other crime). Symptoms commonly include flashbacks or dreams of the original trauma, a state of autonomic hyperarousal with hypervigilance, an enhanced startle reaction, and insomnia.

• *Generalized anxiety disorder (GAD).* Recurrent or persistent excessive worry about everyday, routine life events and activities, lasting at least six months. Freud called this "free-floating" anxiety. It is the most prevalent type of anxiety disorder; it is accompanied by fatigue, trembling, muscle tension, headaches, or nausea.

Diagnostic Guidelines

SOCIAL PHOBIAS

All the following criteria should be fulfilled for a diagnosis of social phobia:

- The psychological, behavioral, or autonomic symptoms must be primarily manifestations of anxiety and not secondary to other symptoms such as delusions or obsessional thoughts.
- The anxiety must be restricted to or predominate in particular social situations.
- Avoidance of the phobic situations must be a prominent feature.

PANIC DISORDER (EPISODIC PAROXYSMAL ANXIETY)

Panic disorder should be the main diagnosis only in the absence of any of the phobias. For a definite diagnosis, several severe attacks of autonomic anxiety should have occurred within a period of about one month

- in circumstances where there is no objective danger,
- without being confined to known or predictable situations, and
- with comparative freedom from anxiety symptoms between attacks (although anticipatory anxiety is common).

OBSESSIVE-COMPULSIVE DISORDER

Obsessional symptoms or compulsive acts, or both, must be present on most days for at least two successive weeks and must be a source of distress or interference with activities. The obsessional symptoms should have the following characteristics:

- They must be recognized as the individual's own thoughts or impulses.
- There must be at least one thought or act that is still resisted unsuccessfully, even

though others may be present that the sufferer no longer resists.

- The thought of carrying out the act must not in itself be pleasurable (simple relief of tension or anxiety is not regarded as pleasure in this sense).
- The thoughts, images, or impulses must be unpleasantly repetitive.

POST–TRAUMATIC STRESS DISORDER

This disorder should not generally be diagnosed unless there is evidence that it arose within six months of a traumatic event of exceptional severity. In addition to evidence of trauma, there must be a repetitive, intrusive recollection or reenactment of the event in memories, daytime imagery, or dreams. Conspicuous emotional detachment, numbing of feeling, and avoidance of stimuli that might arouse recollection of the trauma are often present but are not essential for the diagnosis. Autonomic disturbances, mood disorder (e.g., depression, dramatic bursts of fear or panic), and behavioral abnormalities (aggression disorder, alcohol abuse) all contribute to the diagnosis but are not key.

GENERALIZED ANXIETY DISORDER

Primary symptoms of anxiety must be present most days for at least several weeks at a time and usually for several months. These symptoms should usually involve elements of

- apprehension (worries about future misfortunes, feeling "on edge," difficulty concentrating, etc.),
- motor tension (restless fidgeting, tension headaches, trembling, inability to relax), and
- autonomic overactivity (lightheadedness, sweating, tachycardia or tachypnea, epigastric discomfort, dizziness, dry mouth, etc.).

In children, frequent need for reassurance and recurrent somatic complaints may be prominent.

WHO 1992.

Magnitude of the Problem

Anxiety disorders are the most common mental illnesses in the United States, affecting about 23 million people (4% of women and 2% of men)

each year. Anxiety disorders in the United States accounted for $46.6 billion in direct and indirect costs in 1990 (DuPont et al. 1996). As is the case with depression, young people tend to have more anxiety than do older people. People in the

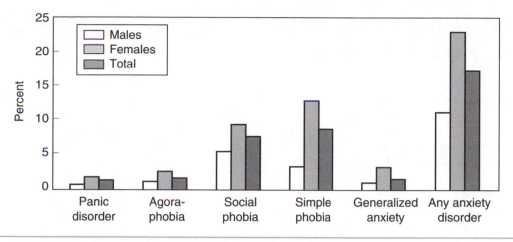

Figure 13.15 Twelve-month prevalence of anxiety disorders.

Data from Kessler et al., 1994. Reprinted, by permission, from J. Buckworth and R.K. Dishman, 2001, *Exercise psychology* (Champaign, IL: Human Kinetics), 115.

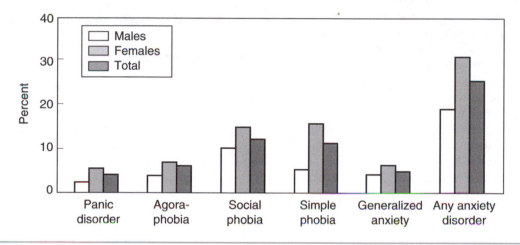

Figure 13.16 Lifetime prevalence of anxiety disorders.

Data from Kessler et al., 1994. Reprinted, by permission, from J. Buckworth and R.K. Dishman, 2001, *Exercise psychology* (Champaign, IL: Human Kinetics), 119.

age group of 15 to 24 years experience episodes of anxiety about 40% more often than people 25 to 54 years old, regardless of race. Figures 13.15 and 13.16 illustrate the annual and lifetime prevalence rates of anxiety disorders in the United States.

Etiology of Anxiety Disorders

Just as people can have a depressive **temperament,** people can also, through genetics and early experiences, have an anxious temperament. Fluctuations in anxiety are a major part of most people's emotional lives, even those who do not have an anxiety disorder. Anxiety, like depression, is a stress emotion. Uncertainties about important events can lead to worry and apprehension, especially when a person feels a lack of control over how the event is going to turn out. Life events such as romance, divorce, paying bills, making good grades, making a good impression on others, and getting a good job contribute to anxieties that affect the quality of life. Smaller hassles of daily living, such as catching the bus on time, making it to class on time, and dealing with a noisy neighbor or a nagging friend or relative, can also add to stress emotions, including anxiety.

Anxiety can also be more subconscious, leading to tension, digestion problems, headaches, high blood pressure, and sleep problems, even when people do not report feeling worried. Feelings of helplessness or loss of control can lead to anxiety, as they do to depression.

Brain Neurobiology in Anxiety Disorders

A neurobiological perspective of anxiety integrates cognitive and neurological theories. For example, neural circuits involved in the experience of anxiety must include **afferent nerve** fibers that allow potentially threatening stimuli to be sensed so that they can be interpreted as threatening by higher brain areas. These brain areas must appraise the input and integrate it with relevant memories. If the stimuli are then interpreted as representing a threat, the response depends on **efferent nerves** that generate a coordinated endocrine, autonomic, and muscular response. The effects of these different neural systems depend on several neurotransmitters, which have been targets for the pharmacologic treatment of anxiety disorders.

As is the case for depression, there is evidence from human and animal research that the amygdala, locus coeruleus, midbrain, **thalamus,** right hippocampus, anterior cingulate cortex, insular cortex, and the right prefrontal cortex (shown previously in figure 13.2) are involved in the genesis and expression of anxiety (Goddard and Charney 1997; Reiman 1997). The amygdala seems to be the critical central neural structure involved in the psychophysiological components of fear and anxiety responses (Goddard and Charney 1997; LeDoux 1998). The amygdala receives input from the thalamus and locus coeruleus and from sensations that have been integrated in higher cortical areas. Other key brain regions involved in anxiety include the hypothalamus and the **periaqueductal gray area,** which is a doughnut-shaped region that surrounds the cerebrospinal fluid channel between the third and fourth ventricles of the brain. The periaqueductal gray processes neuronal signals associated with pain and aversive behavior.

Each of those brain regions is modulated by the actions of serotonin (mainly originating from the dorsal raphe nuclei), norepinephrine (mainly originating from the locus coeruleus), and the inhibitory neurotransmitter **gamma-aminobutyric acid (GABA).** Several **anxiolytic** drugs affect serotonergic systems by blocking serotonin reuptake or by acting on serotonergic receptors as agonists or antagonists. The brain noradrenergic system is also involved in anxiety (O'Connor, Raglin, and Martinsen 2000). Inhibiting the effects of norepinephrine with β-adrenergic blockers, which

down-regulate the norepinephrine receptor-effector system, has been shown to be efficacious in the treatment of social phobia (Gorman and Gorman 1987). However, GABA is the major neural inhibitory brain neurotransmitter involved in anxiety disorders. GABA neurons and receptors are widely distributed in brain areas thought to be important for the expression of anxiety (Menard and Treit 1999).

Treatment of Anxiety Disorders

Anxiety disorders can be treated with psychotherapy or medications. Among antianxiety drugs, benzodiazepines are most commonly used to treat short-term symptoms, although SSRIs are also used to treat certain anxiety disorders.

Psychotherapy

The two most effective forms of psychotherapy used to treat anxiety disorders are behavioral and cognitive-behavioral therapy. Behavioral therapy helps patients change their actions through breathing techniques or through gradual exposure to what is frightening them. Cognitive-behavioral therapy, in addition to these techniques, teaches patients to understand their thinking patterns so that they can react differently to the situations that cause them anxiety.

Pharmacotherapy

A classification of drugs called the benzodiazepines provides the most effective short-term treatment of several anxiety disorders, especially generalized anxiety (Ballenger 2001). Benzodiazepines bind to the $GABA_A$ receptor and inhibit activity of neurons in the brain by opening a chloride channel and hyperpolarizing the cell. Benzodiazepines vary in the strength of their CNS depressant and muscle-relaxing effects, but they all are less sedating and hypnotic than barbiturates, which were commonly used to treat anxiety before benzodiazepines. The benzodiazepines are effective in treating generalized anxiety disorder, and the benzodiazepine receptor inverse agonists (e.g., the beta-carbolines) produce strong anxiety reactions. The four benzodiazepines currently widely prescribed for treatment of anxiety disorders are diazepam, lorazepam, clonazepam, and alprazolam (J.R. Davidson 1998). Alprazolam and lorazepam have a relatively short period of action (i.e., a few hours), whereas diazepam and clonazepam have half-lives up to 24 h. Diazepam also has multiple active metabolites, which increase its side effects.

Benzodiazepines are only weakly effective in the treatment of obsessive-compulsive disorder and post–traumatic stress disorder, which are more effectively treated by SSRI antidepressants. There is a high risk of relapse of symptoms in these disorders when benzodiazepine treatment is ceased. Nonetheless, because benzodiazepines can be mildly addicting, their use is usually tapered after a few months of treatment. For example, treatment of panic disorder and generalized anxiety disorder typically involves a combination therapy of acute benzodiazepine treatment followed by antidepressants.

Excessive responses by nerves that manufacture and release noradrenaline contribute to signs and symptoms of anxiety, especially panic. Drugs that block receptors for noradrenaline, called beta-blockers (e.g., propranolol), help reduce panic symptoms, especially rapid heartbeat and palpitations.

In contrast, inadequate responses by brain neurons that manufacture and release serotonin also play a role in anxiety disorders, especially obsessive-compulsive disorder. SSRI antidepressants are clinically effective in treating anxiety. The tricyclic SSRI clomipramine is especially effective in treating obsessive-compulsive disorder because it has antiobsessional effects (March et al. 1997).

According to the Surgeon General's report on mental health (U.S. Department of Health and Human Services 1999), the current practice guidelines rank the tricyclic antidepressants below the five most popular SSRIs (i.e., fluoxetine, sertraline, paroxetine, fluvoxamine, and citalopram) for treatment of anxiety disorders, mainly because SSRIs have fewer side effects (American Psychiatric Association 1998; Ballenger et al. 1998; Kent, Coplan, and Gorman 1998; March et al. 1997; Westenberg 1996). In addition to their efficacy in treating obsessive-compulsive disorder (Micallef and Blin 2001), SSRIs also have efficacy for treating panic disorder and other anxiety disorders (American Psychiatric Association 1998; Kent, Coplan, and Gorman 1998). Other, newer antidepressants that combine SSRIs and SNRIs also appear to have antianxiety effects for social phobia (e.g., paroxetine) and post–traumatic stress disorder (e.g., nefazodone and sertraline; American Psychiatric Association 1998; March et al. 1997).

Common Drugs Used to Treat Anxiety

Benzodiazepines

Ativan® (lorazepam)

Centrax® (prazepam)

Paxipam® (halazepam)

Serax® (oxazepam)

Valium® (diazepam)

Xanax® (alprazolam)

Barbiturates

Librium® (chlordiazepoxide)

Tranxene® (clorazepate)

Serotonin antagonist

BuSpar® (buspirone)

Selective Serotonin Reuptake Inhibitors

Celexa™ (citalopram)

Luvox® (fluvoxamine)

Paxil™ (paroxetine)

Zoloft® (sertraline)

Side effects: sedation; low muscle tone; anticonvulsant effects; tolerance or dependence and withdrawal may develop

---

Buspirone (BuSpar) is an atypical antianxiety drug that does not block the neuronal reuptake of monoamines. Rather, it binds with brain D_2 dopamine receptors, where it acts as an antagonist and agonist, and with 5-HT_{1A} receptors, where it acts as an agonist (Stahl 1996). Like tricyclic and SSRI antidepressants, buspirone takes about a month to be effective for treating generalized anxiety disorder, especially when combined with SSRIs, but it is not effective alone for the treatment of panic, obsessive-compulsive disorder, or post–traumatic stress disorder (Stahl 1996).

Physical Activity and Anxiety: The Evidence

The 1996 U.S. Surgeon General's report on physical activity and health (U.S. Department of Health and Human Services 1996) concluded that regular physical activity reduces feelings of anxiety. However, unlike the study of physical activity and depression, virtually no epidemiologic studies have examined the association between physical activity and anxiety, in either patient or normal populations. An exception is the Canada Fitness Survey, which asked 22,000 Canadians over age 10 questions about anxiety and exercise (Stephens 1988). Those reporting little or no activity had more symptoms of anxiety than those reporting moderate or very active lifestyles. Most studies have been experimental studies of the effects of acute exercise on state anxiety or chronic exercise on trait anxiety among people without anxiety disorders. A few randomized controlled trials of the effects of exercise on panic disorder and on generalized anxiety disorder also have been reported.

State Anxiety

The first modern-day, controlled study of exercise and state anxiety was reported by William P. Morgan (1973) of the University of Wisconsin. He measured state anxiety in 40 men before, shortly after, and 20 to 30 min after 45 min of vigorous exercise. There was a slight increase in anxiety immediately after exercise, but a significant decrease below preexercise anxiety 20 to 30 min later. In a subsequent study, the reduction in state anxiety after 20 min of exercise at 70% of aerobic capacity was comparable to reductions after meditation or quiet rest in a group of 75 middle-aged men (Bahrke and Morgan 1978). That study was especially important because it generated the **distraction hypothesis,** the hypothesis that the key feature common to each of the conditions was time out, or diversion, from the source or symptoms of anxiety and that distraction might be a plausible explanation for anxiety reduction after exercise. This hypothesis recently has found support (Breus and O'Connor 1998).

Since Morgan's seminal studies, a large body of research has shown reductions in self-rated anxiety after aerobic exercise in adults without anxiety disorders (e.g., Landers and Petruzzello 1994; Petruzzello et al. 1991). Studies have reported an average reduction ranging from one-fourth standard deviation (McDonald and Hodgdon 1991; Petruzzello et al. 1991) to one-half standard deviation (Landers and Petruzzello 1994), with larger changes typically occurring 5 to 30 min after exercise that lasted about 20 to 30 min. Several studies have suggested that acute exercise is as effective as meditation (Bahrke and Morgan 1978) and biofeedback and drugs (Broocks et al.

1998) but no more effective than quiet rest or distraction in decreasing state anxiety (Bahrke and Morgan 1978; Breus and O'Connor 1998). However, the anxiolytic effects of exercise apparently last longer than rest or distraction, and short periods of exercise have been associated with decreases in state anxiety that have persisted up to several hours after exercise. For example, Raglin and Wilson (1996) reported that state anxiety remained decreased up to 2 h after 20 min of cycling at either 40%, 60%, or 70% of $\dot{V}O_2$max.

Trait Anxiety

Petruzzello et al. (1991) and later Landers and Petruzzello (1994) concluded from meta-analyses of exercise and anxiety research that the typical reduction in trait anxiety after exercise training was about one-third to nearly one-half standard deviation, a change of about 3 to 5 points on the most common rating scale used in the studies, Spielberger's state-trait anxiety inventory, which ranges from 20 (almost never anxious) to 80 (almost always anxious). Despite the fact that virtually none of the people studied had diagnosed anxiety disorders, greater reductions were seen among people who had higher trait anxiety. Effects for exercise were as good as other active treatments and better than control conditions. However, all studies were conducted on people who did not have diagnosed anxiety disorders.

Exercise Training by Patients With Anxiety Disorders

Few training studies have been conducted with people diagnosed with anxiety disorders, but generally there are reductions in anxiety regardless of training intensity or changes in aerobic capacity. Early randomized controlled trials with anxiety patients were conducted by Norwegian psychiatrist Egil Martinsen at the Modum Bads Nervesanatorium in the mid-1980s. Martinsen, Hoffart, and Solberg (1989a) examined the effects of aerobic (walking, jogging) and nonaerobic (strength, flexibility, relaxation) exercise on 79 inpatients with various anxiety disorders. Patients were randomly assigned to the groups and exercised for 1 h three days per week. After eight weeks of training, patients in both groups showed similar and significant reductions in anxiety regardless of changes in aerobic capacity. Benefits of exercise training were also documented in another study of 44 inpatients with a variety of anxiety disorders (Martinsen, Sandvik, and Kolbjørnsrud 1989). Patients performed 1 h of aerobic exercise five times a week for eight weeks. All of them exhibited improvements in anxiety symptoms during the study, except those diagnosed with social phobia. Patients with generalized anxiety disorder and agoraphobia without panic attacks maintained their improvements at follow-up one year later. Sexton, Mære, and Dahl (1989) also reported persistence in anxiety reduction six months after hospitalized patients had participated in eight weeks of moderate or low-intensity aerobic exercise training. In addition, improvements in psychological symptoms were similar for both intensities.

Most of the clinical research on anxiety and exercise has focused on panic disorders, in part because of a concern in psychiatry since the 1960s that vigorous exercise poses a risk of inducing panic attacks in patients diagnosed with panic disorder, presumably resulting from hypersensitivity to bodily symptoms induced from blood lactate (O'Connor, Raglin, and Martinsen 2000). Contrary to that concern, empirical evidence from 15 studies conducted since 1987 refutes the association between exercise and panic attacks; only five panic attacks were reported during exercise involving 444 exercise bouts performed by 420 panic disorder patients (O'Connor, Smith, and Morgan 2000). Research has also shown that lactate accumulation resulting from exercise is not related to increased risk of panic attacks among patients with panic disorder (Martinsen et al. 1998) or postexercise anxiety in normal individuals (e.g., Garvin, Koltyn, and Morgan 1997). Moreover, a small, randomized clinical trial recently showed that 10 weeks of aerobic exercise training was effective in reducing symptoms of anxiety among patients with panic disorder and agoraphobia, though not as effective as drug therapy (Broocks et al. 1998). In that study, 46 outpatients suffering from moderate to severe panic disorder with agoraphobia (4 did not have agoraphobia) were randomly assigned to a 10-week treatment consisting of regular aerobic exercise (running), the serotonin reuptake inhibitor clomipramine (112.5 mg/day), or placebo pills. The dropout rate was 31% for the exercise group, 27% for the placebo group, and 0% for the clomipramine treatment group. Compared with placebo, both exercise and clomipramine were accompanied by a significant decrease in symptoms, but clomipramine treatment improved anxiety symptoms sooner and more effectively. Though some evidence has suggested that individuals with panic disorders are physically inactive and actually avoid exercise (Broocks et al. 1997), there is no scientific consensus that patients diagnosed with panic disorder avoid physical activity because of fear (O'Connor, Smith, and Morgan 2000).

Most research on anxiety and exercise has examined the effects of aerobic, low-resistance exercises such as swimming, cycling, or running at moderate or high intensities. Anxiety reductions following high-resistance exercise such as weightlifting have been examined less frequently. In 1993, Raglin, Turner, and Eksten found no decrease in state anxiety after weight training but significant decreases after leg cycle exercise. Focht and Koltyn (1999) found a reduction in state anxiety after resistance exercise at 50% but not 80% of 1RM, although this effect was delayed by more than 60 min after exercise. In another study, anxiety reductions after resistance exercise were delayed until 1.5 to 2 h after exercise (O'Connor, Bryant et al. 1993). Bartholomew and Linder (1998) found decreased state anxiety after 20 min of resistance exercise at 40% to 50% of 1RM, and this effect occurred 15 and 30 min after exercise. They also found that anxiety was increased 5 and 15 min after 20 min of high-intensity resistance exercise (75%–85% of 1RM).

Strength of the Evidence

There is no compelling evidence that increased physical activity or fitness changes a person's temperament from anxious to calm and relaxed. However, studies have shown that a single session of physical activity can reduce state anxiety and that regular exercise can reduce trait anxiety. Because there is no evidence that physical activity causes the underlying sources of anxiety to disappear or causes people to perceive events as less threatening, how can these reductions in anxiety be explained?

Temporal Sequence

Controlled prospective cohort studies of the association between physical activity and anxiety symptoms or the risk of developing anxiety disorders have yet to be reported. About 100 experimental studies, which have the proper temporal sequence to establish cause and effect, of the effects of acute exercise on state anxiety and of chronic exercise on trait anxiety in people without anxiety disorders have generally agreed that exercise decreases self-rated symptoms of anxiety to a small to moderate degree.

Strength of Association

About 150 small-sample studies cumulatively have shown a small to moderate reduction either in self-rated state anxiety after acute exercise (about 0.25–0.50 SD) or in trait anxiety after chronic exercise (about 0.33–0.40 SD). Reductions in trait anxiety averaging 1 to 2 SD have been found after four to five months of exercise training, rivaling the size of symptom reduction after psychotherapy. A handful of studies show similar reductions in symptoms among patients diagnosed with panic disorders or generalized anxiety disorder, but it is not yet known whether such reductions in symptoms are sufficiently large to alter clinical diagnosis.

Consistency

As was the case for studies of depression, most studies of anxiety and exercise were not designed to compare demographic groups on their anxiety responses to exercise and were limited to ages younger than 55 years or arbitrarily used middle age (e.g., 40 or 45 years) as a criterion for aging effects. There have been very few controlled studies of children and people over age 65. Quantitative reviews concluded that age did not moderate reductions in self-ratings of state anxiety and trait anxiety (e.g., Landers and Petruzzello 1994; Petruzzello et al. 1991). Neither men nor women had reduced state anxiety in one review (Schlict 1994), but the small number of studies

reviewed led to low statistical power, and it appears that sampling errors prevented powerful tests of age in both analyses. Another quantitative review found that state anxiety was reduced after exercise among men but not women. Reductions in physiological variables under nonstress conditions were significant for subjects under 45 years but not over 45 years.

Although it is likely that sociocultural factors differently influence the ways in which women and men of different ages, education levels, races, or ethnicities perceive exercise, its outcomes, and its context, the current evidence does not permit conclusions about whether the association of exercise with anxiety is consistent across demographic groups.

Dose Response

Despite biological reasons to expect that the effects of physical activity on anxiety would vary according to exercise intensity (e.g., body temperature, the relevance of which for anxiety is explained later in this chapter, and endocrine and metabolic responses increase with increasing exercise intensity, depending on training history), available data do not show dose-dependent reductions in anxiety with increasing exercise intensity (figure 13.17). Changes in state anxiety after exercise reported in studies published before 1993 did not differ significantly among exercise intensities expressed as percentages of

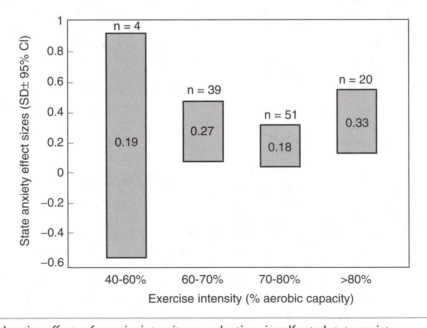

Figure 13.17 Moderating effects of exercise intensity on reductions in self-rated state anxiety.

Reprinted from Physical activity and mental health, R.K. Dishman. In *Encyclopedia of mental health*, H.S. Friedman (ed), 171-188, Copyright 1998, with permission from Elsevier. Data from Petruzzello et al. 1991.

$\dot{V}O_2$peak (Landers and Petruzzello 1994; Petruzzello et al. 1991), but most of those studies did not quantify relative exercise intensity according to different levels of cardiorespiratory fitness nor compare intensities within the same participants. Often, aerobic capacity was estimated based on submaximal fitness tests or heart rate, which can be up to 20% off from actual aerobic capacity. Accurate assessment of exercise intensity is critical for determining the necessary or optimal exercise intensity for reducing anxiety for prescribing a training program. Studies published since 1993 typically have used standard methods for quantifying exercise intensity. They reported decreased or unchanged anxiety after intensities ranging from 40% to 70% $\dot{V}O_2$peak (Breus and O'Connor 1998; Dishman, Farquhar, and Cureton 1994; Garvin, Koltyn, and Morgan 1997; Koltyn and Morgan 1992; O'Connor and Davis 1992; Raglin and Wilson 1996) and increased, decreased, or unchanged anxiety after maximal exercise testing with different samples of participants (Koltyn, Lynch, and Hill 1998; O'Connor et al. 1995).

Also, too few studies have been conducted to permit a statistically powerful quantitative analysis of the concomitant effects of intensity and duration. It appears that moderate intensities of exercise lasting up to about 30 min generally are associated with the largest reductions (about 0.75 SD) in self-rated state anxiety (figure 13.18), but there have been few studies of short durations (e.g., 5–10 min) or intermittent sessions. A few studies have specifically contrasted the effects of different intensities or durations of exercise on anxiety, but they confounded intensity and duration and used only slightly different intensities or used intensities too high and durations too short for clinical applications.

With the exception of one report (Pronk et al. 1994), studies examining dose–response effects of acute exercise on state anxiety have not attempted to equate the total energy expenditure of exercise conditions of varying intensity and duration. Thus, the effects of different total energy expenditures may be falsely attributed to varying the intensity or duration of the activity. Substantial reductions (about 1.0–2.0 SD) in trait anxiety reportedly require about four to five months of exercise training (figure 13.19).

Plausibility

As was the case for depression, biological plausibility is not the only concept that can explain mental health outcomes of physical activity. Several of the most popular cognitive and social explanations are discussed first, followed by a traditional examination of biological plausibility.

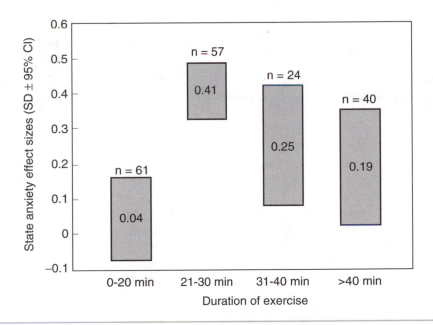

Figure 13.18   Moderating effects of exercise duration on reductions in self-rated state anxiety. The reduction for durations of 21 to 30 min were larger than for durations up to 20 min. Reductions did not differ among exercise intensities.

Reprinted from Physical activity and mental health, R.K. Dishman. In *Encyclopedia of mental health*, H.S. Friedman (ed), 171-188, Copyright 1998, with permission from Elsevier. Data from Petruzzello et al. 1991.

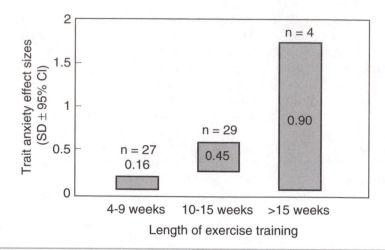

Figure 13.19   Moderating effects of the length of exercise training on reduction in self-rated trait anxiety. The reduction in trait anxiety was greater after 15 weeks compared to 4 to 9 weeks. The reduction in depression after 20 weeks was greater than periods less than 20 weeks.

Reprinted from Physical activity and mental health, R.K. Dishman. In *Encyclopedia of mental health,* H.S. Friedman (ed), 171-188, Copyright 1998, with permission from Elsevier. Data from Petruzzello et al. 1991.

Cognitive and Social Factors.   It is important to determine whether reduced anxiety after acute exercise or an exercise training program can be explained by a direct effect of exercise or merely by other aspects of the exercise setting. It is unlikely that exercise would directly decrease the occurrence of some forms of anxiety. For example, there is no reason to expect that exercise would reduce simple phobias. A person afraid of spiders will experience anxiety when exposed to one whether he or she is active and fit or sedentary. However, physical activity might help people cope with the experience of anxiety, distract them from worry, or reduce some symptoms.

Physiological sensations from exercise might help redefine the subjective meaning of arousal and could thus compete with the perception of anxiety symptoms. This has been proposed as a way that exercise could help panic patients who are very sensitive to somatic symptoms of arousal. Repeated exercise might help people with panic disorder learn to perceive arousal as less threatening. Sensations of the heart pounding during exercise can be reinterpreted as a sign of a good workout rather than a symptom of anxiety.

Exercise can also distract attention from anxiety-provoking thoughts and provides a time-out from cares and worries (Bahrke and Morgan 1978). Breus and O'Connor (1998) tested this distraction hypothesis by measuring state anxiety in 18 highly trait-anxious college women before and after exercise at moderate intensity (40% of aerobic capacity), exercise while studying, studying only, and quiet rest. There was no change in anxiety after exercise while studying, studying only, or quiet rest. There was a significant decrease in anxiety after the exercise-only condition, which indicates that the anxiolytic effect of exercise (exercise as a distraction from worries and concerns) was blocked by studying.

> ••• *The distraction hypothesis states that exercise distracts attention from anxiety-provoking thoughts and provides a time-out from cares and worries.*

Biological Plausibility.   Physical activity is unique among behavioral treatments for mental health. The increased metabolism of physical exertion produces several acute responses during exercise and more long-lasting adaptations to chronic exercise that appear to improve mental health. Possible explanations for reduced anxiety after exercise include body warming, alterations in endorphins, reduced arousal, altered brain electrocortical activity, changes in the brain noradrenaline and serotonin systems, and influences on the brain GABA/benzodiazepine system.

• *Body warming.* Increases in body temperature in the range that occurs with moderate to intense exercise (about 1–1.5 °C) at normal environmental temperatures have been associated with reduced muscle tension. The speculation that reduced anxiety after exercise depends on increased body temperature is biologically plausible, but the dozen or so studies that tested the idea did not support it (Koltyn 1997). Changes in anxiety after acute exercise have not corresponded with manipulations of body temperature before or during exercise. However, the studies that simulated natural exercise (e.g., underwater finning exercise with or without a wet suit) did an incomplete job of controlling temperature or used inadequate nonexercise control conditions. A study that effectively controlled temperature during exercise did so in an unnatural exercise setting: Subjects cycled in shoulder-deep water (Youngstedt et al. 1993). It remains plausible that increased temperature during typical exercise contributes to reduced anxiety, but body warming probably is not the sole or direct cause of the reduced anxiety or improved mood.

• *Endorphins.* For the same reasons discussed earlier regarding depression, endorphins could plausibly be involved with anxiety reduction after acute exercise, but there currently is no compelling evidence to support that idea. Studies in humans that used opioid-blocking drugs during exercise still found that people reported reduced state anxiety or feelings of tension (e.g., Farrell et al. 1982). Other research has shown that men who had the largest increases in blood levels of β-endorphin during cycling exercise also had the largest increase in state anxiety, exactly the converse of the endorphin hypothesis.

• *Physiological arousal.* A few early studies reviewed by de Vries (1981) and a recent study (Smith et al. 2002) have shown that acute and chronic exercise can reduce muscle reflexes and tension. It is not yet clear, though, whether reduced muscle tension after exercise is part of anxiety reduction or is a biological response to exercise that is independent of anxiety. Recent research on the **Hoffmann reflex,** which has been presumed to be an objective index of relaxation after acute exercise (Bulbulian and Darabos 1986; de Vries et al. 1981; Petruzzello et al. 1991), has shown that reductions in the Hoffman reflex after mild or vigorous cycling exercise were not related to reductions in self-rated state anxiety (Motl, O'Connor, and Dishman 2003).

Likewise, reductions in blood pressure after exercise have been interpreted by some investigators as indirect evidence of an anxiolytic effect of exercise (e.g., Petruzzello et al. 1991; Raglin, Turner, and Eksten 1993). However, postexercise hypotension (i.e., lowered blood pressure for up to 2 h after exercise) is a well-known physiological phenomenon that occurs even when anxiety is not lowered after exercise (e.g., Youngstedt et al. 1993).

In contrast, one modern theory proposes that an **electromyogram (EMG)** measure of the startle response provides an index of people's predisposition to interpret environmental events as negative or threatening (Lang, Bradley, and Cuthbert 1998). A recent study showed that a reduction in startle response was related to reduced self-ratings of state anxiety after both quiet rest and moderate-intensity cycling exercise (Smith et al. 2002).

• *Brain electrocortical activity.* Another contemporary theory of emotional response proposes that **electroencephalograms (EEGs)** of **hemispheric asymmetry** in brain waves provide another index of a predisposition to interpret environmental events as negative or threatening (R.J. Davidson 1998). Recently, EEG asymmetry in the alpha frequency band has been shown to be related to self-ratings of anxiety after moderately intense treadmill and cycling exercise (Crabbe, Smith, and Dishman 1999; Petruzzello and Landers 1994; Petruzzello and Tate 1997).

However, moderate to large increases in the alpha brain wave frequency band measured by EEG are common during and after exercise (Crabbe and Dishman 2000; Kubitz and Mott 1996; Petruzzello et al. 1991; figure 13.20). Increased alpha activity is traditionally viewed as an index of relaxed wakefulness, but this view is not universally held by EEG experts, and the exercise studies did not show that the increased alpha activity was caused by the exercise or related to reduced anxiety; other brain wave frequencies presumably unrelated to anxiety also increase after exercise (Crabbe and Dishman 2000).

• *Brain neurotransmitters: serotonin, norepinephrine, and GABA.* Animal studies have found increased activity of serotonin neurons in the raphe nucleus during treadmill running (Jacobs and Fornal 1999), increased brain release of serotonin during treadmill running (Wilson and Marsden 1996), and increased release of serotonin and increased levels of serotonin in several brain regions after exercise training (Dunn and Dishman 1991; Meeusen and De Meirleir 1995). There is also indirect evidence of effects of exercise on central serotonergic systems based on measures of tryptophan disposition in the blood and concentrations of 5-HIAA (a serotonin metabolite) in

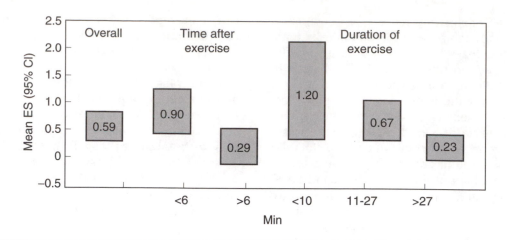

Figure 13.20   Results for encephalogram α brain wave band frequency after exercise.

Reprinted, by permission, from J. Buckworth and R.K. Dishman, 2001, *Exercise psychology* (Champaign, IL: Human Kinetics), 123.

cerebrospinal fluid (Chaouloff 1997a). One mechanism for increased brain levels of serotonin with exercise is the effect of exercise on increasing the transport of the amino acid tryptophan from the bloodstream into the brain. Exercise induces increased lipolysis, or the breakdown of triglycerides into free fatty acids, which are used to fuel increased levels of muscular contraction. Increased serum levels of free fatty acids compete with tryptophan for binding with albumin, leading to increases in free tryptophan. This increase in free tryptophan stimulates an influx of tryptophan into the brain and thus the potential for increased synthesis of serotonin.

Chronic activity-wheel running and treadmill exercise training increase levels of norepinephrine in the locus coeruleus, amygdala, hippocampus, and hypothalamus (Dishman, Renner et al. 2000) and decrease the number of β-adrenoreceptors in the frontal cortex (Yoo, Tackett et al. 2000). Chronic activity-wheel running also reduces the release of norepinephrine in the frontal cortex during stress (Soares et al. 1999), possibly by up-regulating the expression of genes for neuropeptides such as galanin and **neuropeptide Y** that inhibit locus coeruleus activity (O'Neal et al. 2001). All those changes are similar to some of the actions of antidepressant drugs that presumably underlie their therapeutic effects. Chronic activity-wheel running also increases levels of GABA and decreases the number of GABA$_A$ receptors in the corpus striatum, consistent with an anxiolytic effect (Dishman et al. 1996). The explanation for the anxiolytic effect of exercise based on GABA may be the effects of exercise on

central cholinergic function, which is inhibited by benzodiazepine receptor agonists.

An increase in locomotion usually reflects an adaptive motivational state in rats, indicating reduced behavioral inhibition (e.g., less freezing; Dishman 1997a). An increase in open-field locomotion has been reported in rats following forced exercise swimming and after motorized treadmill running. Locomotion by the rat in an open field is associated inversely with observer ratings of anxiety when the locomotion appears purposeful and the animal exhibits other exploratory behaviors such as rearing or approaching the center of the open field. In contrast, low levels of locomotion, few approaches to the center of the open field, freezing, defecation, urination, and shivering are conventionally regarded as isomorphic with the hypervigilance, hesitancy, fear, and autonomic activation common in human anxiety. Under certain circumstances of threat, increased locomotion seems to indicate panic (e.g., the flight response to a predator). A study conducted at the University of Georgia found that chronic activity-wheel running led to increased open-field locomotion and changes in GABA receptor binding, consistent with an anxiety-reducing effect (Dishman et al. 1996).

Summary

Despite imperfect methods, there are enough population-based prospective cohort studies to conclude that physical inactivity is associated with a small to moderate increase in the risk of depression symptoms among adults. Similarly, there are enough randomized controlled trials to conclude that regular exercise can reduce symptoms among patients diagnosed with mild to moderate unipolar depression. Some studies have shown that the effects of exercise are similar, but not additive, to the effects of psychotherapy and drug therapy. However, it has not yet been possible to conclude that the reduction in symptoms is large enough for an improved clinical diagnosis of remission. Also, studies have not yet completely shown that exercise alone was responsible for the effects, independently of increased social contact or light exposure. Many studies have shown that acute exercise reduces self-rated anxiety and that regular exercise reduces trait anxiety in young to middle-aged adults without anxiety disorders, but there is virtually no population-based evidence that such effects prevent future anxiety disorders. Only a few randomized controlled trials have been conducted to show that regular exercise reduces symptoms among anxiety patients. Contrary to popular clinical opinion, exercise does not appear to pose a risk for panic patients.

At this point, more prospective, large cohort studies are needed that include enough people of varying ages and races or ethnicities to permit comparisons of the effects of physical activity on the risk of depression and anxiety disorders among subgroups of the population. Ideally, such studies would include measures across several time periods to permit an examination of whether naturally occurring changes in physical activity precede changes in the risk of depression and anxiety disorders. Also, more randomized controlled trials that include diverse ethnic groups of all ages are needed to clarify the true role of physical activity in mental health.

In addition to that type of evidence, many advances are needed in understanding the biological mechanisms of the antidepressant and antianxiety effects of exercise. A recent body of evidence has clearly shown that chronic activity-wheel running in rats increased gene expression for brain neurotrophins, especially brain-derived neurotrophic factor (BDNF) in the hippocampus (Cotman and Engesser-Cesar 2002), similar to the effects of the tricyclic antidepressant drug imipramine (Russo-Neustadt, Beard, and Cotman 1999; Russo-Neustadt et al. 2001). Though neurotrophins are cell growth factors that help protect brain neurons from damage, their potential role in helping to explain the antidepressant effects of exercise has not yet been confirmed using a valid animal model of depression (Russo-Neustadt et al. 2001; Van Hoomissen et al. 2003; Yoo, Bunnell et al. 2000). No human studies as yet have tested whether neurobiological responses and adaptations can help explain the antidepressant and antianxiety effects of physical activity. Technological advances and increasing accessibility of brain neuroimaging will likely soon lead to such studies by permitting objective measurements of functional changes in brain metabolism and neurotransmission that can be compared to changes in symptoms of anxiety and depression after exercise (Nemeroff, Kilts, and Berns 1999). Until such human studies are done, animal models of depression and anxiety offer a complementary, but not widespread, approach.

Bibliography

Aksiskal, H.S., and W.T. McKinney. 1975. Overview of recent research in depression: Integration of ten conceptual models into a comprehensive clinical frame. *Archives of General Psychiatry* 32: 285–305.

American Psychiatric Association. 1998. Practice guidelines for the treatment of patients with panic disorder. *American Journal of Psychiatry* 155 (Suppl. 12): 1–34.

———. 2000a. *Diagnostic and statistical manual of mental disorders.* 4th ed., text revision. Washington, DC: American Psychiatric Association.

———. 2000b. Practice guidelines for the treatment of patients with major depressive disorder (revision). *American Journal of Psychiatry* 157 (4): 1–45.

Babyak, M., J.A. Blumenthal, S. Herman, P. Khatri, M. Doraiswamy, K. Moore, W.E. Craighead, T.T. Baldewicz, and K.R. Krishnan. 2000. Exercise treatment for major depression: Maintenance of therapeutic benefit at 10 months. *Psychosomatic Medicine* 62: 633–638.

Bahrke, M.S., and W.P. Morgan. 1978. Anxiety reduction following exercise and meditation. *Cognitive Therapy and Research* 2 (4): 323–333.

Baldessarini, R.J. 1989. Current status of antidepressants: Clinical pharmacology and therapy. *Journal of Clinical Psychiatry* 50 (4): 117–126.

Baldessarini, R.J., L. Tondo, J. Hennen, and A.C. Viguera. 2002. Is lithium still worth using? An update of selected recent research. *Harvard Review of Psychiatry* 10 (2): 59–75.

Ballenger, J.C. 2001. Overview of different pharmacotherapies for attaining remission in generalized anxiety disorder. *Journal of Clinical Psychiatry* 62 (Suppl. 19): 11–19.

Ballenger, J.C., J.R. Davidson, Y. Lecrubier, D.J. Nutt, J. Bobes, D.C. Beidel, Y. Ono, and H.G. Westenberg. 1998. Consensus statement on social anxiety disorder from the International Consensus Group on Depression and Anxiety. *Journal of Clinical Psychiatry* 59 (Suppl. 17): 54–60.

Barlow, D.H., and C.L. Lehman. 1996. Advances in the psychosocial treatment of anxiety disorders. *Archives of General Psychiatry* 53: 727–735.

Bartholomew, J.B., and D.E. Linder. 1998. State anxiety following resistance exercise: The role of gender and exercise intensity. *Journal of Behavioral Medicine* 21 (2): 205–219.

Beck, A.T. 1976. *Cognitive therapy and the emotional disorders.* New York: International Universities Press.

Beck, A.T., A.J. Rush, and B.F. Shaw. 1979. *Cognitive therapy of depression.* New York: Guilford Press.

Blumenthal, J.A., M.A. Babyak, K.A. Moore, W.E. Craighead, S. Herman, P. Khatri, R. Waugh, M.A. Napolitano, L.M. Forman, M. Appelbaum, et al. 1999. Effects of exercise training on older patients with major depression. *Archives of Internal Medicine* 159: 2349–2356.

Bouchard, C., R. Shephard, and T. Stephens, eds. 1994. *Physical activity, fitness, and health: International proceedings and consensus statement.* Champaign, IL: Human Kinetics.

Breus, M.J., and P.J. O'Connor. 1998. Exercise-induced anxiolysis: A test of the "time out" hypothesis in high anxious females. *Medicine and Science in Sports and Exercise* 30 (7): 1107–1112.

Broocks, A., B. Bandelow, G. Pekrun, A. George, T. Meyer, U. Bartmann, U. Hillmer-Vogel, and E. Rüther. 1998. Comparison of aerobic exercise, clomipramine, and placebo in the treatment of panic disorder. *American Journal of Psychiatry* 155: 603–609.

Broocks, A., T.F. Meyer, B. Bandelow, U. Bartmann, E. Rüther, and U. Hillmer-Vogel. 1997. Exercise avoidance and impaired endurance capacity in patients with panic disorder. *Neuropsychobiology* 36: 182–187.

Broocks, A., T. Meyer, A. George, U. Hillmer-Vogel, D. Meyer, B. Bandelow, G. Hajak, U. Bartmann, C.H. Gleiter, and E. Rüther. 1999. Decreased neuroendocrine responses to meta-chlorophenylpiperazine (m-CPP) but normal responses to ipsapirone in marathon runners. *Neuropsychopharmacology* 20 (2): 150–161.

Brown, S.W., M.C. Welsh, E.E. Labbe, W.F. Vitulli, and P. Kulkarni. 1992. Aerobic exercise in the psychological treatment of adolescents. *Perceptual and Motor Skills* 74: 555–560.

Buckworth, J.B., and R.K. Dishman. 2002. *Exercise psychology.* Champaign, IL: Human Kinetics.

Bulbulian, R., and B.L. Darabos. 1986. Motor neuron excitability: The Hoffmann reflex following exercise of low and high intensity. *Medicine and Science in Sports and Exercise* 18: 697–702.

Bunney, W.E. Jr., and J.M. Davis. 1965. Norepinephrine in depressive reactions: A review. *Archives of General Psychiatry* 13: 483–494.

Burton, R. 1632. *The anatomy of melancholy.* Oxford: Printed by Ion Lichfield for Henry Cripps.

Calfas, K.J., and W.C. Taylor. 1994. Effects of physical-activity on psychological variables in adolescents. *Pediatric Exercise Science* 6: 406–423.

Camacho, T.C., R.E. Roberts, N.B. Lazarus, G.A. Kaplan, and R.D. Cohen. 1991. Physical activity and depression: Evidence from the Alameda County Study. *American Journal of Epidemiology* 134: 220–231.

Campbell, D.D., and J.E. Davis. 1939–1940. Report of research and experimentation in exercise and recreational therapy. *American Journal of Psychiatry* 96: 915–933.

Chambliss, H.O., and R.K. Dishman. 2004. Physical activity and depression: A quantitative synthesis. Unpublished manuscript, The University of Georgia, Athens.

Chaouloff, F. 1989. Physical exercise and brain monoamines: A review. *Acta Physiologica Scandinavica* 137: 1–13.

———. 1994. Influence of physical exercise on 5-HT$_{1A}$ receptor- and anxiety-related behaviours. *Neuroscience Letters* 176 (2): 226–230.

———. 1997a. Effects of acute physical exercise on central serotonergic systems. *Medicine and Science in Sports and Exercise* 29: 58–62.

———. 1997b. The serotonin hypothesis. In *Physical activity and mental health,* edited by W.P. Morgan, pp. 179–198. Washington, DC: Hemisphere.

Charney, D.S. 1998. Monoamine dysfunction and the pathophysiology and treatment of depression. *Journal of Clinical Psychiatry* 59 (Suppl. 14): 11–14.

Charney, D.S., S.W. Woods, W.K. Goodman, and G.R. Heninger. 1987. Serotonin function in anxiety: II. Effects of the serotonin agonist MCPP in panic disorder patients and healthy subjects. *Psychopharmacology* 92 (1): 14–24.

Charney, D.S., S.W. Woods, J.H. Krystal, L.M. Nagy, and G.R. Heninger. 1992. Noradrenergic neuronal dysregulation in panic disorder: The effects of intravenous yohimbine and clonidine in panic disorder patients. *Acta Psychiatrica Scandinavica* 86 (4): 273–282.

Chrousos, G.P. 1998. Stressors, stress, and neuroendocrine integration of the adaptive response. *Annals of the New York Academy of Sciences* 851: 311–335.

Cooper-Patrick, L., D.E. Ford, L.A. Mead, P.P. Chang, and M.J. Klag. 1997. Exercise and depression in midlife: A prospective study. *American Journal of Public Health* 87: 670–673.

Coryell, W., R. Noyes, and J. Clancy. 1982. Excess mortality in panic disorder: A comparison with primary unipolar depression. *Archives of General Psychiatry* 39 (6): 701–703.

Cotman, C.W., and C. Engesser-Cesar. 2002. Exercise enhances and protects brain function. *Exercise and Sport Sciences Reviews* 30 (2): 75–79.

Crabbe, J.B., and R.K. Dishman. 2000. Exercise and brain electrocortical activity: A quantitative synthesis. *Medicine and Science in Sports and Exercise* 32 (Suppl. 5): S43.

Crabbe, J.B., J.C. Smith, and R.K. Dishman. 1999. EEG and emotional response after cycling exercise. *Medicine and Science in Sports and Exercise* 31 (Suppl. 5): S173.

Craft, L.L., and D.M. Landers. 1998. The effect of exercise on clinical depression and depression resulting from mental illness: A meta-analysis. *Journal of Sport and Exercise Psychology* 20: 339–357.

Davidson, J.R. 1998. Pharmacotherapy of social anxiety disorder. *Journal of Clinical Psychiatry* 59 (Suppl. 17): 47–53.

Davidson, R.J. 1998. Anterior electrophysiological asymmetries, emotion, and depression: Conceptual and methodological conundrums. *Psychophysiology* 35: 607–614.

Davidson, R.J., and W. Irwin. 1999. The functional neuroanatomy of emotion and affective style. *Trends in Cognitive Sciences* 3 (1): 11–21.

Davidson, R.J., W. Irwin, M.J. Anderle, and N.H. Kalin. 2003. The neural substrates of affective processing in depressed patients treated with venlafaxine. *American Journal of Psychiatry* 160: 64–75.

Desharnais, R., J. Jobin, C. Cote, L. Levesque, and G. Godin. 1993. Aerobic exercise and the placebo effect: A controlled study. *Psychosomatic Medicine* 55: 149–154.

DeVane, C.L. 2000. Pharmacologic characteristics of ideal antidepressants in the 21st century. *Journal of Clinical Psychiatry* 61 (Suppl. 11): 4–8.

de Vries, H.A. 1981. Tranquilizer effect of exercise: A critical review. *The Physician and Sportsmedicine* 9: 47–55.

de Vries, H.A., R.A. Wiswell, R. Bulbulian, and T. Moritani. 1981. Tranquilizer effect of exercise. Acute effects of moderate aerobic exercise on spinal reflex activation level. *American Journal of Physical Medicine* 60: 57–66.

Dishman, R.K. 1997a. Brain monoamines, exercise, and behavior stress: Animal models. *Medicine and Science in Sports and Exercise* 29 (1): 63–74.

———. 1997b. The norepinephrine hypothesis. In *Physical activity and mental health,* edited by W.P. Morgan, pp. 199–212. Washington, DC: Hemisphere.

———. 1998. Physical activity and mental health. In *Encyclopedia of mental health,* edited by H.S. Friedman, vol. 3, pp. 171–188. San Diego: Academic Press.

Dishman, R.K., A. Dunn, S. Youngstedt, J.M. Davis, M.L. Burgess, S.P. Wilson, and M.A. Wilson. 1996. Increased open-field locomotion and decreased striatal GABA$_A$ binding after activity wheel running. *Physiology and Behavior* 60: 699–705.

Dishman, R.K., R. Farquhar, and K.J. Cureton. 1994. Responses to preferred intensities of exertion in men differing in activity levels. *Medicine and Science in Sports and Exercise* 26: 783–790.

Dishman, R.K., S. Hong, J.M. Warren, S.D. Youngstedt, H. Yoo, B.N. Bunnell, E.H. Mougey, J.L. Meyerhoff, L. Jaso-Friedmann, and D.L. Evans. 2000. Treadmill exercise training blunts suppression of natural killer cell activity after footshock. *Journal of Applied Physiology* 83: 1547–1554.

Dishman, R.K., K.J. Renner, J.E. White-Welkley, and B.N. Bunnell. 2000. Treadmill exercise training augments brain norepinephrine response to familiar and novel stress. *Brain Research Bulletin* 52: 337–342.

Dishman, R.K., K.J. Renner, S.D. Youngstedt, T.G. Reigle, B.N. Bunnell, K.A. Burke, H.S. Yoo, E.H. Mougey, and J.L. Meyerhoff. 1997. Activity wheel running reduces escape latency and alters brain monoamine levels after footshock. *Brain Research Bulletin* 42 (5): 399–406.

Dishman, R.K., J.M. Warren, S.D. Youngstedt, H. Yoo, B.N. Bunnell, E.H. Mougey, J.L. Meyerhoff, L. Jaso-Friedmann, and D.L. Evans. 1995. Activity wheel running attenuates suppression of natural killer cell activity after footshock. *Journal of Applied Physiology* 78: 1547–1554.

Doyne, E.J., D.J. Ossip-Klein, E.D. Bowman, K.M. Osborn, I.B. McDougall-Wilson, and R.A. Neimeyer. 1987. Running versus weight lifting in the treatment of depression. *Journal of Consulting and Clinical Psychology* 55 (5): 748–754.

Drevets, W.C. 1998. Functional neuroimaging studies of depression: The anatomy of melancholia. *Annual Review of Medicine* 49: 341–361.

Dunn, A.L., and R.K. Dishman. 1991. Exercise and the neurobiology of depression. *Exercise and Sport Sciences Reviews* 19: 41–98.

Dunn, A.L, T.G. Reigle, S.D. Youngstedt, R.B. Armstrong, and R.K. Dishman. 1996. Brain norepinephrine and metabolites after treadmill training and wheel running in rats. *Medicine and Science in Sports and Exercise* 28: 204–209.

Dunn, A.L., M.H. Trivedi, and H.A. O'Neal. 2001. Physical activity dose–response effects on outcomes of depression and anxiety. *Medicine and Science in Sports and Exercise* 33 (Suppl. 6): S587–S597.

DuPont, R.L., D.P. Rice, L.S. Miller, S.S. Shiraki, C.R. Rowland, and H.J. Harwood. 1996. Economic cost of anxiety disorders. *Anxiety* 2: 167–172.

Ernst, E., J.I. Rand, and C. Stevinson. 1998. Complementary therapies for depression: An overview. *Archives of General Psychiatry* 55: 1026–1032.

Farmer, M.E., B.Z. Locke, E.K. Moscicki, A.L. Dannenberg, D.B. Larson, and L.S. Radloff. 1988. Physical activity and depressive symptoms: The NHANES I epidemiologic follow-up study. *American Journal of Epidemiology* 128: 1340–1351.

Farrell, P.A., W.K. Gates, M. Maksud, and W.P. Morgan. 1982. Increases in plasma b-endorphin/b-lipotropin immunoreactivity after treadmill running in humans. *Journal of Applied Physiology* 52: 1245–1249.

Focht, B.C., and K.F. Koltyn. 1999. Influence of resistance exercise of different intensities on state anxiety and blood pressure. *Medicine and Science in Sports and Exercise* 31 (3): 456–463.

Fox, K.E. 2000. Self-esteem, self-perceptions and exercise. *International Journal of Sport Psychology* 31: 228–240.

Franz, S.I., and G.V. Hamilton. 1905. The effects of exercise upon the retardation in conditions of depression. *American Journal of Insanity* 62: 239–256.

Fremont, J., and L.W. Craighead. 1987. Aerobic exercise and cognitive therapy in the treatment of dysphoric moods. *Cognitive Therapy and Research* 11 (2): 241–251.

Garvin, A.W., K.F. Koltyn, and W.P. Morgan. 1997. Influence of acute physical activity and relaxation on state anxiety and blood lactate in untrained college males. *International Journal of Sports Medicine* 18: 1–7.

Goddard, A.W., and D.S. Charney. 1997. Toward an integrated neurobiology of panic disorder. *Journal of Clinical Psychiatry* 58 (Suppl. 2): 4–12.

———. 1998. SSRIs in the treatment of panic disorder. *Depression and Anxiety* 8 (Suppl. 1): 114–120.

Gold, P.W., and G.P. Chrousos. 1998. The endocrinology of melancholic and atypical depression: Relation to neurocircuitry and somatic consequences. *Proceedings of the Association of American Physicians* 111 (1): 22–34.

Gorman, J.M., and L.K. Gorman. 1987. Drug treatment of social phobia. *Journal of Affective Disorders* 13 (2): 183–192.

Greenberg, P.E., L.E. Stiglin, S.N. Finkelstein, and E.R. Berndt. 1993. The economic burden of depression in 1990. *Journal of Clinical Psychiatry* 54 (11): 405–418.

Greist, J.H., M.H. Klein, R.R. Eischens, J. Faris, A.S. Gurman, and W.P. Morgan. 1978. Running through your mind. *Journal of Psychosomatic Research* 22: 259–294.

Gruber, J. 1986. Physical activity and self-esteem development in children: A meta-analysis. In *Effects of physical activity on children: Papers of the American Academy of Physical Education,* edited by G.A. Stull and H.M. Eckhardt, vol. 19, pp. 30–48. Champaign, IL: Human Kinetics.

Harris, S.S., C.J. Caspersen, G.G. DeFriese, and E.J. Estes. 1989. Physical activity counseling for healthy adults as a primary preventive intervention in the clinical setting: Report for the U.S. Preventive Services Task Force. *Journal of the American Medical Association* 261: 3588–3598.

Hirschfeld, R.M.A., M.B. Keller, S. Panico, B.S. Arons, D. Barlow, F. Davidoff, J. Endicott, J. Froom, M. Goldstein, J.M. Gorman, et al. 1997. The National Depressive and Manic-Depressive Association consensus statement on the undertreatment of depression. *Journal of the American Medical Association* 277: 333–340.

Hoffman, P. 1997. The endorphin hypothesis. In *Physical activity and mental health,* edited by W.P. Morgan, pp. 163–177. Washington, DC: Hemisphere.

Jacobs, B.L., and C.A. Fornal. 1999. Activity of serotonergic neurons in behaving animals. *Neuropsychopharmacology* 21 (Suppl. 2): 9–15.

James, H. 1926. *The letters of William James.* Boston: Little Brown.

James, W. 1899. *Talks to teachers on psychology: And to students on some of life's ideals.* New York: Holt.

Jefferson, J.W., J.H. Greist, P.J. Clagnze, R.R. Eischens, W.C. Marten, and M.A. Evenson. 1982. Effects of strenuous exercise on lithium level in man. *American Journal of Psychiatry* 139: 1593–1595.

Kalin, N.H., R.J. Davidson, W. Irwin, G. Warner, J.L. Orendi, S.K. Sutton, B.J. Mock, J.A. Sorenson, M. Lowe, and P.A. Turski. 1997. Functional magnetic resonance imaging studies of emotional processing in normal and depressed patients: Effects of venlafaxine. *Journal of Clinical Psychiatry* 58 (Suppl. 16): 32–39.

Kandel, E.R. 1998. A new intellectual framework for psychiatry. *American Journal of Psychiatry* 155 (4): 457–469.

Kelly, J.P., A.S. Wrynn, and B.E. Leonard. 1997. The olfactory bulbectomized rat as a model of depression: An update. *Pharmacology and Therapeutics* 74 (3): 299–316.

Kent, J.M., J.D. Coplan, and J.M. Gorman. 1998. Clinical utility of the selective serotonin reuptake inhibitors in the spectrum of anxiety. *Biological Psychiatry* 44: 812–824.

Kessler, R.C., P. Berglund, O. Demler, R. Jin, D. Koretz, K.R. Merikangas, A.J. Rush, E.E. Walters, and P.S. Wang. 2003. The epidemiology of major depressive disorder: Results from the National Comorbidity Survey Replication (NCS-R). *Journal of the American Medical Association* 289: 3095–3105.

Kessler, R.C., K.A. McGonagle, S. Zhao, C.B. Nelson, M, Hughes, S. Eshleman, H.U. Wittchen, and K.S. Kendler. 1994. Lifetime and 12-month prevalence of DSM-III-R psychiatric disorders in the United States: Results from the National Comorbidity Survey. *Archives of General Psychiatry* 51 (1): 8–19.

King, A.C., R.F. Oman, G.S. Brassington, D.L. Bliwise, and W.L. Haskell. 1997. Moderate-intensity exercise and self-rated quality of sleep in older adults: A randomized controlled trial. *Journal of the American Medical Association* 227: 32–37.

King, A.C., C.B. Taylor, and W.L. Haskell. 1993. Effects of differing intensities and formats of 12 months of exercise training on psychological outcomes in older adults. *Health Psychology* 12 (4): 292–300.

Koltyn, K. 1997. The thermogenic hypothesis. In *Physical activity and mental health,* edited by W.P. Morgan, pp. 213–226. Washington, DC: Hemisphere.

Koltyn, K., N.A. Lynch, and D.W. Hill. 1998. Psychological responses to brief exhaustive cycling exercise in the morning and evening. *International Journal of Sport Psychology* 29: 145–156.

Koltyn, K.F., and W.P. Morgan. 1992. Influence of underwater exercise on anxiety and body temperature. *Scandinavian Journal of Medicine and Science in Sports* 2: 249–253.

Krause, N., L. Goldenhar, J. Liang, G. Jay, and D. Maeda. 1993. Stress and exercise among the Japanese elderly. *Social Science Medicine* 36: 1429–1441.

Kubitz, K.A., D.M. Landers, S.J. Petruzzello, and M. Han. 1996. The effects of acute and chronic exercise on sleep: A meta-analytic review. *Sports Medicine* 21: 277–291.

Kubitz, K.A., and A.A. Mott. 1996. EEG power spectral densities during and after cycle ergometer exercise. *Research Quarterly for Exercise and Sport* 67: 91–96.

Kugler, J., H. Seelbach, and G.M. Kruskemper. 1994. Effects of rehabilitation exercise programmes on anxiety and depression in coronary patients: A meta-analysis. *British Journal of Clinical Psychology* 33: 401–410.

Kupfer, D.J. 1991. Long-term treatment of depression. *Journal of Clinical Psychiatry* 52 (Suppl. 5): 28–34.

Landers, D.M., and S.J. Petruzzello. 1994. Physical activity, fitness, and anxiety. In *Physical activity, fitness, and health: International proceedings and consensus statement,* edited by C. Bouchard, R.J. Shephard, and T. Stephens, pp. 868–882. Champaign, IL: Human Kinetics.

Lang, P.J., M.M. Bradley, and B.N. Cuthbert. 1998. Emotion, motivation, and anxiety: Brain mechanisms and psychophysiology. *Biological Psychiatry* 44: 1248–1263.

Lawlor, D.A., and S.W. Hopker. 2001. The effectiveness of exercise as an intervention in the management of depression: Systematic review and meta-regression analysis of randomised controlled trials. *British Medical Journal* 322: 1–8.

Layman, E.M. 1960. Contributions of exercise and sports to mental health and social adjustment. In *Science and medicine of exercise and sports,* edited by W.R. Johnson. New York: Harper.

LeDoux, J.E. 1998. Fear and the brain: Where have we been, and where are we going? *Biological Psychiatry* 44 (12): 1229–1238.

Lehtinen, V., and M. Joukamaa. 1994. Epidemiology of depression: Prevalence, risk factors and treatment situation. *Acta Psychiatrica Scandinavica* 377 (Suppl.): 7–10.

Lydiard, R.B., O. Brawman-Mintzer, and J.C. Ballenger. 1996. Recent developments in the psychopharmacology of anxiety disorders. *Journal of Consulting and Clinical Psychology* 64: 660–668.

Maas, J.W. 1979. Neurotransmitters and depression: Too much, too little, or unstable? *Trends in the Neurosciences* 2: 306–308.

Maas, J.W., and J.F. Leckman. 1983. Relationships between central nervous system noradrenergic function and plasma and urinary MHPG and other norepinephrine metabolites. In *MHPG: Basic mechanisms and psychopathology,* pp. 33–43. New York: Academic Press.

March, J.S., A. Frances, D. Carpenter, and D.A. Kahn. 1997. Treatment of obsessive-compulsive disorder: The expert consensus panel for obsessive-compulsive disorder. *Journal of Clinical Psychiatry* 58: 2–72.

Martinsen, E.W. 1994. Physical activity and depression: Clinical experience. *Acta Psychiatrica Scandinavica* 377 (Suppl.): 23–27.

Martinsen, E.W., S. Friis, and A. Hoffart. 1995. Assessment of depression: A comparison between Beck Depression Inventory and Comprehensive Psychopathological Rating Scale. *Acta Psychiatrica Scandinavica* 92: 460–463.

Martinsen, E.W., A. Hoffart, and Ø.Y. Solberg. 1989a. Aerobic and non-aerobic forms of exercise in the treatment of anxiety disorders. *Stress Medicine* 5: 115–120.

———. 1989b. Comparing aerobic with nonaerobic forms of exercise in the treatment of clinical depression: A randomized trial. *Comprehensive Psychiatry* 30 (4): 324–331.

Martinsen, E.W., and A. Medhus. 1989. Adherence to exercise and patients' evaluation of physical exercise in a comprehensive treatment programme for depression. *Nordisk Psykiatrisk Tidsskrift* 43: 411–415.

Martinsen, E.W., A. Medhus, and L. Sandvik. 1985. Effects of aerobic exercise on depression: A controlled study. *British Medical Journal* 291: 109.

Martinsen, E.W., J.S. Raglin, A. Hoffart, and S. Friis. 1998. Tolerance to intensive exercise and high levels of lactate in panic disorder. *Journal of Anxiety Disorders* 12 (4): 333–342.

Martinsen, E.W., L. Sandvik, and O.B. Kolbjørnsrud. 1989. Aerobic exercise in the treatment of nonpsychotic mental disorders: An exploratory study. *Nordisk Psykiatrisk Tidsskrift* 43: 521–529.

Mazzeo, R.S. 1991. Catecholamine responses to acute and chronic exercise. *Medicine and Science in Sports and Exercise* 23 (7): 839–845.

McCulloch, T.L., and J.S. Bruner. 1939. The effect of electric shock upon subsequent learning in the rat. *Journal of Psychology* 7: 333–336.

McDonald, D.G., and J.A. Hodgdon. 1991. *Psychological effects of aerobic fitness training: Research and theory.* New York: Springer-Verlag.

McNeil, J.K., E.M. LeBlanc, and M. Joyner. 1991. The effect of exercise on depressive symptoms in the moderately depressed elderly. *Psychology and Aging* 6: 487–488.

Meeusen, R., and K. De Meirleir. 1995. Exercise and brain neurotransmission. *Sports Medicine* 20 (3): 160–188.

Meeusen, R., M.F. Piacentini, and K. De Meirleir. 2001. Brain microdialysis in exercise research. *Sports Medicine* 31 (14): 965–983.

Meeusen, R., I. Smolders, S. Sarre, K. De Meirleir, H. Keizer, M. Serneels, G. Ebinger, and Y. Michotte. 1997. Endurance training effects on neurotransmitter release in rat striatum: An in vivo microdialysis study. *Acta Physiologica Scandinavica* 159 (4): 335–341.

Menard, J., and D. Treit. 1999. Effects of centrally administered anxiolytic compounds in animal models of anxiety. *Neuroscience and Biobehavioral Review* 23 (4): 591–613.

Micallef, J., and O. Blin. 2001. Neurobiology and clinical pharmacology of obsessive-compulsive disorder. *Clinical Neuropharmacology* 24 (4): 191–207.

Morgan, W.P. 1973. Influence of acute physical activity on state anxiety. In *Proceedings, annual meeting of the College Physical Education Association for Men,* edited by C.E. Mueller, pp. 113–121. Minneapolis: University of Minnesota.

———. 1979. Anxiety reduction following acute physical activity. *Psychiatric Annals* 9 (3): 36–41.

———. 1994. Physical activity, fitness, and depression. In *Physical activity, fitness and health,* edited by C. Bouchard, R.J. Shephard, and T. Stephens, pp. 851–867. Champaign, IL: Human Kinetics.

———, ed. 1997. *Physical activity and mental health.* Washington, DC: Taylor and Francis.

Morgan, W.P., D.R. Brown, J.S. Raglin, P.J. O'Connor, and K.A. Ellickson. 1987. Psychological monitoring of overtraining and staleness. *British Journal of Sports Medicine* 21: 107–114.

Morgan, W.P., and S.E. Goldston. 1987. *Exercise and mental health.* Washington, DC: Hemisphere.

Morgan, W.P., J.A. Roberts, F.R. Brand, and A.D. Feinerman. 1970. Psychological effect of chronic physical activity. *Medicine and Science in Sports* 2: 213–217.

Motl, R.W., A.S. Birnbaum, M.Y. Kubik, and R.K. Dishman. 2003. Naturally occurring changes in physical activity are inversely related to depressive symptoms during early adolescence. Unpublished manuscript, The University of Georgia, Athens.

Motl, R.W., P.J. O'Connor, and R.K. Dishman. 2003. Effects of cycling exercise on state anxiety and the soleus H-reflex among males with low or high trait anxiety. *Psychophysiology,* in press.

Murray, C.J., and A.D. Lopez. 1997. Alternative projections of mortality and disability by cause 1990–2020: Global Burden of Disease Study. *Lancet* 349 (9064): 1498–1504.

Nemeroff, C.B. 1998. Psychopharmacology of affective disorders in the 21st century. *Biological Psychiatry* 44: 517–525.

Nemeroff, C.B., C.D. Kilts, and G.S. Berns. 1999. Functional brain imaging: Twenty-first century phrenology or psychobiological advance for the millennium? *American Journal of Psychiatry* 156: 671–673.

Norris, R., D. Carroll, and R. Cochrane. 1992. The effects of physical activity and exercise training on psychological stress and well-being in an adolescent population. *Journal of Psychosomatic Research* 36: 55–65.

North, T.C., P. McCullagh, and V.T. Zung. 1990. Effect of exercise on depression. *Exercise and Sport Sciences Reviews* 18: 379–415.

O'Connor, P.J., L.E. Aenchbacher, and R.K. Dishman. 1993. Physical activity and depression in the elderly. *Journal of Aging and Physical Activity* 1: 34–58.

O'Connor, P.J., C.X. Bryant, J.P. Veltri, and S.M. Gebhardt. 1993. State anxiety and ambulatory blood pressure following resistance exercise in females. *Medicine and Science in Sports and Exercise* 25: 516–521.

O'Connor, P.J., and J.C. Davis. 1992. Psychobiologic responses to exercise at different times of the day. *Medicine and Science in Sports and Exercise* 24: 714–719.

O'Connor, P.J., S.J. Petruzzello, K.A. Kubitz, and T.L. Robinson. 1995. Anxiety responses to maximal exercise testing. *British Journal of Sports Medicine* 29: 97–102.

O'Connor, P.J., J.S. Raglin, and E.W. Martinsen. 2000. Physical activity and anxiety disorders. *International Journal of Sport Psychology* 31: 136–155.

O'Connor, P.J., J.C. Smith, and W.P. Morgan. 2000. Physical activity does not provoke panic attacks in patients with panic disorder: A review of the evidence. *Anxiety, Stress, and Coping* 13: 333–353.

O'Neal, H.A., A.L. Dunn, and E.W. Martinsen. 2000. Depression and exercise. *International Journal of Sport Psychology* 31: 110–135.

O'Neal, H.A., J.D. Van Hoomissen, P.V. Holmes, and R.K. Dishman. 2001. Prepro-galanin messenger RNA levels are increased in rat locus coeruleus after exercise training. *Neuroscience Letters* 299 (1–2): 69–72.

Orwin, A. 1974. Treatment of a situational phobia: A case for running. *British Journal of Psychiatry* 125: 95–98.

Paffenbarger, R.S., I.-M. Lee, and R. Leung. 1994. Physical activity and personal characteristics associated with depression and suicide in American college men. *Acta Psychiatrica Scandinavica* 377 (Suppl.): 16–22.

Pagliari, R., and L. Peyrin. 1995a. Norepinephrine release in the rat frontal cortex under treadmill exercise: A study with microdialysis. *Journal of Applied Physiology* 78 (6): 2121–2130.

———. 1995b. Physical conditioning in rats influences the central and peripheral catecholamine responses to sustained exercise. *European Journal of Applied Physiology* 71: 41–52.

Perry, P.J., T. Sanger, and C. Beasley. 1997. Olanzapine plasma concentrations and clinical response in acutely ill schizophrenic patients. *Journal of Clinical Psychopharmacology* 17: 472–477.

Petruzzello, S.J., and D.M. Landers. 1994. State anxiety reduction and exercise: Does hemispheric activation reflect such changes? *Medicine and Science in Sports and Exercise* 26 (8): 1028–1035.

Petruzzello, S.J., D.M. Landers, B.D. Hatfield, K.A. Kubitz, and W. Salazar. 1991. A meta-analysis on the anxiety reducing effects of acute and chronic exercise: Outcomes and mechanisms. *Sports Medicine* 11 (3): 143–182.

Petruzzello, S.J., and A.K. Tate. 1997. Brain activation, affect, and aerobic exercise: An examination of both state-independent and state-dependent relationships. *Psychophysiology* 34: 527–533.

Pollock, M.L., G.A. Glaser, J.D. Butcher, J.P. Despre, R.K. Dishman, B.F. Franklin, and C.E. Garber. 1998. The recommended quantity and quality of exercise for developing and maintaining cardiorespiratory and muscular fitness, and flexibility in healthy adults. *Medicine and Science in Sports and Exercise* 30 (6): 975–991.

Prange, A.J. 1964. The pharmacology and biochemistry of depression. *Diseases of the Nervous System* 25: 217–221.

Pronk, N.P., A.F. Jawad, S.F. Crouse, and J.J. Rohack. 1994. Acute effects of walking on mood profiles in women: Preliminary findings in postmenopausal women. *Medicine, Exercise, Nutrition, and Health* 3: 148–153.

Raglin, J.S. 1997. Anxiolytic effects of physical activity. In *Physical activity and mental health,* edited by W.P. Morgan, pp. 107–126. Washington, DC: Taylor and Francis.

Raglin, J.S., P.E. Turner, and F. Eksten. 1993. State anxiety and blood pressure following 30 min of leg ergometry or weight training. *Medicine and Science in Sports and Exercise* 25: 1044–1048.

Raglin, J.S., and M. Wilson. 1996. State anxiety following 20 minutes of bicycle ergometer exercise at selected intensities. *International Journal of Sports Medicine* 17: 467–471.

Rajala, U., A. Uusimaki, S. Keinanen-Kiukaanniemi, and S.L. Kivela. 1994. Prevalence of depression in a 55-year-old Finnish population. *Society of Psychiatry and Psychiatric Epidemiology* 29: 126–130.

Rasmussen, K., D.A. Morilak, and B.L. Jacobs. 1986. Single unit activity of locus coeruleus neurons in the freely moving cat: I. During naturalistic behaviors and in response to simple and complex stimuli. *Brain Research* 371: 324–334.

Regier, D.A., J.H. Boyd, J.D. Burke Jr., D.S. Rae, J.K. Myers, M. Kramer, L.N. Robins, L.K. George, M. Karno, and B.Z. Locke. 1988. One-month prevalence of mental health disorders in the United States. *Archives of General Psychiatry* 45: 977–986.

Regier, D.A., D.S. Rae, W.E. Narrow, C.T. Kaelber, and A.F. Schatzberg. 1998. Prevalence of anxiety disorders and their comorbidity with mood and addictive disorders. *British Journal of Psychiatry* 34 (Suppl.): 24–28.

Reiman, E.M. 1997. The application of positron emission tomography to the study of normal and pathologic emotions. *Journal of Clinical Psychiatry* 58 (Suppl. 16): 4–12.

Rice, D.P., and L.S. Miller. 1995. The economic burden of affective disorders. *British Journal of Psychiatry* 166 (Suppl. 27): 34–42.

Rudorfer, M.V., M.E. Henry, and H.A. Sackheim. 1997. Electroconvulsive therapy. In *Psychiatry,* edited by A. Tasman, J. Kay, and J.A. Lieberman, pp. 1535–1556. Philadelphia: Saunders.

Rushton, J.L., M. Forcier, and R.M. Schectman. 2002. Epidemiology of depressive symptoms in the National Longitudinal Study of Adolescent Health. *Journal of the American Academy of Child and Adolescent Psychiatry* 41: 199–205.

Russo-Neustadt, A., R.C. Beard, and C.W. Cotman. 1999. Exercise, antidepressant medications, and enhanced brain derived neurotrophic factor expression. *Neuropsychopharmacology* 21 (5): 679–682.

Russo-Neustadt, A., T. Ha, R. Ramirez, and J.P. Kesslak. 2001. Physical activity–antidepressant treatment combination: Impact on brain-derived neurotrophic factor and behavior in an animal model. *Behavioural Brain Research* 120 (1): 87–95.

Schildkraut, J.J. 1965. The catecholamine hypothesis of affective disorders: A review of the supporting evidence. *American Journal of Psychiatry* 122: 509–522.

Schildkraut, J.J., P.J. Orsulak, A.F. Schatzberg, and A.H. Rosenbaum. 1983. Relationship between psychiatric diagnostic groups of depressive disorders and MHPG. In *MHPG basic mechanisms and psychopathology,* edited by J.W. Maas, pp. 129–144. New York: Academic Press.

Schlict, W. 1994. Does physical exercise reduce anxious emotions? A meta-analysis. *Anxiety, Stress, and Coping* 6: 275–288.

Segar, M.L., V.L. Katch, R.S. Roth, A.W. Garcia, T.I. Portner, S.G. Glickman, S. Haslinger, and E.G. Wilkins. 1998. The effect of aerobic exercise on self-esteem and depressive and anxiety symptoms among breast cancer survivors. *Oncology Nursing Forum* 25: 107–113.

Sexton, H., A. Mære, and N.H. Dahl. 1989. Exercise intensity and reduction in neurotic symptoms. *Acta Psychiatrica Scandinavica* 80: 231–235.

Singh, N.A., K.M. Clements, and M.A. Fiatarone. 1997a. A randomized controlled trial of the effects of exercise on sleep. *Sleep* 20: 40–46.

———. 1997b. A randomized controlled trial of progressive resistance training in depressed elders. *Journal of Gerontology* 52A (1): M27–M35.

Smith, J.C., P.J. O'Connor, J.B. Crabbe, and R.K. Dishman. 2002. Emotional responsiveness after low- and moderate-intensity exercise and seated rest. *Medicine and Science in Sports and Exercise* 34: 1158–1167.

Soares, J., P.V. Holmes, K.J. Renner, G.L. Edwards, B.N. Bunnell, and R.K. Dishman. 1999. Brain noradrenergic responses to footshock after chronic activity-wheel running. *Behavioral Neuroscience* 113: 558–566.

Sonstroem, R.J. 1998. Physical self-concept: Assessment and external validity. *Exercise and Sport Sciences Reviews* 26: 133–164.

Sonstroem, R.J., and W.P. Morgan. 1989. Exercise and self-esteem: Rationale and model. *Medicine and Science in Sports and Exercise* 21: 329–337.

Sothmann, M.S., J. Buckworth, R.P. Claytor, R.H. Cox, J.E. White-Welkley, and R.K. Dishman. 1996. Exercise training and the cross-stressor adaptation hypothesis. *Exercise and Sport Sciences Reviews* 24: 267–287.

Stahl, S.M. 1996. *Essential psychopharmacology: Neuroscientific basis and clinical applications.* New York: Cambridge University Press.

Stephens, T. 1988. Physical activity and mental health in the United States and Canada: Evidence from four population surveys. *Preventive Medicine* 17: 35–47.

Tantillo, M., C.M. Kesick, G.W. Hynd, and R.K. Dishman. 2002. The effects of exercise on children with attention-deficit hyperactivity disorder. *Medicine and Science in Sports and Exercise* 34: 203–212.

U.S. Department of Health and Human Services. 1996. *Physical activity and health: A report of the Surgeon General.* Report DHHS publication no. (PH5) 017-023-00196-5. Atlanta: U.S. Department of Health and Human Services, Centers for Disease Control and Prevention, National Center for Chronic Disease Prevention and Health Promotion.

———. 1999. *Mental health: A report of the Surgeon General— executive summary.* Rockville, MD: U.S. Department of Health and Human Services, Substance Abuse and Mental Health Services Administration, Center for Mental Health Services, National Institutes of Health, National Institute of Mental Health.

Van Hoomissen, J.D., H.O. Chambliss, P.V. Holmes, and R.K. Dishman. 2003. The effects of chronic exercise and imipramine on mRNA for BDNF after olfactory bulbectomy in rat. *Brain Research* 974: 228–235.

Van Hoomissen, J.D., H.A. O'Neal, J.E. Dishman, P.V. Holmes, and R.K. Dishman. 2000. Serotonin transporter mRNA in dorsal raphe is unchanged by treadmill running. *Medicine and Science in Sports and Exercise* 32 (Suppl. 5): S42.

Van Hoomissen, J.D., H.A. O'Neal, P.V. Holmes, and R.K. Dishman. 2001. The effects of exercise on masculine sexual behavior and BDNF mRNA after olfactory bulbectomy in rats. Abstracts, Society for Neuroscience 31st Annual Meeting, p. 133. San Diego, November 10–15.

Vaux, C.L. 1926. A discussion of physical exercise and recreation. *Occupational Therapy and Rehabilitation* 5: 329–333.

Veale, D., K. Le Fevre, C. Pantelis, V. de Souza, A. Mann, and A. Sargeant. 1992. Aerobic exercise in the adjunctive treatment of depression: A randomized controlled trial. *Journal of the Royal Society of Medicine* 85: 541–544.

Weissman, M.M., R.C. Bland, G.J. Canino, C. Faravelli, S. Greenwald, H.G. Hwu, P.R. Joyce, E.G. Karam, C.K. Lee, J. Lellouch, et al. 1997. The cross-national epidemiology of panic disorder. *Archives of General Psychiatry* 54 (4): 305–309.

Weissman, M.M., J.S. Markowitz, R. Ouellette, S. Greenwald, and J.P. Kahn. 1990. Panic disorder and cardiovascular/ cerebrovascular problems: Results from a community survey. *American Journal of Psychiatry* 147: 1504–1508.

Westenberg, H.G. 1996. Developments in the drug treatment of panic disorder: What is the place of the selective serotonin reuptake inhibitors? *Journal of Affective Disorders* 40: 85–93.

Weyerer, S. 1992. Physical inactivity and depression in the community: Evidence from the Upper Bavarian Field Study. *International Journal of Sports Medicine* 13: 492–496.

White-Welkley, J.E., B.N. Bunnell, E.H. Mougey, J.L. Meyerhoff, and R.K. Dishman. 1995. Treadmill exercise training and estradiol differentially modulate hypothalamic-pituitary-adrenal cortical responses to acute running and immobilization. *Physiology and Behavior* 57: 533–540.

Willner, P. 1995. Animal models of depression: Validity and applications. In *Depression and mania: From neurobiology to treatment,* edited by G. Gessa, W. Fratta, L. Pani, and G. Serra, pp. 19–41. New York: Raven Press.

Wilson, W.M., and C.A. Marsden. 1996. In vivo measurement of extracellular serotonin in the ventral hippocampus during treadmill running. *Behavioural Pharmacology* 7: 101–104.

Workman, E.A, and D.D. Short. 1993. Atypical antidepressants versus imipramine in the treatment of major depression: A meta-analysis. *Journal of Clinical Psychiatry* 54: 5–12.

World Health Organization. 1992. *International classification of diseases-10.* Geneva: World Health Organization.

Yoo, H.S., B.N. Bunnell, J.B. Crabbe, L.R. Kalish, and R.K. Dishman. 2000. Failure of neonatal clomipramine treatment to alter forced swim immobility: Treadmill or activity wheel running and imipramine. *Physiology and Behavior* 70: 407–411.

Yoo, H.S., R.L. Tackett, B.N. Bunnell, J.B. Crabbe, and R.K. Dishman. 2000. Antidepressant-like effects of physical activity vs. imipramine: Neonatal clomipramine model. *Psychobiology* 28: 540–549.

Youngstedt, S.D. 2000. The exercise–sleep mystery. *International Journal of Sport Psychology* 35: 242–255.

Youngstedt, S.D., R.K. Dishman, K.J. Cureton, L.J. Peacock. 1993. Does body temperature mediate anxiolytic effects of acute exercise? *Journal of Applied Physiology* 74: 825–831.

Youngstedt, S.D., P.J. O'Connor, J.B. Crabbe, and R.K. Dishman. 1998. Acute exercise reduces caffeine-induced anxiogenesis. *Medicine and Science in Sports and Exercise* 30 (5): 740–745.

———. 2000. Effects of acute exercise on caffeine-induced insomnia. *Physiology and Behavior* 68: 563–570.

Youngstedt, S.D., P.J. O'Connor, and R.K. Dishman. 1997. The effects of acute exercise on sleep: A quantitative synthesis. *Sleep* 20: 203–213.

Web Site

www.mentalhealth.com. This is the site of Internet Mental Health, a free encyclopedia of mental health information created by a Canadian psychiatrist, Dr. Phillip Long. It provides access to international definitions of affective and anxiety disorders.

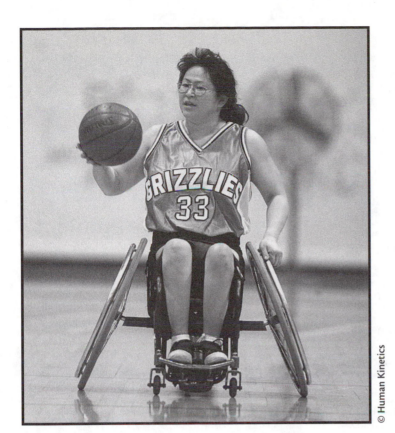

© Human Kinetics

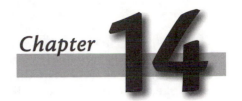

Chapter 14

Physical Activity and Disability

The disparities . . . in men (sic) are superficial . . . Each is incomparably superior to his companion in some faculty. His want of skill in other directions has added to his fitness for his own work. Each seems to have some compensation yielded to him by his infirmity, and every hindrance operates as a concentration of his force.

—*Ralph Waldo Emerson (1844)*

We have to have a way to reduce the potential for future loss of function, particularly in the 10 or 15 percent of the population that use most of our health care dollars and are most vulnerable to loss of function.

—*Gretchen Swanson, Public Hearings of the Subcommittee on Populations, National Committee on Vital and Health Statistics, January 2000*

Disability connotes limitations in ability to perform life activities, including activities of daily living (ADL) and instrumental activities of daily living (IADL), because of an impairment (LaPlante 1991). For example, disability can be characterized by deleterious anatomical or structural changes or the loss of mental or physiological function as a result of active disease, residual losses from formerly active disease, or congenital losses or injury not associated with active disease (LaPlante 1991). The Americans with Disabilities Act (ADA) of

1991 (Public Law 101-336) defines a **person with a disability** as either a person with a physical or mental impairment that substantially limits one or more of the major life activities, a person with a medical record of such impairment, or a person regarded as having such impairment. This definition has been clarified through recent decisions of the U.S. Supreme Court in which a person with a disability is defined as "someone who struggles to do basic tasks that are 'central to daily life,' not the special tasks that go with a particular job" ("Defining disability, court raises bar" 2002). The word disability is derived from the Latin word *dbilis*, meaning to be weak, feeble, or infirm. Though modern use of the term disability continues to denote a limitation in function, its contemporary connotation has evolved to be more consistent with the sentiments expressed in the opening quote by the American essayist, Emerson, recognizing that people with physical or other disabilities or limitations retain the innate capacity to participate fully in human affairs by exerting their capabilities. Just as Emerson recognized the great capacity for humans to compensate for their limitations by strengthening other attributes, we examine in this chapter ways by which physical activity can help restore or preserve physical functions related to the health of people who have a disability. And, as noted in the opening quote by Swanson, the high prevalence of disability in the United States, and worldwide, emphasizes the importance of knowing how physical activity can help reduce the public health burden of disability.

Definitions used for surveillance and assessment of disability are more clearly understood by linking them to a conceptual framework of the consequences of disease and injury. The **International Classification of Functioning, Disability and Health (ICF)** is such a conceptual framework (WHO 2001). In the ICF, the consequences of disease and injury are defined in two parts: (1) functioning and disability, which consists of body functions and structures and activities and participation, and (2) contextual factors, consisting of **environmental factors** and personal factors. Each of the components in both parts of the ICF can be expressed in both positive and negative terms. Within this system, the term *disability* serves as an umbrella term for impairments, **activity limitations,** or participation restrictions (Centers for Disease Control and Prevention 2001).

> ••• *Disability affects more than one in five American adults. Rates of disability are higher among older adults, who also have higher rates of chronic diseases. However, most disability occurs during the working years, which contributes to the high cost of disability.*

Magnitude of the Problem

According to results from the 1997 National Health Interview Survey (NHIS; National Center for Health Statistics 2000, 229–231), 13.3%, or about 40 million, of noninstitutionalized U.S. adults 18 years and older report having a disability (figure 14.1).

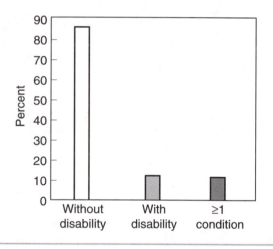

Figure 14.1   The results from the 1997 National Health Interview Survey (NHIS; National Center for Health Statistics 2000) show that 13.3% of the noninstitutionalized U.S. adult (18 years and older) population report having a disability.
Data from National Center for Health Statistics, 2000.

The 40 million people with a disability report 1.6 conditions per person, on average, for a total of 64 million disabling conditions. Heart disease ranks first in causing disability among Americans. Heart disease is followed by back disorders, arthritis, orthopedic impairments of the lower extremity, and asthma. When diseases of the musculoskeletal system and connective tissue are combined (i.e., including back disorders and other musculoskeletal disorders), then the prevalence of this category exceeds the prevalence of disabilities due to heart disease (figure 14.2).

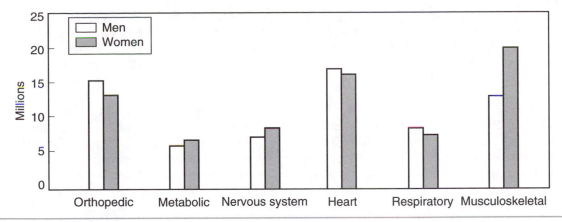

Figure 14.2   Categories of disabilities.

Women are more likely to have a disability than men (13.4% and 13.1%, respectively). American Indians have the highest levels of disability (23.1%), followed by non-Hispanic blacks (17.0%), non-Hispanic whites (13.2%), white Hispanics (12.8%), and Asian and Pacific Islanders (7.5%). The proportion of the population with a disability increases with age (figure 14.3).

The Health and Activity Limitation Surveys (HALS) in Canada reported an estimated 3.3 million people (13%) with some level of disability (Hamilton 1989). The survey also showed a significant increase in disability with age. While 5% of children 14 years old and younger had a disability, 11% of adults ages 15 to 64 had a disability, and 46% of those ages 65 years and older reported a disability. Over 60% of the disabled population 15 years and older had more than one disability. The prevalence of multiple disabilities increased with age. The HALS classified disabilities by function. Disabilities associated with

mobility impairments were the most prevalent (65%), followed by hearing impairment (30%), visual impairment (18%), and impairment of speech or communication (8%).

> ••• *In the United States, the number of people reporting disabling conditions increased from 49 million during 1991 to 1992 to 54 million during 1994 to 1995. During 1996, direct medical costs for people with disabilities were $260 billion.*

Primary Disabling Conditions

A consistent finding across national surveys is that the most prevalent chronic conditions and impairments causing disability include orthopedic

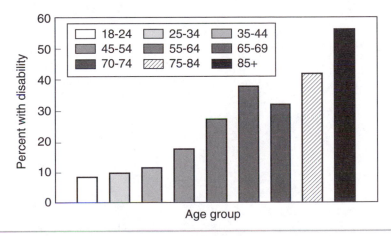

Figure 14.3   Proportion of the population with a disability by age.
Data from National Center for Health Statistics, 2000.

impairments, arthritis, heart disease, hypertension, visual impairments, diabetes, mental disorders, asthma, intervertebral disk disorders, and nervous disorders. In addition, the proportion of people reporting disabilities due to chronic health conditions and impairments appears to have been increasing since the early 1980s (LaPlante and Carlson 1996). Finally, a disproportionate number of people above the age of 65 report having a disability.

Thus, understanding and describing the patterns of regular physical activity, sports, and active recreation among those who report having a disability assumes growing importance. There is little information available to shed light on the question of the extent to which reported disability is a consequence of a chronic condition per se, self-imposed physical inactivity, or a combination of both. Examining the patterns of regular physical activity among people with disabilities not only provides some insight into this question but also helps define the role of physical activity in maintaining function, preventing the progression of the primary disabling condition itself, preventing complications associated with physical inactivity, and preventing compounding of the disability.

In general, people with disabilities are less active and have a lower work capacity than people without disabilities. Figure 14.4 illustrates that Americans who have a disability are less physically active than people without disabilities on each of the major *Healthy People 2010* objectives established by the U.S. Department of Health and Human Services (2000). An inactive lifestyle compounds the effects of the disability itself and makes this a major public health issue. Poor stamina, reduced muscle strength, and limited flexibil-

ity restrict functional ability and therefore personal independence. This loss of autonomy through inactivity deserves attention because there may be an element of functional loss that may not be inevitable and may be in part reversible.

The long-term effects of inactivity among people with disabilities should be a legitimate concern for the public health community. Improvements in medical care and **assistive technology** and the continuing removal of social and environmental barriers have brought the prospect of longer, more satisfying, and more productive lives for those with chronic disabling conditions. Since an inactive lifestyle increases the risk of coronary heart disease (CHD), high blood pressure, thrombosis, osteoporosis, obesity, and type 2 diabetes mellitus among the general population, the importance of regular physical activity among people with disabilities may be even more critical to their health and well-being than to people without disabilities. Persuading people with disabilities to adopt a more active lifestyle poses a major challenge, including the need to raise expectations of the people themselves, their caregivers, and the professional groups that advocate for them.

> ••• *In general, people with disabilities are less active and have lower work capacities than people without disabilities. An inactive lifestyle compounds the effects of the disability itself and makes inactivity a major public health issue.*

Many people expend more energy participating in ADL because of their impairment. The extra metabolic cost of performing physical

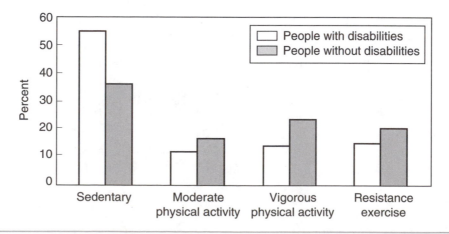

Figure 14.4 Americans who have a disability are less physically active than people without disability.

tasks may arise because of reduced muscle mass, because of inefficient locomotion and abnormal posture attributable to paralysis, or because of high ventilatory effort due to respiratory impairment. For example, a person with an above-the-knee amputation uses about 50% more energy than a person without such an impairment to walk at an average pace (Davis 1993). Although there have been substantial attempts to document fitness levels among people with disabilities (for a review, see Heath and Fentem 1997), very little information exists regarding the physical activity levels and patterns of people with disabilities. Dearwater et al. (1986) recognized the lack of such information and attempted to document the activity levels of people at what they considered the lowest level of the physical activity spectrum, people after spinal cord injuries (SCI). Recognizing the difficulty of using conventional physical activity questionnaires, these investigators employed physical activity movement counters to document the physical activity patterns of people with paraplegia and quadriplegia. The mean counts per hour were 126.7, 33.2, 32.3, 24.2 (wrist), and 4.0 (ankle) for college students, blue-collar men, older women, and people with SCI, respectively. The values obtained using these movement counters may not accurately reflect actual energy expenditure. No subsequent studies among people with disabilities have been conducted using this assessment methodology. Godin et al. (1986) used a questionnaire to assess the physical activity levels of 62 adults with a lower-limb disability and found the cause of disability to be a strong predictor of physical activity. Other studies have attempted to document the physical activity or exercise behavior of people with SCI (Noreau et al. 1993), multiple sclerosis (Ponichtera-Mulcare 1993), mental retardation (Rimmer et al. 1999), and arthritis (Minor and Hewett 1995). Each of these studies documented a lower participation rate in physical activity than for people without these disabilities. Unfortunately, few studies among people with disabilities have used standardized, valid, and reliable measures to assess physical activity, thus leaving little room for comparison with people without disabilities.

Canada and the United States have collected at the national level self-reported information about physical activity and recreational patterns of people with disabilities. The earliest data from Canada were collected in 1981 as part of the Canada Fitness Survey (Dowler and Jordan-Simpson 1990). The prevalence of people with disabilities in this survey was 13.7%. Respondents were asked about selected leisure-time physical activities, and 58% reported walking at least once in the past year, 29% gardening, 24% bicycling, 22% home exercises, 22% swimming, 9% dancing, 9% jogging, 8% skating, 9% individual sports, and 8% team sports. The nature and extent of the disability were not explored in any detail. In a subsequent survey, the Canadian HALS, 65% of respondents with a disability did not report any physical activities such as walking, swimming, bicycling, or jogging on a regular basis—that is, at least once per week (Dowler and Jordan-Simpson 1990; Hamilton 1989). Thirty-five percent of people with disabilities reported that they would have liked to have participated more in walking, swimming, bicycling, or jogging but were prevented by their condition.

In the United States, the results of the NHIS indicate that over 30% of people with disabilities report not doing any leisure-time physical activity. It also indicated that 27% of people with a disability, compared with 37% of people without a disability, engaged in regular moderate physical activity, while 9.6% and 14% of people with and without a disability, respectively, engaged in regular intense or vigorous physical activity (Heath and Fentem 1997). These differences in activity patterns between people with and without disabilities are often confounded by age, socioeconomic status, and health status but suggest several potentially effective physical activity intervention points for people with disabilities. An analysis of the NHIS Health Promotion and Disease Prevention Supplement has determined the physical activity patterns of people with disabilities by type of disability and impairment status (e.g., mobility impairment, sensory impairment; figure 14.5).

••• *Prolonged physical inactivity is associated with long-term risks of disease in people with or without disabilities. Because people with disabilities are often less active, their risk of gaining weight is greater than that of people without disabilities. Excess body weight may itself have a disabling effect, further restricting mobility, particularly when leg muscles are already weak. Regular physical activity can reduce weight among people with and without disabilities.*

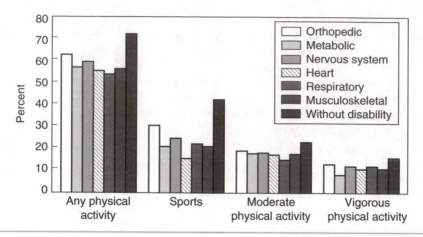

Figure 14.5   An analysis of the NHIS Health Promotion and Disease Prevention Supplement has determined the physical activity patterns among persons with disabilities by the type of disability.

Inactivity and Aging

As mentioned previously, older adults are more likely to experience a disability than younger adults (LaPlante and Carlson 1996). This is due in part to older adults' greater likelihood of having an existing chronic condition or disease that limits their activity (LaPlante and Carlson 1996). Additionally, as people grow older, they generally become less physically active. This reduced activity contributes to a lowering of capacity beyond that related to chronic health condition, disease, or age. A negative spiral of deterioration leads to loss of autonomy and reduction in the quality of life. Cross-sectional (Heath et al. 1981; Larsson et al. 1984) and longitudinal studies (Hagberg 1987; Kasch and Wallace 1976; Pollock et al. 1987) of individuals who have maintained high activity levels over many years provide strong evidence that many of the expected declines in physical capacity with increasing age are not inevitable.

> ••• *Low physical work capacity is reversible. The physiological and biochemical improvements that occur in the muscles, heart, and blood vessels with regular physical activity do not depend on enormous physical effort, only physical effort greater than that to which an individual is accustomed. Although athletes may require work at a high intensity to improve their fitness and performance, sedentary or relatively inactive individuals require little exertion for improvement.*

Several long-term studies of people who remained very active have not shown the expected deterioration in stamina with age (Pollock et al. 1987). Athletes ages 50 to 70 years had a maximum work capacity 60% higher than that of untrained middle-aged men. Physiological changes in cardiovascular function with age limit exercise capacity. Older people do have lower maximal heart rates than younger people (Heath 1994; Rodeheffer et al. 1984), but maximal cardiac output and maximal work rate can, in general, still be preserved through increases in stroke volume, provided that health is good and activity is maintained (Hagberg 1987; Pollock et al. 1987; Rodeheffer et al. 1984). Athletes who have trained to peak capacity may experience a decline as they age, but the majority of active people can certainly maintain work capacity at levels well above the average. With good stamina, a wide range of activities, including the occasional demands of extra exertion, can be continued safely and comfortably. Some deterioration is inevitable. The number of muscle cells decreases with increasing age (Grimby and Saltin 1983). This loss is thought to be due to loss of the motor neurons. The result is that muscles become weaker and contract more slowly (Davies, Thomas, and White 1986). Regular physical activity appears to moderate this loss. In a five-year study of 70-year-olds, those who engaged in moderate physical activity had greater muscle strength and therefore greater reserves of strength than their sedentary peers (Aniansson et al. 1983). A reserve of muscle strength is vital to independent life. To rise from the toilet or a chair, the average healthy 80-year-old woman uses maximum quadriceps strength (Young 1986). If reserve capacity is already close to such a critical threshold, an illness or other period of inactivity can place an individual below the threshold at which independent function can be resumed.

Impaired range of joint movement and pain on movement are the most frequent health problems among older adults. Thirty-one percent of all people classified as having a disability have some form of arthritis or joint disorder (LaPlante 1991). Joints tend to degenerate with age (Bell and Hoshizaki 1981), and there is an average reduction in joint flexibility of 25% to 30% (Adrian 1981). This results in a decline in ability to perform many of the normal ADL. Inability to accomplish such tasks as dressing or climbing onto a bus or entering a vehicle seriously restricts independent life.

Long-term physical activity may reduce the risk of degenerative noninflammatory joint disease, and the resulting severe restrictions on independent life, in later years (Burry 1987). A sedentary occupation and low leisure activity were each associated with greater joint disability in later life (Bergström et al. 1985).

Improvements in stamina, as measured by maximum work capacity, have been documented in older people when they engage in regular physical activity (Seals et al. 1984). Greater functional strength, attributable to either better neural recruitment or intrinsic changes in the exercised muscle cells, is common (Agre et al. 1988; Frontera et al. 1988). Improvements in flexibility resulted from physical activity programs in both older women (Raab et al. 1988) and men (Chapman, de Vries, and Swezey 1972). These improvements have been documented to some extent among the frail elderly as well, leading to the conclusion that frailty itself can possibly be prevented by instituting early remedial programs of physical activity among older adults (Fiatarone et al. 1994).

Most intervention studies involving physical activity exclude older people who have physical impairments arising from chronic and degenerative diseases, but some studies have been conducted exclusively with people representing this subgroup. While the subjects of one study did not demonstrate any significant changes in maximal capacity after 16 weeks of intervention, there were favorable changes in many measured parameters, including workload, strength, blood pressure, and plasma lipids (Thompson et al. 1988). In another study of older men that did not exclude those with disabilities, a four-month-long physical activity program led to significant favorable changes in physical status. Although there was a high dropout rate, 76% of those who completed the program had one or more chronic diseases. Those who completed the program showed increases in treadmill time, abdominal strength, and hip flexibility; decreases in both resting and submaximal heart rate; and a reduction in body fat (Morey et al. 1989). There were no adverse reactions to the program in either study, and participants reported subjective improvements and were enthusiastic about continuing to be physically active (Thompson et al. 1988). Walking by older people is equivalent to jogging by younger people in terms of relative effort. Improvements in stamina are possible with a modest program of walking or some equivalent physical activity for those who cannot use their legs to get about. Walking or its equivalent is also beneficial for maintaining or improving bone density. A prospective study concluded that walking at least 1 mile (1.6 km) three times per week reduced risk of suffering a fracture by a third among older women (Sorock et al. 1988). A program of sitting and standing exercises that load the bones adequately can be devised when walking is impossible (Smith, Reddan, and Smith 1981). Swimming is also beneficial, as it maintains both range of motion and strength of a large number of joints and muscles without loading damaged joint surfaces (Suominen, Heikkinen, and Parkatti 1977). However, as swimming is ineffective for maintaining bone density (Jacobson et al. 1984), some other exercise should also be performed regularly.

> *••• Regular physical activity and exercise cannot completely restore the capacity lost through damage or disease, but some improvement is possible and within the reach of many people with disabilities. The high levels of fitness of participants in the Paralympics and other similar competitions demonstrate what some people with disabilities can achieve (Madorsky and Madorsky 1983; Shephard 1991). However, even small increases in stamina, strength, and flexibility can lead to large improvements in the quality of life of people with disabilities.*

The Disabling Consequences of Inactivity: Conditions Attributable to Inactivity

Prolonged physical inactivity is associated with long-term risks of disease in people with and without disabilities. To date, no studies have been conducted to determine whether the long-term benefits of physical activity seen among people without disabilities—such as lower risks of CHD (Powell et al. 1987), osteoporosis (Chow et al. 1986), and obesity (Bouchard, Depres, and Trembley 1993)—also apply to people with disabilities. It is reasonable to argue that increasing life expectancies for those with even the most severe disabilities now place them at risk from these diseases in later life. Thus, it makes sense for people who have disabilities to protect themselves from inactivity-related conditions that may either exacerbate existing disabilities or contribute to premature death.

Overweight and Obesity

Physical activity is important in preventing weight gain and in reducing weight for those who are overweight. Because people with disabilities are often less active, their risk of gaining weight is greater than that of people without disabilities. Excess body weight may itself have a disabling effect, further restricting mobility, particularly when leg muscles are weak already. Severe obesity—that is, more than 30% above the desirable weight for height—exacerbates the effects of other conditions and increases the risk of death before age 65 (Bouchard, Depres, and Trembley 1993). Regular physical activity can reduce weight. This has been established among people with and without a disability (Findlay et al. 1987; Leon et al. 1979).

Coronary Heart Disease

It has been argued that, for the general population, physical inactivity is as great a risk factor for CHD as hypertension, hypercholesterolemia, or smoking (Powell et al. 1987). Because of increasing longevity, CHD has become a significant cause of death in people who are paraplegic or bilateral lower-limb amputees due to trauma. Physical activity appears to lower risk by its favorable effect on blood lipid levels (Wood et al. 1983), arterial blood pressure (Blair et al. 1984), blood clotting factors (Williams et al. 1980), and glucose tolerance and insulin sensitivity among people without disabilities.

There is strong evidence that high concentrations of high-density lipoprotein (HDL) in the blood are inversely related to the incidence of CHD (Castelli et al. 1986). There is also strong evidence for a positive relationship between levels of physical activity and plasma levels of HDL (Wood et al. 1983). Levels of HDL are generally lower among people who use manual or electric wheelchairs than among people who do not use wheelchairs, and this was shown to be associated with their inactivity (Brenes et al. 1986). Brenes et al. (1986) estimated that among those with SCI, men face a 60% greater and women a 90% greater than average risk of suffering a myocardial infarction. Increased levels of physical activity appear to lead to higher HDL levels among people with SCI (Brenes et al. 1986). This same finding has been demonstrated among people with other disabilities, including those with rheumatoid arthritis (Minor and Hewett 1995). Athletes with visual impairments who train and compete using manual wheelchairs had higher levels of HDL and lower levels of total cholesterol than control subjects who did not participate in regular wheelchair physical activity (Brenes et al. 1986; Shindo, Komagai, and Tanaka 1987). The levels of HDL of the wheelchair athletes were similar to those of active people without disabilities.

Hypertension is the most common manifestation of cardiovascular disease among people with SCI (Cowell, Squires, and Raven 1986). Physical activity has been shown to reduce arterial blood pressure in people without disabilities who have mild or moderate hypertension (Cade et al. 1984; Hagberg et al. 1983). As discussed in chapter 6, while the effects of regular physical activity on arterial blood pressure among people with disabilities have not been reported, it seems plausible to suppose that the effect is similar.

While it seems likely that chronic physical inactivity of people with disabilities contributes to an increased risk of CHD and that increased levels of physical activity can reduce this risk, the role of multiple risk factors for CHD should be acknowledged. As in the population of people without disabilities, moderate-intensity to vigorous physical activity is no absolute guarantee against developing CHD.

Deep-Vein Thrombosis

Prolonged physical inactivity is associated with the development of lower-limb deep-vein thrombosis, making this an important potential complication of prolonged immobility (Housley 1988). Regular physical activity has been shown to reduce this risk and consequently that of pulmonary embolism, a more serious complication.

Osteoporosis

There is strong evidence that bone density and bone mass are partially determined by habitual levels of physical activity in people with disabilities (Cowell, Squires, and Raven 1986), as in people without disabilities (Chow et al. 1986; see chapter 10). Bone is lost rapidly during bed rest or immobility. The rate of loss can be as high as 5% per month (Schneider and McDonald 1984). Studies have shown that moderate physical activity can reverse this loss. Two observations about activity's role in maintaining bone emerge from studies among people without disabilities: (1) The effect appears to be quite specific to the bones that are loaded during the particular physical activity, and (2) gravity and the impact of weight bearing appear to be important factors (Jacobson et al. 1984; Schneider and McDonald 1984). The effects of physical activity on bone density with weight-bearing physical activity among people with disabilities have not been investigated, but it is a reasonable hypothesis that the effect is the same as that observed in older adults (Smith, Reddan, and Smith 1981). Walking appears to be an ideal form of physical activity for the purpose of maintaining bone mass. Walking provides a gravity-dependent stimulus to the bones of the back and lower limbs. These bones are most at risk of osteoporotic fractures. Walking with crutches, braces, or orthoses, even for brief periods, should trigger the osteogenic activity of the bone-building cells and maintain bone density, according to the known mechanisms (Yeh and Rodan 1984). Maintaining bone density presents a particular problem for people who cannot stand. Paralyzed limbs are most at risk of osteoporotic fractures. Their bones can become so fragile that fractures occur with little or no trauma (Cowell, Squires, and Raven 1986). These problems are not insurmountable, however. An ingenious use of a tiltboard to simulate the effects of weight bearing and gravity during strengthening exercises by people with quadriplegia provided a significant reduction in calcium loss (Kaplan et al. 1981). The same strengthening exercises performed without the tiltboard showed no such reduction. The reduction of calcium loss may also reduce the incidence of kidney stones common among people with SCI (Cowell, Squires, and Raven 1986).

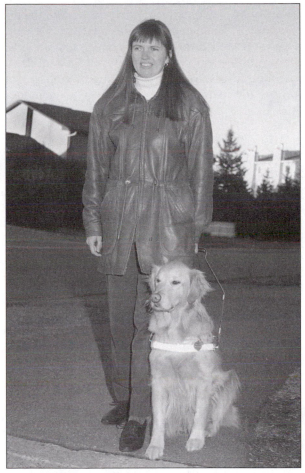

© John T. Fowler

Physical Activity in the Prevention of Disability and Complications

Regular physical activity and exercise training cannot completely restore the capacity lost through damage or disease, but some improvement is possible and within the reach of many people with disabilities and many older adults (Nilsson, Staff, and Pruett 1975; Seals et al. 1984). The high levels of fitness of participants in the Paralympics and other similar competitions demonstrate what can be achieved by some people with disabilities (Madorsky and Madorsky 1983;

Shephard 1991). However, even small increases in stamina, strength, and flexibility can lead to large improvements in the quality of life of people with disabilities. Increases in stamina have been achieved with a modest increase in physical activity by previously inactive older adults who have taken up walking (Frontera et al. 1988). This is equivalent to jogging by younger people in terms of improvement in maximal work capacity (Suominen, Heikkinen, and Parkatti 1977). Given a suitable and interesting physical activity program, people who have a variety of disabilities, including those for whom walking or standing is impossible, can experience such improvements (Hoskins 1975; Nilsson, Staff, and Pruett 1975).

> ••• Regular physical activity, sports participation, and active recreation are essential for the prevention of disease, promotion of health, and maintenance of functional independence for people with and without disabilities.

Physical Work Capacity

Low physical work capacity is reversible. The physiological and biochemical improvements that occur in the muscles, heart, and blood vessels with regular physical activity do not depend on enormous physical effort, only physical effort greater than that to which an individual is accustomed. Although athletes may require work at a high intensity to improve their fitness and performance, sedentary or relatively inactive individuals require little exertion for improvement. Training occurs when the effort of an activity is somewhat greater than that to which the individual is accustomed. The degree of improvement depends on the intensity, duration, and frequency of the activity (Hickson et al. 1982). In people with low exercise tolerance, improvements have resulted from rhythmic physical activity of very short duration (i.e., less than 2 min) performed sufficiently frequently (Harkcom et al. 1985). Greater reserve capacity can compensate for the increased energy expenditure required by a physical impairment. Training can improve the skill with which a maneuver can be performed and reduce inefficiency of movements, thus also reducing the effort to perform them. Training-induced improvements in reserve capacity are especially important for people with mobility impairments.

Muscular Strength

When muscle strength is decreased and the mass of functional muscle is reduced by paralysis or disease, it is a benefit to strengthen the remaining muscle. Indeed, it is vital that residual capacity be increased and maintained. Studies with both older people and people with disabilities demonstrated that brief contractions of the muscles repeated at frequent intervals led to an increase in the size of the muscle cells (Einarsson 1991; Gaffney et al. 1981; Kristensen, Hansen, and Saltin 1980) and the strength of the muscles being used (Gehlsen, Grigsby, and Winant 1984; Nilsson, Staff, and Pruett 1975). Improvements in muscle strength protect joints, ligaments, and the muscles themselves by stabilizing the joints and minimizing the damaging effects of sudden movements and unexpected strain.

Joint Pain and Flexibility

It appears that long-term, regular use of a joint has a beneficial effect. Rather than wearing out joint surfaces, regular movement increases joint nutrition and lubrication, protecting the surfaces and so preventing degenerative joint disease (Ahlqvist 1985; Burry 1987). Gentle motion, by lubricating the joint, makes movement less painful, which is particularly beneficial to those with joint disease (Nordemar et al. 1981; Van Deusen 1987). Suppleness or range of joint movement becomes reduced with inactivity due to joint diseases, paralysis, or aging. Muscles and tendons shorten if the full range of joint movement is not regularly used. Simple daily stretching exercises help to avoid this. Habitual sitting leads to flexion contractures, which make an individual rigid. This rigidity leads to problems in changing position and makes personal hygiene and transfer from bed to chair and similar movements difficult. Walking, or stretching exercises when walking is impossible, appears helpful in avoiding joint contractures (Hardy and Jones 1986). Children with paralysis due to spina bifida who were able to walk and did so had virtually no joint contractures, while contractures were a severe problem for those who consistently used a wheelchair (Agre et al. 1987). Improvements in stamina, strength, and flexibility widen the range of activities an individual can undertake. The importance of being able to walk a bit farther, transfer into and out of a chair, or brush one's own hair cannot be overestimated.

Quality of Life: Psychological Aspects

Success in overcoming physical, psychological, and social barriers helps in adjusting to a disability and improves self-image. In a society that can devalue individuals for having disabilities, an individual with a disability can devalue himself or herself. Physical achievement can provide an important opportunity for people with disabilities to gain more control over their bodies and lives. In doing so, their own perceptions of their disabilities and abilities may change, potentially enhancing mental health (Meyer 1981; Shephard 1991).

Function for Daily Living

For people with disabilities who are not interested in sports or exercise, a physical activity plan can be based on customary activities (Gloag 1985). For example, getting out of a chair with minimal use of the arms can maximize quadriceps strength. Many such activities have been designed for older adults and can be adapted for use by people with disabilities (Fentem 1992).

In addition to the risk of decline in physical capacity due to a gradual decline in physical activity, there is risk of deterioration with even relatively brief periods of bed rest (Coyle et al. 1985; Siegel, Blomqvist, and Mitchell 1970). Bed rest must be kept as short as an impairment or illness allows, and subsequent rehabilitation needs to be energetic.

> ••• *Many people with a variety of disabilities can adapt to increased levels of physical activity, as evidenced by alterations in various components of physical fitness. More important, participation in regular physical activity by people with some disabilities improves functional status and quality of life.*

Summary

Regular physical activity and active recreation are essential for the prevention of disease, promotion of health, and maintenance of functional independence for people with and without disabilities. Population-based surveys have consistently demonstrated that people with disabilities are less likely to be physically active than people without such limitations. However, this observation is based on a relatively few surveys and on physical activity assessment methods that may not be sensitive and specific enough for people with disabilities.

Studies demonstrate that many people with a variety of disabilities can adapt to increased levels of physical activity, as evidenced by alterations in various components of physical fitness. More important, studies provide consistent evidence that participation in regular physical activity by people with some disabilities improves functional status and quality of life. Some areas where more research is needed include children with disabilities and accessibility and safety of physical activity programs for people with disabilities (Cooper et al. 1999). Improved methodology is critically needed in the area of physical activity assessment for people with disabilities. These methods are needed to enable survey researchers and those in public health surveillance to measure and monitor the activity patterns of people with disabilities. This information is important not only for public health officials but also health policy analysts, service providers, disability advocacy groups, and people with disabilities. The role of physical activity in the maintenance of function and independence among people with disabilities needs to be better understood. Finally, the environmental and social barriers to physical activity and the determinants of physical activity among people with disabilities need to be further examined, including the use of assistive technology to maximize intrinsic anatomical and physiological functional capacity.

Bibliography

Adrian, M.J. 1981. Flexibility in the aging adult. In *Exercise and aging: The scientific basis,* edited by E.L. Smith and R.C. Serfass, pp. 45–57. Hillside, NJ: Enslow.

Agre, J.C., T.W. Findley, M.C. McNally, R. Habeck, A.S. Leon, L. Stradel, R. Birkebak, and R. Schmalz. 1987. Physical activity capacity in children with myelomeningocele. *Archives of Physical Medicine and Rehabilitation* 68: 372–377.

Agre, J.C., L.E. Pierce, D.M. Raab, M. McAdams, and E.L. Smith. 1988. Light resistance and stretching exercise in elderly women: Effect upon strength. *Archives of Physical Medicine and Rehabilitation* 69: 273–276.

Ahlqvist, J. 1985. On the structural and physiological basis of the influence of exercise, movement and immobilization in inflammatory joint diseases. *Annales Chirurgiae et Gynaecologiae* 198 (Suppl.): 10–18.

Aniansson, A., L. Sperling, K. Rundgren, and E. Lehnberg. 1983. Muscle function in 75-year-old men and women: A longitudinal study. *Scandinavian Journal of Rehabilitation Medicine Supplement* 9: 92–102.

Bell, R.D., and T.B. Hoshizaki. 1981. Relationships of age and sex with range of motion of seventeen joint actions in humans. *Canadian Journal of Applied Sport Sciences* 6: 202–206.

Bergström, G., A. Aniansson, A. Bjelle, G. Grimby, B. Lundgren-Lindquist, and A. Svanborg. 1985. Functional consequences of joint impairment at age 79. *Scandinavian Journal of Rehabilitation Medicine* 17: 183–190.

Blair, S.N., N.N. Goodyear, L.W. Gibbons, and K.H. Cooper. 1984. Physical fitness and incidence of hypertension in healthy normotensive men and women. *Journal of the American Medical Association* 252: 487–490.

Bouchard, C., J.P. Depres, and A. Trembley. 1993. Exercise and obesity. *Obesity Research* 1: 133–147.

Brenes, G.S., S. Dearwater, R. Shapera, R.E. LaPorte, and E. Collin. 1986. High density lipoprotein cholesterol concentrations in physically active and sedentary spinal cord injured patients. *Archives of Physical Medicine and Rehabilitation* 67: 445–450.

Breslow, L., and N. Breslow. 1993. Health practices and disability: Some evidence from Alameda County. *Preventive Medicine* 22: 86–95.

Burry, H.C. 1987. Sport, exercise and arthritis. *British Journal of Rheumatology* 26: 386–388.

Cade, R., D. Mars, H. Wagemaker, C. Zauner, D. Packer, M. Privette, M. Cade, J. Peterson, and D. Hood-Lewis. 1984. Effect of aerobic exercise training on patients with systemic arterial hypertension. *American Journal of Medicine* 77: 785–790.

Castelli, W.P., R.J. Garrison, P.W.F. Wilson, R.D. Abbott, S. Kalousdian, and W.B. Kannel. 1986. Incidence of coronary heart disease and lipoprotein cholesterol levels: The Framingham Study. *Journal of the American Medical Association* 256: 2835–2838.

Centers for Disease Control and Prevention. 1993. Prevalence of mobility and self-care disability—United States, 1990. *Morbidity and Mortality Weekly Report* 42: 760–768.

———. 2001. Prevalence of disabilities and associated health—United States, 1999. *Morbidity and Mortality Weekly Report* 50: 120–125.

Chapman, E.A., H.A. de Vries, and R. Swezey. 1972. Joint stiffness: Effects of exercise on young and old men. *Journal of Gerontology* 27: 218–221.

Chow, R.K., J.E. Harrison, C.F. Brown, and V. Hajek. 1986. Physical fitness effect on bone mass in postmenopausal women. *Archives of Physical Medicine and Rehabilitation* 67: 231–234.

Compton, D.M., P.A. Eisenman, and H.L. Henderson. 1989. Exercise and fitness for persons with disabilities. *Sports Medicine* 7: 150–162.

Cooper, R.A., L.A. Quatrano, P.W. Axelson, W. Harlan, M. Stineman, B. Franklin, J.S. Krause, J. Bach, H. Chambers, E.Y. Chao, et al. 1999. Research on physical activity and health among people with disabilities: A consensus statement. *Journal of Rehabilitation Research and Development* 36 (2): 142–154.

Cowell, L.L., W.G. Squires, and P.B. Raven. 1986. Benefits of aerobic exercise for the paraplegic: A brief review. *Medicine and Science in Sports and Exercise* 18: 501–508.

Coyle, E.F., W.H. Martin, S.A. Bloomfield, O.H. Lowry, and J.O. Holloszy. 1985. Effects of detraining on responses to submaximal exercise. *Journal of Applied Physiology* 59: 853–859.

Crespo, C.J., S.J. Keteyian, G.W. Heath, and C.T. Sempos. 1996. Leisure-time physical activity among U.S. adults: Results from the third National Health and Nutrition Examination Survey. *Archives of Internal Medicine* 156: 93–98.

Davies, C.T.M., D.O. Thomas, and M.J. White. 1986. Mechanical properties of young and elderly human muscle. *Acta Medica Scandinavica* 220 (Suppl. 711): 219–226.

Davis, G.M. 1993. Exercise capacity of individuals with paraplegia. *Medicine and Science in Sports and Exercise* 25: 423–432.

Dearwater, S.R., R.E. LaPorte, R.J. Robertson, G. Brenes, L.L. Adams, and D. Becker. 1986. Activity in the spinal cord-injured patient: An epidemiologic analysis of metabolic parameters. *Medicine and Science in Sports* 18: 541–544.

Defining disability, court raises bar. 2002. *Atlanta Journal and Constitution,* January 9.

de Vries, H.A. 1979. Physiological effects of an exercise training regimen upon men aged 52–88. *Journal of Gerontology* 4: 325–336.

Dowler, J.M., and D.A. Jordan-Simpson. 1990. Participation of people with disabilities in selected activities. *Health Reports* 2: 269–277.

Einarsson, G. 1991. Muscle adaptation and disability in late poliomyelitis. *Scandinavian Journal of Rehabilitation Medicine Supplement* 25: 1–76.

Emerson, R.W. 1844. New England reformers: A lecture read before the society in Amory Hall on Sunday, March 3, 1844. Essays and English traits. Selected by C.W. Eliot, ed. *The Harvard Classics. Vol. 5, 1914.* New York: P.F. Collier and Son.

Fentem, P.H. 1992. Exercise in the prevention of disease. *British Medical Bulletin* 48: 630–650.

———. 1994. Benefits of exercise in health and disease. *British Medical Journal* 308: 1291–1295.

Fentem, P.H., and E.J. Bassey. 1985. *50+ All to play for: A guide for those in charge of activity groups.* London: Sports Council.

Fiatarone, M.A., E.F. O'Neill, N.D. Ryan, K.M. Clements, G.R. Solares, M.E. Nelson, S.B. Roberts, J.J. Kehayias, L.A. Lipsitz, and W.J. Evans. 1994. Exercise training and nutritional supplementation for physical frailty in very elderly people. *New England Journal of Medicine* 330: 1769–1775.

Findlay, I.N., R.S. Taylor, H.J. Dargie, S. Grant, A.R. Pettigrew, J.T. Wilson, T. Aitchison, J.G. Cleland, A.T. Elliott, B.M. Fisher, et al. 1987. Cardiovascular effects of training for a marathon run in unfit middle aged men. *British Medical Journal* 295: 521–524.

Frontera, W.R., C.N. Meredith, K.P. O'Reilly, H.G. Knuttgen, and W.J. Evans. 1988. Strength conditioning in older men: Skeletal muscle hypertrophy and improved function. *Journal of Applied Physiology* 64: 1038–1044.

Gaffney, F.A., G. Grimby, B. Danneskiold-Samsøe, and O. Halskov. 1981. Adaptation to peripheral muscle training. *Scandinavian Journal of Rehabilitation Medicine* 13: 11–16.

Gehlsen, G.M., S.A. Grigsby, and D.M. Winant. 1984. Effects of an aquatic fitness program on the muscular strength and endurance of patients with multiple sclerosis. *Physical Therapy* 64: 653–657.

Gloag, D. 1985. Rehabilitation in rheumatic diseases. *British Medical Journal* 290: 132–136.

Godin, G., A. Colantonio, G.M. Davis, R.J. Shephard, and C. Simard. 1986. Prediction of leisure time exercise behavior among a group of lower-limb disabled adults. *Journal of Clinical Psychology* 42: 272–279.

Grimby, G., G. Einarsson, M. Hedberg, and A. Aniansson. 1989. Muscle adaptive changes in post-polio subjects. *Scandinavian Journal of Rehabilitation Medicine* 21: 19–26.

Grimby, G., and B. Saltin. 1983. The ageing muscle: Mini-review. *Clinical Physiology* 3: 209–218.

Hagberg, J.M. 1987. Effect of training on the decline of $\dot{V}O_2$ max with aging. *Federation Proceedings* 46: 1830–1833.

Hagberg, J.M., D. Goldring, A.A. Ehsani, G.W. Heath, A. Hernandez, K. Schechtman, and J.O. Holloszy. 1983. Effect of exercise training on the blood pressure and hemodynamic features of hypertensive adolescents. *American Journal of Cardiology* 52: 763–768.

Hamilton, M.K. 1989. The health and activity limitation survey. *Health Reports* 1: 175–187.

Hardy, L., and D. Jones. 1986. Dynamic flexibility and proprioceptive neuromuscular facilitation. *Research Quarterly for Exercise and Sport* 57: 150–153.

Harkcom, T.M., R.M. Lampman, B.F. Banwell, and C.W. Castor. 1985. Therapeutic value of graded aerobic exercise training in rheumatoid arthritis. *Arthritis and Rheumatism* 28: 32–39.

Heath, G.W. 1994. Physical fitness and aging: Effects of deconditioning. *Science and Sports* 9: 197–200.

———. 2000. Epidemiologic research: A primer for the clinical exercise physiologist. *Clinical Exercise Physiology* 2: 60–67.

Heath, G.W., and P.H. Fentem. 1997. Physical activity among persons with disabilities: A public health perspective. *Exercise and Sport Sciences Reviews* 25: 195–234.

Heath, G.W., J.M. Hagberg, A.A. Ehsani, and J.O. Holloszy. 1981. A physiological comparison of young and older endurance athletes. *Journal of Applied Physiology* 51: 634–640.

Hickson, R.C., C. Kanakis Jr., J.R. Davis, A.M. Moore, and S. Rich. 1982. Reduced training duration effects on aerobic power, endurance, and cardiac growth. *Journal of Applied Physiology* 53: 225–229.

Hoskins, T.A. 1975. Physiologic responses to known exercise loads in hemiplegic patients. *Archives of Physical Medicine and Rehabilitation* 56: 544.

Housley, E. 1988. Treating claudication in five words. *British Medical Journal* 296: 1483.

Hubert, H.B., D.A. Bloch, and J.F. Fries. 1993. Risk factors for physical disability in an aging cohort: The NHANES I Epidemiologic Follow-Up Study. *Journal of Rheumatology* 20: 480–488.

Jacobson, P.C., W. Beaver, S.A. Grubb, T.N. Taft, and R.V. Talmage. 1984. Bone density in women: College athletes and older athletic women. *Journal of Orthopaedic Research* 2: 328–332.

Kaplan, P.E., W. Roden, E. Gilbert, L. Richards, and J.W. Goldschmidt. 1981. Reduction of hypercalciuria in tetraplegia after weight-bearing and strengthening exercises. *Paraplegia* 19: 289–293.

Kasch, F.W., and J.P. Wallace. 1976. Physiological variables during 10 years of endurance exercise. *Medicine and Science in Sports* 8: 5–8.

Kinne, S., D.L. Patrick, and E.J. Maher. 1999. Correlates of exercise maintenance among people with mobility impairments. *Disability and Rehabilitation* 21: 15–22.

Kovar, P.A., I.P. Allegrante, C.R. MacKenzie, M.G.E. Peterson, B. Gutin, and M.E. Charlson. 1992. Supervised walking in patients with osteoarthritis of the knee: A randomized controlled trial. *Annals of Internal Medicine* 116: 529–534.

Kristensen, J.H., T.I. Hansen, and B. Saltin. 1980. Cross-sectional and fiber size changes in the quadriceps muscle of man with immobilization and physical training. *Muscle and Nerve* 3: 275–276.

LaPlante, M.P. 1991. Medical conditions associated with disability. In *Disability in the United States: A portrait from national data*, edited by S. Thompson-Hoffman and I. Fitzgerald Storck, pp. 34–72. New York: Springer.

LaPlante, M.P., and D. Carlson. 1996. *Disability in the United States: Prevalence and causes, 1992*. Disability Statistics Report No. 7. Washington, DC: U.S. Department of Education, National Institute of Disability and Rehabilitation Research.

LaPlante, M.P., G.W. Heath, N. Barker, and M.H. Chang. 1996. Prevalence of leisure-time physical activity among people with and without disability: United States, 1990–1991. *Proceedings of the Paralympic Scientific Congress*, Atlanta, GA.

Larsson, B., P. Renstrom, K. Svardsudd, L. Welin, G. Grimby, H. Eriksson, L.-O. Ohlson, L. Wilhelmsen, and P. Bjorntorp.

1984. Health and ageing characteristics of highly physically active 65-year-old men. *European Heart Journal* 5 (Suppl. E): 31–35.

Laukkanen, P., E. Heikkinen, and M. Kauppinen. 1995. Muscle strength and mobility as predictors of survival in 75–84-year-old people. *Age and Ageing* 24: 468–473.

Launer, L.J., T. Harris, C. Rumpel, and J. Madans. 1994. Body mass index, weight change, and risk of mobility disability in middle-aged and older women: The epidemiologic follow-up study of NHANES I. *Journal of the American Medical Association* 271: 1093–1098.

Lee, P., A. Helewa, H.A. Smythe, C. Bombardier, and C.H. Goldsmith. 1985. Epidemiology of musculoskeletal disorders (complaints) and related disability in Canada. *Journal of Rheumatology* 12: 1169–1173.

Leon, A.S., J. Conrad, D.B. Hunninghake, and R. Serfass. 1979. Effect of a vigorous walking program on body composition, and carbohydrate and lipid metabolism of obese young men. *American Journal of Clinical Nutrition* 33: 1776–1787.

Madorsky, J.G., and A. Madorsky. 1983. Wheelchair racing: An important modality in acute rehabilitation after paraplegia. *Archives of Physical Medicine and Rehabilitation* 64: 186–187.

Meyer, C.M.H. 1981. Sport and recreation for the severely disabled. *South African Medical Journal* 60: 868–871.

Minor, M.A., and J.E. Hewett. 1995. Physical fitness and work capacity in women with rheumatoid arthritis. *Arthritis Care and Research* 8: 146–154.

Morey, M.C., P.A. Cowper, J.R. Feussner, R.C. DiPasquale, G.M. Crowley, D.W. Kitzman, and R.J. Sullivan. 1989. Evaluation of a supervised exercise program in a geriatric population. *Journal of the American Geriatric Society* 37: 348–354.

National Center for Health Statistics. 2000. *Health, United States, 2000 with adolescent health chartbook*. Hyattsville, MD: National Center for Health Statistics.

Nilsson, S., P.H. Staff, and E.D.R. Pruett. 1975. Physical work capacity and the effect of training on subjects with long-standing paraplegia. *Scandinavian Journal of Rehabilitation Medicine* 7: 51–56.

Nordemar, R., U. Berg, B. Ekblom, and L. Edstrom. 1976. Changes in muscle fibre size and physical performance in patients with rheumatoid arthritis after 7 months' physical training. *Scandinavian Journal of Rheumatology* 5: 233–238.

Nordemar, R., B. Ekblom, L. Zachrisson, and K. Lundqvist. 1981. Physical training in rheumatoid arthritis: A controlled long-term study. *Scandinavian Journal of Rheumatology* 10: 17–23.

Noreau, L., R.J. Shephard, C. Simard, G. Pare, and P. Pomerleau. 1993. Relationship of impairment and functional ability to habitual activity and fitness following spinal cord injury. *International Journal of Rehabilitation Research* 16: 265–275.

Painter, P., and G. Blackburn. 1988. Exercise for patients with chronic disease. *Postgraduate Medicine* 83: 185–196.

Phillips, W.T., and W.L. Haskell. 1995. "Muscular fitness"—Easing the burden of disability for elderly adults. *Journal of Aging and Physical Activity* 3: 261–289.

Pollock, M.L., C. Foster, D. Knapp, J.L. Rod, and D.H. Schmidt. 1987. Effect of age and training on aerobic capacity and body composition of master athletes. *Journal of Applied Physiology* 62: 725–731.

Ponichtera-Mulcare, J.A. 1993. Exercise and multiple sclerosis. *Medicine and Science in Sports and Exercise* 25: 451–465.

Powell, K.E., P.D. Thompson, C.J. Casperson, and J.S. Kendrick. 1987. Physical activity and the incidence of coronary heart disease. *Annual Review of Public Health* 8: 253–287.

Raab, D.M., J.C. Agre, M. McAdams, and E.L. Smith. 1988. Light resistance and stretching exercise in elderly women: Effect upon flexibility. *Archives of Physical Medicine and Rehabilitation* 69: 268–272.

Rimmer, J.H., D. Braddock, and K.H. Pitetti. 1996. Research on physical activity and disability: An emerging national priority. *Medicine and Science in Sports and Exercise* 28: 1366–1372.

Rimmer, J.H., S.S. Rubin, and D. Braddock. 2000. Barriers to exercise in African-American women with physical disabilities. *Archives of Physical Medicine and Rehabilitation* 81: 182–188.

Rimmer, J.H., S.S. Rubin, D. Braddock, and G. Hedman. 1999. Physical activity patterns of African-American women with physical disabilities. *Medicine and Science in Sports and Exercise* 31: 613–618.

Rodeheffer, R.J., G. Gerstenblith, L.C. Becker, J.L. Fleg, M.L. Weisfeldt, and E.G. Lakatta. 1984. Exercise cardiac output is maintained with advancing age in healthy human subjects: Cardiac dilatation and increased stroke volume compensate for a diminished heart rate. *Circulation* 69: 203–213.

Santiago, M.C., C.P. Coyle, and W.B. Kinney. 1993. Aerobic exercise effect on individuals with physical disabilities. *Archives of Physical Medicine and Rehabilitation* 74: 1192–1198.

Schneider, V.S., and J. McDonald. 1984. Skeletal calcium homeostasis and countermeasures to prevent disuse osteoporosis. *Calcified Tissue International* 36 (Suppl.): S151–S154.

Seals, D.R., J.M. Hagberg, B.F. Hurley, A.A. Ehsani, and J.O. Holloszy. 1984. Endurance training in older men and women: I. Cardiovascular responses to exercise. *Journal of Applied Physiology* 57: 1024–1029.

Shephard, R.J. 1991. Benefits of sport and physical activity for the disabled: Implications for the individual and for society. *Scandinavian Journal of Rehabilitation Medicine* 23: 51–59.

Shindo, M., S. Komagai, and H. Tanaka. 1987. Physical work capacity and effect of endurance training in visually handicapped boys and young male adults. *European Journal of Applied Physiology* 56: 501–507.

Siegel, W., G. Blomqvist, and J.H. Mitchell. 1970. Effects of a quantitated physical training program on middle-aged sedentary men. *Circulation* 41: 19–29.

Smith, E.L. Jr., W. Reddan, and P.E. Smith. 1981. Physical activity and calcium modalities for bone mineral increase in aged women. *Medicine and Science in Sports and Exercise* 13: 60–64.

Sorock, G.S., T.L. Bush, A.L. Golden, L.P. Fried, B. Breuer, and W.E. Hale. 1988. Physical activity and fracture risk in a free-living elderly cohort. *Journal of Gerontology* 43: M134–M139.

Suominen, H., E. Heikkinen, and T. Parkatti. 1977. Effect of eight weeks' physical training on muscle and connective tissue of the m. vastus lateralis in 69-year-old men and women. *Journal of Gerontology* 32: 33–37.

Taylor, W.C., T. Baranowski, and D.R. Young. 1998. Physical activity interventions in low-income, ethnic minority, and populations with disability. *American Journal of Preventive Medicine* 15: 334–343.

Thompson, R.F., D.M. Crist, M. Marsh, and M. Rosenthal. 1988. Effects of physical exercise for elderly patients with physical impairments. *Journal of the American Geriatric Society* 36: 130–135.

U.S. Department of Health and Human Services. 2000. *Healthy people 2010.* 2nd ed. 2 vols. Washington, DC: U.S. Government Printing Office.

Van Deusen, J. 1987. The efficacy of ROM dance program for adults with rheumatoid arthritis. *American Journal of Occupational Therapy* 41: 90–95.

Williams, R.S., E.E. Logue, J.L. Lewis, T. Barton, N.W. Stead, A.G. Wallace, and S.V. Pizzo. 1980. Physical conditioning augments the fibrinolytic response to venous occlusion in healthy adults. *New England Journal of Medicine* 302: 987–991.

Wood, P.D., W.L. Haskell, S.N. Blair, P.T. Williams, R.N. Krauss, F.T. Lindgren, J.J. Albers, P.H. Ho, and J.W. Farquhar. 1983. Increased exercise level and plasma lipoprotein concentrations: A one-year, randomized, controlled study in sedentary, middle-aged men. *Metabolism* 32: 31–39.

World Health Organization. 2001. *International classification of functioning, disability, and health, ICF.* Geneva: World Health Organization.

Yeh, C.-K., and G.A. Rodan. 1984. Tensile forces enhance prostaglandin E synthesis in osteoblastic cells grown on collagen ribbons. *Calcified Tissue International* 36 (Suppl.): S67–S71.

Young, A. 1986. Exercise physiology in geriatric practice. *Acta Medica Scandinavica Supplementum* 711: 227–232.

Web Site

www.ncpad.org. Home page of the National Center on Physical Activity and Disability, funded by the Centers for Disease Control and Prevention and part of the Department of Disability and Human Development in the College of Applied Health Sciences at the University of Illinois at Chicago.

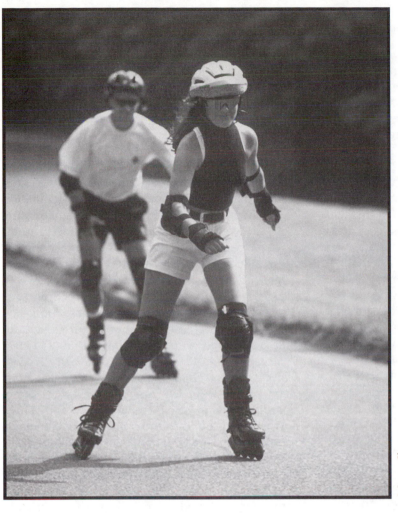

Chapter 15

© SportsChrome

Hazards of Physical Activity

Both excessive and defective exercise destroys the strength.

—*Aristotle, Eudemian Ethics, 384–322 B.C.*

The secret of my abundant health is that whenever the urge to exercise comes upon me, I lie down for a while and it passes.

—*R.M. Hutchins, President, University of Chicago, 1929–1951*

Contrary to the satirical wit of R.M. Hutchins, this book has confirmed that leisure-time physical activity, rather than sedentariness, is associated with lower risk of premature death and several chronic diseases. Nonetheless, there is an ironic grain of truth in the opening quote by Aristotle; vigorous physical activity is not without increased risk of **injury,** and even sudden death, in some circumstances. Just as the precise dose–response relationship between physical activity and lowered health risk is not yet known for most chronic diseases, neither are the types, amounts, and settings of physical activity that increase its hazards fully known. Nonetheless, it is likely that the golden mean of Aristotle, "All things in moderation," holds for many of the health benefits of exercise. More is not always better. Knowledge about the association between injury and exposure to different types of physical activity is necessary to identify activities that optimize long-term health benefits while minimizing injury and sudden death.

The epidemiologic study of the hazards of occupational physical activity can be traced to the observations of Bernardino Ramazzini in the late 1600s. In his 1713 book *De Morbis Artificum Diatriba* (The Diseases of Workers), Ramazzini recommended moderation to prevent illness in jobs that required severe muscular exertion such as that performed by bricklayers, woodworkers, and printers: "Therefore in work so taxing moderation would be the best safeguard against these maladies, for men and women alike; for the common maxim 'nothing in excess' is one of which I excessively approve" (Ramazinni 1983). However, the modern study of the hazards of leisure-time physical activity did not get organized until about 250 years later, as described by Dr. Jeffrey Koplan, immediate past director of the Centers for Disease Control and Prevention: "If we are to continue advocating exercise as a health-promoting activity, it is our responsibility as advocates and health professionals to provide the public with information that presents a full and balanced view of exercise, namely, its benefits and risks" (Koplan, Siscovick, and Goldbaum 1985).

> ••• *In 1713, Bernardino Ramazzini, possibly the first injury epidemiologist, recommended moderation to prevent illness in jobs that required severe muscular exertion.*

Magnitude of the Problem

Few estimates of the incidence of injuries during leisure-time physical activity among adults of different ages and exposure are available, either worldwide or in the United States. The 1994 Injury Control and Risk Survey (ICARIS) interviewed over 5,000 English-speaking adults by telephone after random-digit dialing of U.S. residential households (Powell et al. 1998). The 30-day injury rates reported among participants in five activities were then estimated for the

period of late spring and early summer of 1994 and extrapolated to the U.S. adult population ages 18 years and older. Prevalence rates and numbers were 0.9% (330,000 people) for outdoor bicycling, 1.4% (1,877,000) for walking, 1.4% (2,131,000) for gardening and yard work, 1.6% (394,000) for aerobics, and 2.4% (964,000) for weightlifting.

According to estimates from the National Hospital Ambulatory Care Survey (NHACS) conducted between 1997 and 1998, about 1.1 million adults over 24 years of age and 2.6 million children and young adults who played sports or otherwise exercised visited an emergency room as the result of an activity-related injury (Burt and Overpeck 2001). According to that study, 25% of all emergency-room injuries among people ages 5 to 24 years result from sport participation. The most common emergency-room injuries seen in that age range were from basketball (447,000 visits), cycling (421,000 visits), football (271,000 visits), and baseball or softball (245,000). Other risky sports were ice- and roller-skating, skateboarding, gymnastics, and water and snow sports. Playground injuries led to 137,000 emergency-room visits (Burt and Overpeck 2001).

Recent analyses by the CDC of data from the National Electronic Injury Surveillance System All Injury Program (NEISS-AIP) indicate higher rates of sports- and recreation-related injuries in the U.S. population than estimated by the earlier NHAMCS. During the period of July 2000 to June 2001, the rate of sports- and recreation-related injuries treated in U.S. hospital emergency rooms was estimated to be 4.3 million cases (1.54% of the population), accounting for 16% of all **unintentional injury**-related visits (Gotsch, Annest, and Holmgreen 2002).

Head injury during competitive sport participation has reached epidemic status of an estimated 300,000 cases annually in the United States (CDC 1997). Among competitive sports, American football has the highest rate of head injuries in the United States; an estimated 4% to 20% of all participants suffer a mild traumatic brain injury (a concussion) each season (Bailes and Cantu 2001). Additionally, there are approximately four deaths per year that can be attributed to participation in organized football. The annual rates (%) of concussion in other sports include: hockey (7%), rugby (6%), basketball (2%), and baseball (1%) (Bailes and Cantu 2001). According to the National Center for Catastrophic Sports Injury Research (NCCSIR), between 1982 and 1996 high school fall sports resulted

Eleven Riskiest Activities in the United States

The percentage of all unintentional injury-related visits that were sports- and recreation-related was highest for people aged 10 to 14 years (51.5% for boys, 38.0% for girls), and lowest for persons aged >45 years (6.4% for men, 3.1% for women). Types of sports- and recreation-related activities where the injuries occurred varied by age and sex. Among people aged up to 9 years, the leading types were playground- and bicycle-related injuries. Scooter- and trampoline-related injuries ranked among the top seven types of injuries for both boys and girls aged up to 9 years. For males aged 10 to 19 years, football-, basketball-, and bicycle-related injuries were most common. For females aged 10 to 19 years, basketball-related injuries ranked highest. Among people aged 20 to 24 years, basketball- and bicycle-related injuries ranked among the three leading types of injuries. Basketball-related injuries ranked highest for men aged 25 to 44 years. Exercise (e.g., weightlifting, aerobics, stretching, walking, jogging, and running) was the leading injury-related activity for women aged >20 years and ranked among the top four types of injuries for men aged >20 years.

Data from Gotsch, Annest, and Holmgreen 2002.

Males (2,978,423 total cases)	Females (1,272,299 total cases)
Basketball 520,032 (17.5%)	Bicycling 163,012 (12.8%)
Bicycling 434,371 (14.6%)	Basketball 114,644 (9%)
Football 374,072 (12.6%)	Playground 108,023 (8.5%)
Exercise 140,661 (4.7%)	Exercise 98,475 (7.7%)
Baseball 136,632 (4.6%)	Gymnastics 73,405 (5.8%)
Playground 127,028 (4.3%)	Soccer 60,987 (4.8%)
Soccer 104,775 (3.5%)	Softball 56,759 (4.5%)
Skateboarding 84,457 (2.8%)	Horseback riding 45,336 (3.6%)

The number (percentage of total) of injury cases from the eight riskiest activities for males and females who received emergency room treatment in the United States from July 2000 to June 2001.

---

in 387 direct deaths (caused by performing the sport) and catastrophic injuries, with 374 (97%) related to football. Indirect deaths (secondary to overexertion while playing a sport) totaled 115, of which 89 (77%) were related to football. Though football had the highest death rates, the incidence rate was less than 1 player per 100,000 participants. High school winter sports during the same period resulted in 70 direct deaths and catastrophic injuries. Direct death rates were highest in wrestling (33 deaths) and basketball (7 deaths) but were less than 1 per 100,000 participants.

••• *In the United States nearly 1.5 million adults over 20 years of age and 3 million children and youth visit an emergency room each year as a result of an injury from sports or other leisure-time physical activities.*

Most Frequent Types and Sites of Injury in the United States

Type of injury	Site of injury
Strain/sprain (29.1%)	Ankle (12.1%)
Fracture (20.5%)	Finger (9.5%)
Contusion/abrasion (20.1%)	Face (9.2%)
Laceration (13.8%)	Head (8.2%)
	Knee (8.1%)

The most frequent types and body parts of injuries diagnosed during emergency room treatment in the United States from July 2000 to June 2001 (% of total cases)

Data from Gotsch, Annest, and Holmgreen 2002.

Another recent study described the types and frequencies of musculoskeletal injuries among a cohort of 5,028 men and 1,285 women 20 to 85 years of age who were participants in the Aerobics

Center Longitudinal Study and had above average levels of physical activity (Hootman, Macera, Ainsworth, Addy et al. 2002). The participants reported detailed information about their physical activity levels and injuries between 1970 and 1982, when their initial clinical examinations occurred, and 1986 when they responded to a mailed survey about their physical activity habits and history of orthopedic injuries. An injury was defined as any self-reported soft tissue or bone injury that occurred during the 12 months preceding the survey. Injuries that participants said occurred as a result of their participation in a formal exercise program were classified as activity-related injuries. Twenty-five percent of the cohort reported that they had experienced musculoskeletal injury during the past year, and 83% of those injuries were activity-related, mainly coming from sports participation. More than two thirds of the activity-related injuries occurred in the lower extremities, especially the knee. Men and women had similar rates of injuries, which are depicted in figure 15.1.

The population-based, observational studies discussed so far used cross-sectional or retrospective designs. Other studies have examined incidence rates over time in a population cohort. For example, Koplan, Rothenberg, and Jones (1995) conducted a 10-year follow-up of a cohort of participants in Atlanta's Peachtree Road Race, the world's largest 10-km race, with over 50,000 runners and walkers each year. During the year following the 1980 race, 37% of about 1,400 runners reported that they had suffered an injury that required a reduction in their running distance for at least a week; 14% needed medical treatment (Koplan et al. 1982). About 500 of 1,400 runners surveyed initially were surveyed 10 years later by mail regarding physical characteristics, smoking status, education, running and other exercise, BMI, injuries, and treatment. Injury was defined as a musculoskeletal ailment that caused respondents to limit or eliminate exercise or that disrupted school or work attendance. Results indicated that 56% of the respondents were still running and 81% continued to exercise in some form. Among men, 31% who no longer ran reported injury as the main reason for stopping. More than 50% of those surveyed reported at least one injury, most of which (32% for men, 28% for women) were to the knee. An inverted-U relationship existed between injuries and weekly distance (in which those who ran median distances had the most injuries). Overall, injury incidence was 1.02 per 10 person-years for all injuries, and 0.58 for those requiring medical attention.

Evaluating Risk

Consistent with the concept of the epidemiologic triangle of host, agent, and environment introduced in chapter 2, before determining whether physical activity represents an independent haz-

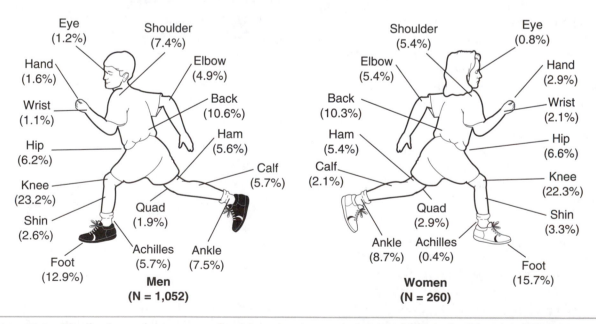

Figure 15.1 Distribution and percentage of activity-related musculoskeletal injuries by body part and gender.

Adapted, by permission, from J.M. Hootman et al., 2002, "Epidemiology of musculoskeletal injuries among sedentary and physically active adults," *Medicine and Science in Sports and Exercise* 34(5): 838–844.

ard, it is necessary to consider people's prior risk of injury or death, the type of physical activity, and the environment where activity takes place. Factors that might affect the risk of injury during swimming, for example, are age, sex, or whether the ear is predisposed to infection and such attributes of the activity itself as type of stroke, frequency, speed, distance, and warm-up. For example, someone who swims freestyle often and has a flawed stroke might have increased risk for shoulder problems. A person with a vulnerable ear canal who swims in a warm lake might be at risk for an inner-ear infection. The risk of injury during swimming depends not just on time of exposure but also features of the swimmer and where and how the swimming occurs. About one fourth of nonfatal heart attacks occur during some form of physical activity. However, the risk of serious cardiovascular complications during exercise is higher in people who have had a prior heart attack than in apparently healthy people. Contributing factors include uncontrolled hypertension, a recent heavy meal, emotional excitement, and prolonged activity without adequate preparation.

Given that exposure is a fundamental risk factor for disease and accidents, it is logical that the most prevalent physical activities should be associated with the highest rates of injury and sudden death. The National Health Interview Survey published in 1991 estimated that, based on percentage of participation, the most popular activities reported by adults 18 years of age or older in the United States were walking (44%), gardening or yard work (29%), stretching exercises (26%), riding a bicycle or stationary exercise cycle (15%), resistance exercise (e.g., weightlifting; 14%), stair climbing (11%), jogging or running (9%), aerobics and aerobic dance (7%), and swimming (6%) (National Center for Health Statistics 1991). Of those activities, evidence about rates and risk factors of injury or death is available only for jogging or running and aerobic dance.

Host Factors

Age

The NEISS-AIP study of U.S. emergency room visits found that unintentional injury-related visits that were sports- and recreation-related were highest for people aged 10 to 14 years (51.5% for boys, 38.0% for girls), and lowest for persons aged >45 years (Gotsch, Annest, and Holmgreen 2002). However, those rates were not adjusted for time of exposure during participation in risky

sports among younger people. Hence, injury rates were likely confounded by sport participation rates. In an early review of running injury studies, van Mechelen (1992) concluded that age was not independently associated with injury. That conclusion was supported by Koplan, Rothenberg, and Jones (1995), who found only a minor increase in the rate of injury among male runners over the age of 50. No other age-related differences were found. Population-based studies that examined multiple sports found that sport participants ages 20 to 24 (Kujala et al. 1995; Sandelin et al. 1988; Sandelin and Santavirta 1991) or 16 to 25 (Nicholl, Coleman, and Williams 1995) had a higher incidence of injury than other age groups. However, it may be that people of this age group are more likely to be involved in sports in which injury incidence is high.

> ••• *Injury during vigorous physical activity appears to be independent of age from youth through middle age; it is an equal-opportunity hazard. However, aging becomes a key risk factor among the elderly.*

Some studies have looked at injury incidence in particular age groups, namely, school-aged youths and the elderly. Many children's primary exposure to physical activity is in organized sport and physical education classes.

Sex

Data from the National Collegiate Athletic Association Injury Surveillance System were used to compare the five-year rate (1989–1993) of knee injuries among 300,000 male and female collegiate athletes participating in soccer and basketball (Arendt and Dick 1995). The incidence of knee injuries among soccer players was higher in females (1.6 cases per 1,000 athletes) than males (1.3 cases per 1,000 athletes) or as a percentage of all injuries, when compared with male soccer players over the five-year (1989–1993) time period. The rate of injury (expressed as a percentage of athletes) to the anterior cruciate ligament (ACL) of the knee in women's soccer (0.31%) was double the rate in men's soccer (0.13%), or one ACL injury per 385 activity sessions in men compared to one ACL injury per 161 activity sessions in women. Likewise, in basketball the ACL injury rate of 0.29% (one injury per 247 activity sessions) in women was four times higher than the rate of 0.07% (one injury per 952 activity sessions) in men. Rates of other types of knee injuries did not differ between men and women.

With the exception of higher rates of tears of the anterior cruciate ligament (ACL) in the knee among females (Kirkendall and Garrett 2000), other information on sex differences in exercise-related injury rates is inconclusive. Some studies that investigated sex differences showed that males are at higher risk for injury (Garrick, Gillien, and Whiteside 1986; Nicholl, Coleman, and Williams 1995; Sandelin et al. 1988), others reported higher injury incidence in females (Koplan, Rothenberg, and Jones 1995), and still others showed no differences between the sexes (Backx et al. 1991; de Loes, Jacobsen, and Goldie 1990; Kujala et al. 1995; Zebas et al. 1995). For runners, there appear to be no sex differences in injury risk, though few studies included enough women to allow accurate comparisons (van Mechelen 1992). More injury risk studies are needed that have equivalent participation rates by men and women.

> ••• *Other than higher rates of tears of the anterior cruciate ligament (ACL) at the knee among females, information available on sex differences in injury rates during vigorous physical activity is sparse or inconclusive.*

A recent prospective, cohort analysis of data from the Aerobics Center Longitudinal Study examined whether sex-specific predictors of lower extremity injury could be identified among 5,028 men and 1,285 women who participated in running, walking, or jogging for exercise (Hootman, Macera, Ainsworth, Martin et al. 2002). Possible predictor variables included height, weight, and cardiorespiratory fitness measured at an initial physical examination conducted between 1970 and 1981. Other predictors, along with self-reports of lower extremity (i.e., legs and feet) musculoskeletal injuries and physical activity levels, were obtained from a follow-up mail survey whereby participants were asked to recall over two preceding time periods, 5 years and 12 months. An injury was defined as any lower extremity injury that required a consultation with a physician. Among men, previous lower extremity injury was the strongest predictor of lower extremity injury (RR = 1.93–2.09), regardless of recall period. Among women, mileage ex-

ceeding 20 miles/wk was the strongest predictor for the 5-year period (RR = 2.08), and previous lower extremity injury was the strongest predictor for the 12-month period (RR = 2.81). Injury rates during standard U.S. Army combat training were compared between 756 men and 474 women (Knapik et al. 2001). A subsample of 182 men and 168 women completed fitness tests and questionnaires about physical activity and smoking before combat training began. All subjects were administered the Army Physical Fitness test consisting of push-ups, sit-ups, and a 3.2-km run. Injuries were registered from medical records. Women had over twice the injury rate of men. For men and women, fewer push-ups, slower 3.2-km run times, lower peak VO_2, and cigarette smoking were risk factors for time-loss injury. Among the men only, lower levels of physical activity before combat training commenced and both high and low levels of flexibility were also time-loss injury risk factors. Lower peak VO_2 and cigarette smoking were independent risk factors for time-loss injury for both men and women.

However, the sex difference in injury rates among soldiers does not appear to be independent of differences in fitness among men and women (Bell et al. 2000). Among 861 trainees observed during their 8-week basic training course, women experienced twice as many injuries as men and had 2.5 times higher risk of time-loss injuries than men. However, when the lower fitness and higher fatness of women at the beginning of training were adjusted for, sex was no longer an independent predictor of injury risk.

Though the explanation is not yet known, males appear to be at higher risk of nontraumatic sport-related death among competitive athletes. In an analysis of data from the National Center for Catastrophic Sports Injury Research (NCCSIR) over a 10-year period from July 1983 to June 1993, there were nontraumatic sports deaths reported in 126 high school athletes (115 males and 11 females) and 34 college athletes (31 males and 3 females) (Van Camp et al. 1995). Estimated annual death rates in male athletes (7.5 per million athletes) were five times higher than in female athletes (1.33 per million athletes). Cardiovascular conditions (especially hypertrophic cardiomyopathy and congenital coronary artery anomalies) were the most common causes of death.

Physical Activity Experience

Van Mechelen (1992) reported that men with less running experience may be more likely to suffer an acute injury when running, but results have been inconclusive. Macera et al. (1989) found that runners with less than three years' running experience had an injury odds ratio of 2.2 compared with runners with more than three years' experience. Among students 14 to 19 years of age, those who were more physically active outside of school (2 or more hours per week) were less likely to be injured than their sedentary peers (de Loes, Jacobsen, and Goldie 1990). Risk factors of exercise injuries during 12 weeks of army infantry training were evaluated among 303 young men (Jones et al. 1993). Physical training was documented on a daily basis, and injuries were registered by medical records. One or more lower extremity injuries (mainly muscle strains, ankle and knee sprains, and overuse syndrome of the knee) accounted for 80% of the injuries. Risk factors were: older age, smoking, previous injury (sprained ankles), low levels of previous occupational and physical activity, low frequency of running before entry into the army, flexibility (both high and low), low physical fitness at entry, and high running mileage during training.

••• *Though exposure is a risk factor for hazards during physical activity, previous experience in physical activity or sports seems to reduce the risk of injury.*

Injury History

Several epidemiological studies have found a greater risk for injury during physical activity among people who previously suffered an exercise-related injury, especially among runners (Jacobs and Berson 1986; Koplan et al. 1982; Macera et al. 1989; Marti et al. 1988; Walter et al. 1989). Van Mechelen (1992) concluded that previous running injuries were an independent risk factor for future running injuries, and Marti et al. (1988) found a 65% increase in risk of injury for previously injured runners. In studies of marathon running, those who needed treatment during and immediately after the marathon were more likely to have had an injury before the race (Kretsch et al. 1984). In earlier studies this effect was not adjusted for other running characteristics such as running distance, and it was not clear whether a previous injury represented additional risk for future injuries after adjusting for distance. However, several studies found a previous injury to be a significant predictor of injury during follow-up, even after controlling for distance (Macera et

al. 1989; Marti et al. 1988; Walter et al. 1989). It is not clear whether this finding suggests incomplete healing of the original injury, a susceptibility for injury recurrence, or an uncorrected flaw in running gait.

Garrick, Gillien, and Whiteside (1986) reported that participants in group aerobics who had previously experienced a knee, leg, or ankle injury were twice as likely to have a subsequent, similar injury as their peers without a history of orthopedic injury during physical activity. Among men and women participants in the Aerobics Center Longitudinal Study, previous lower extremity injury was one of the strongest predictors of lower extremity injury during the past year (Hootman, Macera, Ainsworth, Martin et al. 2002).

••• *A history of previous injury is a risk factor for future injury.*

Body Mass

The effects of high or low weight or percent body fat on injury rates have been examined in several ways. Pollock et al. (1977) found that among those beginning a running program, those with a high percentage of body fat had more injuries. However, in this study, as is the case in all studies of regular runners, there were very few obese individuals. Some studies found no convincing evidence that body composition moderated injury rates (Koplan et al. 1982; Macera et al. 1989), whereas other studies reported a U-shaped relationship whereby both the lightest and heaviest groups were at increased risk for injuries compared to groups having average weight (Marti et al. 1988). However, population studies of the effects of body mass or fatness have not yet adequately controlled for the confounding of body mass and running experience and the sampling bias that most long-term runners have low body mass.

Preexercise Stretching

Although stretching is often recommended as a safety measure for preventing injuries (James, Bates, and Osternig 1978), there is a paucity of evidence from population-based studies about its protective effects. Several studies of runners found no difference in injury rates between participants who stretch before running and those who don't stretch (Koplan et al. 1982; Macera et al. 1989), especially after controlling for weekly running distance and previous injury (Walter et al. 1989).

Features of the Agent: Physical Activity

Paradoxically, the same features of physical activity that are believed to reduce health risks for mortality and chronic diseases (namely the frequency, duration, intensity, and type of physical activity) also may increase the risk of injury. To date, however, the feature of physical activity most consistently reported as an injury risk factor is total exposure to physical activity (Jones, Cowan, and Knapik 1994).

Total Exposure

Studies in different populations with different definitions of injury have consistently reported an increase in injuries with an increase in distance run, with risk increasing after about 33 km (20 miles) per week. This factor remained a strong predictor of injury even after adjusting for other running-related practices. Lysholm and Wiklander (1987) also found a positive association between the injury rate during any given month and the training distance covered during the previous month among marathon runners.

Cumulative distance is more associated with injury than is the lack of rest between runs (James, Bates, and Osternig 1978). For example, Marti (1988) found no differences in injury rates among runners who ran similar overall weekly distances but ran the distance in two, three, or four training sessions per week.

> ••• *Weekly mileage is the main risk factor for running injuries, more so than running surface, time of day, or warm-up stretching.*

Epidemiologic investigations consistently find that total exposure to physical activity is more strongly associated with increased injury incidence than specific features of the intensity, frequency, or duration of physical activity (Backx et al. 1991; Jones, Cowan, and Knapik 1994; Koplan, Rothenberg, and Jones 1995; Marti et al. 1988; van Mechelen 1992). However, total exposure is easier to estimate than its specific features, so more studies have used total exposure, rather than its features, as the dose measure. Hence, the evidence about the dose–response relationships between physical activity and injury risk may be biased by the methods used to define physical activity exposure.

Frequency

The number of exercise sessions per week has been weakly related to physical activity injury incidence; but its influence has been poorly defined in population-based studies. Marti et al. (1988) found that injury rates during running were similar for weekly frequencies of two, three, or four sessions, after adjusting for total running distance. Conversely, Garrick, Gillien, and Whiteside (1986) reported that aerobics participants who attended only one class per week had twice the injury incidence of those attending four classes per week, when injury rates were expressed relative to time of total exposure. In a randomized controlled trial, Pollock et al. (1977) found that when distance, duration, and relative intensity were controlled, running injuries occurred twice as often among those who ran five days per week compared with those running one or three days per week.

Duration

The epidemiologic data on exercise duration and musculoskeletal injury are sparse. In the articles examined for this chapter, no data regarding duration of exercise sessions were given. Total exposure (e.g., person-hours or person-years of participation) was provided and, in studies of walking or running, a relative index of miles per week was commonly used (Backx et al. 1991; Koplan, Rothenberg, and Jones 1995; Kujala et al. 1995). Pollock et al. (1977) examined the influence of exercise duration on injury incidence while running frequency was held constant at three days per week. Participants who ran for a longer duration (45 min vs. 15 or 30 min) had a greater injury incidence rate.

Intensity

The only sport for which data on exercise intensity (in this case, speed) have been consistently recorded is running. For example, Marti et al. (1988) reported that a runner's best time on a 16-km (10-mile) run was associated with increased risk for running injury. However, running pace was not an important risk factor after adjusting for total distance. The paucity of data on the intensity of other types of physical activity prevents clear conclusions about the influence of the intensity of physical activity on injury risk (van Mechelen 1992).

Type of Physical Activity

Regardless of method used to define and measure types of physical activity, it is clear that injury rates differ according to types of physical activity (Backx et al. 1991; de Loes, Jacobsen, and Goldie 1990; Kujala et al. 1995; Nicholl, Coleman, and Williams 1995; Sandelin and Santavirta 1991). Individual and team sports that have high occurrences of physical contact between participants (e.g., soccer, rugby, basketball, ice hockey, karate, judo) have higher injury rates than physical activities that involve less contact. Furthermore, more injuries occur during competition than during practice (Kujala et al. 1995). Organized sports were responsible for a greater percentage (62%) of the total injuries incurred than physical education and nonorganized sports (Backx et al. 1991). Unfortunately, several popular types of physical activity such as golf, swimming, walking, cycling, and calisthenics remain understudied (Koplan, Siscovick, and Goldbaum 1985). Population studies that compared injury rates among many types of physical activity (e.g., Burt and Overpeck 2001; Gotsch, Annest, and Holmgreen 2002) did not control for time of exposure and features of the participants, activities, and environments sufficiently to permit direct comparisons of independent risks among activities.

Environmental Factors

Even when host factors and features of physical activity are controlled, aspects of the environment where physical activity occurs can affect the risk of injury. Little is yet known about the influence of the myriad potential environmental influences on injury (e.g., street and bike lane design in urban areas).

Exercise Surface

Although clinical studies suggest that a hard running surface or running in the morning is associated with an increased risk of injuries (James, Bates, and Osternig 1978), population studies have not found such differences, especially after controlling for weekly running distance (Macera et al. 1989; Marti et al. 1988; Walter et al. 1989).

In a review of running injury studies, van Mechelen (1992) found no differences, at least for men, in injury incidence among running surfaces. Sixty-five percent of injuries sustained by adolescents during skateboarding occur on public roads, footpaths, and parking lots (Fountain and Meyers 1996). Studies have found conflicting results about the influence of type of floor surface injury risk during aerobic dance (Garrick, Gillien, and Whiteside 1986; Richie, Kelso, and Bellucci 1985).

Temperature

The influence of environmental temperature on injury risk was indirectly tested by examining seasonal differences in injury incidence during U.S. Army basic combat training, which is similar at all times of the year (Knapik et al. 2002). Injury data were retrieved retrospectively from medical records of 1,543 men and 1,025 women who trained for 8 weeks in two separate groups in the summer and two groups in the fall. Among men, the relative risk of a time-loss injury (one that required time away from activity) was 2.5 times higher in the summer than in the fall. Among women, the relative risk of suffering a time-loss injury was 1.7 times higher in the summer than the fall. The injury rates were unchanged after adjustment for age, BMI, and physical fitness (push-ups, sit-ups, and 2-mile run). Daily temperature was strongly correlated with injury rates ($r = 0.92$ to 0.97), suggesting that environmental temperature is a strong, independent risk factor of injury during strenuous exercise training.

Urban Environment Features

A recent descriptive epidemiological study of pedestrian injuries among children and adolescents examined environmental and pedestrian factors associated with all motor vehicle crashes occurring in New York City between 1991 and 1997 (DiMaggio and Durkin 2002). Among 693,283 crashes, 97,245 resulted in injuries to 32,578 youth under the age of 20. The rate of pedestrian injuries was 246 per 100,000 people in the population per year, and the fatality rate was 6 per 1,000. Younger children (6–14 years) were more likely to be struck mid-block, during daylight hours, and during the summer. Adolescents were more likely to be struck at intersections and at night. Road and weather conditions did not influence injury risk.

Methods of Research

Knowledge about the incidence rates and causes of injury during exercise is limited by the methods used by researchers. A mail survey or personal interview has the potential to provide more detailed and accurate information about injuries that do not require medical attention and about the circumstances in which injuries occur than retrospective examination of hospital or doctor records. However, medical records provide more objective information about injury diagnosis, severity, and treatment than self-reports by participants about their injuries.

A popular method of epidemiologic investigation of injuries has been a mail survey of a selected population (Koplan, Siscovick, and Goldbaum 1985; Nicholl, Coleman, and Williams 1991, 1995;

Sandelin et al. 1988). Rates of injuries or illnesses related to physical activity in the United Kingdom were estimated from 17,654 people who responded to a survey mailed to a sample of 28,857 adult inhabitants of England and Wales between the ages of 16 and 45 years during 1989 and 1990 (Nicholl, Coleman, and Williams 1995). The survey asked questions about sport participation, injuries, and general background and habits (e.g., age, weight, smoking, education) during the preceding month. Participation was defined as involvement in "sports or other recreational activities involving physical exercise." Injury was defined as any "injury or illness, however minor, through taking part in any of the activities [you] listed." Injuries were further classified as "trivial" or "substantive," which were defined as those that restricted the participant from taking part in usual activities, including work, for a minimum of one day and those for which treatment had been sought. Information was also obtained on whether the injury was new or recurring. Respondents reported 1,803 new or recurring injuries. Soccer accounted for more than 25% of all injuries but the risk of a substantive injury in rugby (96.7 injuries per 1,000 occasions of participation and an attributable risk of 29%) for all new injuries was three times higher than in soccer. Over a third of injuries occurred in men aged 16 to 25 years. The most frequently reported injuries were sprains and strains of the lower limbs. Treatment was sought in approximately 25% of the injury cases, and 7% of all new injuries were followed by a visit to a hospital emergency room. After soccer, three fitness activities—running, weight training, and "keeping fit" (i.e., swimming, aerobics, or using an exercise bike)—accounted for most of the injuries. Running accounted for 15.3 injuries per 1,000 occasions of participation.

The interview is another frequently used method of inquiry about injuries (Garrick, Gillien, and Whiteside 1986; Sandelin et al. 1988). In 1980, the Central Statistical Office of Finland interviewed 10,405 persons in the Greater Helsinki area (a total population of about 600,000) between the ages of 15 and 75 years about injury occurrence during sports, regardless of severity or treatment, during the preceding year (Sandelin et al. 1988). Injuries were classified into three categories: minor, absence from sport for less than one week; moderate, absence for one to three weeks; and severe, absence for more than three weeks. Results indicated that 75% of those interviewed

participated in physical activity for health reasons, and of those participants, 40% said they practiced sports involving large muscle groups and leading to sweating and breathlessness, requiring approximately 50% of cardiorespiratory capacity. The most popular forms of exercise were walking, cycling, and jogging. About 40,000 sports-related injuries were reported, an annual incidence rate of about 670 per 10,000 people. About 70% of the injuries were classified as minor sprains. However, 9% (an estimated 4,000 cases) were severe enough to require a visit to a hospital emergency room.

Another method used to assess injury incidence is to retrospectively examine archives of hospital or insurance company records (de Loes, Jacobsen, and Goldie 1990; Kujala et al. 1995; Scheiber and Branche-Dorsey 1995; Zebas et al. 1995). For example, national sports injury insurance registry data in Finland during the period of 1987 to 1991 were retrieved to determine incident rates for 62,169 person-years of exposure among participants in soccer, ice hockey, volleyball, basketball, judo, or karate, sports that required insurance enrollment prior to participation. Acute sports injuries that required medical treatment and were reported to the insurance company were analyzed. The age and sex of the person injured and the type of injury, anatomical location, and injury circumstances were described. A total of 54,186 sports injuries were recorded. Injury rates were low in athletes aged under 15, while 20- to 24-year-olds had the highest rates. Results indicated that, despite more time being spent in training than in competition, 46% to 59% of injuries occurred during competition. Also, injury rates were highest in sports that involved body contact. For example, ice hockey had the highest injury incidence. Most injuries occurred to the lower limbs and mainly involved sprains, strains, and contusions.

The Injury Definition Problem

A problem common to the various methods used to measure injury incidence is the general absence of standardization of the definitions of injury (de Loes 1997) and the measures of physical activity or exercise. Definition of injury by a visit to a health care professional is likely not equivalent to injury defined as disruption in regular physical activity. Likewise, the challenge of measuring physical activity in population-based studies described in chapter 2 has impeded standardization of features of physical activity that may alter injury risks. Thus, decisions made about definitions differ among investigators and undoubtedly influence conclusions about rates of injury and their risk factors.

> ••• *Standardized definitions of injury and physical activity are needed to accurately compare estimates of risk among groups of people and types of physical activity.*

The method of reporting injury incidence varies among studies. Incidence rates have been reported as absolute numbers and as rates expressed per person and per time of exposure. As was the case for evaluating the protective effects of physical activity against chronic diseases, the most informative expression of injury rates is injury incidence per time of exposure because using the common denominator of exposure permits a direct comparison of injury rates between different types of physical activity and different participants. It is also important, however, to also include properly matched, nonactive controls in order to determine whether injury risk factors are independent influences on injury rates (Koplan, Siscovick, and Goldbaum 1985). These issues are illustrated in the following section about the denominator problem in studies of physical activity injury risks.

> ••• *The most accurate method of expressing injury rates is injury incidence per time of exposure. This allows direct comparisons among different types of physical activity and different people.*

The Denominator Problem

Clinical studies have reported high numbers of patients seeking treatment of injuries associated with exercise. However, clinical studies cannot provide information on the prevalence or incidence of exercise-related injuries in a population. Hence, clinical studies suffer from a "nondenominator" problem (Castelli and Adams 1990; de Loes 1997; Garrick, Gillien, and Whiteside 1986). Conclusions cannot be reached about the public health impact of a series of cases seen by physicians without knowing the size of the population from which the clinical cases were drawn. Without such a denominator, the rate of occurrence cannot be computed. Also, it is critical that the appropriate denominator be chosen for comparison. Otherwise, a distorted picture of risk can result. For example, an estimated 300,000 cases of traumatic brain injuries occur during sport participation each year in the United States (Sosin, Sniezek, and Thurman 1996). Though about a third of all deaths from injury each year in the United States are attributable to traumatic brain injuries (Sosin, Sniezek, and Waxweiler 1995), most brain injuries during vigorous physical activity are mild to moderate concussions. Mild concussions are seldom fatal, though when repeated over months or years, they can lead to neurological and cognitive **impairment.** Thus, relating sport brain injuries to fatal brain injuries would misleadingly inflate the negative health impact of traumatic brain injury during sport participation.

> ••• *About a third of all deaths from injury each year in the United States are attributable to traumatic brain injuries, but most brain injuries during vigorous physical activity are mild-to-moderate concussions, which are seldom fatal. Thus, equating sport brain injuries to fatal brain injuries would yield an overly alarming incidence rate of the negative health impact of traumatic brain injury during sport participation.*

The incidence of death during physical activity has been estimated in various population subgroups, including Finnish cross-country skiers; British, American, Finnish, and Israeli military personnel; participants in fitness facilities; and the general young and adult population bases in several countries. Unfortunately, studies have used such varying definitions of injury and such different methods to determine rates that it is difficult to compare their results and reach general conclusions. For example, the definition of a physical activity–related injury varied, and some studies included cases that occurred up to 24 h after participation. The choice of the denominator for computing **death rates** also differed widely among studies.

Coronary heart disease is the main contributing **cause of death** attributable to physical activity, but incidence figures have varied widely, depending on the prevalence of coronary heart disease in the population being studied. For example, the comparatively low rates of sudden death during physical activity among military personnel might be explained by their young ages, their low prevalence of coronary heart disease, and the fact that screening exams exclude from military service or training people who are at cardiac risk because they have potentially fatal malformations of the heart such as aortic stenosis, hypertrophic cardiomyopathy, or Marfan's syndrome. Even among military personnel, however, the incidence of exercise deaths varies among the groups that are studied. During six weeks of basic training among air force recruits, for example, 17 of 19 sudden cardiac deaths occurred during physical activity (M. Phillips et al. 1986). Autopsy revealed myocarditis in four of the deaths. That rate of myocarditis (20%) was higher than reported in other studies of military personnel. It might have resulted from viral infections spread by barracks living or recent vaccinations, which are common in recruits but not in older military personnel.

When comparing injury rates among sports, it is necessary to have accurate descriptions of exposure and injuries, including total injury numbers, injury diagnoses, time of injury occurrence, and follow-up treatment. An early review of sport injury studies found that just 11 of 88 studies had used a measure of incidence (Kennedy, Vanderfield, and Kennedy 1977). A few studies of communities have provided better estimates of the incidence or prevalence of activity-related injury. For example, about 670 sport injuries per 10,000 people, 14% of all injuries, were reported in Helsinki, Finland, in 1980 (Sandelin et al. 1988). In a rural city of about 31,000 residents in Sweden, the sport injury rate observed during a year was 150 per 10,000 people, 17% of all injuries, and accounted for 3% of all visits to hospital emergency rooms (de Loes 1990; de Loes and Goldie 1988).

In Rochester, Minnesota, an overall incidence rate of 187 ankle fractures was reported per 100,000 person-years of exposure (Daly et al. 1987); 36% of the fractures occurred during sport participation. About 38% of knee surgeries to repair a torn meniscus were attributed to sport injury in another study (Hede et al. 1990).

Consensus Guidelines for the Measurement of Injury Incidence

1. Provide carefully developed and precisely presented definitions of *injury*.
2. Include denominator data so that injury cases can be related to an at-risk population.
3. Make every effort to minimize selection bias.
4. Monitor injury experience, activity behavior, and other potential behavioral risk factors concurrently.
5. Employ prospective research designs.

Myocardial Infarction and Sudden Death

The cardiovascular complications of vigorous physical activity include cerebrovascular accidents, symptomatic cardiac arrhythmias, aortic dissection, myocardial infarction, and sudden cardiac death (Thompson 1996). The main causes of exercise-related cardiovascular complications are congenital abnormalities in young subjects and atherosclerotic coronary disease in adults. The incidence of exercise deaths is low; about 7.5 and 1.3 per million young male and female athletes and 60 per million middle-aged men die during exertion per year (Thompson 1996). Thus, though the risk of cardiac events is transiently increased during exercise, the absolute risk is low, especially, as will be shown later in this chapter, when compared to the overall risk of cardiac events among people who are sedentary.

In Helsinki, Finland, 3.7% of sudden cardiac deaths (within 1 h of onset of symptoms), 6.3% of delayed cardiac deaths, and 6.8% of nonfatal cardiac events were associated with physical activity (Romo 1972). Furthermore, an additional 9% of sudden cardiac deaths occurred immediately after snow shoveling, sport, or other exceptional physical activity so that physical activity contributed to approximately 14% of all sudden cardiac deaths. Nonetheless, these figures probably underestimate the percentage of exercise events, because unwitnessed deaths, such as those during sleep, were not included in the numerator.

Another study of patients in cardiac exercise rehabilitation programs estimated that the risks during exercise were 1 in 112,000 h of participation for cardiac arrest, 1 in 294,000 h of participation for heart attack, and 1 in 784,000 h of participation for cardiac death (Van Camp and Peterson 1986).

Dr. William Castelli, former medical director of the Framingham Heart Study, used two early epidemiologic studies of jogging deaths to illustrate how important it is to use the correct denominator when computing the hazards of physical activity (Castelli and Adams 1990). The first study was conducted by cardiologist Paul D. Thompson and colleagues (1982), who reported on 12 men ages 30 to 64 years who died while jogging in Rhode Island during a five-year period from 1975 to 1980. To express the number of jogging deaths as an incidence rate, the investigators surveyed the state using a random telephone sample to determine that, among men aged 30 through 64 years, about 7.4% reported jogging at least twice a week. Using that group as the denominator, the incidence of death during jogging for men of that age group was one death per year for every 7,620 joggers, or about one death per 400,000 person-hours of jogging. Though very low, this mortality rate during jogging was about seven times the estimated death rate during sedentary activities. However, that increased risk was not fully independent of other factors. Resting electrocardiograms were on file for 5 of the 12 runners, and most were abnormal, so the risk of sudden death during jogging was not completely independent of existing heart disease. A more accurate odds ratio would have used the total number of joggers in Rhode Island who had heart disease in the denominator.

A subsequent study conducted in King County, Washington, illustrates this point about the importance of choosing the proper denominator (figure 15.2; Siscovick et al. 1984). The physical activity history prior to and during a fatal heart attack was obtained by interview with the wives of 133 men ages 25 to 75 years. Wives of a group of apparently healthy men were similarly questioned about their husbands' exercise habits, which provided the denominator. Among sedentary men, the odds of dying were increased six times during exercise (from a rate of 5 to a rate of 30 cases per 100 million person-hours of exposure). However, the overall 24-h rate of death from any cause among the regular exercisers (about 7 cases) was half that of the sedentary men (about 15 cases). Thus, even though exercise carried a short-term risk, its long-term benefits still outweighed the risks of being sedentary.

> ••• *Though the odds that men with coronary disease will die suddenly of a heart attack are increased about six times during exercise, the overall 24-h rate of death from any cause among the regular exercisers is half that of sedentary men. So, even though exercise carries a short-term risk, its long-term benefits still outweigh the risks of being sedentary.*

An important question is whether someone who has had an exercise-related coronary event

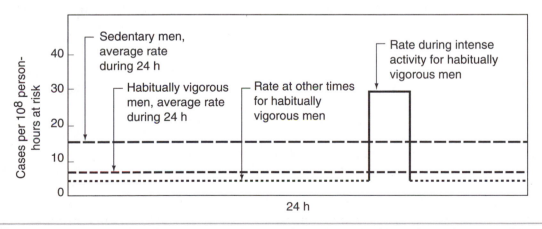

Figure 15.2   A study conducted in King County, Washington, shows the odds of dying from a heart attack in sedentary and physically active men.

Data from D.S. Siscovick et al., 1984.

would have encountered a similar fate in the near future if he or she had not exercised. Vuori, Makarainen, and Jaaskelainen (1978) were among the first to notice that sudden deaths were more frequent during physical activity. Their observation raised the possibility that the increased metabolic demand placed on the heart during exercise is responsible for the increased fatality rate of any coronary events that happen during exertion. Another view is that physical exertion only hastens the inevitable, as illustrated by a study of the February 1978 Rhode Island blizzard (Faich and Rose 1979). On the day of this storm, the death rate from ischemic heart disease nearly doubled compared with the February average for the previous five years. The death rate remained elevated for several days but then decreased below the usual February average so that the overall death rate in February 1978 was similar to that for the preceding five years. This suggests that the physical and emotional stress of the storm only hastened deaths that would have occurred anyway. However, such a conclusion is tenuous because it is based on the same type of logic described in chapter 2 for the problem of the ecological fallacy, whereby causes of death are inferred from trends of co-occurring events.

Most reported sudden deaths during jogging are due to cardiac arrhythmias secondary to underlying coronary artery disease. People at elevated risk include experienced runners, often who undertake considerable weekly running distance, who have one or more major coronary risk factors, who started jogging later in life (probably after the development of significant underlying coronary artery disease), and who often ignore prodromal symptoms (i.e., advance warning signs such as chest pain). Other reported causes of death during exercise include myocarditis, idiopathic hypertrophic cardiomyopathy, congenital anomalies of the heart or blood vessels, rupture of the heart or a major blood vessel, heart failure, and heatstroke.

Haskell (1978) surveyed 30 cardiac rehabilitation programs in North America about cardiovascular problems among a cumulative 14,000 patients and 1.6 million patient-hours of exercise exposure. There was one cardiac arrest, one myocardial infarction, and one death for each 33,000, 233,000, and 116,000 patient-hours of participation, respectively. The rehabilitation programs also reported a 4% annual mortality rate, which was the expected rate for postinfarction patients regardless of whether they exercised.

Because of potential cardiac problems during physical exertion, many experts and groups that promote exercise, including the American College of Sports Medicine, recommend a multistage exercise ECG test as part of the medical screening program prior to beginning a strenuous exercise program for sedentary people 45 (men) to 55 (women) years of age or older and for younger people estimated to be at high coronary risk because of family history, premature coronary heart disease, cigarette smoking, obesity, high blood pressure, or elevated levels of serum cholesterol.

Joint and Muscle Injury

Orthopedic and musculoskeletal injuries are much more common than cardiovascular accidents during exercise, especially during running or jogging, yet little is known about the rates and risk factors for activities such as resistance exercise training and stretching for flexibility.

Running and Jogging

Population-based studies of runners have consistently reported annual rates of musculoskeletal injuries that range from 35% (Koplan et al. 1982) to 65% (Lysholm and Wiklander 1987). This variation in injury rates may be due to the diversity of populations studied and the different definitions of injury applied among the studies. Most injuries occur to the lower extremities, especially the knee, foot, and ankle. The most frequently reported types of musculoskeletal injuries are sprains, strains, stress fractures, and various overuse injuries (e.g., patellar or Achilles tendonitis).

Despite poor standardization of methods used to document injury rates and severity, van Mechelin (1992) concluded that the annual incidence rate of running injuries varied from 37% to 56% for the average recreational runner who trains regularly. Expressed as incidence relative to exposure time, those rates approximated a range of 2.5 to 12.1 injuries per 1,000 hours of running exposure. Most running injuries (70%–80% of the total) involved the lower extremities, and the most common injuries among different subgroups of runners were tendonitis (competitive runners), stress fractures (boys and girls), and strains and tendonitis (general population). The studies found that injuries led to a reduction or temporary curtailment of running in about 30% to 90% of all injuries; about 20% to 70% of all injuries required medical attention, and less than 5% resulted in lost time from work.

Potential Risk Factors for Running Injury

Increased risk	No effect	Weak or mixed evidence
Previous injury	Age	Warming up
Lack of running experience	Gender	Stretching exercises
Running to compete	BMI	Body height
Excessive weekly running distances	Hill running	Malalignment
	Running on hard surfaces	Restricted range of motion
	Participation in other sports	Running frequency
	Time of the year	Intensity of performance
	Time of the day	Stability of running pattern
		Shoes and orthotics
		Running on one side of the road

van Mechelen 1992.

Walking

Walking is the most prevalent form of exercise among adults in North America. The 1994 Injury Control and Risk Survey (ICARIS) of U.S. residential households estimated that 1.4% of adults 18 years or older (about 1,877,000 people) had sustained a walking injury during the preceding month in early summer (Powell et al. 1998). Though walking would seem to have few hazards, injury rates during walking have not been studied much. In a study of injuries associated with physical activity in Helsinki, Finland (Sandelin et al. 1988), walking was the most popular activity, practiced by 75% of the sample surveyed, but it was not listed as having a noteworthy percentage of the observed injuries. Among 698 men and 169 women participants in the Aerobics Center Longitudinal Study who reported a physical activity-related injury requiring physician visits in the previous year, walkers had 25% lower risk of injury than runners among men younger than 45 years and a 33% lower risk among men 45 years or older. Regardless of age, women who walked had about a 25% reduction in risk compared to women who ran, but the reduction wasn't statistically significant because of the small number of women studied. Injury rates were adjusted for age, body mass index, previous injury, and strength training, and they were unrelated to the amount of walking (Colbert, Hootman, and Macera 2000).

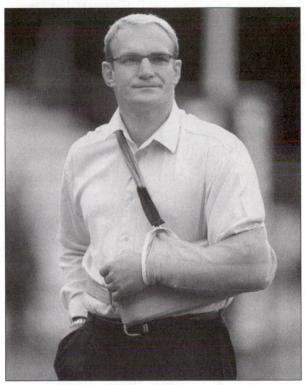

© Empics

Bicycling

The 1994 ICARIS study found that less than 1% of adults aged 18 years or older in the United States (an estimated 330,000 people) reported a bicycling accident during the preceding month of early summer (Powell et al. 1998). Other injury rate estimates have come from clinical studies of cumulative visits to physicians for treatment of injuries from bicycling (though not from stationary cycling). Most of these reports have been of head trauma (Guichon and Myles 1975; Sacks et al. 1991; R.S. Thompson, Rivara, and Thompson 1989). Injury rates ranged from 4.6% (Kiburz et al. 1986) to 13% (Kruse and McBeath 1980), but injuries were minor and required no treatment or only self-treatment. A study of urban cyclists found that increased cycling distance and length of cycling time were associated with increased accidents (Sgaglione, Suljaga-Petchell, and Frankel 1982). The difficulty in comparing injury rates and risk factors among the various studies is that the study population varies by type of cycling (recreation, transportation, and sport), and the equipment and riding environment associated with each type of cycling can vary a great deal.

The most common type of cycling injury requiring hospitalization is head trauma (Guichon and Myles 1975). A case–control study of head trauma among bicyclists demonstrated the effectiveness of safety helmets in reducing the severity of head trauma (Thompson, Rivara, and Thompson 1989). Other studies have similarly concluded that safety helmets are effective in preventing severe injury and even death (Sacks et al. 1991).

Aerobics

Aerobics include a variety of group exercise programs that vary in intensity. The most common feature involves rhythmic movements set to music. The ICARIS study found that less than 1.6% of adults aged 18 years or older in the United States (an estimated 394,000 people) reported an accident associated with aerobics participation during the preceding month (Powell et al. 1998). Cross-sectional and prospective clinical studies of injuries among aerobic dance participants have yielded consistent results. Overall, about 45% of students and 75% of instructors report injuries (Garrick, Gillien, and Whiteside 1986; Richie, Kelso, and Bellucci 1985; Rothenberger, Chang, and Cable 1988). In one study, the annual injury incidence rate was 2.33 injuries per individual (233 per 100 person-years) (Requa, DeAvilla, and Garrick 1993), similar to the rate of 2.1 injuries per person per year among competitive Irish dancers (Watson 1993). In another study, almost half of the women currently in a program reported having had a previous injury; 23% of these injuries required a visit to a physician (Rothenberger, Chang, and Cable 1988). Although the absolute injury rate for aerobic dance seems high, the rate of long-term limitations on activity appears low. Garrick, Gillien, and Whiteside (1986) reported that 80% of the injuries affected the participant only during the aerobics class. The most common site of injury is the shin, consistently accounting for over 20% of the injuries for both instructors and students.

The only risk factor that has been consistently identified among studies on aerobic dance is frequency of dance class participation. Those participating more than four times per week had a higher injury rate than those participating fewer than four times per week. However, the rate of injury per hour of aerobics decreased as the number of hours of participation increased, similar to results for running discussed earlier for the Carolina Runners Study and the Peachtree Road Race follow-up study. Higher injury rates also were found in people who had a history of leg and joint problems and who were inexperienced in other types of fitness activities.

Resistance Exercise Training

Injury associated with resistance exercise, like the preceding activities, has been understudied by epidemiological methods. The ICARIS study estimated that 2.4% of U.S. adults 18 years or older (an estimated 964,000 people) had suffered a weightlifting injury during the past month (Powell et al. 1998). Other clinical studies have recently described the types and impact of such injuries in select subgroups of the population. Among 45 women who participated in a 24-week training program of weightlifting, running, sprint running, backpacking, and lift and carry drills, 22 (49%) had at least one injury, an injury rate of 2.8 cases per 1,000 hours of exposure. Total visits to a physician and days lost from training were 89 and 69, respectively. Most were overuse injuries of the lower back, knees, and feet (Reynolds et al. 2001).

A clinical, case–control study examined the long-term effects of power weightlifting on spinal disk degeneration in 12 pairs of monozygotic (i.e., identical) male twins aged 35 to 69 years who differed according to lifetime histories of participation (on average, 2,300 hours vs. 200 hours of weightlifting). Though twins who differed in endurance exercise participation did not differ in spinal disk degeneration, the men who had more participation in power weightlifting had greater disk degeneration in the thoracic vertebrae T6-T12 but not in the lumbar spine. Adjustment of the injury rate comparisons for previous back injuries, loading of the spine during occupational work, smoking, and time spent driving did not change the results (Videman et al. 1997).

Injury Features

In assessing the impact of injuries on the health of an individual as well as society as a whole, it is important to characterize injuries by type, location, severity, and consequences.

Type and Location

The most common type of activity-related injuries are sprains and strains of the lower limbs, particularly the knee and ankle (Kallinen and Markku 1995; Nicholl, Coleman, and Williams 1995; Zebas et al. 1995). Runners are prone to tendonitis as well (Koplan, Rothenberg, and Jones 1995; van Mechelen 1992). Contact sports have a higher incidence of fractures, contusions, and upper-body injuries (Backx et al. 1991; Sandelin et al. 1988).

Severity and Consequences

The majority of physical activity injuries are classified as minor and require little or no medical treatment. Sandelin et al. (1988) reported that out of 40,380 total sport injuries, 53% required an adhesive bandage and only 25% necessitated medical treatment involving painkillers. Backx et al. (1991) reported that 175 of 399 recorded sport injuries among schoolchildren ages 8 to 17 were not serious enough to report to physicians. Marti et al. (1988) investigated lifestyle disruption resulting from running injuries and found that 44% of 1,994 running injuries resulted in cessation of training for an average of 4.8 weeks, 31% required medical treatment, and 5% led to absence from work. Van Mechelen (1992) concluded that 20% to 70% of all running injuries need medical attention and 30% to 90% result in cessation of training.

Risk of Physical Activity Injuries: The Evidence

To judge the health risks of exercise, it is necessary to use Mill's canons of causality to judge the strength of evidence for a cause-and-effect relationship between exercise and the incidence of musculoskeletal injury. Most studies have not used an appropriate control group to provide base rates of injury among people who are sedentary, so the magnitude of the risk ratios reported in many studies is not an accurate indicator of the strength of association between physical activity and injury rates. Dose dependency has been demonstrated in that greater total exposure (frequency × duration × intensity) is associated with increased risk for injury, but the independent effects of specific features of physical activity on injury risk are as yet unestablished. A few longitudinal and prospective cohort studies have demonstrated a temporal sequence appropriate for a causal relationship between exercise and injury. Consistency has been established in studies examining a large, representative, random sample of people from population bases, although there are relatively few such studies. The moderating effect of age as a risk factor for injury during exercise has been established in several studies, findings for sex are conflicting, and few other factors (e.g., fitness level, sport skill, race, socioeconomic status) have been shown to have moderating effects on injury risk. The independence of features of physical activity and its settings, from other confounders of injury risk, has been incompletely tested in observational studies. Clinical studies have provided some experimental confirmation of biologically plausible mechanisms of injury, but specific features of people, the environment, and physical activity that influence the rates and severity of injuries have been poorly defined and understudied for most types of physical activity injuries in population-based studies.

Other Medical Hazards

Various other hazards have been associated with participation in physical activity for some people (table 15.1). They represent a clinical problem for those who suffer and require medical treatment. The prevalence and incidence rates of these hazards in the general population have not been determined, though, so at this point it is not clear how large or widespread a problem they are.

Psychological Hazards

There is some concern among mental health professionals that the disciplined training and social climate in some sports and leisure-time

TABLE 15.1 MEDICAL HAZARDS OF VIGOROUS PHYSICAL ACTIVITY	
Type	**Hazard**
Cardiovascular	Cardiac arrest in heart patients
	Ruptured aorta
Musculoskeletal	Muscle injury (including delayed onset muscle soreness)
	Tendon strains
	Ligament tears (sprains)
	Exertional rhabdomyolysis (myoglobin in urine)
	Joint inflammation
Pulmonary	Exercise-induced bronchospasm
Gastrointestinal	Irritable bowel
	GI blood loss in runners
Allergic	Exercise-induced anaphylaxis
	Skin welts
Gynecologic	Delayed menarche
	Amenorrhea
	Oligomenorrhea
Endocrinologic	Hypoglycemia in diabetics
Renal	Hematuria (blood in urine)
	Proteinuria (protein in urine)
Hematologic	Anemia (usually false anemia due to plasma volume expansion, but normal red blood cell count)
	GI blood loss in runners
Thermal	Heat cramps
	Heat exhaustion
	Heatstroke
	Frostbite
	Hypothermia

From Gotsch et al., 2002.

fitness activities that emphasize lean body composition and dietary restriction can increase the risk of eating problems or add to existing eating problems among participants. Attention has also been recently drawn to the problem of potential steroid and substance abuse among some weightlifters who have a distorted body image. Despite the recognition over 20 years ago that exercise can, like food or drugs, be abused (Dishman 1985; Morgan 1979), it is still not known whether excessive exercise and disordered eating share a common course that is motivated by common goals and followed by common medical outcomes.

Disordered Eating

Clinical parallels, including elevated anxiety and depression, have been drawn between highly committed runners and patients diagnosed as suffering from anorexia nervosa (i.e., self-starvation). Although some studies of small samples of elite ballet dancers, gymnasts, and wrestlers show higher than expected rates of eating problems, how long they persist and whether they represent goal-appropriate behaviors for the sport rather than medical or psychological pathology have not been established (Dishman 1985). It has been proposed that anorexia athletica (defined as increased risk factors for eating disorders common among some sport groups) is a subclinical syndrome of anorexia nervosa (Sundgot-Borgen 1994). Though 22% of a sample of over 500 elite Norwegian female athletes were judged to be at risk for an eating disorder (Sundgot-Borgen 1994), the prevalence of disordered eating and the independent risk caused by sport and exercise have not yet been established by controlled epidemiologic and clinical studies. In most cases, the eating behaviors of athletes do not appear to signal anorexia nervosa or bulimia (i.e., bingeing and purging; O'Connor and Smith 1999), which have prevalence rates in the United States of about 1% and 4%, respectively.

Results from more than 50 studies on the topic are inconclusive because the studies merely described symptoms among different groups of active or inactive people without fully considering attributes other than activity history that might account for eating problems (Davis 2000). The studies often lacked standard definitions or valid measures of physical activity or disordered eating. For example, many runners cover 50 miles (80 km) or more each week with no problems at all, whereas other people might not tolerate 20 miles (32 km) a week. Though anorexics often augment food restriction by hyperactivity, because of muscle wasting and anemia, their aerobic fitness ($\dot{V}O_2$max) is well below average, in contrast to the above-average aerobic fitness of habitual runners and overtrained athletes. In addition, cross-sectional studies have not revealed a common psychopathology between obligatory (i.e., excessively committed) runners and anorexic patients (table 15.2).

TABLE 15.2 ANOREXIC VS. ATHLETIC FEMALE
Shared features
Dietary faddism
Controlled calorie consumption
Specific carbohydrate avoidance
Low body weight
Resting bradycardia and low blood pressure
Increased physical activity
Amenorrhea or oligomenorrhea
Anemia (may or may not be present)
Distinguishing features
Athlete
Purposeful training
Increased exercise tolerance
Good muscular development
Accurate body image
Body fat level within defined normal range
Anorexic
Aimless physical activity
Poor or decreasing exercise performance
Poor muscular development
Flawed body image (patient believes herself to be overweight)
Body fat level below normal range
Biochemical abnormalities if abusing laxatives and/or diuretics

Reprinted, by permission, from J.A. McSherry, 1984, "The diagnostic challenge of anorexia nervosa," *American Family Physician* 29(2): 144.

Researchers who believe that sport participation increases risk for disordered eating have typically studied small groups of athletes without fully considering the ways that different sports, levels of competition, behaviors of coaches or teammates, eating or activity histories, and socioeconomic backgrounds affect eating problems. Comparisons of the rates of disordered eating or its risk factors among sports or athletes are not meaningful when other influences on eating behaviors, such as age, personal and family history, personality, or socioeconomic status, are not controlled for. Athletes' risk profiles have not been evaluated against those of nonathletes from the same academic, socioeconomic, or psychological backgrounds. These scientific limitations prevent conclusions that differences or similarities in eating behaviors or attitudes between athletes and patients diagnosed with eating disorders result from involvement in sport or exercise rather than from attributes that existed prior to their becoming anorexic, bulimic, athletic, or physically active.

Muscle Dysmorphia

Harvard-affiliated researchers K.A. Phillips, O'Sullivan, and Pope (1997) proposed a form of body dysmorphic disorder that they have termed **muscle dysmorphia,** in which a person develops a pathological preoccupation with his or her muscularity. They presented case studies in which they concluded that muscle dysmorphia was associated with severe subjective distress, impaired social and occupational functioning, and abuse of anabolic steroids and other substances (Gruber and Pope 2000; Pope et al. 1997).

> ### *Diagnostic Criteria for Body Dysmorphic Disorder*
>
> - Preoccupation with an imagined defect in appearance. If a slight physical anomaly is present, the person's concern is excessive.
> - The preoccupation causes clinically significant distress or impairment in social, occupational, or other important areas of functioning.
> - The preoccupation is not better accounted for by another mental disorder (e.g., the dissatisfaction with body shape and size as in anorexia nervosa).
>
> American Psychiatric Association 2000 (468).

The investigators next tested the hypothesis that men in Western societies would desire to have a leaner and more muscular body than they had or perceived that they had (Pope et al. 2000). The height, weight, and body fat of college-aged men in Austria (*n* = 54), France (*n* = 65), and the United States (*n* = 81) were measured. Each man chose pictures that he believed represented (1) his own body, (2) the body he ideally would like to have, (3) the body of an average man of his age, and (4) the male body he believed women would prefer. The men's actual body fatness and muscularity were compared with that of the four images chosen. Despite modest differences between measured fat and the fatness of the images chosen, men from all three countries chose an ideal body that was an average of 28 lb (12.7 kg) more muscular than their own bodies. The men also believed that women prefer a male body about 30 lb (13.6 kg) more muscular than themselves, even though women in fact said they preferred an average looking male body. The investigators speculated that the wide discrepancy between men's ideal body image and actual muscularity might help explain muscle dysmorphia and some anabolic steroid abuse.

In another study, 24 men classified as having muscle dysmorphia reportedly had higher body dissatisfaction, riskier eating attitudes, higher prevalence of anabolic steroid use, and greater lifetime prevalence of mood, anxiety, and eating disorders when compared with 30 normal comparison weightlifters recruited from gymnasiums in Boston (Olivardia, Pope, and Hudson 2000). The men with muscle dysmorphia said they frequently experienced shame, embarrassment, and impaired function at work and in social situations. Several cases of body dysmorphia were also reported among 75 women bodybuilders recruited from Boston area gymnasiums (Gruber and Pope 2000). Though these studies suggest that a clinically meaningful hazard of distorted body image exists, there have not been any population-based studies to determine its prevalence nor any prospective cohort studies or randomized clinical studies to determine whether either muscle dysmorphia or body dysmorphia results from participation in resistance exercise training or whether people who have existing vulnerability to a distorted body image and self-concept are drawn to weightlifting.

Exercise Abuse

There have been case reports of excessive involvement with or dependence on leisure exercise training. William P. Morgan (1979) of the University of Wisconsin first described eight cases of "running addiction," in which commitment to running exceeded prior commitments to work, family, social relations, and medical advice. Similar cases have been labeled *positive addiction, runner's gluttony, fitness fanaticism, athlete's neurosis, obligatory running,* and *exercise abuse.* However, little is understood about the origins, valid diagnosis, or mental health impact of exercise abuse (Davis 2000; Dishman 1985).

Though exercise abuse or addiction is a problem requiring medical treatment for some people, its prevalence is probably not high enough to warrant population interventions. The problem in the United States is too little, not too much, physical activity!

> *••• Though abusive or addictive exercise exists as a problem requiring medical treatment for some people, its prevalance is probably not high enough to warrant population interventions. The problem in the U.S. is too little, not too much, physical activity!*

Summary

Knowledge about the risks of injury during prevalent types of physical activity, such as walking and gardening, is very sparse. The common perception is that walking and gardening involve minimal risks of musculoskeletal injury aside from muscle soreness and joint pain. Whether that is true remains to be determined by proper epidemiologic studies. Likewise, resistance exercise, weightlifting, aerobic dance, and cycling have become increasingly popular in recent years, yet relatively little is known about the risk factors for injury among participants in these activities. Finally, it is also important to consider that risks to mental health or social adjustment can be associated with extreme dedication to exercise or preoccupation with fitness or physique. Conditions such as anorexia athletica, muscle dysmorphia, and exercise abuse are not recognized as psychiatric diagnoses, and no controlled prospective studies have yet been conducted to show that they directly result from participation in leisure-time exercise by healthy people. Nonetheless, their appearance in clinical and scientific literature illustrates that their measurement, prevalence, and health consequences require epidemiologic study.

Bibliography

American Psychiatric Association. 2000. *Diagnostic and statistical manual of mental disorders.* 4th ed. Text revision. Washington, DC: American Psychiatric Association.

Arendt, E., and R. Dick. 1995. Knee injury patterns among men and women in collegiate basketball and soccer. *The American Journal of Sports Medicine* 23: 694–701.

Backx, F.J., H.J. Beijer, E. Bol, and W. Erich. 1991. Injuries in high-risk persons and high-risk sports. A longitudinal study of 1818 school children. *American Journal of Sports Medicine* 19: 124–130.

Backx, F.J., W.B. Erich, A.B. Kemper, and A.L. Verbeek. 1989. Sports injuries in school-aged children. An epidemiologic study. *American Journal of Sports Medicine* 17: 234–240.

Bailes, J.E., and R.C. Cantu. 2001. Head injuries in athletes. *Neurosurgery* 48: 26–46.

Bell, N.S., T.W. Mangione, D. Hemenway, P.J. Amoroso, B.H. Jones. 2000. High injury rates among female army trainees: A function of gender? *American Journal of Preventive Medicine* 18 (3 Suppl.): 141–146.

Blair, S.N., H.W. Kohl, and N.N. Goodyear. 1987. Rates and risks for running and exercise injuries: Studies in three populations. *Research Quarterly in Exercise and Sports* 58 (3): 221–228.

Blumenthal, J.A., S. Rose, and J.L. Chang. 1985. Anorexia nervosa and exercise. *Sports Medicine* 2: 237–247.

Bovens, A.M., G.M.E. Janssen, H.G.W. Vermeer, J.H. Hoeberigs, M.P.E. Janssen, and F.T.J. Verstappen. 1989. Occurrence of running injuries in adults following a supervised training program. *International Journal of Sports Medicine* 10: S186–S190.

Burt, C.W., and M.D. Overpeck. 2001. Emergency visits for sports-related injuries. *Annals of Emergency Medicine* 37: 301–308.

Castelli, W.P., and D.G. Adams. 1990. Running doesn't kill people with healthy hearts. *Your Patient and Fitness* 2 (2): 12–17.

Centers for Disease Control and Prevention. 1997. Sports-related recurrent brain injuries, United States. *Morbidity and Mortality Weekly Report* 46: 224–227.

Colbert, L.H., J.M. Hootman, and C.A. Macera. 2000. Physical activity-related injuries in walkers and runners in the Aerobics Center Longitudinal Study. *Clinical Journal of Sports Medicine* 10: 259–263.

Daly, P.J., R.H. Fitzgerald, L.J. Melton, and D.M. Ilstrip. 1987. Epidemiology of ankle fractures in Rochester, Minnesota. *Acta Orthopaedica Scandinavica* 58: 539–544.

Davis, C. 2000. Exercise abuse. *International Journal of Sport Psychology* 31: 278–304.

de Loes, M. 1997. Exposure data. Why are they needed? *Sports Medicine* 24: 172–175.

de Loes, M. 1990. Medical treatment and costs of sports-related injuries in a total population. *International Journal of Sports Medicine* 11: 66–72.

de Loes, M., and I. Goldie. 1988. Incidence rate of injuries during sport activity and physical exercise in a rural Swedish municipality: Incidence rates in 17 sports. *International Journal of Sports Medicine* 9 (6): 461–467.

de Loes, M., B. Jacobsen, and I. Goldie. 1990. Risk exposure and incidence of injuries in school physical education at different activity levels. *Canadian Journal of Sport Science* 15 (2): 131–136.

DiMaggio, C., and M. Durkin. 2002. Child pedestrian injury in an urban setting: Descriptive epidemiology. *Academy of Emergency Medicine* 9: 54–62.

Dishman, R.K. 1985. Medical psychology in exercise and sport. *Medical Clinics of North America* 69: 123–143.

Einerson, J., A. Ward, and P. Hanson. 1988. Exercise responses in females with anorexia nervosa. *International Journal of Eating Disorders* 7: 253–260.

Faich, G., and R. Rose. 1979. Blizzard morbidity and mortality: Rhode Island, 1978. *American Journal of Public Health* 69: 1050–1052.

Fountain, J.L., and M.C. Meyers. 1996. Skateboarding injuries. *Sports Medicine* 22: 360–366.

Garrick, J.G., D.M. Gillien, and P. Whiteside. 1986. The epidemiology of aerobic dance injuries. *American Journal of Sports Medicine* 14 (1): 67–72.

Gotsch, K., J.L. Annest, and P. Holmgreen. 2002. Nonfatal sports- and recreation-related injuries treated in emergency departments—United States, July 2000–June 2001. *Morbidity and Mortality Weekly Report* 51 (33): 736–740.

Gruber, A.J., and H.G. Pope. 2000. Psychiatric and medical effects of anabolic-androgenic steroid use in women. *Psychotherapy and Psychosomatics* 69: 19–26.

Guichon, D.M.P., and S.T. Myles. 1975. Bicycle injuries: One year sample in Calgary. *Journal of Trauma* 15 (6): 504–506.

Haskell, W.L. 1978. Cardiovascular complications during exercise training of cardiac patients. *Circulation* 57: 920–924.

Heath, G.W., and J.S. Kendrick. 1989. Outrunning the risks: A behavioral risk profile of runners. *American Journal of Preventive Medicine* 5 (6): 347–352.

Hede, A., D.B. Jensen, P. Blyme, and S. Sonne-Holm. 1990. Epidemiology of meniscal lesions in the knee. *Acta Orthopaedica Scandinavica* 61 (5): 435–437.

Holmich, P., S.W. Christensen, E. Darre, F. Jahnsen, and T. Hartvig. 1989. Non-elite marathon runners: Health, training and injuries. *British Journal of Sports Medicine* 23 (3): 177–178.

Hootman, J.M., C.A. Macera, B.E. Ainsworth, C.L. Addy, M. Martin, and S.N. Blair. 2002. Epidemiology of musculoskeletal injuries among sedentary and physically active adults. *Medicine and Science in Sports and Exercise* 34: 838–844.

Hootman, J.M., C.A. Macera, B.E. Ainsworth, M. Martin, C.L. Addy, and S.N. Blair. 2002. Predictors of lower extremity injury among recreationally active adults. *Clinical Journal of Sport Medicine* 12: 99–106.

Jacobs, S.J., and B.L. Berson. 1986. Injuries to runners: A study of entrants to a 10,000 meter race. *American Journal of Sports Medicine* 14: 151–155.

James, S.L., B.T. Bates, and L.R. Osternig. 1978. Injuries to runners. *American Journal of Sports Medicine* 6 (2): 40–50.

Jones, B.H., D.N. Cowan, and J.J. Knapik. 1994. Exercise training and injuries. *Sports Medicine* 18 (3): 202–214.

Jones, B.H., D.N. Cowan, J.P. Tomlison, J.R. Robinson, D.W. Polly, and P.N. Frykman. 1993. Epidemiology of injuries associated with physical training among young men in the army. *Medicine and Science in Sports and Exercise* 25 (2): 197–203.

Kallinen, M., and A. Markku. 1995. Aging, physical activity and sports injuries: An overview of common sports injuries in the elderly. *Sports Medicine* 20 (1): 41–52.

Kennedy, M.C., G.K. Vanderfield, and J.R. Kennedy. 1977. Sport: Assessing the risk. *Medical Journal of Australia* 2: 253–254.

Kiburz, D., R. Jacobs, F. Reckling, and J. Mason. 1986. Bicycle accidents and injuries among adult cyclists. *American Journal of Sports Medicine* 14 (5): 416–419.

Kirkendall, D.T., and W.E. Garrett Jr. 2000. The anterior cruciate ligament enigma: Injury mechanisms and prevention. *Clinical Orthopaedics and Related Research* 372: 64–68.

Knapik, J.J., M. Canham-Chervak, K. Hauret, M.J. Laurin, E. Hoedebecke, S. Craig, and S.J. Montain. 2002. Seasonal variations in injury rates during US Army Basic Combat Training. *Annals of Occupational Hygiene* 46: 15–23.

Knapik, J.J., M.A. Sharp, M. Canham-Chervak, K. Hauret, J.F. Patton, and B.H. Jones. 2001. Risk factors for training-related injuries among men and women in basic combat training. *Medicine and Science in Sports and Exercise* 33: 946–954.

Koplan, J.P., K.E. Powell, R.K. Sikes, R.W. Shirley, and C.C. Campbell. 1982. An epidemiologic study of the benefits and risks of running. *Journal of the American Medical Association* 248 (23): 3118–3121.

Koplan, J.P., R.B. Rothenberg, and E.L. Jones. 1995. The natural history of exercise: A 10-year follow up of a cohort of runners. *Medicine and Science in Sports and Exercise* 27 (8): 1180–1184.

Koplan, J.P., D.S. Siscovick, and G.M. Goldbaum. 1985. The risks of exercise: A public health view of injuries and hazards. *Public Health Reports* 100 (2): 189–195.

Kretsch, A., R. Gragan, P. Duras, F. Allen, J. Sumner, and I. Gillam. 1984. 1980 Melbourne marathon study. *Medical Journal of Australia* 141: 809–814.

Kruse, D.L., and A.A. McBeath. 1980. Bicycle accidents and injuries. *American Journal of Sports Medicine* 8 (5): 342–344.

Kujala, U.I., S. Taimela, I. Antti-Poika, S. Orava, R. Tuominen, and P. Myllynen. 1995. Acute injuries in soccer, ice hockey, volleyball, basketball, judo, and karate: Analysis of national registry data. *British Medical Journal* 311: 1465–1468.

Lysholm, J., and J. Wiklander. 1987. Injuries in runners. *American Journal of Sports Medicine* 15 (2): 168–171.

Macera, C.A., R.R. Pate, K.E. Powell, K.L. Jackson, J.S. Kendrick, and T.E. Craven. 1989. Predicting lower-extremity injuries among habitual runners. *Archives of Internal Medicine* 149: 2565–2568.

Marti, B. 1988. Benefits and risks of running among women: An epidemiologic study. *International Journal of Sports Medicine* 9 (2): 92–98.

Marti, B., J.P. Vader, C.E. Minder, and T. Abelin. 1988. On the epidemiology of running injuries: The 1984 Bern Grand-Prix study. *American Journal of Sports Medicine* 16 (3): 285–294.

McSherry, J.A. 1984. The diagnostic challenge of anorexia nervosa. *American Family Physician* 29: 141–145.

Morgan, W.P. 1979. Negative addiction in runners. *Physician and Sportsmedicine* 7 (2): 57–70.

Morgan, W.P., D.R. Brown, J.S. Raglin, P.J. O'Connor, and K.A. Ellickson. 1987. Psychological monitoring of overtraining and staleness. *British Journal of Sports Medicine* 21: 107–114.

National Center for Health Statistics, P.F. Adams, and V. Benson. 1991. *Current estimates for the National Health Interview Survey, 1990. Vital and Health Statistics, Series 10, No. 181.* Hyattsville, MD: U.S. Department of Health and Human Services, Centers for Disease Control, National Center for Health Statistics. DHHS Publication No. (PHS) 92-1509.

Nicholl, J.P., P. Coleman, and B.T. Williams. 1991. Pilot study of the epidemiology of sports injuries and exercise-related morbidity. *British Journal of Sports Medicine* 25: 61–66.

———. 1995. The epidemiology of sports and exercise related injury in the United Kingdom. *British Journal of Sports Medicine* 4: 232–238.

O'Connor, P.J., and J.C. Smith. 1999. Physical activity and eating disorders. In *Lifestyle medicine,* edited by J.M. Rippe, pp. 1005–1015. Cambridge, MA: Blackwell Science.

Olivardia, R., H.G. Pope, and J.I. Hudson. 2000. Muscle dysmorphia in male weightlifters: A case–control study. *American Journal of Psychiatry* 157: 1291–1296.

Phillips, K.A., R.L. O'Sullivan, and H.G. Pope. 1997. Muscle dysmorphia. *Journal of Clinical Psychiatry* 58: 361.

Phillips, M., M. Robinowitz, J.R. Higgins, K.J. Boran, T. Reed, and R. Virmani. 1986. Sudden cardiac death in Air Force recruits. *Journal of the American Medical Association* 256: 2696–2699.

Pollock, M.L., L.R. Gettman, C.A. Milesis, M.D. Bah, L. Durstine, and R.B. Johnson. 1977. Effects of frequency and duration of training on attrition and incidence of injury. *Medicine and Science in Sports* 9 (1): 31–36.

Pope, H.G., A.J. Gruber, P. Choi, R. Olivardia, and K.A. Phillips. 1997. Muscle dysmorphia: An underrecognized form of body dysmorphic disorder. *Psychosomatics* 38: 548–557.

Pope, H.G., A.J. Gruber, B. Mangweth, B. Bureau, C. deCol, R. Jouvent, and J.I. Hudson. 2000. Body image perception among men in three countries. *American Journal of Psychiatry* 157: 1297–1301.

Powell, K.E., G.W. Heath, M.J. Kresnow, J.J. Sacks, and C.M. Branche. 1998. Injury rates from walking, gardening, weightlifting, outdoor bicycling, and aerobics. *Medicine and Science in Sports and Exercise* 30 (8): 1246–1249.

Powell, K.E., H.W. Kohl, C.J. Casperson, and S.N. Blair. 1986. An epidemiological perspective on the causes of running injuries. *Physician and Sportsmedicine* 14 (6): 100–114.

Ramazzini, B. 1983. *Diseases of workers: Latin text of 1713 revised with translation and notes by Wilmer Cave Wright.* New York: Classics of Medicine Library, Division of Gryphon Editions.

Requa, R.K., L.N. DeAvilla, and J.G. Garrick. 1993. Injuries in recreational adult fitness activities. *American Journal of Sports Medicine* 21: 461–467.

Reynolds, K.L., E.A. Harman, R.E. Worsham, M.B. Sykes, P.N. Frykman, and V.L. Backus. 2001. Injuries in women associated with a periodized strength training and running program. *Journal of Strength and Conditioning Research* 5 (1): 136–143.

Richie, D.H., S.F. Kelso, and P.A. Bellucci. 1985. Aerobic dance injuries: A retrospective study of instructors and participants. *Physician and Sportsmedicine* 13 (2): 130–140.

Romo, M. 1972. Factors related to sudden death in acute ischaemic heart disease. *Acta Medica Scandinavica* 547 (Suppl. I): 1–92.

Rothenberger, L.A., J.I. Chang, and T.A. Cable. 1988. Prevalence and types of injuries in aerobic dancers. *American Journal of Sports Medicine* 16: 403–407.

Sacks, J.J., P. Holmgreen, S.M. Smith, and D.M. Sosin. 1991. Bicycle-associated head injuries and deaths in the United States from 1984 through 1988. *Journal of the American Medical Association* 266: 3016–3018.

Samet, J.M., T.W. Chick, and C.A. Howard. 1982. Running-related morbidity: A community survey. *Annals of Sports Medicine* 1 (1): 30–34.

Sandelin, J., and S. Santavirta. 1991. Occurrence and epidemiology of sports injuries in Finland. *Annals of Chir Gynaecology* 80: 95–99.

Sandelin, J., S. Santavirta, R. Lattila, P. Vuolle, and S. Sarna. 1988. Sports injuries in a large urban population: Occurrence and epidemiological aspects. *International Journal of Sports Medicine* 9 (1): 61–66.

Scheiber, R.A., and C.M. Branche-Dorsey. 1995. In-line skating injuries: Epidemiology and recommendations for prevention. *Sports Medicine* 19 (2): 427–432.

Sgaglione, N.A., K. Suljaga-Petchell, and V.H. Frankel. 1982. Bicycle-related accidents and injuries in a population of urban cyclists. *Bulletin of the Hospital for Joint Diseases Orthopaedic Institute* 42 (1): 80–91.

Siscovick, D.S., N.S. Weiss, R.H. Fletcher, and T. Lasky. 1984. The incidence of cardiac arrest during vigorous exercise. *New England Journal of Medicine* 311: 874–877.

Sosin, D.M., J.E. Sniezek, and D.J. Thurman. 1996. Incidence of mild and moderate brain injury in the United States, 1991. *Brain Injury* 10: 47–54.

Sosin, D.M., J.E. Sniezek, and R.J. Waxweiler. 1995. Trends in death associated with traumatic brain injury, 1979 through 1992: Success and failure. *Journal of the American Medical Association* 273: 1778–1780.

Sundgot-Borgen, J. 1994. Risk and trigger factors for the development of eating disorders in female elite athletes. *Medicine and Science in Sports and Exercise* 26: 414–419.

Thompson, P.D. 1996. The cardiovascular complications of vigorous physical activity. *Archives of Internal Medicine* 156: 2297–2302.

Thompson, P.D., E.J. Funk, R.A. Carleton, and W.Q. Sterner. 1982. Incidence of death during jogging in Rhode Island from 1975 through 1980. *Journal of the American Medical Association* 247: 2535–2538.

Thompson, P.D., M.P. Stern, P. Williams, K. Duncan, W.L. Haskell, and P.D. Wood. 1979. Death during jogging or running: A study of 18 cases. *Journal of the American Medical Association* 242: 1265–1267.

Thompson, R.S., F.P. Rivara, and D.C. Thompson. 1989. A case–control study of the effectiveness of bicycle safety helmets. *New England Journal of Medicine* 320 (21): 1361–1367.

U.S. Department of Health and Human Services. 1991. *Healthy people 2000: National health promotion and disease prevention objectives.* Washington, DC: U.S. Department of Health and Human Services.

Van Camp, S.P. 1987a. The hazards of exercise. *Your Patient and Fitness* 1 (4): 18–21.

———. 1987b. The hazards of exercise (conclusion). *Your Patient and Fitness* 1 (5): 15–17.

Van Camp, S.P., C.M. Bloor, F.O. Mueller, R.C. Cantu, and H.G. Olson. 1995. Nontraumatic sports death in high school and college athletes. *Medicine and Science in Sports and Exercise* 27: 641–647.

Van Camp, S.P., and R.A. Peterson. 1986. Cardiovascular complications of outpatient cardiac rehabilitation programs. *Journal of the American Medical Association* 256: 1160–1163.

van Mechelen, W. 1992. Running injuries: A review of the epidemiological literature. *Sports Medicine* 14: 320–335.

Videman, T., M.C. Battie, L.E. Gibbons, H. Manninen, K. Gill, L.D. Fisher, and M. Koskenvuo. 1997. Lifetime exercise and disk degeneration: An MRI study of monozygotic twins. *Medicine and Science in Sports and Exercise* 29: 1350–1356.

Vuori, I., M. Makarainen, and A. Jaaskelainen. 1978. Sudden death and physical activity. *Cardiology* 63: 287–304.

Walter, S.D., L.E. Hart, J.M. McIntosh, and J.R. Sutton. 1989. The Ontario cohort study of running-related injuries. *Archives of Internal Medicine* 149: 2561–2564.

Watson, A.W. 1993. Incidence and nature of sports injuries in Ireland: An analysis of four types of sport. *American Journal of Sports Medicine* 21: 137–143.

Yates, A., K. Leehey, and C. Shisslak. 1983. Running—an analogue of anorexia? *New England Journal of Medicine* 308: 251–255.

Zebas, C.J., K. Louden, M. Chapman, L. Magee, and S. Bowman. 1995. Musculoskeletal injuries in a college-age population during a 1-semester term. *Journal of American College Health* 44 (1): 32–34.

Web Sites

www.cdc.gov/health/injuries.htm. A site maintained by the Centers for Disease Control and Prevention dedicated to surveillance of selected injury rates in the U.S. population.

www.mentalhealth.com. This is the site of Internet Mental Health, a free encyclopedia of mental health information created by a Canadian psychiatrist, Dr. Phillip Long. It provides access to international definitions of disorders relating to eating and body image.

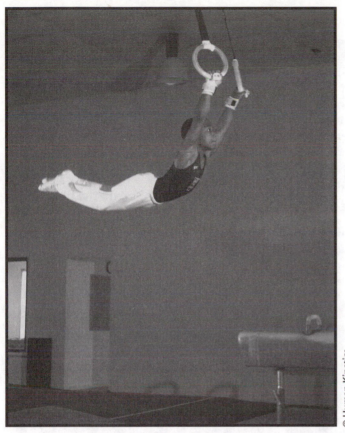
© Human Kinetics

Chapter 16

Adopting and Maintaining a Physically Active Lifestyle

I noticed when I taught slow, heavy, fancy . . . gymnastics, athletics, etc., that I would have a very large membership at the first of the year, but that they would soon drop out.

—*Robert Jeffries Roberts, Director of Physical Education, YMCA, Springfield, Massachusetts, 1887–1889 (quoted in Leonard and Affleck 1947, 315–319)*

Train up a child in the way he should go; and when he is old, he will not depart from it.

—*Holy Bible, King James Version, Book of Proverbs, chapter 22 verse 6*

Despite the cumulative evidence presented in this book that physical activity promotes health, most Americans are not sufficiently physically active. The full magnitude of the physical inactivity problem in the United States and other developed nations was clearly illustrated in chapter 3. Getting people to adopt and then maintain a regular physical activity program are two of the biggest challenges facing public health in developed nations, including the United States. Today, national estimates indicate that 60% of American adults are not sufficiently active, and 28% get no leisure-time physical activity (U.S. Department of Health and Human Services 1999). Depending on the strictness of the definitions of sedentariness and vigorous activity, 25% to 40% are not active at all, and only 10% to 25% are active at levels known to increase or maintain cardiorespiratory and muscular fitness. A dramatic decrease in physical activity occurs during adolescence, in the last years of high school. It can be even harder for many young adults to stay physically active when they enter the workforce. Seventy percent of 12-year-old children report vigorous physical activity (Centers for Disease Control and Prevention [CDC] 2000; Kann et al. 2000), but by age 21, only 40% of men and 30% of women continue vigorous activity (CDC 2001b). The participation rate continues to decline with increasing age until retirement, after which leisure activity tends to increase (Caspersen, Pereira, and Curran 2000). Physical inactivity represents a public health burden that is virtually worldwide in scope; it was the centerpiece for World Health Day in 2002. The most recent estimates of the prevalence of leisure-time physical inactivity and the objectives for changing those rates by the year 2010 (discussed in chapter 3) are summarized in table 16.1.

Research suggests that only about 20% of the variation in people's physical activity is explainable by genetic inheritance (Perusse et al. 1989), though families also can transmit a home culture that promotes or hinders physical activity. Social cultures outside the home also can create learned and physical barriers to physical activity, which can offset the effectiveness of interventions that focus on a person's individual motivation. Therefore, it is important to understand the physical and social environmental influences that might be changed to increase physical activity.

> ••• *Only about 20% of the variation in people's physical activity is explainable by genetics, so it is important to identify and change the key environmental factors that influence people's decision to be physically active during their leisure time.*

TABLE 16.1   SELECTED OBJECTIVES FOR INCREASING PHYSICAL ACTIVITY—*HEALTHY PEOPLE 2010*

Objective	Population	PERCENTAGE OF TOTAL U.S. POPULATION	
		Baseline*	2010 objective
No leisure-time physical activity	Adult	40% (1997)	Reduce to 20%
Moderate physical activity for ≥30 min regularly, preferably daily**	Adult	15% (1997)	Increase to 30%
Moderate physical activity for ≥30 min on ≥5 of previous 7 days	Adolescents	27% (1999)	Increase to 35%
Vigorous physical activity that promotes development and maintenance of cardiorespiratory fitness on ≥3 days/wk for ≥20 min/occasion	Adult	23% (1997)	Increase to 30%
Vigorous physical activity that promotes development and maintenance of cardiorespiratory fitness on ≥3 days/wk for ≥20 min/occasion	Adolescents	65% (1999)	Increase to 85%
Daily school physical education	Adolescents	29% (1999)	Increase to 50%
View television for ≤2 hours on a school day	Adolescents	57% (1999)	Increase to 75%
Trips of ≤1 mile made by walking	Adults	17% (1995)	Increase to 25%
Trips to school of ≤1 mile made by walking	Children and adolescents	31% (1995)	Increase to 50%
Trips of ≤5 miles made by bicycling	Adults	0.6% (1995)	Increase to 2.0%
Trips to school of ≤2 miles made by bicycling	Children and adolescents	2.4% (1995)	Increase to 5.0%

U.S. Department of Health and Human Services. Healthy people 2010. 2nd ed. Understanding and improving health. 2 vol. Washington, DC: U.S. Government Printing Office, 2000b.

*Years indicate when the data were analyzed to establish baseline estimates. Certain estimates are age-adjusted to the year 2000 standard population.

**This objective has been redefined by CDC/NCHS to recommend either moderate or vigorous physical activity. For tracking purposes the baseline rate of moderate or vigorous physical activity is 32% and the 2010 objective is 50%. http://wonder.cdc.gov/data2010/focus.htm

The problem of leisure-time physical inactivity is not just motivating people to try. In the absence of successful behavioral intervention, the average dropout rate from exercise programs has remained at about 50% across the first 6 to 12 months of participation (shown in figure 16.1) since the first studies were published about exercise **adherence** over 30 years ago (Dishman 1982; Oldridge et al. 1983; Sanne et al. 1973).

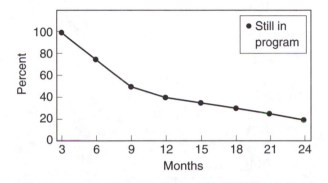

Figure 16.1 Average dropout rate from exercise programs.

Understanding the knowledge, **attitudes,** and behavioral and social skills associated with adopting and maintaining a regular exercise program was a priority identified in *Healthy People 2000,* the U.S. national health goals (U.S. Department of Health and Human Services 1991), and the promotion of physical activity is a key aspect of the new national health goals, *Healthy People 2010* (U.S. Department of Health and Human Services 2000a). As figure 16.2 depicts, this chapter describes the features of people, environments, and behavior (including physi-

cal activity itself) that are potential causes of or barriers to physical activity participation. Theories and interventions that have been used to understand physical inactivity and to increase moderate to vigorous physical activity and exercise are discussed.

Physical activity is not a single behavior. Figure 16.3 illustrates that it is a complex set of distinct acts that include, for example, planning for participation, initial **adoption of physical activity,** continued participation or **maintenance,** and overall periodicity of participation (e.g., relapse, resumption of activity, and seasonal variation). Such a complex behavior has many influences and requires multiple interventions directed at specific features of people and their environments. Studies have identified about 50 different potential reasons for leisure-time physical inactivity (Dishman and Sallis 1994; Sallis, Prochaska, and Taylor 2000) (see tables 16.2 to 16.5 later in this chapter); each can influence the decision to increase moderate lifestyle physical activity or to begin or stay with a vigorous exercise program under certain circumstances. Although it is not yet clear which factors are most critical, it appears that for many people **beliefs** about physical activity (e.g., false expectations of a quick and easy impact on body weight and shape) combine with poor self-control skills to make sustaining an exercise program difficult for many people. Those factors, coupled with social and physical environments that impede physical activity or reinforce other, sedentary behaviors that compete with physical activity when people make choices about how to spend their leisure time, make it easy to understand why so many people in the United States and other economically developed nations are too inactive.

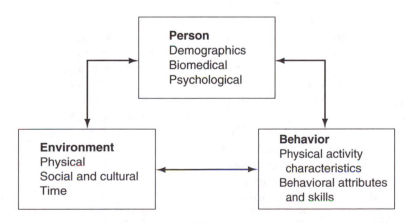

Figure 16.2 Determinants of exercise behavior.

Reprinted, by permission, from J. Buckworth and R.K. Dishman, 2001, *Exercise psychology* (Champaign, IL: Human Kinetics), 196.

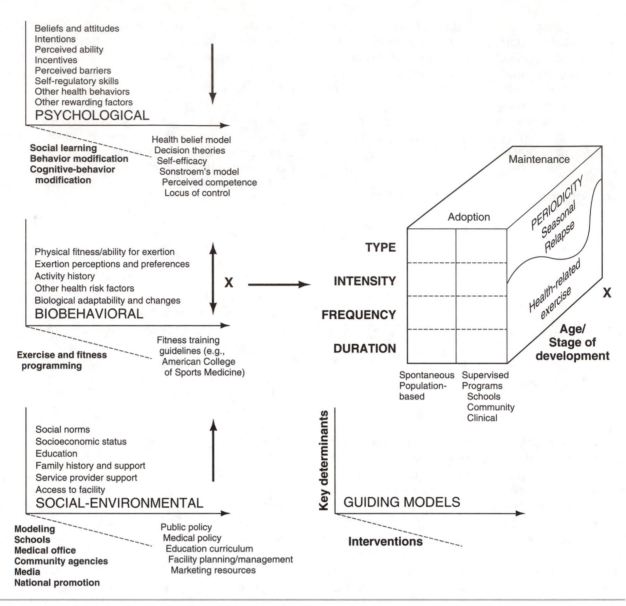

Figure 16.3　A lifespan interactional model for exercise adherence.

Reprinted, by permission, from R.K. Dishman and A.L. Dunn, 1988, Exercise adherence in children and youth. In *Exercise adherence: Its impact on public health*, edited by R.K. Dishman (Champaign, IL: Human Kinetics), 185.

No single variable can predict or fully explain participation in physical activity and exercise. The significance of each potential **determinant** of physical activity has to be viewed in the context of other personal and environmental characteristics, other behavioral choices, as well as features of physical activity. An overarching idea that encompasses these many factors and their interactions is **reciprocal determinism** (Bandura 1997b), which is the cornerstone to contemporary theories of behavior change such as **social cognitive theory** (Bandura 1986) and **social ecology** (Bookchin 1982, 1995; Stokols 1992), discussed later in this chapter. Reciprocal determin-ism describes a mutually influencing relationship among two or more factors. In this view, determinants of physical activity are not isolated variables. As illustrated in figure 16.3, they interact dynamically to influence behavior, and the pattern of this interaction among variables changes over time and age or stage in life. For example, a person's attitudes and physical activity history can interact with environmental variables, such as social support and the weather. After physical activity becomes an established habit, though, the negative influence of bad weather, and the positive influence of social support, on physical activity might become less important.

Most research on understanding the personal determinants of physical activity has been cross-sectional or prospective rather than experimental (Dishman 1994b). Few controlled studies have been conducted to experimentally manipulate variables presumed to operate as causal determinants. Therefore, throughout this chapter we use the term *determinant* to refer to variables that have established reproducible associations or predictive relationships, rather than proven cause-and-effect connections. Later, however, we introduce the concepts of **mediators** and **moderators** of physical activity and discuss some new studies conducted with adolescent girls that confirm that changes in such mediators by interventions indeed result in increased physical activity.

> ••• *Determinants denote established, reproducible associations that are potentially causal rather than proven cause-and-effect relationships. Mediators denote variables that explain the effect of an intervention to increase physical activity or variables that explain the effect of another variable in the causal chain of influence on physical activity. Moderators denote variables that modify the effect of an intervention or another variable on physical activity.*

Motivation is typically synonymous with needs, drives, incentives or an impetus to action. Many approaches toward understanding and increasing physical activity have focused on motivation without proper attention toward understanding how barriers detract from and interact with motivation to determine the direction, intensity, and persistence of human physical activity. Given the high prevalence of sedentariness in developed nations despite widespread attempts to promote physical activity, an alternative focus on barriers can help sharpen thinking about the best ways to intervene in the future.

Barriers to Physical Activity

Costs and barriers associated with a behavior have been recognized as important influences on that behavior since theories about how people make decisions began to proliferate in the 1950s (Janis and Mann 1977). Some barriers to physical activity differ among children and youths, the middle-aged, and older adults and between women and men (Godin et al. 1994). For example, pregnancy and early child rearing can present unique barriers to physical activity for mothers. Nonetheless, not enough is known about the roles of costs and barriers in determining physical activity. Most barriers that are known can be categorized as personal factors, environmental factors, social factors, or features of physical activity (Dishman and Sallis 1994).

Personal Barriers

The descriptive epidemiology of physical activity in the United States that was presented in chapter 3 illustrated that racial and ethnic minorities, people who have less formal education or low-income jobs, and people who live in rural areas are least physically active during their leisure time. The highest prevalence of physical inactivity is found in the southeastern region of the United States, which is heavily rural. Women and girls are less likely to be active than men and boys, regardless of age or race or ethnicity but not physical activity intensity. Generally, participation in moderate intensity activity is similar for males and females, but the rate of participation in vigorous physical activity is lower among females (U.S. Department of Health and Human Services 2000b).

Several personal factors are targets of interventions to increase physical activity because they are potential mediators of people's behavioral choices regarding physical activity. Key personal factors are listed in table 16.2. These include people's beliefs about the outcomes of being physically active or inactive (Steinhardt and Dishman 1989), the **values** they place on those outcomes (Godin and Shephard 1990) compared with other behaviors, satisfaction with their current status and physical activity goals (Dzewaltowski 1994), confidence about being physically active (McAuley and Blissmer 2000) or ability to change their current level of physical activity (Sallis et al. 1988), **behavioral intentions** about being active (Godin 1994), and enjoyment of physical activity (Kendzierski and DeCarlo 1991; Motl et al. 2001), among many other factors.

Other personal attributes may be related to levels of physical activity but are not changeable (e.g., age and sex). Nonetheless, such attributes are important to identify and consider when designing physical activity programs or behavioral interventions, because they may moderate

TABLE 16.2 PERSONAL FACTORS INFLUENCING PHYSICAL ACTIVITY	
Factor	**Influence**
Demographics	
Increasing age	Negative
Blue-collar occupation	Negative
Higher level of education	Positive
Gender (male)	Positive
High risk for heart disease	Negative
Higher socioeconomic status	Positive
Injury history	Unclear
Overweight/obesity	Negative
Race (nonwhite)	Negative
Pregnancy and early child rearing	Negative
Cognitive variables	
Positive attitude	Positive
Perceived barriers to exercise	Negative
Self-efficacy	Positive
Enjoyment of exercise	Positive
Expected benefits	Positive
Value of expected outcomes	Positive
Self-instruction	Positive
Intention to exercise	Positive
Knowledge of health and exercise	Neutral

the effects of interventions to increase physical activity. They can serve as sentinel markers of people who have high risk for being sedentary or who may need special interventions. The personal characteristics that have been considered in determinants research have been organized into demographic factors and social-cognitive factors.

Demographic Barriers

Occupation, ethnicity, smoking, education, income, age, and obesity are examples of personal attributes that can present barriers to physical activity or are signals of underlying habits or circumstances that reinforce sedentary living.

Occupation. Hourly workers in low-exertion blue-collar occupations are among the least-active Americans in their leisure time and have high risk of dropping out of an exercise program (Oldridge et al. 1983). In one study of a period eight years after graduation from high school, people who held blue-collar jobs or were unemployed had lower cardiorespiratory fitness than classmates who became civil servants, white-collar workers, or students, even though both groups had similar fitness levels at the end of high school (Andersen 1996). Many blue-collar or hourly workers may have the attitude that their job requires enough physical activity for health and fitness, but with the use of technology in today's industry, most workers do not expend much energy compared with workers 50 years ago.

Socioeconomic Status. Socioeconomic status is mainly determined by years of formal education and income in adults, both of which are positively associated with physical activity of adults (Sallis et al. 1986, 1992) and children (Sallis, Prochaska, and Taylor 2000). For children and adolescents, higher socioeconomic status of their parents means more access to physical activity programs in and out of school. Transportation to facilities and events influences accessibility and represents an important form of direct support from parents and responsible adults. The association between parents' activity level and the activity level of their children is mixed. The relationship is stronger for females but less significant for adolescents in general (Kohl and Hobbs 1998). For adolescents, peer pressure is a stronger social determinant of physical activity level than family support, although in youths (Sallis, Simons-Morton et al. 1992) and college students (Wallace et al. 2000), family support for exercise is more important for young women and peer support is more important for young men.

Age. Overall participation in physical activity decreases with increasing age, but age has less of an impact on moderate-intensity activity (U.S. Department of Health and Human Services 2000a). Physical activity declines with age during adolescence, but the age at which the decline begins and the pattern of decline is not clear (Stone et al. 1998). A decline in physical activity of about 1.8% to 2.7% per year among boys between ages 10 and 17 years has been reported (Sallis 1993).

The decline in physical activity among girls between ages 10 and 17 years has been estimated to be 2.6% to 7.4% per year (Sallis 1993). Results from the 1999 Youth Risk Behavior Surveillance indicate that vigorous physical activity decreases significantly from grades 9 to 12, more so for girls (Kann et al. 2000). In the 9th grade, 77% of the boys and 68.0% of the girls reported vigorous activity, compared with 70.7% of the boys and 52.3% of the girls in the 12th grade. Lower levels of moderate-intensity activity were reported, but the declines were not as great as for vigorous activity (28.3% in 9th grade and 26.7% in 12th grade).

Among 1,213 black girls and 1,166 white girls enrolled in the National Heart, Lung, and Blood Institute Growth and Health Study who were followed for about 10 years from the ages of 9 or 10 to the ages of 18 or 19 years, the median level of leisure-time physical activity declined by 64% for white girls and by 100%, to zero, among black girls (Kimm et al. 2002). By the age of 16 or 17 years, 56 percent of the black girls and 31 percent of the white girls reported no regular leisure-time activity. Higher BMI was associated with a greater decline in physical activity. Lower levels of parental education were associated with greater decline in activity for white girls at all ages, but only for the older black girls. Pregnancy was associated with decline in activity among black girls but not white girls, whereas cigarette smoking was associated with decline in activity among white girls but not black girls.

Though older people have similar attitudes toward physical activity as younger adults, as many as half have no intentions to become more physically activity (Stephens and Craig 1990). A number of barriers can restrict physical activity as individuals age. After middle age, increasing age is associated with deteriorating health that can limit physical activity (Cooper et al. 2001). Older individuals may lack knowledge of the benefits of physical activity. Perceived control over exercise and health is slightly lower in older persons. Access to activity programs is a barrier that often results in exercising alone at home. Older men perceive a lack of support for participation in a program of activity (Stephens and Craig 1990). Another factor is the extent to which older persons view exercise as an appropriate activity for their age (Melillo et al. 2001) or have high self-efficacy about their ability to exercise (Brassington et al. 2002). Although activity tends to decline with advancing age, age does not necessarily predispose an individual to lower activity. For example, factors associated with a person's job (e.g., conflicts with leisure time or a false perception of adequate physical activity at work) or disposable income (e.g., leisure physical activity may be a low-priority expense) that created barriers to exercise during middle age may diminish during retirement.

Lack of access to facilities is an especially important barrier to physical activity among older adults (Booth et al. 2000). Older people are more likely to exercise alone at home rather than in a supervised and monitored environment. Access to facilities is even more of a problem for people who depend on others for transportation or who have health conditions that limit their mobility, (e.g., those who are disabled or institutionalized).

Studies have examined personal determinants of physical activity in younger age groups. A recent review of 108 studies published between 1970 and 1999 examined determinants of physical activity in children (ages 3–12) and adolescents (ages 13–18; Sallis, Prochaska, and Taylor 2000). Among children, negative associations with physical activity were found for female sex, previous physical inactivity, lack of access to program or facilities, and time spent indoors. Some of the variables negatively associated with physical activity in adolescents were female sex, ethnicities other than white European, nonparticipation in community sports, being sedentary after school and on weekends, sibling's nonparticipation in physical activity, previous physical inactivity, lack of parents' support or support from significant others, and lack of opportunities to exercise or access to facilities or programs.

Obesity. Excessive body mass can make activities that require weight bearing physically harder than for people of normal weight (Wilfley and Brownell 1994). Also, a history of bad experiences with physical activity, including embarrassment, can contribute to bad attitudes toward physical activity, especially exercise classes with participants of normal weight. An obese person may be less confident about exercising successfully. Indeed, the high failure rate of maintaining weight loss after a diet among people who are obese may lead to lower confidence about staying with an exercise program too. The typical obese person regains one third of an average 22-lb (10-kg) weight loss within the year after a diet, with all the weight regained within three to five years (Foreyt and Goodrick 1993, 1994).

Psychological Barriers

Psychological factors can help explain why physical activity varies even among people whose age, education, income, social circumstance, and other demographic factors are very similar. In other words, psychological attributes are important for explaining why some people are active despite circumstances that predict they would be sedentary and why others are sedentary even though they have many opportunities and resources available to them that support physical activity. Put another way, there are senior citizens who are active despite their age, high school dropouts who are active despite their lack of education, and smokers who exercise.

Social Cognitive Determinants of Physical Activity

Social cognitive factors are psychological variables that are transmitted to people from society by learning and **reinforcement** history. Attitudes toward exercising and, to a lesser extent, social norms about exercise influence intention to exercise, but intentions are often fleeting, influenced by changing priorities and personality factors such as will power or self-motivation. The intention to exercise can also be influenced by actual (e.g., available leisure time or access to facilities) and perceived personal control over the ability to exercise, especially **self-efficacy.**

How Do People Decide to Be Active?

Several theories about how people make decisions to be physically active include barriers to behavior. These theories are discussed and their usefulness for explaining physical activity evaluated in the following sections.

Health Belief Model

The health belief model proposes that when people believe that the benefits of exercise in reducing their vulnerability to disease outweigh its costs, they are motivated to exercise (Rosenstock 1974). The model has not been very useful in explaining physical activity (Biddle and Nigg 2000; Dishman 1990). Paradoxically, people who feel unhealthy are less active even when they believe exercise is beneficial. Also, physical activity is viewed by most people as requiring more time and effort than other health behaviors and is only weakly associated with other health behaviors (Norman 1986), suggesting that physical activity is unique among health-related behaviors. The model was designed to describe risk-avoidance behavior, not health-promotive behavior. Thus, it may apply less to those who view physical activity as a health-promotive behavior than to those who see physical activity as an illness-reducing behavior. The possibility that people do not view physical activity as a risk-avoidance behavior is supported by the results of a large population-based study conducted in five northern California cities (Meyer et al. 1980; Young et al. 1996). Several health risk behaviors were favorably influenced by an educational media campaign, while self-reported physical activity remained unchanged for five years.

Though results from health risk appraisals and fitness tests provide a starting point for planning a physical activity program and for goal setting, the boost in motivation from those tests usually does not last very long (Dishman 1993). In one study of the impact of a physician-supervised graded treadmill test on the one-year exercise habits, of the 2,001 who responded to a mail questionnaire, 50% of the 1,384 men who had been sedentary at the time of the test reported that the exercise test motivated them to increase daily exercise (Bruce, DeRouen, and Hossack 1980). No objective measurement of actual physical activity was obtained, however. It was not shown that their increased motivation actually led to increased physical activity. A more controlled study later demonstrated that exercise stress testing had no influence on health behavior, attitudes, objective health measures, or self-reported exercise. Another study examined the effects of exercise testing on physical activity three weeks after a heart attack. The patients' confidence increased when performing activities similar to the treadmill exercise (e.g., walking, stair climbing, and running), and increased self-ratings of activity were verified by daily heart rate monitoring and by decreased heart rate response to standard exercise after training.

A common finding is that intentions to be active initially increase after fitness testing and health risk appraisal, but neither intentions to be active nor actual physical activity remains changed after a few months. One shortcoming of health risk appraisals and fitness testing is that they do not teach the behavioral skills needed to translate intentions into actions.

Theory of Planned Behavior

According to the theory of planned behavior, attitudes toward physical activity and social norms about physical activity influence the intention to be physically active (Ajzen 1985), which is the main factor leading to physical activity (Hausenblaus, Carron, and Mack 1997). Intention can be transient, though, and it is also influenced by personality factors such as self-motivation or will power and by actual or perceived personal control over physical activity and over the barriers that reduce or prevent it. Intentions seem largely necessary but not sufficient to predict physical activity. Many people who are physically active seem to be past the point of actively planning for exercise; their past habits and their perceived control over being active are the best predictors of their future physical activity (Godin 1994).

Self-Efficacy Theory

Self-efficacy theory, which developed from social learning theory, proposes that a person's perceived capability to be physically active is composed of more specific components: expectancies about valued outcomes of physical activity and self-efficacy (i.e., self-confidence) regarding control of physical activity or barriers to being active (Bandura 1986). Self-efficacy develops by (1) actual success, (2) watching others like oneself succeed, (3) being persuaded by someone, and (4) emotional or perceived signs of coping ability (e.g., lowered **perceived exertion** after increasing fitness; Bandura 1997b). Of course, self-efficacy is not a major influence on behavior when goals or incentives are not present. That is, believing that you can accomplish something is not important when you have no reason to try.

According to self-efficacy theory, self-change operates through self-initiated reactions that are stimulated by a discrepancy between a person's goals or standards and knowledge of personal achievement. Individuals who are dissatisfied with their current exercise or fitness, who adopt challenging goals, and who are confident that they can attain their goals and overcome barriers would presumably have optimal motivation for maintaining exercise (Dzewaltowski 1994).

Psychological factors such as beliefs, values, expectations, and intentions influence people's

---

Perceived Benefits of and Barriers to Physical Activity

While the aforementioned theoretical models differ according to their pivotal, causal variable, they all include **outcome-expectancy values** as a cornerstone component. In common language, outcome-expectancy values are similar to attitudes; they refer to the importance people place on their beliefs about the benefits and barriers they hold regarding physical activity. They provide a basis of people's intentions to behave and people's goals. These can vary in specific ways according to age, sex, or other personal circumstances (e.g., pregnancy, illness, change in work schedule), but the general categories of perceived benefits of and perceived barriers to physical activity are remarkably similar for men and women from college age through middle age (Steinhardt and Dishman 1989) and old age (Stephens and Craig 1990).

Perceived benefits	*Perceived barriers*
1. Stay in shape	1. Lack of motivation
2. Feel better in general	2. Too lazy
3. Maintain good health	3. Too busy
4. Maintain proper body weight	4. Not enough time
5. Improve appearance	5. Interference with school
6. Enhance self-image and confidence	6. Too tired
7. Achieve a positive psychological effect	7. Interference with work
8. Reduce stress and relax	8. Too inconvenient
9. Fun and enjoyment	9. Bad weather
10. Help cope with life's pressures	10. Lack of facilities
11. Lose weight	11. Bored by exercise
12. Companionship	12. Fatigued by exercise
13. Family obligations	
14. Limiting health	

Adapted from Steinhardt and Dishman 1989.

behavior and are especially important for motivating people to take the first steps toward being physically active (e.g., thinking about and planning physical activity or starting a new exercise program). These factors can be changed by personal experience and social norms. Other factors such as **self-motivation** (Dishman and Ickes 1981) are related to skills for regulating personal behavior once the decision to try to be more active has been made. Skills involved with **self-regulation** of behavior include effective **goal setting, self-monitoring** of progress, and self-reward and self-punishment. These skills are important for maintaining physical activity when goals are not easily reached and barriers arise that make physical activity difficult. Exercise programs that provide strong social support or social reinforcement in settings that do not demand high frequency or high intensity of physical activity can minimize the importance of self-motivation (Wankel, Yardley, and Graham 1985). Nonetheless, it remains an important factor to help offset the waxing and waning of good intentions to be active. Factors related to knowledge, beliefs, and values are more responsive to educational and persuasive campaigns designed to alter health behaviors.

Physically inactive members of minority and low socioeconomic groups are relatively uninformed about the health benefits of exercise and its appropriate forms or amounts. In one U.S. population survey, only 5% of the U.S. population accurately identified all three of optimal intensity, duration, and frequency of physical activity for cardiorespiratory fitness, though 70% knew the recommended duration and intensity (Caspersen, Christenson, and Pollard 1985). A lack of knowledge about appropriate physical activity and negative or indifferent beliefs and attitudes about the benefits of being physically active certainly can hinder physical activity for many people, but knowledge and positive attitudes about the healthy **consequences** of being physically active alone are not enough to guarantee that a person will start or stay with a regular exercise program (Sallis et al. 1986). Expectations of benefits from being physically active often motivate someone to start exercising, but personal goal attainment, satisfaction, and enjoyment of activities seem to be stronger reinforcers of physical activity maintenance. Though education about physical activity and personal fitness is important in helping form attitudes and plans for increasing physical activity, it does not directly lead to increased physical activity. Knowing does not directly lead

to doing. Undoubtedly, there are cancer researchers who smoke, nutritionists who are obese, safety engineers who do not wear seat belts, and physical education teachers who do not exercise. Nonetheless, education about the benefits of physical activity and about the best way to be active is the first step toward forming positive attitudes about being active and planning how to get started. Education might more effectively increase physical activity if it dispels misinformation promising greater and quicker benefits from exercise than are realistic.

Because most people who join an exercise program share similarly positive attitudes and beliefs about outcomes from exercise, those attitudes and beliefs do not explain why half stop exercising within a few months. Positive attitudes about being active and confidence about controlling one's behavior influence a person's intention to be active (Godin 1994; Godin and Shephard 1990; Hausenblaus, Carron, and Mack 1997), but intentions explain at best only about 25% of people's actual physical activity (Dishman 1994b; Hausenblaus, Carron, and Mack 1997).

Self-efficacy has been the most consistent psychological correlate of physical activity in adults (McAuley and Blissmer 2000) and youths (Sallis, Prochaska, and Taylor 2000). In early studies, the self-efficacy that heart (Ewart et al. 1983) and lung (Kaplan, Atkins, and Reinsch 1984) patients had in their ability to exercise was correlated to their following an exercise program prescribed by a physician. Confidence about staying active was also a predictor of leisure physical activity in a large community in Southern California (Sallis et al. 1986). Recently, self-efficacy about physical activity was the strongest predictor of change in physical activity among adolescent girls (Dishman, Motl, Saunders, Felton et al. in press; Motl et al. 2002).

Environmental Barriers

Environmental barriers to physical activity can be divided into physical barriers and social barriers, although the two types interact. In early studies of supervised exercise programs, dropouts reported that program inconvenience was a barrier (e.g., facilities were not easily accessible, the exercise schedule conflicted with other commitments such as work) (see Dishman 1994b for a review). Though about 20% to 30% of heart patients dropped out from exercise programs for medical reasons, nonmedical barriers such as work conflicts, relocation, and inaccessibility of exercise facilities accounted for 10% to 40% of dropouts (Andrew and Parker 1979; Oldridge et al. 1983). Today, estimates indicate that people tend to be more physically active if recreational facilities are near their homes, and nearly twice as many people choose to walk or cycle in neighborhoods that are designed for self-powered transportation compared with those designed mainly for automobile transportation (Cervero and Gorham 1995).

Although the impact of the social environment on physical activity is still incompletely understood, one of the earliest studies of **compliance** with a cardiac rehabilitation exercise program found that one of the best predictors of compliance by the men was the attitude that their wives had toward the men's participation, which was a better predictor than the attitudes held by the men themselves (Heinzelmann and Bagley 1970).

Physical Environment

Climate or season is associated with overall level of physical activity (table 16.3). Activity levels by children and adolescents are lowest in the winter and highest in the summer. From observational studies, the time spent outdoors is one of the best correlates of physical activity in preschool children (Kohl and Hobbs 1998). Financial costs of programs and home exercise equipment demonstrate no consistent association with supervised or overall physical activity. Access to exercise facilities has been found to influence participation (Sallis, Hovell, Hofstetter, Elder, Hackley et al. 1990; Teraslinna et al. 1969; Troped et al. 2001), although the relationship is complicated. Access can be considered in terms of geography, economics, and safety. For example, running in some urban neighborhoods is risky because of air pollution and high crime

rates. However, access can also be considered in terms of perception. When access to facilities has been measured by objective methods (e.g., distance), access typically is related to both the adoption and maintenance of supervised and overall physical activity. However, perceived access is associated mainly with participation in supervised programs (Dishman 1994b).

> ••• *One of the first clinical studies of the use of exercise to rehabilitate a group of Swedish heart patients found that allowing the men to exercise at home increased their amount of exercise (Sanne et al. 1973), a finding replicated recently by researchers at Stanford University (King et al. 1991). In a study of a community in Southern California, half the adults reported exercising at home (Sallis et al. 1986).*

Though home exercise adds convenience, it alone is not the answer to America's inactivity. According to figures compiled by the National Sporting Goods Manufacturing Association, wholesale revenues spent in the United States on exercise machines nearly tripled from 1986 to 1996, from about $1.2 billion to about $3 billion. Television shoppers spent $100 million dollars on exercise equipment in 1994. During the abdominal machine craze of late 1996 and early 1997, peak sales of these machines were about $3 million a week. During the 10-year period from 1986 to 1996, however, Americans increased their actual participation in moderate and vigorous physical activity by only 2%; a lot of that equipment ended up in closets, garages, and second-hand stores. The recent fad of electrical stimulators, which promised abdominal fitness without physical exertion, had peak sales of a million dollars a week in 2001 and 2002 before consumer protection complaints stemmed sales.

Nonetheless, access to physical activity settings remain an important area of research and public policy. In a study of a community in Southern California, adults who had more commercial exercise facilities located within 1 km (0.6 mile) of their home were more likely to report that they exercised at least three times a week, regardless of age, education, and income (Sallis, Hovell, Hofstetter, Elder, Hackley et al. 1990). Another more recent study found that access and perceived access to hiking and biking trails were positively related to their use (Troped et al. 2001).

TABLE 16.3 ENVIRONMENTAL FACTORS INFLUENCING PHYSICAL ACTIVITY	
Factor	**Influence**
Climate/season	Negative
Perceived lack of time	Negative
Easy access to facilities	Positive
Home equipment	Unknown

Reprinted, by permission, from A. Jackson, J. Morrow Jr., D. Hill, and R.K. Dishman, 1999, *Physical activity for health and fitness* (Champaign, IL: Human Kinetics), 324.

In contrast, other studies have shown that dropouts from exercise programs actually had more leisure time and lived closer to the exercise facilities than did their peers who remained active (Gettman, Pollock, and Ward 1983). Such findings suggest that removing barriers related to time and place (e.g., by providing flexible scheduling or home programs) does not guarantee an increase in physical activity. Changing perceptions about barriers or teaching time-management skills may help. However, barriers such as time and inconvenience reported by the inactive may actually reveal that physical activity is a low-priority choice for using leisure time. Hence, tactics for reducing the reported barriers to physical activity must also consider alternative behaviors that compete with physical activity for the use of people's leisure time.

Lack of time can represent a true barrier, merely a perceived barrier, a lack of skills (e.g., time-management) for controlling one's own behavior, or merely an excuse for a lack of motivation to be active. A good way to tell the difference is to ask someone which of their current leisure activities they are willing to give up to be replaced by exercise. Adding exercise to an already busy schedule merely invites a schedule conflict or makes lack of time an easy excuse. Unwillingness to replace a current activity with exercise probably signals that exercise is not a priority.

Raynor, Coleman, and Epstein (1998) considered the interaction between accessibility and the reinforcing value of the alternatives in a study of 34 sedentary men. Accessibility was defined as physical proximity to physically active and sedentary alternatives. Amount of time that participants spent exercising out of a possible 20 min was compared among four conditions that differed in accessibility to active and sedentary alternatives. The most time (20 min) was spent exercising when the active alternatives were near (in the same room) and the sedentary alternatives were far (a 5-min walk away). Regardless of the accessibility of the active alternatives, if the sedentary alternatives were near, less than 1 min on average was spent exercising. Participants were active 42% of the time when both alternatives were less accessible. Raynor, Coleman, and Epstein (1998) concluded that sedentary men are more physically active if the physical activities are more convenient and the sedentary activities are less convenient.

The long-term decline of self-powered transportation shown in figure 16.4 and the steady increase in transportation by automobile shown in figure 16.5 signal a key problem for planning urban communities that accommodate physical activity. The U.S. Department of Transportation (1997) estimates that one fourth of the trips that people make today are a mile (1.6 km) or less in distance, but three fourths of those trips are made by car. Children ages 5 to 15 walk and ride bicycles 40% less today than they did 25 years ago. Fewer than a third of trips to school that are less than a mile (1.6 km) are walked by children; just 2% of trips to school of 2 miles (3.2 km) or less are made by bicycle.

Most modern communities in the United States were designed to accommodate automotive travel and neglected the building of sidewalks and bicycle trails or lanes. Recognition of these trends led to the creation of the Active Community Environments project by the CDC, discussed later in this chapter.

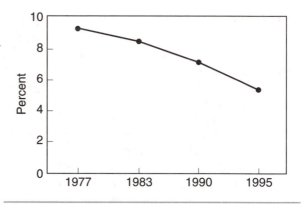

Figure 16.4   Between 1977 and 1995, trips made by walking declined. This trend poses an important public health problem when the effects of physical inactivity and excess weight are considered.

Data from U.S. Department of Transportation. 1997. *Nationwide personal transportation survey.* Lanham, MD: Federal Highway Commission.

Notwithstanding the transportation barriers to physical activity, other data indicate that the degree of urbanization is complexly associated with the level of leisure-time physical activity in the United States. Data from the 1996 Behavioral Risk Factor Surveillance Survey indicate that the overall prevalence of physical inactivity is lowest in central metropolitan areas (27.4%) and in the western United States (21.1%) (CDC 1998). Physical inactivity is highest (36.6%) in rural areas, particularly in the southeastern United States (43.7%). The inverse relationship between degree of urbanization and physical inactivity is relative-

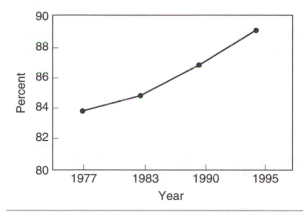

Figure 16.5 Between 1977 and 1995, trips made by automobile increased. Studies show that one fourth of all trips people make are 1 mile or less, but three fourths of these short trips are made by car.

Data from U.S. Department of Transportation. 1997. *Nationwide personal transportation survey.* Lanham, MD: Federal Highway Commission.

ly consistent when data are stratified by age, sex, level of education, and household income.

Social Environment

Relationships and interactions with others can have a strong impact on behavior. They can create or resolve barriers to physical activity, as shown in table 16.4. Through words and deeds, family and friends can help or hinder efforts to be physically active. For example, in a large Canadian study, lack of wives' support for exercise involvement was associated with a threefold increase in the dropout rate by men who were

TABLE 16.4 SOCIAL FACTORS INFUENCING PHYSICAL ACTIVITY

Factor	Influence
Class size	Unknown*
Exercise role models	Unknown*
Good group cohesion	Positive*
Physician influence	Positive
Past family influences	Positive
Social support (friends/peers)	Positive
Social support (spouse/family)	Positive
Social support (staff/instructor)	Positive

*Experts predict the influence of these factors, but not enough research has been done to draw firm conclusions.

Reprinted, by permission, from A. Jackson, J. Morrow Jr., D. Hill, and R.K. Dishman, 1999, *Physical activity for health and fitness* (Champaign, IL: Human Kinetics), 325.

recovering from a heart attack (Andrew and Parker 1979; Andrew et al. 1981; Oldridge et al. 1983). Encouragement, praise, sharing chores to free time for exercise, or being an exercise companion can help encourage physical activity. Family and friends can also sabotage efforts by excessive nagging or by distracting a person from personal goals or tempting him or her with other activities that are appealing but sedentary. Family and friends also can influence another's behavior less directly; a person learns attitudes and habits from watching and listening to other people.

In a meta-analysis of studies that examined social influences on exercise, Carron, Hausenblas, and Mack (1996) examined the separate effects of social variables on exercise behavior, beliefs, satisfaction, and attitude. Overall effects were small to medium in size, but moderately large **effect sizes** of 0.62 to 0.69 were found for the influence of support by family and important others on attitudes about exercise and for the influence of family support and of task cohesion on exercise behavior. Social support from family and friends has consistently been related to physical activity in cross-sectional and prospective studies. Support from a spouse also appears to be reliably correlated with exercise participation. Individuals who join a fitness center with their spouses demonstrate better exercise adherence than married individuals whose spouses do not join (Wallace, Raglin, and Jastremski 1995). Social interactions and social influences appear to be more important for exercise behavior in women. For example, adherence to a structured exercise program was predicted by women's perception that they received adequate guidance and reassurance of worth, but social provisions did not predict adherence in men (Duncan, Duncan, and McAuley 1993). In contrast, participation in supervised exercise programs is weakly associated with class size, group cohesion, and social support from staff or instructor. No consistent association has been found between exercise models or past family influence and exercise or physical activity.

••• Social support is related to physical activity, but this influence is modified by sex.

Behavioral Barriers

Past habits can also be a barrier to a new physical activity program (Godin 1994; Sallis, Hovell, Hofstetter, Elder, Faucher et al. 1990). For example, people who choose not to be physically active in their leisure tend to choose very sedentary leisure alternatives, such as watching television, surfing the Internet, watching movies, or reading, and too often eating extra calories while doing so. On the positive side, the best predictor of someone's future physical activity is his or her past leisure physical activity (table 16.5). However, playing school sports does not seem to influence leisure physical activity after the school years. Men who were athletes in high school or college are not more physically active than former nonathletes during middle age (Dishman 1988). In contrast, one study of alumnae from 10 different colleges found that the women who had played college athletics or participated in intramural sports said they were more active after college compared with nonparticipants (Frisch et al. 1985). The women surveyed in that study went to school from the 1920s to 1950s, so cultural changes regarding sports and changing opportunities for widespread sport participation by boys and girls may paint a different picture for today's young people.

TABLE 16.5   EXERCISE HISTORY AND EXERTION FACTORS INFUENCING PHYSICAL ACTIVITY

Factor	Influence
Past adult activity	Positive
Diet	Unclear
Television watching	Negative
Past childhood activity	Unknown
School sports	Neutral
School sports	Unrelated (men) Positive (women)
Smoking	Unclear
Exercise intensity	Negative
Exercise frequency	Negative
Exercise duration	Negative
Perceived effort of exercise	Negative

Reprinted, by permission, from A. Jackson, J. Morrow Jr., D. Hill, and R.K. Dishman, 1999, *Physical activity for health and fitness* (Champaign, IL: Human Kinetics), 326.

Although organized sport experience might contribute knowledge, attitudes, skills, and habits useful for leisure physical activity in later years, youth sport experiences can also be overshadowed by other personal and environmental

influences that exert a more immediate effect in adulthood. Luckily, past habits are not perfect predictors of future habits. People can change their physical activity.

The type of leisure activity performed by people without major physical or medical limitations to their activity tends to change with increasing age. Activities with low energy requirements, such as walking and gardening, are more popular among older individuals; bicycling, swimming, and dancing become less prevalent.

Competing Versus Reinforcing Behaviors

As noted earlier in this chapter, physical activity likely competes with attractive, sedentary behaviors when people make priority decisions about how to spend their leisure time. Studies of physical activity decision making haven't done a complete job of considering such behaviors (Epstein 1998), though recent studies suggest that reducing sedentary behaviors increases physical activity among children (Epstein and Roemmich 2001; Epstein et al. 1997).

Past studies have relied heavily on theories of behavior change that assume physical activity has similar barriers and reinforcers as do other behaviors, without first establishing whether physical activity is inversely associated with sedentary behaviors and positively associated with other health behaviors, especially among adults. For example, television watching, along with other sedentary behaviors such as working on the computer, is typically viewed as part of the lowest end of the physical activity continuum. However, Dietz (1996) and others have proposed the independence of sedentary behaviors and physical activity behaviors, which deserves further examination. High levels of physical activity are not necessarily correlated with low levels of sedentary behaviors. For example, a marathon runner may have a sedentary job and spend hours each evening using a computer to surf the Internet.

Weak associations have been found between level of physical activity and other health behaviors, such as health protective behaviors, dietary habits, and smoking (Blair, Jacobs, and Powell 1985; Norman 1986). Pate and colleagues (1996) examined associations between physical activity and other health behaviors in data from the 1990 Youth Risk Behavior Survey. Data from over 11,000 youths ages 12 to 18 indicated that little or no involvement in physical activity was associated with cigarette smoking, marijuana use, poor dietary habits, television watching, failure to wear seat belts, and self-rated low academic performance. Level of physical activity was not associated with cocaine use, sexual activity, physical fighting, or self-perception of weight. Steptoe et al. (1997) assessed prevalence of physical activity and other health habits over the previous two weeks of 7,302 men and 9,181 women ages 18 to 30 in 21 European countries. For the whole sample, physical inactivity was significantly associated with smoking, unsatisfactory sleep time, and no desire to lose weight. Inconsistent relationships were found between physical activity and alcohol consumption.

The variety of forms of physical activity provides a broad menu of choices that potentially increases the odds that people will find the form they most enjoy. However, this variety also makes physical activity a complex behavior for beginners and can make it harder to establish a habit early on. Habits are easier to form when a single behavior is reinforced in a specific place and time.

Unique Features of Physical Activity As a Target for Change

- The goal is to increase a positive health behavior, rather than decrease a negative behavior.
- Physical activity is a biologically based behavior; no other health behavior requires exertion several times greater than rest.
- Physical activity is complex, preceded by chains of psychological, behavioral, and environmental events that require multiple decisions and actions.
- The type and quantity of physical activity varies according to its purpose. This variety can make it harder to form a habit early on.

Environmental Intervention and Self-Regulation

The preceding theories and models of how people reach a decision to be physically active view behavior as influenced by expectations that valued outcomes outweigh anticipated costs or barriers to a given behavior. However, those theoretical models do not necessarily do a good job of explaining why such choices often do not result in sustainable behavior change. The models do not adequately address how features of the environment impede or foster physical activity nor do they consider how people can use behavioral skills such as decision making, self-monitoring, goal setting, stimulus control, and reinforcement control to prompt and reinforce their own behavior. The following sections describe how social ecology, behavior modification, and cognitive behavior modification address the ways that the environment and self-regulation can influence physical activity.

People often must make several attempts at behavior change before they experience success. For these reasons, successful behavior change must be viewed as an ongoing endeavor. Increasing the physical activity of Americans requires interventions at the community level (including physicians' offices, schools, churches, families, and local government) with approaches that span multiple levels of change (personal, interpersonal, organizational, environmental, institutional, and legislative) and aim to reach diverse segments of the population otherwise missed by traditional health care.

Social Ecology

Ecology is the study of how systems of nature function. Social ecology is the study of human and natural ecosystems, the interrelationships of culture and nature, and how people function in natural systems, especially during change. Social ecology is a model, more than a theory, for implementing social equity in public policy (Bookchin 1982, 1995). Its guiding principles are unity in diversity and complexity, complementary rather than hierarchical relationships, and active, participatory democracy. Social ecology emphasizes the integration of personal, social, political, and environmental aspects of social concerns, including well-being and health, equity and social justice, and sustainable ecosystems.

In social ecology each person is viewed as valuable to the community and worthy of community respect and support. Social ecological theory suggests that physical activity interventions should integrate personal and environmental resources and focus on developing social support networks, exercise groups, and exercise partnerships (DeJoy and Southern 1993; Stokols 1992). This theory also holds that activity history and habit are strong predictors of current physical activity levels in social contexts. A major objective is to investigate how different social environments (e.g., family, school, workplace) affect human behavior throughout life.

Behavior Modification

Behavior modification is the planned, systematic application of principles of learning to the modification of behavior. According to behavior modification theory, changes in behavior result from associations between external stimuli and the consequences of a specific behavior. The role of people's thoughts, motives, and perceptions is minimized. What precedes and what follows a behavior influence the frequency of that behavior; that is, behavior is cued and reinforced. According to behavior modification, the key to behavior change lies in the identification of the target behavior (e.g., walking at lunch or stationary cycling while studying) and effective cues and reinforcers for it. Behavioral approaches, such as written agreements, behavioral contracts, lotteries, and stimulus and reinforcement control have been successful in exercise intervention studies.

Cognitive Behavior Modification

Many people seem to lack the behavioral skills needed to pursue their commitments to long-range physical activity goals. They may be valued goals, but they are remote and require diligence for many weeks or months before rewarding changes are seen. Also, later gains occur more slowly than initial ones. This is very frustrating when constant improvements are expected. The daily pleasures of sedentary behaviors can erode the good intentions of pursuing physical activity goals.

Cognitive behavior modification is based on the assumption that people can learn behavioral skills that help them self-regulate their behavior. Hence, psychological variables are viewed as key links between the environment and behavior. A wide range of maladaptive behaviors result from an individual's irrational, unproductive thoughts. Learning or insight can serve to restructure, augment, or replace faulty thoughts with behaviorally effective beliefs and skills. Simply put, thoughts and feelings moderate behavior, and they can be changed. People are educated about the relationship of cognitions, feelings, and be-

haviors and are taught skills to identify and control antecedents and consequences that prompt and reinforce behavior. Cognitive-behavioral approaches, including self-monitoring, goal setting, feedback, and decision making, have been effective in increasing exercise adherence when used alone or in combination.

Self-monitoring is keeping and displaying an objective record of behavior (e.g., frequency, time, and place). This objective measure of actual behavior can be compared with goals and gains. It also reduces people's rationalizations that they are already sufficiently physically active when they are not.

Stimulus control involves manipulating antecedent conditions, or cues, that can prompt a behavior. Prompts can be verbal, physical, or symbolic. The goal is to increase cues for the desired behavior and decrease cues for competing behaviors. Examples of cues to increase exercise behavior are posters, slogans, notes, placement of exercise equipment in visible places, recruiting social support, and exercising at the same time and place every day. Before going home after work or first thing in the morning are times when distracting cues are lessened.

Reinforcement control entails understanding and modifying the consequences of a target behavior to increase or decrease its occurrence. Reinforcement is commonly thought of as rewarding a behavior to increase its frequency. Positive reinforcement is the addition of a stimulus that leads to increased frequency of behavior. Negative reinforcement increases behavior by the removal of a stimulus from the environment. In contrast, **punishment** is the addition or removal of a stimulus, after which the frequency of behavior is reduced.

Goal setting is used to accomplish a specific task in a specific period of time. Goals can be simple and time-limited or complex and long-term. Goals serve as immediate regulators of human behavior, providing direction, mobilizing effort, and fostering persistence in the search for task strategies. Goal setting provides a plan of action that focuses and directs activity and emphasizes a clear link between behavior and outcome. Specific, measurable goals make it easier to monitor progress, make adjustments, and know when the goal has been attained. Goals must be reasonable and realistic. A goal might be achievable, but personal and situational constraints can make it unrealistic. For example, losing 2 lb (0.9 kg) a week through diet and exercise is reasonable for many people but almost impossible for a working mother of three who has minimal time for exercise and cooking. Unrealistic goals set the participant up to fail, which can damage self-efficacy and adherence to the program of behavior change.

Stage Theory

Exercise behavior theorists began to recognize the need for dynamic models of exercise that include the idea of stages over 20 years ago (Dishman 1982; Godin, Valois, Desharnais 1995; Sallis and Hovell 1990; Sonstroem 1988). However, those ideas didn't have much impact on interventions designed to increase physical activity. In the early 1990s, Marcus and others (e.g., Marcus et al. 1992; Marcus and Simkin 1993) began applying the **transtheoretical model (TTM) of stages of change** to the study of physical activity.

The TTM is a general model of intentional behavior change that includes a temporal com-

ponent as a critical factor in describing and predicting behavior. Prochaska and DiClemente (1983) observed smokers trying to quit without professional intervention and found that these self-changers passed through specific stages as they tried to decrease or eliminate this health-related behavior. Informed by these observations, Prochaska and DiClemente developed the transtheoretical model in the late 1970s and early 1980s based on an analysis of 18 leading systems of psychotherapy, including psychoanalysis, existentialism, client-centered therapy, gestalt therapy, Adlerian therapy, rational-emotive therapy, transactional analysis, emotional flooding therapies, systems therapies, and **behaviorism.**

The transtheoretical model describes health behavior adoption and maintenance as a process that occurs through a series of behaviorally and motivationally defined stages. The model asserts that change is not linear for most individuals but, rather, involves cycling through the stages at different rates of progression (figure 16.6). The

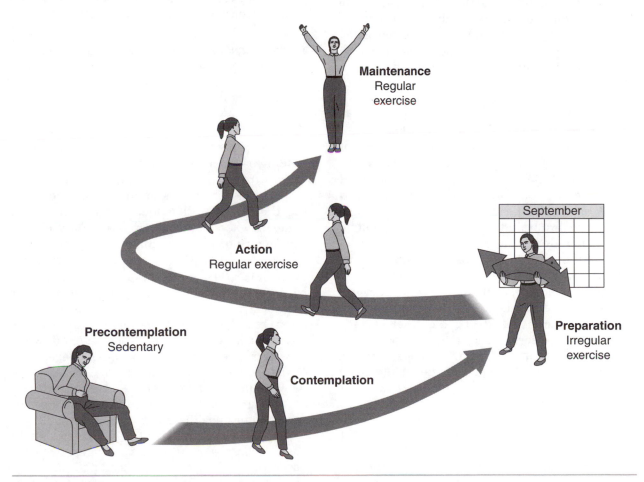

Figure 16.6 Stages of change model.

Reprinted, by permission, from J. Buckworth and R.K. Dishman, 2001, *Exercise psychology* (Champaign, IL: Human Kinetics), 220.

model proposes that each time individuals re-cycle through the stages, they learn from their experiences and are able to move to a higher level of change in future behavior modification attempts. The framing of behavior change as nonlinear provides a context for describing re-lapse and re-adoption.

Although the transtheoretical model was developed to describe changes in addictive behavior, it has expanded to include the adop-tion of preventive health behaviors and the use of medical services, including physical activity (Prochaska et al. 1994).

There are three levels to the transtheoretical model: stages of change, constructs hypothesized to influence behavior change, and level of change. Level of change has not been addressed in the ex-ercise literature, and many studies that applied or tested the transtheoretical model with exer-cise use only the first level of this model—that is, stage of change. Stage is the temporal dimen-sion in which change unfolds. Empirical analysis established five distinct stages that are relatively stable but open to change. A six-month time pe-riod is typically used to define stages, assuming that six months is about as far in the future as people can anticipate making changes. A sixth stage, termination, has been proposed as a point at which there is 100% confidence in ability to maintain the behavior change and there is no risk of a relapse to previous stages (Cardinal 1999), but as yet there is no scientific consensus about the validity of exercise stages and processes.

The second level of the transtheoretical model includes three constructs that are hypothesized to influence behavior change. They include self-efficacy, incorporated from the social cognitive theory; **decisional balance,** which is the evalu-ation of the benefits and costs of the target be-havior; and **processes of change,** which are the strategies used for changing behavior. Several studies have examined exercise stage and self-efficacy for exercise, and, in general, self-efficacy is lowest in the early stages (e.g., precontempla-tion) and higher in each adjacent stage, with the highest exercise self-efficacy in the maintenance stage. There is some longitudinal evidence that exercise self-efficacy increases as a person moves from an established sedentary lifestyle to long-term maintenance of regular exercise (Marcus et al. 1994; Sallis, Hovell, and Hofstetter 1992). How-ever, these data cannot tell us whether people are more active because they have higher self-efficacy or whether they have higher self-efficacy

---

Exercise Stages

Precontemplation stage: Individuals are inactive and have no intention to start exercising. They are not seriously thinking about changing their level of exercise within the next six months, or they deny the need to change.

Contemplation stage: Individuals are also inac-tive, but they intend to start regular exercise within the next six months.

Preparation stage: Individuals are active below a criterion level (typically defined as at least three times per week for 20 min or longer) but intend to become more active in the near fu-ture (within the next 30 days).

Action stage: Individuals have engaged in regular exercise at the criterion level for less than six months. Motivation and investment in behavior change are sufficient at this stage, and the perceived benefits are greater than the perceived cost. However, this is the least stable stage. Individuals in the action stage are at greatest risk of a relapse.

Maintenance stage: Individuals have been exer-cising regularly for more than six months. Ex-ercise behavior is more established than in the other stages, and the risk of a relapse is low.

---

because of past success with exercise, in which case their experience is the true determinant of their current behavior (Dishman 1994b).

Decisional balance is another construct from the transtheoretical model that is believed to influence exercise behavior. Based on the deci-sion theory of Janis and Mann (1977), perceived costs and benefits to oneself and significant others are considered important influences on behavior change. There is good evidence that two constructs (i.e., pros and cons) are adequate for exercise. Pros tend to increase up through the action stage of change and then level off, while cons decrease with each subsequent stage. Most of the evidence also indicates that the balance between pros and cons for exercise shifts during the preparation stage, which is consistent with several other health behaviors.

Prochaska and DiClemente (1983) identified 10 basic processes or strategies to change behavior based on an analysis of the leading systems of psychotherapy. The development of a scale to measure strategies associated with exercise behavior change revealed a 10-factor model with two higher-order general factors representing cognitive/experiential and behavioral processes of change. Cognitive/experiential processes are the processes whereby an individual's own actions or experiences generate relevant information. An example of a cognitive process is self-reevaluation, in which values regarding inactivity are reappraised. Behavioral processes are the processes whereby environmental events and behaviors, such as **stimulus control** and **reinforcement control,** generate information.

The level-of-change dimension is the context in which the target behavior occurs. These levels include symptom/situational, maladaptive cognitions, current interpersonal conflicts, family/systems conflicts, and intrapersonal conflicts. Although not typically applied to exercise, the level of change should be identified to guide interventions. For example, the level of change for someone who wants to begin strength training but does not have access to a fitness center would be situational. Setting up a home exercise program would have more efficacy for this person than targeting his or her cognitions.

Stages of change and processes of change are the components of the transtheoretical model that have been used to develop and implement interventions to enhance the adoption and maintenance of regular exercise. Different strategies are applied based on an individual's stage of change. For example, cognitive strategies, such as increasing knowledge about personal benefits of physical activity, can be directed toward someone in the precontemplation or contemplation stages. Someone in the preparation or action stages might benefit more from behavioral strategies such as reinforcement management and stimulus control.

The key tactic for moving people from precontemplation to contemplation is to get their attention using messages that show relevance. Beliefs about the benefits of exercise should be strengthened and perceived costs reduced. Health risk appraisals and fitness testing are examples of interventions that can prompt contemplation, even though they don't directly lead to long-term behavior change.

The goal with contemplators and people in the preparation stage is to help them take action. Marketing and media campaigns promoting exercise, as well as accurate, easy-to-understand information about how to start an exercise program geared toward people's goals, can help move people into the action stage by increasing knowledge, improving attitudes, and increasing intentions to adopt physical activity.

Initial goals should thus be challenging but realistic in order to foster exercise self-efficacy. Environmental and social supports and barriers should also be evaluated and modified to promote the new behaviors.

Individuals in the action phase are still at high risk of dropping out of an exercise program. Social support is critical in this stage. Instruction in self-regulatory skills, such as stimulus control, reinforcement management, and self-monitoring of progress, and training in relapse prevention are also useful strategies. Relapse prevention is based on the premise that the impact of interruptions and life events on exercise can be diminished if the individual anticipates and plans for their occurrence, recognizes them as only temporary obstructions, and develops self-regulatory skills for preventing relapses to inactivity.

Movement from the action phase to the maintenance phase follows a decrease in the risk of relapse and an increase in self-efficacy. Interventions are more effective if they involve reevaluation of rewards and goals and strategies to cope with potential lapses caused by life events. Social support, self-motivation, self-regulatory skills, and relapse prevention seem necessary to maintain or resume exercise.

Despite its appeal as a model for exercise behavior change and its application in several intervention studies, some uncertainty remains about whether the transtheoretical model has stages and processes that are applicable to understanding exercise behavior change (Dishman 1991; Rosen 2000; Weinstein, Rothman, and Sutton 1998). Indeed, Bandura (1997a) raised several concerns and criticisms of the transtheoretical model in general, such as a lack of adherence to basic tenets of traditional stage theory (e.g., qualitative transformations across stages and invariant sequence of change). A recent meta-analysis of the literature on the transtheoretical model examined the sequencing of processes of change across stages for different health behaviors (Rosen 2000). Experiential and behavioral processes of change were applied sequentially across stage transitions for smoking cessation but were employed concomitantly by people trying to adopt regular exercise, which suggests that readiness for exercise may not be a discrete variable but a continuous variable (Rosen 2000).

If so, stage models in general may not have an advantage over continuum models, such as social cognitive theory, for conceptualizing exercise behavior change. The usefulness of the transtheoretical model for exercise interventions has been mixed. Targeting specific processes of change to facilitate progression of exercise behavior across stages is based on the assumption that differences between adjacent stages (found in cross-sectional studies) point to processes that need to be changed in order to progress to the next stage. However, the efficacy of targeting specific processes to promote stage progression has yet to be adequately tested. There have been few longitudinal prospective designs, and the instruments to measure stages of change and processes of change have been poorly validated for exercise (e.g., Dishman 1991, 1994c; Reed 1999; Rosen 2000).

Readiness for change does not explain why people have difficulty maintaining a change. Even among people who are habitually active, unexpected changes in activity routines or settings can interrupt or end a previously continuous exercise program. Relocation, medical events, and travel can disrupt the continuity of activity and create new activity barriers. Interventions may be needed until physical activity becomes intrinsically rewarding (e.g., fun) to the person.

Relapse Prevention

Most of the theories described so far can be applied to the adoption and maintenance of behavior change. The **relapse prevention** model focuses exclusively on the maintenance of voluntary self-control efforts. The goal of the model is to help people who are attempting to modify their behavior to cope effectively with situations that could tempt them to return to the old, undesired behavior pattern. Marlatt and Gordon (1985) originally designed the model to enhance abstinence from high-frequency, undesired, addictive behaviors such as smoking, substance abuse, and overeating, but the model has also been used to change physical activity (A.L. King and Frederiksen 1984; Knapp 1988). In the model, maintenance of behavioral change is focused on a person's ability to cope with relapses cognitively and behaviorally.

Relapse begins with a **high-risk situation,** which is a situation that challenges a person's confidence in his or her ability to adhere to a desired behavioral change. An adequate coping response leads to increased self-efficacy and de-

> ### Components of Relapse Prevention
>
> - Identifying situations that put a person at high risk for relapse
> - Revising plans to avoid or cope with high-risk situations (e.g., time management, relaxation training, confidence building, reducing barriers to activity)
> - Correcting positive outcome expectancies for inactivity so that consequences of not exercising are placed in proper perspective
> - Expecting and planning for lapses, such as scheduling alternative activities while on vacation or after injury
> - Minimizing the abstinence violation effect, whereby a temporary lapse is catastrophized into feelings of total failure, which lead to loss of confidence and complete cessation
> - Correcting a lifestyle imbalance where "shoulds" outweigh "wants"
> - Avoiding urges to relapse by blocking self-dialogues and images of the benefits of not exercising

creased probability of relapse. Inadequate coping or no coping leads to decreased self-efficacy and possibly positive expectations of what will happen if the behavioral change is skipped. For example, people tired at the end of the workday may expect to feel refreshed if they rest rather than exercise. They actually may feel guilty, however, while the activity would likely have been invigorating. The more rigid the "rule" is, the more obvious the slip. For example, if the rule is to exercise three days per week at 6:15 A.M. for 35 min, starting 10 min late can be perceived as a slip. Perception of slipping may lead to the **abstinence violation effect**, which has both cognitive and emotional components. This effect includes cognitive dissonance, in which there is an incongruity between thoughts or feelings and behavior. For example, the slip behavior does not match the self-concept of being in control of exercise behavior. Another cognitive component of the abstinence violation effect is all-or-nothing thinking, such as defining oneself as either a success or a failure, which also can increase emotional stress. The emotional components of abstinence violation include a sense of failure, self-blame, lowered self-esteem, guilt, and perceived loss of control, which can set the stage for relapse.

> ••• **High-risk situations and rigid rules increase the risk of relapse.**

A lifestyle imbalance in which "shoulds" exceed "wants" also predisposes a person to relapse. Someone who spends more time doing what should be done at the expense of doing what he or she wants to do feels deprived, and the desire for indulgence or self-gratification increases. Exercise might be viewed not as pleasurable but as another obligation. Thus, positive expectations of not adhering to the behavioral change make relapse more attractive.

Conceptually, the relapse prevention model seems useful for exercise adherence, given that 50% of those who begin a regular exercise program drop out within the first six months, most within the first three months. However, the model was developed for maintaining cessation of high-frequency, undesired behaviors, and exercise is a low-frequency, desired behavior. It is clear when someone relapses from smoking cessation, but it is hard to operationally define a slip from regular exercise and identify when a slip becomes relapse. An exercise lapse may be hard to recognize or deal with in time to forestall relapse. One component of relapse prevention training that does not seem effective with exercise is a planned relapse, in which the individual voluntarily returns to the undesired behavior, in this case inactivity, for a short period of time under controlled conditions. Planned relapse may not be a good strategy for acquisition of behaviors in general, particularly in the early stages of behavioral change. Other strategies from relapse prevention, such as identifying high-risk situations, planning for them, and setting flexible goals (or rules) have been applied to exercise with some success.

Intervention Settings

Settings in which behavior-modification and cognitive-behavior modification interventions can be implemented include the home, medical care facilities, schools, work sites, and the general community. Different settings present different real and perceived barriers and supports for physical activity for different target groups.

> ••• **The setting of an intervention has specific supports and barriers for different target populations and goals.**

The Home

Home-based programs can offer accessibility and convenience to people limited by family commitments, finances, location, or transportation. A home-based program should include initial instruction in self-management strategies and appropriate exercise prescriptions, particularly for those just beginning to exercise. The support that is possible in group exercise programs may be lacking in home-based programs, but regular mailings and phone contacts from providers can supply some social support and feedback. Studies that have compared adherence rates of home-based programs and programs in traditional exercise facilities have generally found better results for the home-based interventions (Garcia and King 1991; Jakicic et al. 1999). Strengths of home-based programs include privacy, low cost for the participant and provider, and the opportunity for the participant to personalize the intervention, as by choosing when to exercise and the type of activity.

Health Care

Health care facilities have great potential as settings in which to promote exercise, particularly for women, who are more likely than men to visit physicians. However, physicians' time constraints, lack of training in medical school regarding exercise behavior, and lack of reimbursement for preventive services have limited the implementation of exercise promotion programs in hospitals, clinics, and private practices. However, some programs have been implemented to address these barriers (Eden et al. 2002). Project PACE (Physician-based Assessment and Counseling for Exercise) is an example of a program that has used stage-matched materials in health care settings to increase exercise adoption and adherence with some success (Calfas et al. 1996). The general format of this program involves administering a brief questionnaire to determine the patient's exercise stage before he or she meets with the physician. The patient receives a stage-matched written program with specific recommendations, which the physician then reviews with the patient. Some type of follow-up, such as booster calls by a health educator or other staff member, is used to monitor progress with the program and to answer questions. The necessity of stage-tailored materials tailored to promote exercise in this setting has been questioned, though. Bull, Jamrozik, and Blanksby (1998) tested the effects on initially sedentary patients of verbal advice from a physician combined with standard or stage-matched supportive written material on exercise 1, 6, and 12 months after the office visit. Compared with a control group that received no materials or advice, more patients who received an intervention were active 1 and 6 months later, regardless of the type of intervention.

Schools

It is alarming that only about 30% of U.S. adolescents receive daily physical education classes (U.S. Department of Health and Human Services 2000a). A recent study of 818 third graders sampled from 684 U.S. elementary schools observed that only 5.9% of the children had daily physical education (The National Institute of Child Health and Human Development Study of Early Child Care and Youth Development Network 2003). On average, the children received only 25 minutes (about 37% of total class time) of moderate to vigorous physical activity each week during school physical education classes, far below the 2010 Healthy People objectives that at least 50% of physical education class time be spent in moderate to vigorous physical activity (U.S. Department of Health and Human Services 2000b). School-based programs are critical for the development of health behaviors, but most physical education classes do not teach the cognitive or behavioral skills necessary to increase activity outside of class or to maintain exercise after graduation. There is some evidence that comprehensive school-based health promotion programs have moderately large effects when a randomized design is used to investigate them, measurements of physical activity are valid and reliable, and the programs use extensive interventions (Stone et al. 1998). The Child and Adolescent Trial for Cardiovascular Health (CATCH) is an example of a randomized trial that targeted children in grades 3, 4, and 5. The intervention, which was based on social cognitive theory and organizational change, was implemented in class, with the family, and through policy changes in schools randomly assigned to an experimental (56 schools) or control group (40 schools). Participants in the CATCH program increased mod-

erate to vigorous physical activity in class and vigorous activity outside of class.

A similar intervention, the Lifestyle Education for Activity Project (LEAP), was carried out in 24 high schools in South Carolina and included nearly 3,000 girls during their 8th and 9th grade years (Pate et al. 2003). This comprehensive intervention emphasized changes in instruction and the school environment. It was designed to increase physical activity in high school girls by creating a school environment that supported the unique physical activity needs and interests of adolescent girls. The intervention adopted a social ecological model that emphasized key features of social cognitive theory to increase girls' self-efficacy for physical activity and their enjoyment of physical activity. The LEAP intervention was organized according to the Coordinated School Health Program (CSHP) model (Allensworth and Kolbe 1987; Davis and Allensworth 1994). Six of eight components from the CSHP model were included in project LEAP: physical education, school environment, health education, school health services, faculty/staff health promotion, and parent and community involvement. The intervention staff assisted teachers in the intervention schools who then developed curricula designed to help adolescent girls (1) enhance physical activity self-efficacy through successful experiences with physical activity both inside and outside of school and (2) develop physical and behavioral skills necessary to adopt a physically active lifestyle during the teenage years and to maintain it through adulthood. Teachers at each school developed behavioral skills instructional units that emphasized the acquisition and practice of self-regulatory behaviors (e.g., goal setting, time management, identifying and overcoming barriers, and self-reinforcement); the units were implemented in health education, biology, family and consumer science, or physical education, depending upon how each school provided health education. The LEAP physical education component, known as LEAP PE, included a one-year curriculum designed by the teachers at each school to develop motor skills in a variety of physical activities that were popular with high-school girls, including aerobics, weight training, dance, and self-defense, using approaches that favored small groups and cooperative and successful learning experiences. In addition to facilitating noncompetitive mastery of skills, instruction also used modeling of success, encouragement, and moderately intense exercise directed toward enhancing self-efficacy and enjoyment.

Most studies of interventions in schools have targeted upper-elementary students. There has been a disturbing national trend toward reduction in required physical education classes with increasing grade during the past decade; daily participation in a PE class by high school students decreased from 42% in 1991 to 27% in 1997 (CDC 1998). As figure 16.7 illustrates, the percentage of high school students not enrolled in PE classes is about 50% in most states in the United States that reported PE enrollment to the Youth Risk Behavior Surveillance System as recently as 1997. Since physical activity significantly declines in adolescence (CDC 1998), more community opportunities for recreational activities and sports should be considered. Other directions for interventions through the schools could include curricula that target behavioral skills necessary for lifelong physical activity, the integration of physical activity in other academic classes (e.g., computing target heart rate zone in math class or

writing essays on making exercise fun in English class), noncompetitive and inclusive after-school recreation programs, and programs that involve parents.

Only 46% of people ages 18 to 35 continue an active lifestyle beyond the school years. Efforts to promote exercise adoption and adherence in college settings could affect this trend. Brynteson and Adams (1993) conducted a survey of the exercise attitudes, knowledge, and habits of alumni of four private, conservative, Christian colleges. Physical education was elective in one school, and physical education requirements ranged from four total credit hours to every semester in the other three schools. They found that the school with a conceptually based physical education program and more required hours produced alumni with better attitudes toward exercise who also reported more physical activity. Pearman et al. (1997) reported that a random survey of college alumni indicated that required physical education in college was associated with better health knowledge, more positive

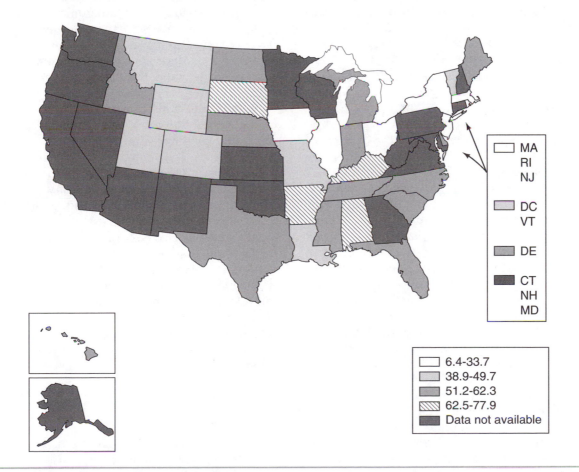

Figure 16.7   Percentage of high school students not enrolled in physical education class in 1997.

CDC, Youth Risk Behavior Surveillance System.

attitudes toward exercise, diet, and smoking, and more exercise behavior after graduation. However, a survey of four-year institutions conducted in 1998 indicated that only 63% required physical education to graduate, down from 67% in 1993 (Hensley 2000). This was the first recorded decline in required college physical education since 1978, and 10% of the schools reported that physical education requirements had been eliminated.

An academic class to teach physical education concepts and self-management skills was developed for college seniors in Project GRAD (Graduate Ready for Activity Daily; Sallis et al. 1999). Postgraduation self-reports of physical activity using the Seven-Day Physical Activity Recall phone interview were compared with control participants who had taken **health education** classes their senior year. There were no effects for men, but initially active women increased total energy expenditure.

Work Sites

The workplace is another setting for exercise interventions, with a "captive audience" for about 40 h per week. The percentage of work sites that offered physical activity and fitness programs increased from 1985 to 1994 (22% to 42%), but these programs varied widely in their available facilities, activities offered, target audiences, costs to employees, and incentives. In general, work-site fitness programs have had equivocal success. On-site fitness facilities may be convenient for some individuals but a barrier to those who have work hours that conflict with scheduled programs, rely on others for transportation home, or simply do not want to spend more time at the work site. Issues in work-site fitness programming include documentation of a favorable cost-benefit ratio, selection of goals and a target audience, institutionalizing the fitness program so that it can sustain changes in corporate culture, implementation of rewards and incentives, and participant recruitment. A meta-analysis of studies published between 1972 and 1997 found a small (0.25 standard deviation) effect size for increases in level of physical activity from work-site interventions (Dishman et al. 1998). Work-site programs may provide information and encouragement to get employees to begin exercising, but additional studies using valid research designs and measures are needed to confirm this.

Communities

The settings for physical activity interventions in communities are diverse (e.g., places of worship, commercial and nonprofit fitness centers, and city or county recreational departments), and types of interventions range from exercise classes to mass media campaigns. Programs in places of worship can provide the impetus to begin exercising, the social support and encouragement to stay active, positive role models, peer-led exercise classes, and information about exercise. For-profit and nonprofit fitness centers, such as the YMCA and YWCA, have been traditional sites for exercise promotion and programs. Comprehensive facilities, flexible hours of operation, classes for beginners, and low-cost or complimentary child care are features that can increase accessibility to regular exercise. Many city or county recreational departments have neighborhood recreational centers and area parks. The effectiveness of their physical activity programs depends on a number of factors, such as safety, privacy, hours of operation, transportation, and child care.

A prime example of a community intervention to increase physical activity at the environmental level is Active Community Environments (ACEs), a CDC-sponsored initiative to promote walking, bicycling, and the development of accessible recreation facilities. ACEs was developed in response to data from a variety of disciplines, including public health, urban design, and transportation planning, that implicated several features of the physical community environment in promoting or impeding physical activity: proximity of facilities, street design, density of housing, availability of public transit, and availability of pedestrian and bicycle facilities.

ACEs encourages environmental and policy interventions that increase levels of physical activity and improve public health. The goals are (1) to encourage the development of pedestrian- and bicycle-friendly environments, (2) to promote active forms of transportation such as walking and bicycling, and (3) to disseminate information about the program. Current activities to promote the goals of the ACEs initiative include

- development of the KidsWalk-to-School program to promote walking and bicycling to school,
- collaboration with public and private agencies to promote National and International Walk-to-School Day,

- development of an ACEs informational sheet,
- development of an ACEs guidebook for public health practitioners to use in collaboration with transportation and city planning organizations to promote walking, bicycling, and close-to-home recreational facilities,
- a partnership with the National Park Services Rivers, Trails, and Conservation Assistance Program to promote the development and use of close-to-home parks and recreational facilities,
- collaboration on an Atlanta-based study to review the relationships among land use, transportation, air quality, and physical activity, and
- collaboration with the Environmental Protection Agency on a national survey to study attitudes of the American public toward the environment, walking, and bicycling.

Although the effectiveness of ACEs-affiliated interventions has not yet been scientifically evaluated, several studies have evaluated the effectiveness of long-term multicommunity interventions that have targeted a number of different health behaviors. For example, the Stanford Five-City Project targeted smoking, nutrition, weight control, blood pressure, and physical activity using a variety of methods, such as applied social learning theory, diffusion of innovations, community organization, and social marketing. There were only modest changes in level of physical activity after six years, but less emphasis was placed on physical activity than the other health behaviors (Young et al. 1996). Problems in detecting changes from large-scale community interventions that last several years are compounded by changes in societal attitudes and norms regarding physical activity and trends in health practices. The Minnesota Heart Health Project used health professionals and community leaders as role models and opinion leaders and implemented personal, intensive, multicontact programs to increase physical activity; however, the small increases in physical activity in treatment groups over the first three years were matched when the control participants also became more active (Luepker et al. 1994).

Levels of Intervention

Interventions can be implemented at different levels within each setting. Programs can be conducted one-on-one with individuals (e.g., Project PACE) or in small groups, such as a strength training class or a walking club. The intervention can also be applied on a broader level, such as in communities (e.g., Stanford Five-City Project) or

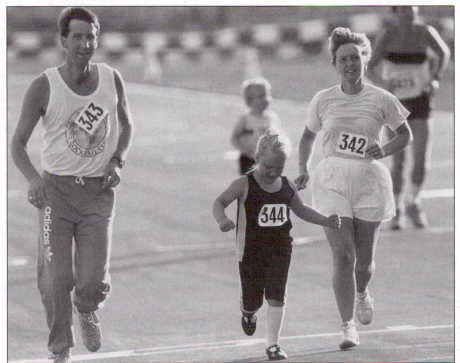

© Sporting Pictures

through legislation supporting increased physical activity (e.g., requiring the construction of bike paths). Program duration can range from one-time events to ongoing programs. Community-based fun runs or walks supporting a local charity may happen only once per year, but they can be opportunities for individuals who primarily want to help the organization to start thinking about exercise for its own sake.

Interest is growing in interventions at the level of the community or society that entail environment engineering, community action, and legislation to support active lifestyles. Local governments and health agencies can develop safe, accessible facilities for exercise with well-equipped buildings with visible stairs and competent staff. Actions can be taken to ensure safe neighborhoods for walking, jogging, and bicycling by improving lighting and adding sidewalks or bike paths that can foster increased physical activity in urban environments.

A highly visible, multilevel community intervention in São Paulo, Brazil, *Agita São Paulo* (Move São Paulo), has targeted the entire state of São Paulo, about 34 million people, since 1995 and served as the main model and venue for the WHO's World Health Day in 2002, *Agita Mundo* (Move the World). Sponsored by the São Paulo Ministry of Health and spearheaded in 1995 by physician Victor Matsudo, the *Agita São Paulo* campaign has successfully penetrated the São Paulo culture with brand recognition of its icon, the 30-Minute Man, a cartoon of an alarm clock that symbolizes the CDC/ACSM recommendations for 30 min of moderate physical activity most days of the week and appears everywhere from billboards to monthly utility bills mailed to individual citizens (Matsudo et al. 2002).

Another extensive public policy initiative for sports and health occurred in Finland during the early 1990s and resulted in two national programs. The initial "Finland on the Move" program was designed to stimulate new local projects by national financial support, training and consultation services, and media promotion. The ongoing "Fit for Life" program is based on the experience gained from the initial intervention but focuses mainly on an intensive mass media approach that targets people ages 40 to 60 years. The Finnish experience has demonstrated that deliberate efforts to communicate scientific knowledge can lead to a better acceptance of physical activity on the national level and that well-planned and sensitive state-level support of grassroots activities can succeed (Vuori, Paronen, and Oja

1998). Some examples of nationally based health initiatives that include the promotion of physical activity are ParticipAction (launched in Canada in 1979), Ireland's National Health Promotion Strategy 2000–2005, the National Assembly for Wales Healthy and Active Lifestyles Task Force, the Northern Ireland Physical Activity Strategy 1998–2002, the National Health Services Framework on Coronary Heart Disease in England, and the National Physical Activity Strategy Task Force in Scotland. The initiatives in the United Kingdom and Ireland include specific goals for increasing physical activity and plan to implement promotional campaigns.

Effectiveness of Physical Activity Interventions

Behavior modification techniques can increase participation rates by about 15% to 35% above the common dropout level of 50% that occurs without behavioral intervention. Nonetheless, long-term maintenance of increased physical activity after the interventions has not been established, and the absolute levels of the increased activity after successful interventions often fall below the frequency, duration, and intensity required to increase physical fitness (Pollock et al. 1998), though, as shown in previous chapters, moderate increases in physical activity can decrease risk for premature death and chronic diseases without necessarily increasing fitness.

The results of a comprehensive review of interventions to increase physical activity suggest that might be the case (Dishman and Buckworth 1996). A quantitative meta-analysis was conducted of 127 studies that examined the efficacy of interventions for increasing physical activity among 131,000 subjects in community, work-site, school, home, and health care settings. The researchers reported 445 effects as Pearson correlation coefficients (r) as they varied according to moderating variables important for community and clinical intervention. The mean effect was moderately large, $r = 0.34$, approximately three fourths of a standard deviation, or an increase in binomial success rate from 50% to 67%. The estimated population effect weighted by sample size was larger, $r = 0.75$, approximately 2 standard deviations, or increased success to 88%. Figures 16.8 through 16.12 illustrate the contrasts between levels of independent moderating variables. Effects were larger when the interventions employed the principles of behavior

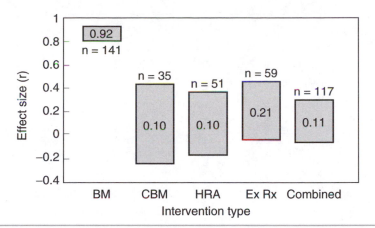

Figure 16.8 Effects of intervention to increase physical activity was largest for behavior modification (BM). CBM = cognitive behavior modification; HRA = health risk appraisal; Ex Rx = traditional exercise prescription; Combined = multiple intervention.

Adapted, by permission, from R.K. Dishman and J. Buckworth, 1996, "Increasing physical activity: A quantitative synthesis," *Medicine and Science in Sports and Exercise* 28: 706-719.

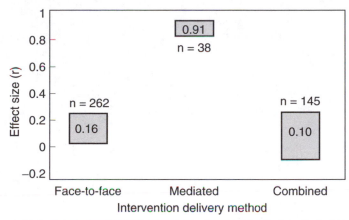

Figure 16.9 The delivery method of physical activity intervention had the largest effect size *r* for mediated interventions; 95% CI excluded zero.

Adapted, by permission, from R.K. Dishman and J. Buckworth, 1996, "Increasing physical activity: A quantitative synthesis," *Medicine and Science in Sports and Exercise* 28: 706-719.

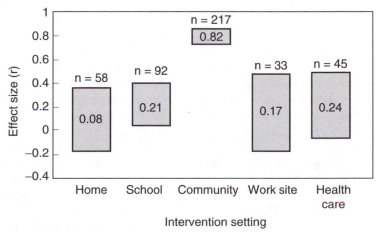

Figure 16.10 The intervention setting of physical activity intervention had an effect size *r* that was largest for community-based interventions; 95% CI excluded zero.

Adapted, by permission, from R.K. Dishman and J. Buckworth, 1996, "Increasing physical activity: A quantitative synthesis," *Medicine and Science in Sports and Exercise* 28: 706-719.

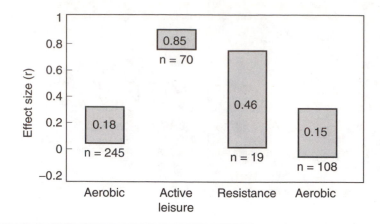

Figure 16.11   The physical activity mode of active leisure had an effect size *r* that was largest for active leisure interventions; 95% CI excluded zero.

Adapted, by permission, from R.K. Dishman and J. Buckworth, 1996, "Increasing physical activity: A quantitative synthesis," *Medicine and Science in Sports and Exercise* 28: 706-719.

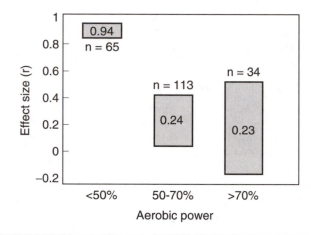

Figure 16.12   Physical activity intervention had an effect size *r* that was largest for low intensity interventions; 95% CI excluded zero.

Adapted, by permission, from R.K. Dishman and J. Buckworth, 1996, "Increasing physical activity: A quantitative synthesis," *Medicine and Science in Sports and Exercise* 28: 706-719.

modification, used a mediated delivery, targeted community groups, and measured active leisure of low intensity. So far, interventions applied in community settings have been the most successful. School-based interventions have had modest success, while the typical interventions conducted at work sites, health care facilities, and home have been virtually ineffective. Also, only about 25% of intervention studies included long-term follow-up to determine whether the interventions had lasting effects once they ended. Therefore, the positive effects of interventions must presently be viewed as short term. The results showed that physical activity *can* be increased by intervention. That is to say, selected interventions have been shown to have efficacy (i.e., they increased physical activity within the context of the experimental intervention and the people who were measured). However, the optimal ways for selecting intervention components, settings, and population segments to maintain increases in physical activity require experimental confirmation through randomized controlled trials. Moreover, the public health significance of an efficacious intervention also depends on whether the intervention reaches a high proportion of the target population, whether it is adopted and implemented fully and well within the target population by the responsible organizations, and whether the effects of the interven-

The RE-AIM Framework for Evaluating Population-Based Behavioral Interventions

Reach: The absolute number, proportion, and population representativeness of people who are willing to participate in an intervention

Efficacy: The impact of an intervention on the primary outcome targeted by the intervention, which can also include desirable secondary outcomes such as quality of life and economic outcomes, as well as undesirable, adverse events such as injury or death

Adoption: The absolute number, proportion, and representativeness of settings and interventionists who are willing to initiate a program

Implementation: The degree of fidelity to the various elements of an intervention's administrative protocol, including consistency of intended delivery and time and cost of the intervention

Maintenance: The extent to which a program or policy becomes institutionalized or part of routine organizational practices and policies or, at the individual level, the long-term effects of a program on outcomes six or more months after the most recent intervention contact

Modified from Glasgow, Vogt, and Boles 1999.

tion are maintained after it ends (Glasgow, Vogt, and Boles 1999; Glasgow et al. 2002).

Recommendations for Community Interventions

The Task Force on Community Preventive Services is an independent, nonfederal panel consisting of 15 members, including a chair, appointed by the director of the CDC. It oversees preparation of *The Guide to Community Preventive Services* (popularly called the Community Guide), a periodic report that provides public health decision makers with recommendations about population-based interventions for the promotion of health and the prevention of disease, injury, disability, and premature death for use by communities and health care systems. Membership in the task force

is multidisciplinary and includes representatives of state and local health departments, managed and primary care practitioners, academics, and professionals in the behavioral and social sciences, communications sciences, mental health, epidemiology, quantitative policy analysis, decision and cost-effectiveness analysis, information systems, and management and policy. The task force determines the scope, topics, and method of evaluation of evidence for the Community Guide and the most appropriate means to assess evidence regarding population-based interventions.

The task force recently reviewed and assessed evidence on the quality and effectiveness of community-based interventions for increasing physical activity (Kahn et al. 2002). Database searches and bibliographic reviews yielded 6,238 potentially relevant titles. After a review of the abstracts and consultation with physical activity specialists, 849 reports were retrieved. Of these, 253 were retained for full review and 94 studies were used for analysis because they were considered to have had good or fair quality of design and execution. Changes in physical activity behavior and aerobic capacity were used to assess effectiveness. A summary of the report indicated that the following types of interventions were effective: (1) informational interventions that used "point-of-decision" prompts to encourage stair use or community-wide campaigns; (2) behavioral or social interventions that used school-based physical education, social support in community settings, or individually-tailored health behavior change; and (3) environmental and policy intervention that created or enhanced access to places for physical activity combined with informational outreach activities.

Because of mixed findings or too few studies, evidence was deemed insufficient to judge the effectiveness of other types of interventions, including (1) classroom-based health education, (2) family-based social support, (3) mass media campaigns, and (4) college-based health education and physical education.

As summarized in table 16.6, the task force used those results as a basis for either recommending or strongly recommending six interventions: two informational approaches (i.e., community-wide campaigns and point-of-decision prompts to encourage use of stairs); three behavioral and social approaches (i.e., school-based physical education, social support interventions in community settings, and individually adapted health

TABLE 16.6   RECOMMENDATIONS FROM THE TASK FORCE ON COMMUNITY PREVENTIVE SERVICES REGARDING USE OF SELECTED INTERVENTIONS TO INCREASE PHYSICAL ACTIVITY BEHAVIORS AND IMPROVE PHYSICAL FITNESS

Interventions (number of qualifying studies)	Task force recommendation for use	Intervention description	Key findings
INFORMATIONAL APPROACHES TO INCREASING PHYSICAL ACTIVITY			
Community-wide campaigns (n = 10)	Strongly recommended	Large-scale, high-intensity, community-wide campaigns with sustained high visibility. Messages regarding physical activity behavior are promoted through television, radio, newspaper columns and inserts, and trailers in movie theaters. Interventions were multicomponent and included support and self-help groups, physical activity counseling, risk factor screening and education, community events, and creation of walking trails. These interventions were evaluated as a combined package because separating out the incremental benefit of each component was impossible.	Effective in increasing measures of physical activity including percentage of persons active (6 studies), estimated energy expenditure (3 studies), time spent in physical activity (3 studies), and scaled activity scores (2 studies). Median net increase: 14.0%; interquartile range: from 3.5% to 21.4%; 10 studies. Median net increase in percentage of persons active: 4.2%; interquartile range: from −1.3% to 8.3%; 5 studies.
Mass media campaigns (n = 3)	Insufficient evidence*	Single-component interventions designed to increase knowledge, influence attitudes and beliefs, and change behavior. These community-wide mass media campaigns include paid advertisements and donated promotions. Messages are transmitted by using channels (e.g., newspapers, radio, television, and billboards) singly or in combination. They do not include other components (e.g., support groups, risk factor screening and education, and community events).	Insufficient evidence on the basis of a minimal number of studies, limitations in the design and execution of available studies, and inconsistent evidence of effectiveness in increasing physical activity behavior.

Point-of-decision prompts to encourage using stairs (n = 6) (This intervention is also included in Environmental and Policy Approaches to Increasing Physical Activity, page 424.)	Recommended	Motivational signs placed close to elevators and escalators encouraging use of nearby stairs for health benefits or weight loss. All interventions evaluated were single component.	Effective in increasing the percentage of persons taking stairs rather than elevators or escalators (median net increase: 53.9%; interquartile range: from 45.4% to 89.5%; 6 studies). Settings in these studies included train, subway, and bus stations; shopping malls; and university libraries. Effective among males and females, overweight or not. All studies excluded children and persons carrying items, children, or both. Evidence from one published study demonstrates that messages tailored to ethnic/racial groups might be more effective than generic messages.
Classroom-based health education focusing on information provision and behavioral skills (n = 6)	Insufficient evidence*	Health education for children in classroom settings. Primary focus on providing information regarding health risks and behavioral risk factors related to physical activity, nutrition, smoking, and alcohol and drug misuse. Methods were primarily didactic with selected behavioral instruction. Did not include interventions to change the way physical education (PE) classes were taught. In the majority of cases, comparison groups received standard health education curriculum.	Inconsistent evidence of effectiveness in increasing physical activity behavior.
BEHAVIORAL AND SOCIAL APPROACHES TO INCREASING PHYSICAL ACTIVITY			
Individually adapted health behavior change programs (n = 18)	Strongly recommended	Programs tailored to the person's readiness for change or specific interests. Designed to help participants incorporate physical activity into their daily routines by teaching them behavioral skills, specifically (a) goal setting and self-monitoring, (b) building social support, (c) behavioral reinforcement through self-reward and positive self-talk, (d) structured problem solving, and (e) relapse prevention. All interventions delivered in group settings or by mail, telephone, or directed media.	Effective in increasing physical activity as measured by minutes spent in activity (median net increase: 35.4%; interquartile range: from 16.7% to 83.3%; 20 studies) and energy expenditure (median net increase: 64.3%; interquartile range: from 31.2% to 85.5%; 11 studies). Effective in increasing aerobic capacity (median net increase: 6.3%; interquartile range: from 5.1% to 9.8%; 13 studies).

(continued)

TABLE 16.6 *(CONTINUED)*

Interventions (number of qualifying studies)	Task force recommendation for use	Intervention description	Key findings
BEHAVIORAL AND SOCIAL APPROACHES TO INCREASING PHYSICAL ACTIVITY			
School-based PE (n = 13)	Strongly recommended	Modified curricula and policies to increase amount of moderate or vigorous activity, increase the amount of time spent in PE class, or increase the amount of time students are active during PE class. Studies designed to modify the amount of physical activity during already scheduled PE. Interventions included changing the activities taught (e.g., substituting soccer for softball) or modifying the rules of the game so that students are more active (e.g., the entire team would run the bases together if the batter made a base hit). Certain interventions also included health education. In the majority of cases, comparison groups received standard health and PE curricula.	Effective in increasing physical activity behavior as measured by minutes per week spent in moderate to vigorous physical activity (MVPA) (4 studies), percentage of class time spent in MVPA (3 studies), and estimated energy expenditure (3 studies). Effective in increasing aerobic capacity (median net increase: 8.4%; interquartile range: from 3.1% to 19.0%; 14 studies). Four studies evaluated interventions in urban settings, and 4 studies evaluated interventions in rural settings. Eight studies evaluated interventions among elementary school students, and 2 studies evaluated interventions among high school students. Evidence of effect was stronger among elementary students than high school students.
Classroom-based health education focusing on reducing television viewing and video game playing (n = 3)	Insufficient evidence*	Classroom-based health education classes that specifically emphasize decreasing the amount of time spent watching television and playing video games. Behavioral strategies included self-monitoring, limiting access, and budgeting time spent watching television and videos. Parental involvement was a prominent part of the strategy, and all households were given automatic television use monitors.	Inconsistent evidence for increases in physical activity behavior and aerobic capacity (3 studies). Consistent evidence for decreases in television viewing, video game playing, and other sedentary behaviors, as well as decreases in adiposity (3 studies). Evidence linking decrease in television viewing to increase in physical activity or fitness was insufficient to make a recommendation.

College-age PE and health education (n = 2)	Insufficient evidence*	Classes taught in university or college settings through physical education or wellness departments, usually for credit or as part of graduation requirements. Components include (a) didactic or lecture session on fitness and health and (b) laboratory-type activities where students engaged in physical activity (e.g., running a specified time or distance or accumulating activity points).	A minimal number of available studies of sufficient quality.
Social support interventions in community settings (n = 9)	Strongly recommended	Focus is on changing physical activity behavior through building, strengthening, and maintaining social networks that provide supportive relationships for behavior change, specifically physical activity. This can be done either by creating new social networks or working within preexisting networks in a social setting outside the family (e.g., the workplace). Interventions involved setting up a buddy system, contracting with another person to complete specified levels of physical activity, or establishing walking groups or other groups to provide friendship and support.	Effective in increasing physical activity as measured by minutes spent in activity (median net increase: 19.6%; interquartile range: from 14.6% to 57.8%; 7 studies) and frequency of exercise episodes (median net increase: 44.1%; interquartile range: from 19.9% to 45.6%; 6 studies). Effective in increasing aerobic capacity (median net increase: 4.0%; interquartile range: from 3.31% to 6.1%; 5 studies).
Social support interventions in family settings (n = 11)	Insufficient evidence*	Changes in social environment that support greater levels of physical activity. Interventions focused on children and families. Intervention components included behavioral contracts among family members, goal setting and problem solving, and other behavioral management techniques. They were usually delivered in joint or separate educational sessions or were adjunct components of school-based interventions, which included take-home packets, reward systems, and family record keeping. Certain interventions also included family-oriented special events.	Inconsistent evidence of effectiveness in increasing physical activity behavior and aerobic capacity (11 studies). Certain studies indicated a more consistent effect on improving strength and flexibility, but recommendations were based on inconsistency of findings for physical activity and aerobic capacity.

(continued)

TABLE 16.6   (CONTINUED)

Interventions (number of qualifying studies)	Task force recommendation for use	Intervention description	Key findings
ENVIRONMENTAL AND POLICY APPROACHES TO INCREASING PHYSICAL ACTIVITY			
Creation of or enhanced access to places for physical activity combined with informational outreach activities (n = 12)	Strongly recommended	Access to places for physical activity can be created or enhanced by building traits or facilities or by reducing barriers to such places (e.g., by reducing fees or providing time for use). Certain programs also provide training in using equipment and incentives (e.g., risk factor screening and counseling or other health education activities). Work-site programs were also included.	Effective in increasing physical activity as measured by percentage of persons exercising on ≥3 days/wk (median net increase: 25.6%; interquartile range: from 10.6% to 50.2%; 4 studies); self-reported exercise score (median net increase: 13.7%; interquartile range: from −1.8% to 69.6%; 6 studies); and energy expenditure (median net increase: 8.2%; interquartile range: from 5.1% to 16.4%; 3 studies). Effective in increasing aerobic capacity (median net increase: 5.1%; interquartile range: from 2.8% to 9.6%; 8 studies).
Point-of-decision prompts to encourage use of stairs (n =6)	See point-of-decision prompts in Informational Approaches to Increasing Physical Activity, page 421.		
Transportation policy and infrastructure changes to promote nonmotorized transit	Pending		
Urban planning approaches, including zoning and land use, neighborhood and street design, and cluster development	Pending		

*A determination that evidence is insufficient should not be regarded as evidence of ineffectiveness. A determination of insufficient evidence assists in identifying (a) areas of uncertainty regarding an intervention's effectiveness and (b) specific continuing research needs. In contrast, evidence of ineffectiveness leads to a recommendation that the intervention not be used.

From MMWR *Recommendations and Reports,* October 26, 2001/50(RR18);1-16. *Increasing Physical Activity: A Report on Recommendations of the Task Force on Community Preventive Services.*

behavior change programs); and one intervention to increase physical activity by using environmental and policy approaches (i.e., creation of or enhanced access to places for physical activity, combined with informational outreach activities).

Because of inconsistent findings, the task force did not recommend classroom-based health education focused on information provision, behavioral skills, or social support interventions in family settings. The task force found an insufficient number of studies of mass media campaigns, college physical education, and health education. They could not recommend classroom-based health education focusing on reducing television viewing and video game playing because no link was demonstrated between reduced television watching or video game playing and increased physical activity.

Future experimental research using valid measures of physical activity are needed in most of the areas reviewed in order to determine whether the recommended types of interventions and their settings will truly lead to sustainable increases in physical activity in the population and among its subgroups. Also, other types of interventions not yet supported by sufficient evidence may prove to be effective upon further study.

Mediators of Physical Activity Interventions

It has been disappointing that cognitive behavior modification and health education interventions designed to increase physical activity have usually been ineffective, but this may partly be explained by poor methods used to implement or evaluate those types of interventions (Dishman and Buckworth 1996; Dishman et al. 1998). Also, nearly all these types of interventions did not clearly target and actually measure changes in the cognitive variables that were presumably targeted by the intervention (Baranowski, Anderson, and Carmack 1998; Dishman 1991; Lewis et al. 2002). But implementation is beginning to improve. Results from a recent study of about 2,000 black and white adolescent girls confirmed that self-efficacy and **perceived behavioral control** (Motl et al. 2002), self-motivation (Motl et al. 2003), as well as enjoyment (Motl et al. 2001) were each positively related to physical activity. Subsequent prospective findings from that study, shown in figures 16.13 and 16.14, indicate that increases in self-efficacy (Dishman, Motl, Saunders,

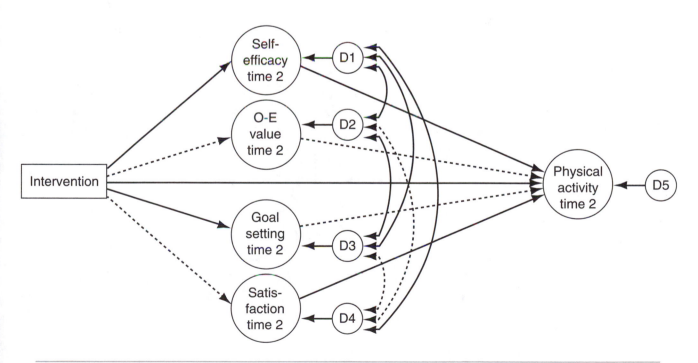

Figure 16.13 Increases in self-efficacy partly explained the effectiveness of a school-based intervention to increase physical activity among adolescent girls. Solid lines denote significant relationships. Broken lines denote nonsignificant relationships. Time 2 = scores in 9th grade.

Felton et al. 2003) and enjoyment (Dishman, Motl, Saunders, Dowda et al. 2003) partly mediated the effectiveness of a school-based intervention designed to increase the girls' leisure-time physical activity during the 8th and 9th grades, a period when physical activity begins to decline among adolescent girls.

Features of Physical Activity That Promote Adoption and Maintenance

In addition to establishing national or international standards for physical activity participation based on epidemiologic evidence for the dose–response relationship between physical activity and health or guidelines for increasing or maintaining fitness (e.g., Pollock et al. 1998), it is important to determine whether activity characteristics encourage or impede participation by the general population or by specific population segments in specific settings.

Most studies of supervised exercise programs in adults do not show an association between dropout rates and exercise intensity. Intensity in these studies is relative to each person's maximal aerobic capacity or maximal strength, thus minimizing the variation among people in the physical strain of exercise and the role of intensity as a determinant. Regardless of exercise intensity, injuries from weight-bearing exercise, including running, can lead directly to dropouts. However, injuries typically do not occur often until durations of 45 min or frequencies of five days per week are approached by previously untrained individuals (Pollock 1988). Dropouts resulting from injuries are not more prevalent in the elderly when walking is the physical activity (Pollock et al. 1991). However, the impact of injury on subsequent physical activity has not been established in population-based studies.

As noted earlier, the typical exercise program based on standard guidelines in sports medicine (e.g., Pollock et al. 1998) has been ineffective in promoting sustained participation, and behavior modification has been most successful when the physical activities targeted were leisure-time activities at intensities of less than 50% of aerobic capacity (Dishman

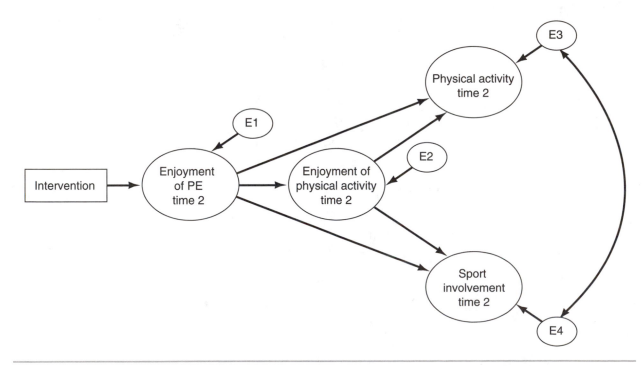

Figure 16.14　Increases in enjoyment of physical education and physical activity partly explained the effectiveness of a school-based intervention to increase physical activity among adolescent girls. Time 2 = scores in 9th grade.

and Buckworth 1996). Only 10% to 25% of U.S. adults follow the typical **exercise prescription,** the exercise intensity, duration, and frequency optimal for fitness.

For example, in a study of California adults, more men (11%) than women (5%) adopted vigorous exercise such as running during a year, but a comparatively higher proportion of women (33%) than men (26%) took up moderate activities such as routine walking, stair climbing, and gardening (Sallis et al. 1986). Both sexes were more likely to adopt regular activities of a moderate intensity than high-intensity fitness activities. Moderate activities showed a dropout rate of 25% to 35%, roughly half that seen for vigorous exercise (50%). Hence, if large numbers of people are unwilling or unable to participate with the frequency or at the duration or intensity recommended by professional consensus for fitness, it is possible that other guidelines for participation could complement fitness standards to increase the activity of a population by reducing total sedentariness.

With this in mind, in 1993 the ACSM and the CDC began promoting an active lifestyle program as a complement to exercise prescription. The recommendation to accumulate 30 min or more of moderate-intensity physical activity most days of the week was designed to encourage sedentary people to pursue activities such as walking, gardening, and household chores (Pate et al. 1995), possibly in multiple (three to five) bouts of short duration (e.g., 5–10 min) daily. This approach could reduce some currently perceived barriers to participation, such as time, effort, and injury. However, experimental evidence is lacking to demonstrate that this approach actually increases physical activity participation. Two randomized controlled trials compared the effects of multiple, short bouts of exercise (i.e., intermittent 10-min sessions totaling about 40 min each day) with traditional long sessions (i.e., 40 min each session) on physical activity, weight loss, and fitness during 20-week (Jakicic et al. 1995) and 18-month (Jakicic et al. 1999) weight-loss interventions among overweight and obese middle-aged women. In general, the multiple short bouts led to similar, but not greater, long-term increases in physical activity, cardiorespiratory fitness, and weight loss compared to traditional long sessions. Regardless of approach, weight loss at 18 months was directly related to the average amount of time spent exercising each week. Women who exercised more than 200 min each week lost an average of 13 kg, compared with an 8.5-kg loss in women who exercised 150 to 200 min, and a 3.5-kg loss in those who exercised less than 150 min each.

Consistent with those findings, the Food and Nutrition Board of the Institute of Medicine recently recommended that adults and children spend at least 1 h each day participating in moderately intense physical activity in order to maintain optimal cardiovascular health regardless of body weight (Couzin 2002). Though that recommendation is similar to the upper end of the amounts of weekly physical activity recommended by the ACSM for weight loss and maintenance among adults (i.e., 300 min each week) (Jakicic et al. 2001), it is more than double the ACSM recommendation that significant health benefits occur with a minimum of 150 min of moderate physical activity each week (Jakicic et al. 2001; Pate et al. 1995).

The ACSM subsequently expressed concerns that the focus on 60 min per day might confuse people, causing them to doubt whether 30 min a day, or shorter bursts of activity such as three 10-min walks, provides any health benefit, perhaps discouraging many sedentary people from adopting any program of moderate activity because they view 60 min each day as an insurmountable goal.

The actual impact of these different recommendations requires experimental comparison in randomized clinical trials. Currently, assumptions about the superiority of one approach over the others for increasing and maintaining physical activity in the population are based on expert opinion not fact. For example, though some health outcomes of physical activity do not require much time and effort among previously sedentary people, other outcomes of exercise valued by many people, such as weight loss or maintenance and improved body image, require more time and effort. Thus, there may be a time–effort paradox in sustaining an exercise program for some people: People who are sedentary may be more apt to adopt an exercise recommendation that requires little time and effort. However, if they expect high fitness or large improvements in physique, they may drop out after becoming frustrated by little or no gain, which is likely if they have invested little time or effort in the exercise program.

Perceived Exertion

When the goal of an exercise program is to promote regular participation, traditional exercise prescriptions and programming should be modified by considerations such as perceived exertion and preferred activities (Dishman 1994c). The limitations of using heart rate as the only index of appropriate exercise intensity among people without heart disease have been recognized for many years. The ACSM recommends using rating of perceived exertion (RPE) among healthy adults to complement the monitoring of heart rate for deciding the appropriate intensity of aerobic exercise for each person (see table 16.7).

Swedish psychologist Gunnar Borg conceived of RPE as a subjective integration of many sensory and physiological responses to exercise (including sensations of muscular force, strain, pain, heavy breathing, body and skin temperature, and sweat). He developed rating scales for

practical measurement of perceived exertion (Borg 1962, 1998). RPEs between 11 and 16 on Borg's 6-to-20 category rating scale usually correspond with exercise intensities between 50% to 75% of maximum METs or 50% to 85% of heart rate (HR) reserve. After people learn to use their whole perceptual range, from no exertion to the highest level they can imagine, the use of RPE permits the exercise intensity to be adjusted to that recommended by target heart rate.

Because perceived exertion is more closely linked in most circumstances with relative oxygen consumption than with relative heart rate (Robertson and Noble 1997), the subjective strain associated with a typical target heart rate can vary widely. Hence, it is not surprising that some participants given age-predicted heart rate ranges frequently complain that the exercise intensity is either too easy or too hard. Studies show that when most people exercise at a pace that feels "somewhat hard," their breathing is not too labored and their pulse rates are likely to be

TABLE 16.7   CLASSIFICATION OF PHYSICAL ACTIVITY INTENSITY BASED ON PHYSICAL ACTIVITY LASTING UP TO 60 MINUTES

	ENDURANCE-TYPE ACTIVITY							RESISTANCE-TYPE EXERCISE
	RELATIVE INTENSITY			ABSOLUTE INTENSITY (METS) IN HEALTHY ADULTS (AGE IN YEARS)				RELATIVE INTENSITY*
Intensity	VO_2R (%) heart rate reserve (%)	Maximal heart rate (%)	RPE†	Young (20-39 years)	Middle-aged (40-64 years)	Old (65-79 years)	Very old (80+ years)	Maximal voluntary contraction (%)
Very light	<20	<35	<10	<2.4	<2.0	<1.6	1.0	<30
Light	20-39	35-54	10-11	2.4-4.7	2.0-3.9	1.6-3.1	1.1-1.9	30-49
Moderate	40-59	55-69	12-13	4.8-7.1	4.0-5.9	3.2-4.7	2.0-2.9	50-69
Hard	60-84	70-89	14-16	7.2-10.1	6.0-8.4	4.8-6.7	3.0-4.25	70-84
Very hard	85	90	17-19	10.2	8.5	6.8	4.25	85
Maximal∞	100	100	20	12.0	10.0	8.0	5.0	100

*Based on 8-12 repetitions for persons under age 50–60 years and 10–15 repetitions for persons aged 50–60 years and older.

†Borg Rating of Perceived Exertion 6-20 scale (Borg 1962).

∞Maximal values are mean values achieved during maximal exercise by healthy adults. Absolute intensity (MET) values are approximate mean values for men. Mean values for women are approximately 1–2 METs lower than those for men; VO_2R = oxygen uptake reserve.

Reprinted, by permission, from M.L. Pollock et al., 1998, "The recommended quantity and quality of exercise for developing and maintaining cardiorespiratory and muscular fitness, and flexibility in healthy adults," *Medicine and Science in Sports and Exercise* 30: 978.

in a range of 120 to 150 beats/min. At this level, most healthy people can safely increase fitness and health while avoiding discomfort.

The Accuracy of RPE for Relative Exercise Intensity

The errors of using RPE to reproduce a level of oxygen consumption of 50% and 70% $\dot{V}O_2$max during exercise are not greater than the errors that occur using target HR (Dunbar et al. 1992). Many studies have used percent HR reserve as the standard for judging the accuracy of RPE production in prescribed exercise, based on the assumption that relative HR best yields the rate of energy expenditure that is optimal for increasing aerobic capacity (i.e., $\dot{V}O_2$max). But the only evidence that percent HR reserve and percent$\dot{V}O_2$max are equivalent across exercise intensities came from studies of small groups of highly trained men. Recent research on a large group of men and women of various ages found that a target HR based on percent HR reserve underestimates percent $\dot{V}O_2$max by about 5% to 10% at intensities between 50% to 60% HR reserve, but overestimates percent $\dot{V}O_2$max by about 4% to 8% at intensities between 80% to 85% HR reserve (figure 16.15) (Wier and Jackson 1992).

Hence, for many people, percent HR reserve is an inaccurate index of low and high relative exercise intensities and thus the wrong standard for prescribing exercise intensity. RPE during low-intensity aerobic exercise depends mainly on the perception of force, but as the exercise intensity increases, sensations associated with increasing blood lactate and hyperventilation play a more significant role (Robertson and Noble 1997). This point is illustrated by a study of 20 untrained college women. During cycle exercise testing, nine women exceeded ventilatory threshold (an index linked with very heavy breathing and the rapid onset of lactic acid in the blood) at 75% HR reserve (Dwyer and Bybee 1983). An intensity of 75% HR reserve is commonly recommended for college students, but these findings suggest that this intensity may be perceived as too effortful for many young people who are not already well conditioned. Ventilatory and lactate thresholds have been associated with ratings of 13 to 15, which correspond with subjective categories of "somewhat hard" to "hard," on Borg's 6-to-20 RPE scale. These intensities may be uncomfortable to many beginning exercisers and may discourage them from maintaining a new exercise program.

As fitness level improves after regular exercise, a standard intensity of exercise is perceived as less effortful because it represents a lower percentage of the person's capacity. However, studies show that perceived exertion after exercise training is more closely linked with blood lactate than percent $\dot{V}O_2$max (Boutcher et al. 1989; Demello et al. 1987; Seip et al. 1991). One hallmark of endurance exercise training is that extra lactic acid does not appear in the blood until a higher relative $\dot{V}O_2$max is reached. The extra lactic acid

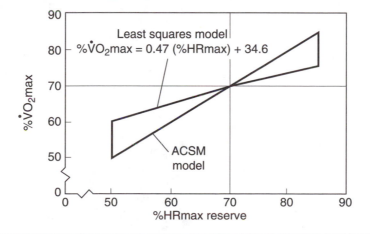

Figure 16.15 Errors of percent heart rate reserve as an estimate of percent aerobic capacity.

Drawn from data in Wier, L.T., and A.S. Jackson. 1992. Percent $\dot{V}O_2$max and percent HRmax reserve are not equal methods of assessing exercise intensity. *Medicine and Science in Sports and Exercise* 24 (Suppl): 105–107.

lowers the pH of muscle and stimulates hyperventilation; each change contributes to pain and perceived exertion. All this means that a person can more comfortably exercise at a higher percentage of aerobic capacity after training because blood lactate levels are lower.

Preferred Exertion

Borg also introduced the idea of **preferred exertion** or "preference level" as the intensity of exercise perceived as being just about right or comfortable (Borg 1962). High physiological strain relative to perceived exertion may increase risks for musculoskeletal and orthopedic injuries that can lead to inactivity. If inactive people select, or are prescribed, an exercise intensity that is perceived as very effortful relative to their physiological responses, they may be less likely to continue participation. Conversely, some individuals prefer to exceed conventional prescriptions. In a recent 1-year randomized exercise trial of middle-aged, sedentary adults, similar adherence was observed for groups assigned to comparatively low (60%–73% HRmax) or high (73%–88% HRmax) intensities (King et al. 1991). However, the authors reported that each group selected intensities during the year that regressed toward a common level corresponding to mean daily exercise RPEs of about 12 to 13. Farrell et al. (1982) instructed trained male runners to run for 30 min at a freely chosen pace and compared responses with 30-min runs at fixed intensities of 60% and 80% $\dot{V}O_2$max. The preferred intensity was approximately 75% $\dot{V}O_2$max and ranged from 65% to 90%. Ratings of perceived exertion during the preferred run initially averaged 9.2 and increased to 11.5. These ratings were between the mean RPE values of 8.8 and 12.3 for the 60% and 80% $\dot{V}O_2$max runs. When we asked young and middle-aged men to select either a power output while cycling or a treadmill speed at zero grade that was comfortable, they chose intensities that were about 60% $\dot{V}O_2$max, with an RPE of 11 to 14, which is moderately hard (Dishman, Farquhar, and Cureton 1994). Trained runners appear to prefer intensities ranging from 65% to 90% $\dot{V}O_2$max.

Summary

It is not easy to alter personal preferences or long-standing habits. For the fortunate, regular, moderate physical activity, or vigorous exercise, is a natural part of the day. For most people, though, changing from a sedentary lifestyle to one that includes regular physical activity is plain hard work and requires planning before a new physical activity habit is formed. Changing physical activity is not like changing most other health behaviors. On the plus side, the variety of forms of physical activity increases the odds that people can find types that they will enjoy. However, this variety also makes physical activity complex for beginners and can make it harder to establish a habit early on. Habits are easier to form when a single behavior is reinforced in a specific place and time. Though replacing sedentary behaviors with physical activity is important, the goal for physical activity is to adopt and maintain a positive health behavior rather than to give up or stop a negative health behavior, such as drinking too much alcohol or smoking cigarettes. The exertional nature of physical activity also makes it unique among health behaviors. No other health behavior requires that metabolism be raised several times higher than rest. The sensations of physical exertion can yield complex interactions with psychological aspects of physical activity. For example, discomfort, fatigue, and soreness are common early outcomes of a new exercise program and can discourage a beginning exerciser.

Recognizing personal and social environmental barriers to physical activity is a first step toward increasing physical activity. This chapter outlined those that have been identified. Until physical activity becomes habitual or enjoyable, sustained participation requires active behavior modification. Most behavior modification techniques for changing physical activity center around (1) goal setting based on initial fitness and desired outcomes, (2) identification of personal costs and expected barriers to adoption and maintenance of an activity routine, (3) strategies for preventing or minimizing the impact of barriers to participation and for increasing support and reinforcement from friends and family, (4) planning a gradual progression of difficulty to optimize success so that the participant has growing confidence in both physical abilities and the ability to maintain the new pattern of activity, (5) feedback from fitness testing and self-monitoring of activity and progress by the participant, and (6) personal strategies for returning to activity after a period of relapse to inactivity due to flagging motivation, injury, vacation, and so on.

An ecological model for understanding and changing physical activity can be added to the traditional approaches to expand our ability to identify and overcome barriers to physical activity, which are also defined on different levels. Personal barriers can be psychological, such as low exercise self-efficacy or perceived lack of time, or physical, such as past injuries. Barriers can also be interpersonal, as when peers support and encourage sedentary behaviors. Environmental barriers can be natural (e.g., inclement weather) or constructed (lack of transportation to an exercise facility or unsafe neighborhoods). Life transitions, such as graduation, marriage, childbirth, or divorce, can interrupt an established physical activity habit, and seasonal variations in opportunities for physical activity require study.

Increasing the physical activity of Americans, and people in other nations, requires interventions at the community level (including physicians' offices, schools, churches, families, and local government) with approaches that span multiple levels of change (personal, interpersonal, organizational, environmental, institutional, and legislative) and aim to reach diverse segments of the population otherwise missed by the traditional health care system (King 1994).

Bibliography

Ajzen, I. 1988. *Attitudes, personality and behavior*. Chicago: Dorsey Press.

———. 1985. From intentions to actions: A theory of planned behavior. In *Action-control: From cognition to behavior*, edited by J. Kuhl and J. Beckman, pp. 11–39. Heidelberg: Springer.

Allensworth, D.D., and L.J. Kolbe. 1987. The comprehensive school health program: Exploring an expanded concept. *Journal of School Health* 57: 409–412.

Andersen, L.B. 1996. Tracking of risk factors for coronary heart disease from adolescence to young adulthood with special emphasis on physical activity and fitness: A longitudinal study. *Danish Medical Bulletin* 43 (December): 407–418.

Andrew, G.M., N.B. Oldridge, J.O. Parker, D.A. Cunningham, P.A. Rechnitzer, N.L. Jones, C. Buck, T. Kavanagh, R.J. Shephard, and J.R. Sutton. 1981. Reasons for dropout from exercise programs in post-coronary patients. *Medicine and Science in Sports and Exercise* 13: 164–168.

Andrew, G.M., and J.O. Parker. 1979. Factors related to dropout of post myocardial infarction patients from exercise programs. *Medicine and Science in Sports and Exercise* 11: 376–378.

Auweele, Y.A., R. Rzewnicki, and V. Van Mele. 1997. Reasons for not exercising and exercise intentions: A study of middle-aged sedentary adults. *Journal of Sports Sciences* 15: 151–165.

Bandura, A. 1986. *Social foundations of thought and action*. Englewood Cliffs, NJ: Prentice Hall.

———. 1997a. Editorial: The anatomy of stages of change. *American Journal of Health Promotion* 12 (1): 8–10.

———. 1997b. *Self-efficacy: The exercise of control*. New York: Freeman.

Baranowski, T., C. Anderson, and C. Carmack. 1998. Mediating variable framework in physical activity interventions: How are we doing? How might we do better? *American Journal of Preventive Medicine* 15: 266–297.

Baron, R.M., and D.A. Kenny. 1986. The moderator–mediator variable distinction in social psychological research: Conceptual, strategic, and statistical considerations. *Journal of Personality and Social Psychology* 51: 1173–1182.

Beunen, G., and M. Thomis. 1999. Genetic determinants of sports participation and daily physical activity. *International Journal of Obesity and Related Metabolic Disorders* 23 (Suppl. 3): S55–S63.

Biddle, S.J.H., and C.R. Nigg. 2000. Theories of exercise behavior. *International Journal of Sport Psychology* 31 (2): 290–304.

Blair, S.N., M. Booth, I. Gyarfas, H. Iwane, B. Marti, V. Matsudo, M.S. Morrow, T. Noakes, and R. Shephard. 1996. Development of public policy and physical activity initiatives internationally. *Sports Medicine* 21 (3): 157–163.

Blair, S.N., D.R. Jacobs, and K.E. Powell. 1985. Relationships between exercise or physical activity and other health behaviors. *Public Health Reports* 100: 172–180.

Blamey, A., N. Mutrie, and T. Aitchison. 1995. Health promotion by encouraged use of stairs. *British Medical Journal* 311: 289–290.

Bookchin, M. 1982. *The ecology of freedom: The emergence and dissolution of hierarchy*. Palo Alto, CA: Cheshire Books.

———. 1995. *The philosophy of social ecology: Essays on dialetical naturalism*. 2nd ed., revised. Montreal: Black Rose Books.

Booth, M.L., N. Owen, A. Bauman, O. Clavisi, and E. Leslie. 2000. Social-cognitive and perceived environmental influences associated with physical activity in older Australians. *Preventive Medicine* 31: 15–22.

Borg, G.A.V. 1962. *Physical performance and perceived exertion*. Vol. 11 of *Studia psychologica et paedagogica. Series altera*. Lund, Sweden: Gleerup.

———. 1998. *Borg's perceived exertion and pain scales*. Champaign, IL: Human Kinetics.

Boutcher, S.H., R.L. Seip, R.K. Hetzler, E.F. Pierce, D. Snead, A. Weltman. 1989. The effects of specificity of training on rating of perceived exertion at the lactate threshold. *European Journal of Applied Physiology and Occupational Physiology* 59: 365–369.

Brassington, G.S., A.A. Atienza, R.E. Perczek, T.M. DiLorenzo, and A.C. King. 2002. Intervention-related cognitive versus social mediators of exercise adherence in the elderly. *American Journal of Preventive Medicine* 23 (2 Suppl.): 80–86.

Brownell, K., A.J. Stunkard, and J. Albaum. 1980. Evaluation and modification of exercise patterns in the natural environment. *American Journal of Psychiatry* 136: 1540–1545.

Bruce, R.A., T.A. DeRouen, and K.F. Hossack. 1980. Pilot study examining the motivational effects of maximal exercise testing to modify risk factors and health habits. *Cardiology* 66 (2): 111–119.

Bruce, E., R. Frederick, R.A. Bruce, and L.D. Fisher. 1976. Comparison of active participants and dropouts in CAPRI cardiopulmonary rehabilitation programs. *American Journal of Cardiology* 37: 53–60.

Brynteson, P., and T.M.I. Adams. 1993. The effects of conceptually based physical education programs on attitudes and exercise habits of college alumni after 2 to 11 years of follow-up. *Research Quarterly for Exercise and Sport* 64: 208–212.

Buckworth, J., and R.K. Dishman. 2001. *Exercise psychology.* Champaign, IL: Human Kinetics.

Bull, F.C., K. Jamrozik, and B.A. Blanksby. 1998. Tailoring advice on exercise: Does it make a difference? *American Journal of Preventive Medicine* 16 (3): 230–239.

Burke, E.J., and M.L. Collins. 1984. Using perceived exertion for the prescription of exercise in healthy adults. In *Clinical sports medicine.* Lexington, MA: Callamore Press.

Calfas, K.J., B.J. Long, J.F. Sallis, W. Wooten, M. Pratt, and K. Patrick. 1996. A controlled trial of physician counseling to promote the adoption of physical activity. *Preventive Medicine* 25 (3): 225–233.

Calfas, K.J., J.F. Sallis, B. Oldenburg, and M. French. 1997. Mediators of change in physical activity following an intervention in primary care: PACE. *Preventive Medicine* 26: 297–304.

Cardinal, B.J. 1999. Extended stage model of physical activity behavior. *Journal of Human Movement Studies* 37: 37–54.

Carron, A.V., H.A. Hausenblas, and D. Mack. 1996. Social influence and exercise: A meta-analysis. *Journal of Sport and Exercise Psychology* 18: 1–16.

Caspersen, C.J., G.M. Christenson, and R.A. Pollard. 1985. Status of the 1990 physical fitness and exercise objectives: Evidence from HNIS 1985. *Public Health Reports* 101: 587–592.

Caspersen, C.J., M.A. Pereira, and K.M. Curran. 2000. Changes in physical activity patterns in the United States, by sex and cross-sectional age. *Medicine and Science in Sports and Exercise* 32 (9): 1601–1609.

Castro, C., J.F. Sallis, S.A. Hickmann, R.E. Lee, and A.H. Chen. 1999. A prospective study of psychosocial correlates of physical activity for ethnic minority women. *Psychology and Health* 14 (2): 277–293.

Centers for Disease Control and Prevention. 2000. *Fact sheet: Youth risk behavior trends from CDC's 1991, 1993, 1995, 1997, and 1999 Youth Risk Behavior Surveys.* Atlanta: U.S. Department of Health and Human Services, Centers for Disease Control and Prevention, National Center for Chronic Disease Prevention and Health Promotion.

———. 1998. Self-reported physical inactivity by degree of urbanization—United States, 1996. *Morbidity and Mortality Weekly Report* 47 (50): 1097–1100.

———. 2001a. Increasing physical activity: A report on recommendations of the Task Force on Community Preventive Services. *Morbidity and Mortality Weekly Report* 50 (RR-18): 1–16.

———. 2001b. Physical activity trends—United States, 1990–1998. *Morbidity and Mortality Weekly Report* 50 (9): 166–169.

Cervero, R., and R. Gorham. 1995. Commuting in transit versus automobile neighborhoods. *Journal of the American Planning Association* 61: 210–225.

Cooper, K.M., D. Bilbrew, P.M. Dubbert, K. Kerr, and K. Kirchner. 2001. Health barriers to walking for exercise in elderly primary care. *Geriatric Nursing* 22: 258–262.

Courneya, K.S., and T.M. Bobick. 2000. Integrating the theory of planned behavior with the processes and stages of change in the exercise domain. *Psychology of Sport and Exercise* 1: 41–56.

Courneya, K.S., and L.M. Hellsten. 1998. Personality correlates of exercise behavior, motives, barriers, and preferences: An application of the five-factor model. *Personality and Individual Differences* 24 (5): 625–633.

Courneya, K.S. and E. McAuley. 1994. Are there different determinants of the frequency, intensity, and duration of physical activity? *Behavioral Medicine* 20 (2): 84–90.

———. 1995. Cognitive mediators of the social influence-exercise adherence relationship: A test of the Theory of Planned Behavior. *Journal of Behavioral Medicine* 18 (5): 499–515.

Couzin, J. 2002. Nutrition research. IOM panel weighs in on diet and health. *Science* 297 (5588): 1788–1789.

Crespo, C.J., E. Smit, R.E. Andersen, O. Carter-Pokras, and B.E. Ainsworth. 2000. Race/ethnicity, social class and their relation to physical inactivity during leisure time: Results from the third National Health and Nutrition Examination Survey, 1988–1994. *American Journal of Preventive Medicine* 18 (1): 46–53.

Davis, T.M., and D.D. Allensworth. 1994. Program management: A necessary component for the comprehensive school health program. *Journal of School Health* 64: 400–404.

DeJoy, D.M., and D.J. Southern. 1993. An integrative perspective on worksite health promotion. *Journal of Occupational Medicine* 35: 1221–1230.

Demello, J.J., K.J. Cureton, R.E. Boineau, and M.M. Singh. 1987. Ratings of perceived exertion at the lactate threshold in trained and untrained men and women. *Medicine and Science in Sports and Exercise* 19: 354–362.

Dennison, B.A., J.H. Straus, E.D. Mellits, and E. Charney. 1988. Childhood physical fitness tests: Predictor of adult physical activity levels? *Pediatrics* 82: 324–330.

Dietz, W.H. 1996. The role of lifestyle in health: The epidemiology and consequences of inactivity. *Proceedings of the Nutrition Society* 55: 829–840.

Dishman, R.K. 1982. Compliance/adherence in health-related exercise. *Health Psychology* 1 (3): 237–267.

———. 1988. Supervised and free-living physical activity: No differences in former athletes and nonathletes. *American Journal of Preventive Medicine* 4: 153–160.

———. 1990. Determinants of participation in physical activity. In C. Bouchard, R.J. Shephard, T. Stephens, J.R. Sutton, and B.D. McPherson, eds., *Exercise, fitness, and health—a consensus of current knowledge,* pp. 78–101. Champaign, IL: Human Kinetics.

———. 1991. Increasing and maintaining exercise and physical activity. *Behavior Therapy* 22: 345–378.

———. 1993. Exercise adherence. In *Handbook of research on sport psychology,* edited by R.N. Singer, M. Murphey, and L.K. Tennant, pp. 779–798. New York: Macmillan.

———, ed. 1994a. *Advances in exercise adherence.* Champaign, IL: Human Kinetics.

———. 1994b. The measurement conundrum in exercise adherence research. *Medicine and Science in Sports and Exercise* 26: 1382–1390.

———. 1994c. Prescribing exercise intensity for healthy adults using perceived exertion. *Medicine and Science in Sports and Exercise* 26: 1087–1094.

Dishman, R.K., and J. Buckworth. 1996. Increasing physical activity: A quantitative synthesis. *Medicine and Science in Sports and Exercise* 28: 706–719.

Dishman, R.K., and A.L. Dunn. 1988. Exercise adherence in children and youth: Implications for adulthood. In *Exercise adherence: Its impact on public health,* edited by R.K. Dishman, pp. 155–200. Champaign, IL: Human Kinetics.

Dishman, R.K., R.P. Farquhar, and K.J. Cureton. 1994. Responses to preferred intensities of exertion in men differing in activity levels. *Medicine and Science in Sports and Exercise* 26: 783–790.

Dishman, R.K., and W.J. Ickes. 1981. Self-motivation and adherence to therapeutic exercise. *Journal of Behavioral Medicine* 4: 421–438.

Dishman, R.K., W.J. Ickes, and W.P. Morgan. 1980. Self-motivation and adherence to habitual physical activity. *Journal of Applied Social Psychology* 10: 115–131.

Dishman, R.K., R.W. Motl, R. Saunders, M. Dowda, G. Felton, D. Ward, and R.R. Pate. 2003. Enjoyment mediates increased physical activity among adolescent girls. Unpublished manuscript, The University of Georgia, Athens.

Dishman, R.K., R.W. Motl, R. Saunders, G. Felton, D. Ward, and R.R. Pate. 2003. Self-efficacy mediates the effect of a school-based physical-activity intervention among adolescent girls. Unpublished manuscript, The University of Georgia, Athens.

Dishman, R.K., B. Oldenburg, H.A. O'Neal, and R.J. Shephard. 1998. Worksite physical activity interventions. *American Journal of Preventive Medicine* 15 (4): 344–361.

Dishman, R.K., and J.F. Sallis. 1994. Determinants and interventions for physical activity and exercise. In *Physical activity, fitness and health: International proceedings and consensus statement,* edited by C. Bouchard, T. Stephens, and R.J. Shephard, pp. 214–238. Champaign, IL: Human Kinetics.

Douglas, K.A., J.L. Collins, C.W. Warren, L. Kann, R. Gold, S. Clayton, J.G. Ross, and L.J. Kolbe. 1997. Results from the 1995 National College Health Risk Behavior Survey. *Journal of American College Health* 46: 55–66.

Dunbar, C.C., R.J. Robertson, R. Baun, M.F. Blandin, K. Metz, R. Burdett, and F.L. Goss. 1992. The validity of regulating exercise intensity by ratings of perceived exertion. *Medicine and Science in Sports and Exercise* 24: 94–99.

Duncan, T.E., S.C. Duncan, and E. McAuley. 1993. The role of domain and gender-specific provisions of social relations in adherence to a prescribed exercise regimen. *Journal of Sport and Exercise Psychology* 15: 220–231.

Duncan, T.E., and E. McAuley. 1993. Social support and efficacy cognitions in exercise adherence: A latent growth curve analysis. *Journal of Behavioral Medicine* 16: 199–218.

Dunn, A.L., R.E. Andersen, and J.M. Jakicic. 1998. Lifestyle physical activity interventions: History, short- and long-term effects, and recommendations. *American Journal of Preventive Medicine* 15: 398–412.

Dunn, A.L., B.H. Marcus, J.B. Kampert, M.E. Garcia, H.W. Kohl III, and S.N. Blair. 1999. Comparison of lifestyle and structured interventions to increase physical activity and cardiorespiratory fitness: A randomized trial. *Journal of the American Medical Association* 281 (4): 327–334.

Dwyer, J., and R. Bybee. 1983. Heart rate indices of the anaerobic threshold. *Medicine and Science in Sports and Exercise* 15: 72–76.

Dzewaltowski, D.A. 1994. Physical activity determinants: A social cognitive approach. *Medicine and Science in Sports and Exercise* 26: 1395–1399.

Dzewaltowski, D.A., J.M. Noble, and J.M. Shaw. 1990. Physical activity participation: Social cognitive theory versus the theories of reasoned action and planned behavior. *Journal of Sport and Exercise Psychology* 12: 388–405.

Eden, K.B, C.T. Orleans, C.D. Mulrow, N.J. Pender, and S.M. Teutsch. 2002. Does counseling by clinicians improve physical activity? A summary of the evidence for the U.S. Preventive Services Task Force. *Annals of Internal Medicine* 137: 208–215.

Edmundson, E., G.S. Parcel, H.A. Feldman, J. Elder, C.L. Perry, C.C. Johnson, B.J. Williston, E.J. Stone, M. Yang, L. Lytle, and L. Webber. 1996. The effects of the Child and Adolescent Trial for Cardiovascular Health upon psychosocial determinants of diet and physical activity. *Preventive Medicine* 25: 442–454.

Epstein, L.H. 1998. Integrating theoretical approaches to promote physical activity. *American Journal of Preventive Medicine* 15: 257–265.

Epstein, L.H, and J.N. Roemmich. 2001. Reducing sedentary behavior: Role in modifying physical activity. *Exercise and Sport Sciences Reviews* 29 (3): 103–108.

Epstein, L.H., B.E. Saelens, M.D. Myers, and D. Vito. 1997. Effects of decreasing sedentary behaviors on activity choice in obese children. *Health Psychology* 16: 107–113.

Estabrooks, P.A. 2000. Sustaining exercise participation through group cohesion. *Exercise and Sport Sciences Reviews* 28: 63–67.

Ewart, C.K., K.J. Stewart, and R.E. Gillilan. 1986. Usefulness of self-efficacy in predicting overexertion during programmed exercise in coronary artery disease. *American Journal of Cardiology* 57: 557–561.

Ewart, C.K., C.B. Taylor, C.B. Reese, and R.F. DeBusk. 1983. Effects of early postmyocardial infarction exercise testing on self-perception and subsequent physical activity. *American Journal of Cardiology* 51: 1076–1080.

Farrell, P.A., W.K. Gates, M.G. Maksud, and W.P. Morgan. 1982. Increases in plasma b-endorphin/b-lipotropin immunoreactivity after treadmill running in humans. *Journal of Applied Physiology* 52: 1245–1249.

Fletcher, G.F., S.N. Blair, J. Blumenthal, C. Casperson, B. Chaitman, and S. Epstein. 1992. Statement on exercise: Benefits and recommendations for physical activity programs for all Americans. *Circulation* 86: 340–344.

Foreyt, J.P., and G.K. Goodrick. 1993. Evidence for success of behavior modification in weight loss and control. *Annals of Internal Medicine* 119: 698–701.

———. 1994. Impact of behavior therapy on weight loss. *American Journal of Health Promotion* 8: 466–468.

Frisch, R.E., G. Wyshak, N.L. Albright, I. Schiff, K.P. Jones, J. Witschi, E. Shiang, E. Koff, and M. Marguglio. 1985. Lower prevalence of breast cancer and cancers of the reproductive system among former college athletes compared to non-athletes. *British Journal of Cancer* 52: 885–891.

Garcia, A.W., and A.C. King. 1991. Predicting long-term adherence to aerobic exercise: A comparison of two models. *Journal of Sport and Exercise Psychology* 13: 394–410.

Gettman, L.R., M.L. Pollock, and A. Ward. 1983. Adherence to unsupervised exercise. *Physician and Sportsmedicine* 11: 56–66.

Glasgow, R.E., S.S. Bull, C. Gillette, L.M. Klesges, and D.H. Dzewaltowski. 2002. Behavior change intervention research in health care settings: A review of recent reports, with emphasis on external validity. *American Journal of Preventive Medicine* 23: 62–69.

Glasgow, R.E., T.M. Vogt, and S.M. Boles. 1999. Evaluating the public health impact of health promotion interventions: The RE-AIM framework. *American Journal of Public Health* 89: 1323–1327.

Godin, G. 1994. Theories of reasoned action and planned behavior: Usefulness for exercise promotion. *Medicine and Science in Sports and Exercise* 26: 1391–1394.

Godin, G., R. Desharnais, P. Valois, L. Lepage, J. Jobin, and R. Bradet. 1994. Differences in perceived barriers to exercise between high and low intenders: Observations among different populations. *American Journal of Health Promotion* 8: 279–285.

Godin, G., and G. Kok. 1996. The theory of planned behavior: A review of its applications to health-related behaviors. *American Journal of Health Promotion* 11: 87–98.

Godin, G., and R.J. Shephard. 1990. Use of attitude–behavior models in exercise promotion. *Sports Medicine* 10 (2) 103–121.

Godin, G., P. Valois, and R. Desharnais. 1995. Combining behavioral and motivational dimensions to identify and characterize the stages in the process of adherence to exercise. *Psychology and Health* 10: 333–344.

———. 2001. A typology of stages of adherence to exercise behavior: A cluster analysis. *Journal of Applied Social Psychology* 31: 1979–1994.

Gordon-Larsen, P., R.G. McMurray, and B.M. Popkin. 1999. Adolescent physical activity and inactivity vary by ethnicity: The National Longitudinal Study of Adolescent Health. *Journal of Pediatrics* 135: 301–306.

Hausenblaus, H.A., A.V. Carron, and D.E. Mack. 1997. Application of the theories and reasoned action and planned behavior to exercise behavior: A meta-analysis. *Journal of Sport and Exercise Psychology* 19: 36–51.

Heinzelmann, F., and R.W. Bagley. 1970. Response to physical activity programs and their effects on health behavior. *Public Health Reports* 86: 905–911.

Hensley, L.D. 2000. State of required physical education in colleges and universities. *Research Quarterly for Exercise and Sport* 71: A71–A72.

Hofstetter, C.R., M.F. Hovell, C. Macera, J.F. Sallis, V. Spry, E. Barrington, and C. Callender. 1991. Illness, injury, and correlates of aerobic exercise and walking: A community study. *Research Quarterly for Exercise and Sport* 62: 1–9.

Hovell, M.F., J.F. Sallis, C.R. Hofstetter, V.M. Spry, J.P. Elder, P. Faucher, and C.J. Caspersen. 1989. Identifying correlates of walking for exercise: An epidemiologic prerequisite for physical activity promotion. *Preventive Medicine* 18: 856–866.

Hoyt, M.F., and I.L. Janis. 1975. Increasing adherence to a stressful decision via a motivational balance-sheet procedure: A field experiment. *Journal of Personality and Social Psychology* 31: 833–839.

Jakicic, J.M., K. Clark, E. Coleman, J.E. Donnelly, J. Foreyt, E. Melanson, J. Volek, and S.L. Volpe. 2001. American College of Sports Medicine position stand: Appropriate intervention strategies for weight loss and prevention of weight regain for adults. *Medicine and Science in Sports and Exercise* 33: 2145–2156.

Jakicic, J.M., R.R. Wing, B.A. Butler, and R.J. Robertson. 1995. Prescribing exercise in multiple short bouts versus one continuous bout: Effects on adherence, cardiorespiratory fitness, and weight loss in overweight women. *International Journal of Obesity Related Metabolic Disorders* 19: 893–901.

Jakicic, J.M., C. Winters, W. Lang, and R.R. Wing. 1999. Effects of intermittent exercise and use of home exercise equipment on adherence, weight loss, and fitness in overweight women. *Journal of the American Medical Association* 282: 1554–1560.

Janis, I.L., and L. Mann. 1977. *Decision making: A psychological analysis of conflict, choice, and commitment.* New York: Free Press.

Kahn, E.B., L.T. Ramsey, R.C. Brownson, G.W. Heath, E.H. Howze, K.E. Powell, E.J. Stone, M.W. Rajab, and P. Corso. 2002. The effectiveness of interventions to increase physical activity. A systematic review. *American Journal of Preventive Medicine* 22 (4 Suppl.): 73–107.

Kann, L., S.A. Kinchen, B.I. Williams, J.G. Ross, R. Lowry, J.A. Grunbaum, and L.J. Kolbe. 2000. Youth risk behavior surveillance—United States, 1999. *Morbidity and Mortality Weekly Reports* 49 (SS-5): 1–96.

Kann, L., S.A. Kinchen, B.I. Williams, J.G. Ross, R. Lowry, C.V. Hill, J.A. Grunbaum, P.S. Blumson, J.L. Collins, and L.J. Kolbe. 1998. CDC surveillance summaries: Youth risk behavior survey—United States, 1997. *Morbidity and Mortality Weekly Reports* 47 (SS-3): 1–89.

Kann, L., C.W. Warren, W.A. Harris, J.L. Collins, B.I. Williams, J.G. Ross, and L.J. Kolbe. 1996. Youth risk behavior surveillance—United States, 1995. *Morbidity and Mortality Weekly Report* 45 (SS-4): 1–83.

Kaplan, R.M., C.J. Atkins, and S. Reinsch. 1984. Specific efficacy expectations mediate exercise compliance in patients with COPD. *Health Psychology* 3: 223–242.

Kendzierski, D., and K.J. DeCarlo. 1991. Physical activity enjoyment scale: Two validation studies. *Journal of Sport and Exercise Psychology* 13 (1): 50–64.

Kimm, S.Y., N.W. Glynn, A.M. Kriska, B.A. Barton, S.S. Kronsberg, S.R. Daniels, P.B. Crawford, Z.I. Sabry, and K. Liu. 2002. Decline in physical activity in black girls and white girls during adolescence. *New England Journal of Medicine* 347: 709–715.

King, A.C. 1994. Community and public health approaches to the promotion of physical activity. *Medicine and Science in Sports and Exercise* 26: 1405–1412.

King, A.C., C. Castro, S. Wilcox, A.A. Eyler, J.F. Sallis, and R.S. Brownson. 2000. Personal and environmental factors associated with physical inactivity among different racial-ethnic groups of U.S. middle-aged and older-aged women. *Health Psychology* 19: 354–364.

King, A.C., W.L. Haskell, H.C. Taylor, and R.F. DeBusk. 1991. Group- vs. home-based exercise training in healthy older men and women. *Journal of the American Medical Association* 266: 1535–1542.

King, A.C., C.B. Taylor, W.L. Haskell, and R.F. DeBusk. 1988. Strategies for increasing early adherence to and long-term maintenance of home-based exercise training in healthy middle-aged men and women. *American Journal of Cardiology* 61: 628–632.

King, A.L., and L.W. Frederiksen. 1984. Low-cost strategies for increasing exercise behavior: Relapse preparation training and support. *Behavior Modification* 3: 3–21.

Knapp, D.N. 1988. Behavioral management techniques and exercise promotion. In *Exercise adherence: Its impact on public health,* edited by R.K. Dishman, pp. 203–236. Champaign, IL: Human Kinetics.

Kohl, H.W., and W. Hobbs. 1998. Development of physical activity behavior among children and adolescents. *Pediatrics* 101 (Suppl. 5): 549–554.

Leonard, F.E., and G.B. Affleck. 1947. *A guide to the history of physical education.* Philadelphia: Lea and Febiger.

Leslie, E., P.B. Sparling, and N. Owen. 2001. University campus settings and the promotion of physical activity in young adults: Lessons from research in Australia and the USA. *Health Education* 3: 116–125.

Lewis, B.A., B.H. Marcus, R.R. Pate, and A.L. Dunn. 2002. Psychosocial mediators of physical activity behavior among adults and children. *American Journal of Preventive Medicine* 23 (2 Suppl.): 26–35.

Lombard, D.N., T.N. Lombard, and R.A. Winett. 1995. Walking to meet health guidelines: The effects of prompting frequency and prompt structure. *Health Psychology* 14 (2): 164–170.

Luepker, R.V., D.M. Murray, D.R. Jacobs, M.B. Mittelmark, N. Bracht, R. Carlaw, R. Crow, P. Elmer, J.R. Finnegan, A.R. Folsom, et al. 1994. Community education for cardiovascular disease prevention: Risk factor changes in the Minnesota Heart Health Program. *American Journal of Public Health* 84: 1383–1393.

Luepker, R.V., C.L. Perry, S.M. McKinlay, P.R. Nader, G.S. Parcel, E.J. Stone, L.S. Webber, J.P. Elder, H.A. Feldman, and C.C. Johnson. 1996. Outcomes of a field trial to improve children's dietary patterns and physical activity: The Child and Adolescent Trial for Cardiovascular Health. *Journal of the American Medical Association* 275: 768–776.

Marcus, B.H., C.A. Eaton, J.S. Rossi, and L.L. Harlow. 1994. Self-efficacy, decision-making and the stages of change: An integrative model of physical exercise. *Journal of Applied Social Psychology* 24: 489–508.

Marcus, B.H., N. Owen, L.H. Forsyth, N.A. Cavill, and F. Fridinger. 1998. Physical activity interventions using mass media, print media, and information technology. *American Journal of Preventive Medicine* 15: 362–378.

Marcus, B.H., V.C. Selby, R.S. Niaura, and J.S. Rossi. 1992. Self-efficacy and the stages of exercise behavior change. *Research Quarterly for Exercise and Sport* 63 (1): 60–66.

Marcus, B.H., and L.R. Simkin. 1993. The stages of exercise behavior. *Journal of Sports Medicine and Physical Fitness* 33: 83–88.

Marcus, B.H., and A.L. Stanton. 1993. Evaluation of relapse prevention and reinforcement interventions to promote exercise adherence in sedentary females. *Research Quarterly for Exercise and Sport* 64: 447–452.

Marlatt, G.A., and J. Gordon. 1985. *Relapse prevention.* New York: Guilford Press.

Martin, J.E., P.M. Dubbert, A.D. Katell, J.K. Thompson, J.R. Raczynski, M. Lake, P.O. Smith, J.S. Webster, T. Sikova, and R.E. Cohen. 1984. The behavioral control of exercise in sedentary adults: Studies 1 through 6. *Journal of Consulting Clinical Psychology* 52: 795–811.

Matsudo, V., S. Matsudo, D. Andrade, T. Araujo, E. Andrade, L.C. de Oliveira, and G. Braggion. 2002. Promotion of physical activity in a developing country: The Agita São Paulo experience. *Public Health Nutrition* 5 (1A): 253–261.

McAuley, E., and B. Blissmer. 2000. Self-efficacy determinants and consequences of physical activity. *Exercise and Sport Sciences Reviews* 28: 85–88.

Melillo, K.D., E. Williamson, S.C. Houde, M. Futrell, C.Y. Read, and M. Campasano. 2001. Perceptions of older Latino adults regarding physical fitness, physical activity, and exercise. *Journal of Gerontology Nursing* 27: 38–46.

Meyer, A., J. Nash, A. McAlister, N. Maccoby, and J.W. Farquhar. 1980. Skills training in a cardiovascular health education campaign. *Journal of Consulting and Clinical Psychology* 48: 129–142.

Motl, R.W., R.K. Dishman, G. Felton, and R.R. Pate. 2003. Self-motivation and physical activity among black and white adolescent girls. *Medicine and Science in Sports and Exercise* 35: 128–136.

Motl, R.W., R.K. Dishman, R. Saunders, M. Dowda, G. Felton, and R.R. Pate. 2001. Measuring enjoyment of physical activity in adolescent girls. *American Journal of Preventive Medicine* 21: 110–117. Erratum in *American Journal of Preventive Medicine* 2001 21: 332.

Motl, R.W., R.K. Dishman, D.S. Ward, R. Saunders, M. Dowda, G. Felton, and R.R. Pate. 2002. Examining social-cognitive determinants of intention and physical activity in adolescent girls using structural equation modeling. *Health Psychology* 21: 459–467.

The National Institute of Child Health and Human Development Study of Early Child Care and Youth Development Network. 2003. Frequency and intensity of activity of third-grade children in physical education. *Archives of Pediatrics and Adolescent Medicine* 157: 185–190.

Norman, R.M.G. 1986. The nature and correlates of health behavior. In *Health promotion studies series,* no. 2, pp. 1–163. Ottawa: Health and Welfare, Canada.

Oldridge, N.B. 1979. Compliance of past myocardial infarction patients from exercise programs. *Medicine and Science in Sports* 11: 373–375.

Oldridge, N.G., A. Donner, C.W. Buck, N.L. Jones, G.A. Anderson, J.O. Parker, D.A. Cunningham, T. Kavanagh, P.A. Rechnitzer, and J.R. Sutton. 1983. Predictive indices for dropout: The Ontario Exercise Heart Collaborative Study Experience. *American Journal of Cardiology* 51: 70–74.

Owen, N., E. Leslie, J. Salmon, and M.J. Fotheringham. 2000. Environmental determinants of physical activity and sedentary behavior. *Exercise and Sport Sciences Reviews* 28: 153–158.

Parcel, G.S., B. Simons-Morton, N.M. O'Hara, T. Baranowski, and B. Wilson. 1989. School promotion of healthful diet and physical activity: Impact on learning outcomes and self-reported behavior. *Health Education Quarterly* 16 (2): 181–199.

Pate, R.R., G.W. Heath, M. Dowda, and S.G. Trost. 1996. Associations between physical activity and other health behaviors in a representative sample of US adolescents. *American Journal of Public Health* 86 (11): 1577–1581.

Pate, R.R., M. Pratt, S.N. Blair, W.L. Haskell, C.A. Macera, C. Bouchard, D. Buchner, W. Ettinger, G.W. Heath, A.C. King, et al. 1995. Physical activity and public health. A recommendation from the Centers for Disease Control and Prevention and the American College of Sports Medicine. *Journal of the American Medical Association* 273: 402–407.

Pate, R.R., D.S. Ward, R. Saunders, G. Felton, M. Dowda, and R.K. Dishman. 2003. Increasing physical activity among adolescent girls using a school-based intervention: Project LEAP. Unpublished manuscript, The University of South Carolina, Columbia.

Pearman, S.N., R.F. Valois, R.G. Sargent, R.P. Saunders, J.W. Drane, and C.A. Macera. 1997. The impact of a required college health and physical education course on the health status of alumni. *Journal of American College Health* 4: 77–85.

Perusse, L., A. Tremblay, C. Leblanc, and C. Bouchard. 1989. Genetic and familial environmental influences on level of habitual physical activity. *American Journal of Epidemiology* 129: 1012–1022.

Pinto, B.M., H. Lynn, B.H. Marcus, J. DePue, and M.G. Goldstein. 2001. Physician-based activity counseling: Intervention effects on mediators of motivational readiness for physical activity. *Annals of Behavioral Medicine* 23: 2–10.

Pollock, M.L. 1988. Prescribing exercise for fitness and adherence. In *Exercise adherence: Its impact on public health,* edited by R.K. Dishman, pp. 259–277. Champaign, IL: Human Kinetics.

Pollock, M.L., J.F. Carroll, J.E. Graves, S.H. Leggett, R.W. Braith, M. Limacher, and J.M. Hagberg. 1991. Injuries and adherence to walk/jog and resistance programs in the elderly. *Medicine and Science in Sports and Exercise* 23: 1194–1200.

Pollock, M.L., G.A. Gaesser, J.D. Butcher, J. Despres, R.K. Dishman, B.A. Franklin, and C.E. Garber. 1998. American College of Sports Medicine position stand: Recommended quantity and quality of exercise for developing and maintaining cardiorespiratory and muscular fitness, and flexibility in healthy adults. *Medicine and Science in Sports and Exercise* 30: 975–991.

Prochaska, J.O., and C.C. DiClemente. 1983. The stages and processes of self-change in smoking: Towards an integrative model of change. *Journal of Consulting and Clinical Psychology* 51: 390–395.

Prochaska, J.O., and B.H. Marcus. 1994. The transtheoretical model: Applications to exercise. In *Advances in exercise adherence,* edited by R.K. Dishman, pp. 161–180. Champaign, IL: Human Kinetics.

Prochaska, J.O., W.F. Velicer, J.S. Rossi, M.G. Goldstein, B.H. Marcus, W. Rakowski, C. Fiore, L.L. Harlow, C.A. Redding, D. Rosenblum, and S.R. Rossi. 1994. Stages of change and decisional balance for 12 problem behaviors. *Health Psychology* 13 (1): 39–46.

Raynor, D.A., K.J. Coleman, and L.H. Epstein. 1998. Effects of proximity on the choice to be physically active or sedentary. *Research Quarterly for Exercise and Sport* 69: 99–103.

Reed, G.R. 1999. Adherence to exercise and the transtheoretical model of behavior change. In S. Bull, ed., *Adherence issues in sport and exercise,* pp. 19–45. New York: John Wiley & Sons.

Robertson, R.J., and B.J. Noble. 1997. Perception of physical exertion: Methods, mediators, and applications. *Exercise and Sport Sciences Reviews* 25: 407–452.

Rosen, C.S. 2000. Is the sequencing of change processes by stage consistent across health problems? A meta-analysis. *Health Psychology* 19 (6): 593–604.

Rosenstock, I.M. 1974. Historical origins of the health belief model. *Health Education Monographs* 2: 1–9.

Rowland, T.W. 1998. The biological basis of physical activity. *Medicine and Science in Sports and Exercise* 30 (3): 392–399.

Sallis, J.F. 1993. Epidemiology of physical activity and fitness in children and adolescents. *Critical Reviews in Food Science and Nutrition* 33: 405–408.

Sallis, J.F., K.J. Calfas, J.F. Nichols, J.A. Sarkin, M.F. Johnson, S. Caparosa, S. Thompson, and J.E. Alcaraz. 1999. Evaluation of a university course to promote physical activity: Project GRAD. *Research Quarterly for Exercise and Sport* 70 (1): 1–10.

Sallis, J.F., R.M. Grossman, R.B. Pinski, T.L. Patterson, and P.R. Nader. 1987. The development of scales to measure social support for diet and exercise behaviors. *Preventive Medicine* 16: 825–836.

Sallis, J.F., W.L. Haskell, S.P. Fortmann, K.M. Vranizan, C.B. Taylor, and D.S. Solomon. 1986. Predictors of adoption and maintenance of physical activity in a community sample. *Preventive Medicine* 15: 331–346.

Sallis, J.F., and M.F. Hovell. 1990. Determinants of exercise behavior. *Exercise and Sport Sciences Reviews* 11: 307–330.

Sallis, J.F., M.F. Hovell, and C.R. Hofstetter. 1992. Predictors of adoption and maintenance of vigorous physical activity in men and women. *Preventive Medicine* 21: 237–251.

Sallis, J.F., M.F. Hovell, C.R. Hofstetter, J.P. Elder, P. Faucher, V.M. Spry, E. Barrington, and M. Hackley. 1990. Lifetime history of relapse from exercise. *Addictive Behaviors* 15: 573–579.

Sallis, J.F., M.F. Hovell, C.R. Hofstetter, J.P. Elder, M. Hackley, C.J. Caspersen, and K.E. Powell. 1990. Distance between homes and exercise facilities related to frequency of exercise among San Diego residents. *Public Health Reports* 105: 179–185.

Sallis, J.F., R.B. Pinski, R.M. Grossman, T.L. Patterson, and P.R. Nader. 1988. The development of self-efficacy scales for health-related diet and exercise behaviors. *Health Education Research* 3: 283–292.

Sallis, J.F., J.J. Prochaska, and W.C. Taylor. 2000. A review of correlates of physical activity of children and adolescents. *Medicine and Science in Sports and Exercise* 32: 963–975.

Sallis, J.F., B.G. Simons-Morton, E.J. Stone, C.B. Corbin, L.H. Epstein, N. Faucette, R.J. Iannotti, J.D. Killen, R.C. Klesges, C.K. Petray, et al. 1992. Determinants of physical activity and interventions in youth. *Medicine and Science in Sports and Exercise* 24 (6): S248–S257.

Sanne, H.M., D. Elmfeldt, G. Grimby, C. Rydin, and L. Wilhelmsen. 1973. Exercise tolerance and physical training of non-selected patients after myocardial infarction. *Acta Medica Scandinavica* 551 (Suppl.): 1–124.

Schmitz, K., S.A. French, and R.W. Jeffery. 1997. Correlates of changes in leisure time physical activity over 2 years: The Healthy Worker Project. *Preventive Medicine* 26: 570–579.

Seip, R.L., D. Snead, E.F. Pierce, P. Stein, and A. Weltman. 1991. Perceptual responses and blood lactate concentration: Effect of training state. *Medicine and Science in Sports and Exercise* 23: 80–87.

Simkin, L.R., and A.M. Gross. 1994. Assessment of coping with high-risk situations for exercise relapse among healthy women. *Health Psychology* 13 (3): 274–277.

Sonstroem, R.J. 1988. Psychological models. In *Exercise adherence: Its impact on public health,* ed. R.K. Dishman. Champaign, IL: Human Kinetics.

Ståhl, T., A. Rutten, D. Nutbeam, A. Bauman, L. Kannas, T. Abel, G. Luschen, D.J. Rodriquez, J. Vinck, and J. van der Zee. 2001. The importance of the social environment for physically active lifestyle: Results from an international study. *Social Science and Medicine* 52: 1–10.

Steinhardt, M.A., and R.K. Dishman. 1989. Reliability and validity of expected outcomes and barriers for habitual physical activity. *Journal of Occupational Medicine* 31: 536–546.

Stephens, T., and C.L. Craig. 1990. *The well-being of Canadians: Highlights of the 1988 Campbell's Survey.* Ottawa: Canadian Fitness and Lifestyle Research Institute.

Steptoe, A., J. Wardle, R. Fuller, A. Holte, J. Justo, R. Sanderman, and L. Wichstrom. 1997. Leisure-time physical exercise: Prevalence, attitudinal correlates, and behavioral correlates among young Europeans from 21 countries. *Preventive Medicine* 26 (6): 845–854.

Stokols, D. 1992. Establishing and maintaining health environments: Toward a social ecology of health promotion. *American Psychologist* 47: 6–22.

Stone, E.J., T.L. McKenzie, G.J. Welk, and M. Booth. 1998. Effects of physical activity interventions in youth: Review and synthesis. *American Journal of Preventive Medicine* 15 (4): 298–315.

Taylor, S.E. 1999. Health behaviors. In *Health psychology,* 4th ed., pp. 50–93. Boston: McGraw-Hill.

Teraslinna, P., T. Partanen, A. Koskela, K. Partanen, and P. Oja. 1969. Characteristics affecting willingness of executives to participate in an activity program aimed at coronary heart disease prevention. *Journal of Sports Medicine and Physical Fitness* 9: 224–229.

Troped, P.J., and R.P. Saunders. 1998. Gender differences in social influence on physical activity at different stages of exercise adoption. *American Journal of Health Promotion* 13: 112–115.

Troped, P.J., R.P. Saunders, R.R. Pate, B. Reininger, J.R. Ureda, and S.J. Thompson. 2001. Associations between self-reported and objective physical environmental factors and use of a community rail-trail. *Preventive Medicine* 32 (2): 191–200.

Turk, D.C., T.E. Rudy, and P. Salovey. 1984. Health protection: Attitudes and behaviors of LPNs, teachers, and college students. *Health Psychology* 3: 189–210.

U.S. Department of Health and Human Services. 1999. *Chronic diseases and their risk factors: The nation's leading causes of death.* Atlanta: Centers for Disease Control and Prevention.

———. 1991. *Healthy people 2000: National health promotion and disease prevention objectives.* DHHS Publication No. [PHS] 91-50212. Washington, DC: Government Printing Office.

———. 2000a. *Healthy people 2010: National health promotion and disease prevention objectives.* DHHS (PHS) 91-50212. Washington, DC: Government Printing Office.

———. 2000b. *Healthy people 2010: Understanding and improving health.* 2nd ed. Washington, DC: Government Printing Office.

———. 1996. *Physical activity and health: A report of the Surgeon General.* Atlanta: U.S. Department of Health and Human Services, Centers for Disease Control, National Center for Chronic Disease Prevention and Health Promotion.

U.S. Department of Transportation. 1997. *Nationwide personal transportation survey.* Lanham, MD: Federal Highway Commission.

Vuori, I.M., P. Oja, and O. Paronen. 1994. Physically active commuting to work—Testing its potential for exercise promotion. *Medicine and Science in Sports and Exercise* 26 (7): 844–850.

Vuori, I., O. Paronen, and P. Oja. 1998. How to develop local physical activity promotion programmes with national support: The Finnish experience. *Patient Education and Counseling* 33 (Suppl. 1): S111–S119.

Wallace, J.P., J.S. Raglin, and C. Jastremski. 1995. Twelve month adherence of adults who joined a fitness program with a spouse vs. without a spouse. *Journal of Sports Medicine and Physical Fitness* 35: 206–213.

Wallace, L.S., J. Buckworth, T.E. Kirby, and W.M. Sherman. 2000. Characteristics of exercise behavior among college students: Application of social cognitive theory to predicting stage of change. *Preventive Medicine* 31: 494–505.

Wankel, L.M., and C. Thompson. 1977. Motivating people to be physically active: Self-persuasion vs. balanced decision-making. *Journal of Applied Social Psychology* 7: 332–340.

Wankel, L.M., J.K. Yardley, and J. Graham. 1985. The effects of motivational interventions upon the exercise adherence of high and low self-motivated adults. *Canadian Journal of Applied Sport Sciences* 10: 147–156.

Ward, A., and W.P. Morgan. 1984. Adherence patterns of healthy men and women enrolled in an adult exercise program. *Journal of Cardiac Rehabilitation* 4: 143–152.

Weinstein, N.D., A.J. Rothman, and S.R. Sutton. 1998. Stage theories of health behavior: Conceptual and methodological issues. *Health Psychology* 17 (3): 290–299.

Whaley, M.H., P.H. Brubaker, L.A. Kaminsky, and C.R. Miller. 1997. Validity of rating of perceived exertion during graded exercise testing in apparently healthy adults and cardiac patients. *Journal of Cardiopulmonary Research* 17 (July–August): 261–267.

Wier, L.T., and A.S. Jackson. 1992. Percent $\dot{V}O_2$max and percent HRmax reserve are not equal methods of assessing exercise intensity. *Medicine and Science in Sports and Exercise* 24 (Suppl. 5): 1057.

Wilfley, D., and K.D. Brownell. 1994. Exercise and weight maintenance. In *Advances in exercise adherence,* edited by R.K. Dishman. Champaign, IL: Human Kinetics.

Young, D.R., W.L. Haskell, C.B. Taylor, and S.P. Fortmann. 1996. Effect of community health education on physical activity knowledge, attitudes, and behavior. *American Journal of Epidemiology* 144: 264–274.

Web Sites

http://apps.nccd.cdc.gov/DNPAProg. This is the site of the State-based Physical Activity Program Directory of the Division of Nutrition and Physical Activity of the CDC's National Center for Chronic Disease Prevention and Health Promotion. It provides information about physical activity programs involving state departments of health.

www.cdc.gov/nccdphp/dnpa/physical/recommendations.htm. This site, maintained by the Division of Nutrition and Physical Activity of the CDC's National Center for Chronic Disease Prevention and Health Promotion, provides evidence-based recommendations for effective population-level interventions to promote physical activity from the *Guide to Community Preventive Services*.

www.cdc.gov/mmwr/preview/mmwrhtml/rr5018a1.htm. This page contains the summary report of the Task Force on Community Preventive Services sponsored by the U.S. Department of Health and Human Services in collaboration with the CDC.

www.re-aim.org. This page describes the RE-AIM (reach, efficacy, adoption, implementation, maintenance) framework designed to guide judgments by researchers, practitioners, and policy makers about the potential impact of behavioral interventions on public health.

Glossary

absolute intensity—Work rate expressed as an absolute value that is the same for all people, for example, running at 6 mi/h (9.7 km/h).

absolute risk—The incidence rate of disease, injury, or death in a group.

abstinence violation effect—When a temporary slip or lapse during an attempt to change a habit is catastrophized by the person into feelings of total failure, lost confidence, and a subsequent relapse to the past habit.

accelerometer—Mechanical device that measures the acceleration and thus movement of the body in one or more planes through use of transducers.

acetylcholine—Neurotransmitter at cholinergic synapses that causes cardiac inhibition, vasodilation, gastrointestinal peristalsis, and other parasympathetic effects; also acts in an excitatory manner between motor neurons and skeletal muscles.

activity limitations—Problems in performance of everyday functions such as communication, self-care, mobility, learning, and behavior.

acute exercise—A single session of exercise, typically short but that can last for 4 h or more (e.g., a marathon).

acute-phase response—Early immune response to an infection, signaled by pro-inflammatory cytokines secreted by monocytes and inflammatory proteins produced by the liver and commonly followed by transient leukocytosis.

adaptive immunity—Acquired memory of the immune system that enhances specific recognition and defense against an antigen, permitting a quicker and larger immune response upon a subsequent exposure.

adherence—In medicine, faithfully following an agreed upon plan of treatment, such as a person's continuation in an exercise program. Otherwise, maintenance of a self-initiated change in behavior.

adhesion molecule—A homing receptor on a lymphocyte that regulates transient adhesion to the blood vascular endothelium. Some examples are called L-selectin, LFA-1, VLA-4, and CD44.

adipose—Composed of fat cells.

adoption of physical activity—Behavioral and cognitive components, including some degree of psychological commitment, of beginning regular, purposeful, structured physical activity.

adrenal cortex—The outer covering of the adrenal gland, which is adjacent to the kidney and secretes glucocorticoid, mineralocorticosteroid, and sex hormones.

adrenaline—See *epinephrine*.

adrenal medulla—The inner core of the adrenal gland; secretes epinephrine, norepinephrine, and enkephalins.

adrenergic receptors—Cells or fibers of the autonomic or central nervous system that use epinephrine as their neurotransmitter.

adrenocorticotropic hormone (ACTH)—A hormone released by the anterior lobe of the hypophysis (anterior pituitary) that controls the production and release of hormones of the adrenal cortex.

afferent nerve—A neural axon that carries nerve impulses away from a sensory organ to the central nervous system.

α_1-receptors—A subclass of α-adrenergic receptors that are widespread, with clinically important concentrations in the liver, heart, vascular, intestinal, and genitourinary smooth muscle and in the central and peripheral nervous systems.

α_2-receptors—A subclass of α-adrenergic receptors found on pancreatic beta cells, platelets, and vascular smooth muscle, as well as both pre- and postsynaptically in the central and peripheral nervous systems.

alpha wave activity—Brain wave activity in the range of 8 to 12 Hz, commonly described as relaxed wakefulness.

amygdala—A group of nuclei located in the limbic system that is involved in the control of appropriate behavior for social situations, emotional memory, and the generation of fear and anger.

angina pectoris—A paroxysmal thoracic pain with a feeling of suffocation and impending death, most often due to anoxia of the myocardium, that is precipitated by effort or excitement.

angiography—Radiographic visualization of blood vessels.

angiotensin I—A physiologically inactive peptide formed from angiotensinogen by the enzyme renin.

angiotensin II—Formed by angiotensin-converting enzyme (ACE) from biologically inactive angiotensin I. Angiotensin II causes contraction of vascular smooth muscle and thus increases blood pressure and stimulates the release of aldosterone from the adrenal gland.

angiotensin-converting enzyme (ACE)—The enzyme that converts angiotensin I to angiotensin II in the lungs by removing two amino acide residues.

angiotensinogen—A peptide produced by the liver that is converted to angiotensin I by renin.

antibody—A protein secreted by plasma cells of the immune system that protects against a specific antigen.

antigen-presenting cell—A cell, such as a macrophage or a dendritic cell, that engulfs antigens and presents them to B or T lymphocytes in a recognizable form (e.g., in an MHC class II molecule).

antioxidant—An enzyme or other organic substance, such as vitamin E or beta-carotene, that is capable of counteracting the damaging effects of oxidation in animal tissue.

anxiety—A response to a perceived threat that consists of feelings of tension, apprehension, and nervousness; unpleasant thoughts or worries; and physiological changes.

anxiety disorder—A mental illness characterized by apprehension or worry that is accompanied by restlessness, muscular tension, elevated heart rate, and breathlessness. Anxiety disorders include phobias, panic disorders, obsessive-compulsive disorders, and generalized anxiety disorder.

anxiolytic—Having the effect of decreasing anxiety.

apoprotein—One of a class of regulatory proteins that combine with enzymes and lipoproteins to regulate their actions.

arteriosclerosis—Induration, or hardening, of arteries.

assistive technology—Under the Assistive Technology Act of 1998 (Public Law 105-394), technology to be utilized in "any item, piece of equipment, or product system, whether acquired commercially, modified, or customized, that is used to increase, maintain, or improve the functional capabilities of individuals with disabilities."

atheroma—A fatty deposit in the inner lining of an artery.

atherosclerosis—Arteriosclerotic disease characterized by deposits of fatty plaques on the inner linings of medium and large arteries.

attitude—An evaluation of and reaction to an object, person, event, or idea, which includes cognitive, affective, and behavioral components.

attributable risk—See *risk difference*.

autonomic nervous system (ANS)—Part of the peripheral nervous system that innervates smooth muscle, cardiac muscle, and glands; composed of the sympathetic, parasympathetic, and enteric divisions.

Ayurveda—Sanskrit for "knowledge of living." The ancient Indian system of medicine.

basophil—Granulocyte containing heparin and histamine that is involved in hypersensitivity responses to an antigen (e.g., allergies). Other than having a segmented nucleus, a basophil's shape and function are similar to a mast cell.

behavioral epidemiology—The observation and study of behaviors, including physical inactivity, that lead to disease, injury, or premature death and the distribution of these behaviors.

behavioral intention—What a person aims to do or accomplish; intention is incremental (e.g., It is somewhat likely that I will do something) rather than dichotomous (e.g., I will or won't do something).

behaviorism—A field of psychology that developed out of learning theory that describes behavior through the associations among observable stimulus, response, and outcome, with no role for personality or mental states in predicting and describing behavior.

beliefs—Expectations, convictions, or opinions.

β_1-receptors—A subclass of β-adrenergic receptors equally sensitive to epinephrine and norepinephrine. They are found in the heart, in juxtoglomerular cells in the kidney, and in the central and peripheral nervous systems.

bias—Any deviation of results or inferences from the truth, or a process leading to such deviations. Bias can result from several sources: systematic variation in measurement from the true value (systematic error), flaws in study design, flawed data, and so on.

biological plausibility—One of Mill's canons, which states that the observed association between a risk factor and a disease outcome must be explainable by existing knowledge about possible biological mechanisms of the disease in order to establish causality.

B lymphocyte—A short-lived lymphocyte not derived in the thymus gland that is a key cell of humoral immunity and a precursor of the plasma cell that secretes immunoglobulins.

body composition—Proportions of fat, water, protein, and mineral that constitute body mass.

body mass index (BMI)—The ratio of body weight (in kilograms) to height (in meters) squared. Individuals with a BMI of 25 to 29.9 are considered overweight, whereas individuals with a BMI of 30 or more are considered obese.

bone involution—The loss of endosteal bone at a faster rate than exosteal bone is deposited, which results in osteopenia, a major risk factor of osteoporosis, and usually begins around age 30 or 40.

breast carcinoma in situ—A cancer that is confined to lobules (milk glands) or ducts (milk passages) and has not spread to surrounding fat cells in the breast or to other organs.

calcitonin—A polypeptide hormone produced by C cells of the thyroid gland that causes a reduction of calcium ions in the blood, inhibits bone resorption, and increases vitamin D receptors in osteoblasts.

calorimetry—A method of measuring energy expenditure by recording increases in temperature in a controlled environment.

cancer—A family of related diseases that result from uncontrolled growth and spread of abnormal cells, which usually become a malignant tumor.

carcinogen—That which causes cancer.

carcinoma—A malignant tumor of epithelial cells.

cardiac arrhythmia—Any variation from the normal rhythm of the heartbeat, including sinus arrhythmia, premature beats, heart block, ventricular fibrillation, and so on.

cardiorespiratory fitness—The capacity of the cardiorespiratory system to take up and use oxygen; the capability to carry out activities that use large muscle groups at moderate intensities, which use oxygen for the production of energy and which can be sustained for more than a few minutes.

case–control study—A research design in which people with a disease or injury or who have died from that condition (i.e., cases) are compared with healthy people (i.e., controls) on the prevalence of a suspected causal risk factor, after matching the cases with controls on exposure to other key risk factors that might be confounders.

catecholamines—Class of synaptic neurotransmitters, including dopamine, norepinephrine, and epinephrine, that also act as hormones and that contain a single amine group (monoamines).

cause of death—A single underlying condition to which a death is attributed, based on information reported on a death certificate and the international rules for selecting the underlying cause of death from reported conditions.

cerebrovascular disease—Any of a variety of diseases that affect the arteries that supply the brain via the obstructive effects of atherosclerosis.

chemokines—A class of pro-inflammatory cytokines released by phagocytes, endothelial cells, fibroblasts, and smooth muscle cells in response to bacteria, viruses, and cell damage at the site of infection; they chemically attract and activate leukocytes in infected tissue.

chemotactic—Facilitating the attraction or repulsion of a cell along a chemical concentration gradient.

cholesterol—The most abundant steroid found in animal tissue. A waxy constituent of cell membranes, hormones, and atheroma.

cholesterol ester transfer protein (CETP)—A protein that regulates the transfer of cholesterol ester from HDL-C to LDL-C, VLDL-C, and chylomicrons in exchange for triglycerides.

chronic exercise—Bouts of exercise that are repeated on a fairly regular basis over a period of time; exercise training or regular exercise that is defined by the type, intensity, duration, weekly frequency, and time period (e.g., weeks, months) of activity.

chylomicron—A very low density lipoprotein, composed of about 95% triglycerides, produced by the small intestine.

cingulate cortex—A band of limbic cortex lying above the corpus collosum and along the lateral walls of the longitudinal fissure that separates the hemispheres of the cerebrum.

clinical trial—A research study conducted with patients, usually to evaluate a new treatment.

clonal expansion—The proliferation of activated, genetically identical B lymphocytes and T lymphocytes; enables the body to have sufficient numbers of antigen-specific lymphocytes to mount an effective immune response.

coagulability—The tendency of a liquid to thicken or to be transformed to a solid, such as the clotting of blood.

cognition—Mental process of knowing, including aspects such as awareness, perception, reasoning, and judgment.

cognitive-behavior therapy—A technique of behavioral change, based on principles from learning theory, that focuses on modifying the cognitions and behaviors related to the target behavior and on cues and reinforcers of the target behavior.

cohort—A large group of individuals identified by a common characteristic that is studied over a period of time as part of a scientific or medical investigation. The term *cohort* is derived from one of the 10 divisions of a Roman legion, consisting of 300 to 600 soldiers.

collagen—The fibrous protein that makes up connective tissue, including bone.

colony stimulating factors—Protein–carbohydrate compounds found in the blood that stimulate the proliferation of bone marrow cells and the formation of colonies of granulocytes and/or macrophages.

complement system—About 20 proteins that augment the action of phagocytic cells by opsonization.

compliance—Following a prescribed standard of behavior, usually related to immediate and short-term health advice to alleviate symptoms, such as taking a specific regimen of medications; a sense of coerced obedience.

confidence interval—A range of values for a variable of interest constructed to have a specified probability of including the true value of the variable.

confounder—An extraneous factor that is not a consequence of exposure to the risk factor under study nor an experimental manipulation but that affects the outcome and thus distorts the study's findings. Confounders are determinants or correlates of the outcome under study that are unequally distributed among the exposed and unexposed individuals, making it difficult or impossible to interpret the relationships among the other variables.

confounding—A situation in which the effects of two or more processes are not separate; the distortion of the apparent effect of an exposure or risk brought about by association with other factors that can influence the outcome.

consequence—Abstract or concrete event that follows a target behavior, either immediately or after some time, and can either reinforce and thus increase the frequency of the target behavior or punish and thus decrease the frequency of the target behavior.

consistency—One of Mill's canons, which states that, to establish causality, the observed association between a risk factor and a disease outcome must always be observed when the risk factor is present.

construct—An abstract idea developed to describe the relationship among phenomena or for other research purposes that exists theoretically but is not directly observable.

control—In experimental research, a group or condition that does not experience the treatment that the researcher is studying, for the sake of comparison with the treatment groups or conditions.

coronary heart disease (CHD)—Atherosclerosis of the medium-sized and large arteries that supply the myocardium (heart muscle).

cortical bone—The superficial thin layer of compact bone found in the shafts of adult long bones; the nontrabecular portion of bone that consists largely of small canals through which blood vessels pass, called osteons, surrounded by concentric layers, or lamellae, of bone.

corticotropin-releasing hormone (CRH)—Hormone released by the paraventricular nucleus (cells separating the lateral ventricles of the brain) of the anterior hypothalamus that controls the diurnal rhythms of adrenocorticotropic hormone release.

cortisol—A steroid hormone; the major glucocorticoid secreted by the adrenal cortex, which plays a primary role in the stress response and in central nervous dysregulation associated with mood disorders and is also involved in stimulating the formation and storage of glycogen and maintenance of blood glucose.

C-reactive protein—An acute phase protein that binds to some bacteria and fungi, serving as both an opsonin and a complement catalyst during inflammation.

cross-sectional study—Research plan in which data are collected at a single point in time and partici-

pants are classified by predictor (independent) and outcome (dependent) variables.

cytokine—Any of a class of antibody proteins released by cells that mediate cellular actions of other cells. Lymphokines and interleukins are specific types found in the immune system.

cytolytic—Pertaining to dissolution of a cell.

cytotoxic—Relating to or producing injury or death of a cell.

death rate—The number of deaths in a population in a given period divided by the total population at the middle of that period.

decisional balance—One of the three components of the transtheoretical model of stages of change; the balance between the perceived benefits of the target behavior and the perceived costs.

dependent variable—A measurable outcome that is influenced by an independent variable.

descriptive epidemiology—The assessment of variation in a behavior or disease prevalence by age, sex, race or ethnicity, health status, geographic location, and so on.

desirable weight—Body weight judged by normative (i.e., averaged among people) weights and associated with socially defined attractiveness, physical performance, or risks for disease and mortality.

determinant—In exercise behavior research, a variable that has an established, reproducible association or predictive relationship with an outcome variable; a correlate, but not necessarily a confirmed cause.

diabetes mellitus—A group of diseases characterized by high levels of blood glucose resulting from defects in insulin production, insulin action, or both.

diapedesis—Transmigration of the leukocyte through the vascular wall into the infected tissue; the last step of extravasation.

disability—The interactions between individuals with health conditions and barriers in their environment.

disease—An interruption, cessation, or disorder of body organs, systems, or functions, usually having a known cause, distinct signs and symptoms, or morphology.

distraction hypothesis—Explanation for the beneficial psychological effects of exercise as time out from worrisome thoughts and daily stressors during exercise.

dopamine—Neurotransmitter that is the precursor for norepinephrine and epinephrine.

dose response—One of Mill's canons, which states that to establish causality the risk of disease associated with a risk factor must be greater with stronger exposure to the risk factor.

doubly labeled water (DLW)—A method of estimating free-living energy expenditure by having subjects ingest a measured amount of water labeled with stable isotopes ($^2H^1H^{18}O$). CO_2 production, and hence energy use, is estimated from the difference in the elimination rates from the body of ^{18}O (which is eliminated as both water and carbon dioxide) and ^2H (which is eliminated only as water) from urine samples obtained over a 7- to 14-day period.

down-regulation—Tolerance developed after repeated administration of a pharmacologically or physiologically active substance or in response to excessively high levels of a substance, which is often characterized by an initial decrease in the affinity of receptors for the substance and a subsequent decrease in the number of receptors.

dual X-ray absorptiometry (DXA)—A radiographic method of determining bone mineral and fat mass by measuring the uptake of radiation energy during a body scan.

dysregulation—Disruption in self-regulation.

dysthymia—Mild, chronic form of major depression.

ecological fallacy—False conclusion that the co-occurrence of a risk factor with a health marker observed in an ecological study indicates cause and effect.

ecological study—Specific type of cross-sectional investigation in which the incidence of a risk factor is observed concurrently with the incidence of a health outcome in a given geographic region.

effectiveness—The ability of an intervention or method to work in other settings, to be practically applied outside of a laboratory setting to yield a successful outcome.

effect modifier—A variable that changes the association between a risk factor and morbidity or mortality. For example, overweight people who are physically fit have less CHD risk than similarly overweight people who are unfit. Thus, physical fitness modifies or moderates the effect of overweight on CHD.

effect size—Measure of the strength of an association or a relationship, often considered an indication of practical significance; the difference in the outcome for the average subject who received a treatment from the outcome for the average subject who did not.

efferent nerve—A neural axon that carries nerve impulses away from the central nervous system to an organ.

efficacy—The ability of an intervention or method to do what it was intended to do.

elastin—The main structural protein that makes up elastic fibers.

electroencephalogram (EEG)—A recording of gross electrical activity of the brain using large electrodes placed on the scalp in a standardized pattern.

electromyogram (EMG)—A recording of the gross electrical activity of muscle contraction.

electrophysiological measure—Measure of neural activity in the brain using electrodes positioned in the brain cortex or in specific regions of brain neurons to record electrical potentials during behavior or in response to stress.

embolism—The sudden blocking of an artery by a clot or foreign material that has been brought to the site by blood flow.

emotion—An intense mental state that arises subjectively rather than through conscious effort and is accompanied by physiological changes related to autonomic activation; brief responses of negative or positive feelings.

endogenous—Produced within the body.

endorphin—Endogenous opioid peptide that can act as a neurotransmitter, neuromodulator, and hormone.

endorphin hypothesis—Proposition that the mood enhancement associated with exercise is due to actions of endorphins, which are secreted during exercise.

endosteum—The layer of vascular connective tissue lining the medullary cavity of bone.

endothelium—The layer of flat cells that line the cavities of the heart and blood vessels and the serous cavities of the body.

enkephalin—An endogenous opioid, a class of compounds that exert effects like those of opium, such as reduced pain sensitivity.

enteric nervous system—The branch of the autonomic nervous system that regulates the intestines.

environmental factors—The policies, systems, social contexts, and physical barriers or facilitators that affect a person's participation in activities, including work, school, leisure, and community events.

eosinophil—Antiparasitic leukocyte.

epidemic—A disease that has a greater than expected frequency in a population during a specific period of time.

epidemiology—The study of the distribution and determinants of health-related states and events in the population.

epinephrine—A compound secreted by the adrenal medulla and by postganglionic sympathetic nerves that acts as a hormone and as a neurotransmitter and plays an important role in preparing to respond to stress. Also known as *adrenaline*.

esterification (of cholesterol)—Removal of water from cholesterol by removing the OH from its acid and alcohol groups. Esterified cholesterol is hydrophobic (i.e., repels water molecules) and moves to the core of the HDL-C molecule, creating a concentration gradient that augments transfer of cholesterol from cell membranes (e.g., endothelial cells) or other lipoproteins to the surface of the HDL-C molecule.

etiology—The causes, development, and pathophysiology of a disease.

exercise—A subset of physical activity consisting of planned, structured, repetitive bodily movements with the purpose of improving or maintaining one or more components of physical fitness or health.

exercise prescription—Recommendation for a specific exercise mode, intensity, duration, and frequency per week to meet specific goals.

exosteum—Bone cells outside the central medullary cavity.

extravasation—Margination and emigration of leukocytes from the blood across vessel walls into infected tissues.

fibrillation—Rapid, asynchronous twitching of individual muscle fibers, commonly in the atria or ventricles of the heart, which causes irregular pulse and can lead to sudden cardiac death.

fibrin—The insoluble protein formed from fibrinogen by the proteolytic action of thrombin during the normal clotting of blood. Fibrin forms the essential portion of the blood clot.

fibrinogenesis—Conversion of the blood protein fibrinogen to fibrin in the presence of ionized calcium by the hydrolytic protease enzyme thrombin.

fibrinolysis—Solubilization of fibrin in blood clots, chiefly by the proteolytic action of plasmin.

fibroblast—A cell that produces connective tissue such as fibrin.

fibrosis—Formation of excessive fibrous tissue.

5-hydroxyindoleacetic acid (5-HIAA)—A major metabolite of serotonin.

flexibility—The range of motion at a specific joint or linked joints during both passive and dynamic movements.

free radical—A chemically active atom or molecular fragment containing a chemical charge due to an excess or deficiency of electrons. Free radicals seek to receive or release electrons to achieve a more stable configuration, a process that can damage the large molecules within cells.

functional magnetic resonance imaging (FMRI)—Method of determining brain activity that applies magnetic resonance to find out which parts of the brain are activated by various types of physical sensations or motor activity.

galanin—Amino acid peptide neurotransmitter that hyperpolarizes noradrenergic neurons and inhibits locus coeruleus firing in vitro.

gamma-aminobutyric acid (GABA)—Major inhibitory transmitter in the nervous system.

generalized anxiety disorder (GAD)—Disorder characterized by excessive or pathologic worry about multiple concerns, exaggerated vigilance, and somatic symptoms of stress and anxiety such as muscular tension.

genotype—The sum of all of the genetic information in an organism.

gestational diabetes—A form of glucose intolerance that occurs in some women during pregnancy. Gestational diabetes occurs more frequently among African Americans, Hispanic Americans, and Native Americans than among non-Hispanic white Americans. It is also more common among obese women and women with a family history of diabetes.

glucocorticoid—Class of hormones that affect carbohydrate metabolism and are released by the adrenal cortex, for example, in response to stress.

goal setting—Process by which specific plans are established in order to achieve a desired outcome.

granulocyte—Any of a class of mature leukocytes having a lobed nucleus, including neutrophils, eosinophils, and basophils.

gymnastics—Subdiscipline of ancient Greek medicine based on therapeutic exercise. It persisted through the European Renaissance.

health—Optimal functioning of an organism without signs of disease or abnormality.

health education—Programs and strategies designed to promote health behavior through educational programs and mass media campaigns.

health-related physical fitness—Components of physical fitness that have been empirically associated with overall health and ability to perform daily tasks and activities, including cardiorespiratory fitness, body composition, flexibility, muscular strength and endurance, and metabolic variables such as glucose tolerance.

hematocrit—Relative volume of blood cells occupied by erythrocytes. An average figure for humans is 45%.

hemispheric asymmetry—Differences in neural circuits between the left and right hemispheres of the brain.

hemostasis—The stoppage of blood flow through a vessel or body part, such as clotting to stop hemorrhage.

hepatic lipoprotein lipase (HPL)—Enzyme that catalyzes the hydrolysis of HDL-C in the liver by the hydrolysis of its triglyceride and phospholipid content. Its net effect is the conversion of HDL2 back to HDL-C in the liver.

high-density lipoprotein cholesterol (HDL-C)—A fraction, about one fourth to one third, of the total blood cholesterol. HDL-C is known as the "good" cholesterol because a high level of it seems to protect against heart attack. Basic studies suggest that HDL-C tends to carry cholesterol away from the arteries and back to the liver to be disposed from the body.

high-risk situation—Any situation that challenges confidence in one's ability to maintain a healthy behavior or to abstain from an unhealthy behavior.

hippocampus—Portion of the limbic system thought to be important in learning and memory.

Hoffmann reflex—A neuromuscular reflex which provides a measure of the efficacy of synaptic transmission between type Ia afferent sensory nerve fibers and alpha motor neurons in the spinal cord. Also termed the H-reflex.

homocysteine—A natural intermediate amino acid formed during the metabolism of an essential amino acid, methionine. A risk factor for atherosclerosis.

homocystinuria—Abnormally high levels of homocysteine because of deficiencies in metabolic enzymes.

hydrolysis—Splitting of a compound into two or more simpler compounds by water.

hygiene—Science or practice of health and its maintenance.

hypercholesterolemia—High levels of blood cholesterol; a risk factor for cardiovascular disease.

hyperglycemia—An abnormally high level of sugar in the blood.

hyperlipidemia—An elevated concentration of any or all of the lipids in the plasma, such as cholesterol, triglycerides, and lipoproteins.

hypertension—Persistently high arterial blood pressure, which may have no known cause (essential or idiopathic hypertension) or may be associated with other primary diseases (secondary hypertension). This condition is considered a risk factor for the development of heart disease, peripheral vascular disease, stroke, and kidney disease.

hypothalamic-pituitary-adrenocortical axis (HPA axis)—The hypothalamus, pituitary gland, and adrenal cortex.

hypothalamus—Part of the diencephalon that controls vegetative functions, regulates hormone balance, and plays a role in emotional behavior.

immune system—An integrated network of molecules, cells, tissues, and organs that defends an organism against infection by foreign substances (e.g., bacteria and viruses) and against mutated native cells (i.e., tumors) and that also helps to repair damaged tissues and to clean up the debris of dead cells.

immunoglobulin (Ig)—Any of a class of antibody proteins secreted by plasma cells formed from B lymphocytes. Immunoglobulins are classified by their relative basal levels in human blood: IgG, 80%; IgA,

10% to 15%; IgM, 5% to 10%; IgD, less than 0.1%; IgE, less than 0.01%.

immunology—The study of the immune system.

impaired fasting glucose—A prediabetic condition, possibly reversible, in which the fasting blood sugar level is elevated to between 110 and 125 mg/dl after an overnight fast but is not high enough to be classified as diabetes.

impaired glucose tolerance (IGT)—A prediabetic condition, possibly reversible, in which the blood sugar level is elevated to between 140 and 199 mg/dl after a 2-h oral glucose tolerance test but is not high enough to be classified as diabetes.

impairment—A chronic physiological, psychological, or anatomical abnormality of bodily structure or function caused by disease or injury.

incident cases—New cases of a disease or condition that occur in a given population during a time frame of interest.

independence—Dissociated from confounders.

independent variable—A measurable factor that is experimentally manipulated, or fluctuates naturally, to influence an outcome (i.e., the dependent variable).

indirect calorimetry—A method of estimating energy expenditure based on the known relationship of oxygen consumption with the caloric output of burning fat, carbohydrate, and protein.

inflammation—A localized response of increased blood flow and capillary permeability in response to injury or an abnormal physical, chemical, or biological stimulus, associated with an influx of neutrophils and macrophages and secretion of cytokines to remove the source of infection and repair the injury. Signs and symptoms include redness, heat, swelling, pain, and impaired function.

injury—Damage to tissue caused by the exchange of kinetic, thermal, chemical, electrical, or radiation energy at levels intolerable to tissue, or the deprivation of oxygen due to suffocation.

innate immunity—Natural, nonspecific recognition and defense against an antigen by the immune system without prior exposure.

insular cortex—An island of involuted cerebral cortex contained beneath the sylvian fissure near the temporal lobe; believed important in regulating emotional responses, especially cardiovascular responses.

integrin molecules—Adhesion receptors expressed on leukocytes that bind with adhesion molecules on the endothelial surface; assists homing of lymphocytes to specific lymphoid sites so that leukocytes stop rolling and become loosely attached to the endothelium, forming the marginal pool.

intensity—How hard a person exerts during physical activity, expressed as force (e.g., Newton-meters), the rate of power output (e.g., watts), as a value relative to maximal capacity (e.g., 70% of maximal aerobic capacity), or as perceived exertion.

interferon-gamma (IFN-γ)—A cytokine produced by activated lymphocytes that plays a major role in antimicrobial, antitumor, and antiviral responses.

interleukins—Generic name for a category of cytokines that are produced by leukocytes and other cell types. Particularly important in cytokine networks that regulate inflammatory and immune responses.

interleukin-1 (IL-1)—A lymphokine and polypeptide hormone produced mainly by macrophages that activates acute-phase responses during the first few hours of infection or tissue damage. Such responses include fever, redistribution of amino acids (including muscle protein catabolism), and increased liver production of antimicrobial plasma proteins. IL-1 also activates the cascade of humoral and cellular immune responses against infection.

interleukin-2 (IL-2)—A lymphokine and polypeptide hormone produced mainly by activated lymphocytes whose main functions are activating other humoral immune cells, clonal expansion of T lymphocytes, increased expression of its receptors, and stimulating the release of other cytokines such as IFN.

interleukin-6 (IL-6)—A lymphokine and polypeptide hormone produced mainly by activated lymphocytes and blood monocytes. Its main functions are to stimulate B and T cells and to induce acute-phase protein synthesis during acute-phase responses, thus regulating the anti-inflammatory response.

interleukin-8 (IL-8)—A chemokine secreted by macrophages and epithelial cells in damaged tissue; attracts neutrophils and fibroblasts involved with healing wounds.

interleukin-10 (IL-10)—An anti-inflammatory cytokine produced by T_{H-2} lymphocytes.

interleukin-12 (IL-12)—A cytokine secreted by macrophages and B cells. Activates T_{H-1} and cytotoxic lymphocytes and natural killer cells.

International Classification of Diseases (ICD-10)—A classification of the nature of illness and injuries, developed by the World Health Organization.

International Classification of Functioning, Disability and Health (ICF)—The World Health Organization's conceptual and coding framework for describing the functioning and disability associated with a person's health condition.

intima—Innermost lining, usually referring to the endothelium of arteries.

invasive breast carcinoma—Cancer cells that spread in the breast and to other parts of the body.

in vitro—Referring to a biological test or procedure done outside the body, as in a laboratory dish.

in vivo—Within a living body, usually in reference to a test or procedure done with intact, live subjects.

ischemia—A low oxygen state, or hypoxia, in the tissue, usually due to obstruction of the arterial blood supply or inadequate blood flow.

isomorphic—Referring to an animal model of disease that evokes the same features as the human disease, which abate after administration of drugs that are clinically useful in humans; the features generated may not have the same etiology or course of development as in the human disease.

ketosis—A toxic, acidotic state resulting from abnormal glucose metabolism, common in uncontrolled diabetes, that leads to cell damage, especially in small blood vessels and nerves.

kyphosis—Exaggeration of the normal posterior curve of the thoracic spine, often caused by compression fractures of the vertebrae.

latency—Length of time between the application of a stimulus and the response.

lecithin—Yellowish or brownish waxy phospholipid that is an essential component of cells and that yields two fatty acids when hydrolyzed.

lecithin:cholesterol acyltransferase (LCAT)—Enzyme that catalyzes the esterification of free cholesterol and the transfer of a free fatty acid from a phospholipid (lecithin) located on the shell of an HDL-C molecule to another cholesterol molecule.

leukocyte—A white blood cell differentiated from stem cells in bone marrow and lymphoid tissue.

leukocytosis—An abnormally high level of leukocytes, most commonly neutrophils, circulating in the blood in response to infection or stress.

lipoprotein—Compound containing lipid (e.g., triglyceride and cholesterol) and protein that is soluble in blood.

lipoprotein lipase (LPL)—Enzyme that catalyzes the hydrolysis of lipoproteins and regulates the concentration of HDL2 in plasma. Increased LPL activity increases the hydrolysis of VLDL and chylomicrons, increasing the formation of lower-density lipoprotein remnants that can be cleared by the liver and can yield cholesterol more easily to HDL-C.

locus coeruleus—Located in the pons, the major brain nucleus for the production of norepinephrine; it has a major role in inhibition of spontaneous firing in areas of the brain that it innervates.

low-density lipoprotein cholesterol (LDL-C)—A fraction of total blood cholesterol that normally circulates in the blood. However, when too much LDL-C is present, it can slowly build up in the walls of the arteries that feed the heart and brain. Together with other substances, it can form a thick, hard deposit called a plaque that can block those arteries.

lymph—A clear, sometimes yellowish fluid containing leukocytes (mainly lymphocytes) collected from bodily tissues and carried through lymphatic vessels and lymph nodes to the venous blood circulation via the thoracic duct.

lymphocyte—A type of leukocyte differentiated from stem cells in lymphatic tissue such as lymph nodes, spleen, thymus gland, tonsils, Peyer's patches, and bone marrow. Lymphocytes make up 20% to 30% of leukocytes in the blood.

lymphoid—Pertaining to the lymph, lymphatic tissue, or the lymphatic system.

lymphokine—Any of a class of cytokines secreted by lymphocytes that augment cellular immunity by activating monocytes, macrophages, lymphocytes, and natural killer cells.

lymph system—Coordinated system composed mainly of lymph, lymphatic tissues (e.g., lymph nodes, spleen, thymus gland, tonsils, Peyer's patches, and bone marrow), lymphocytes, and lymphokines.

lysis—Destruction of a cell.

macrophage—A relatively long-lived phagocytic cell of mammalian tissues derived from blood monocytes.

maintenance—Sustaining a regular exercise program for a specific period of time, usually at least six months.

major depression—One of two major categories of mood disorders (the other being manic-depressive disorder) characterized by depressed mood or loss of interest or pleasure and other behavioral and psychological symptoms.

manic-depressive disorder—One of two major categories of mood disorders (the other being major depression) characterized by periods of depression alternating with periods of elevated mood and associated behavior.

marginal pool—Sequestration of leukocytes in blood vessels by transient adhesion to endothelial cells.

margination—Movement of circulating leukocytes to the edge of the bloodstream, thereby increasing their contact with endothelial cells that line the vessels; facilitates extravasation.

mast cell—Granular, basophilic, connective-tissue cell that contains heparin and histamine and is involved in inflammatory responses, especially in the upper-respiratory system.

maximal aerobic power—The maximal amount of oxygen that the body can take up and use.

mediator—Intervening causal variable necessary to complete a cause–effect pathway between an intervention and physical activity, or a variable that transmits the effects of another variable on physical activity.

melancholia—A severe form of major depressive episode. Key features are a pervasive loss of pleasure or interest in pleasurable activities, dark mood that is worse in the morning, early morning awakening, psychomotor retardation or agitation, weight loss, and extreme feelings of guilt.

melatonin—Hormone released by the pineal gland in a true circadian rhythm that is involved in the sleep–wake cycle.

menarche—The onset of pubertal menstruation.

menopause—Permanent cessation of menses.

messenger RNA—RNA produced by transcription that reflects the exact nucleotide sequence of the genetically active DNA; it carries the code for a particular protein from the nuclear DNA to a ribosome in the cytoplasm, where protein is made in the amino-acid sequences specified by the messenger RNA.

MET—Metabolic equivalent, the energy expended in kilocalories divided by resting energy expenditure in kilocalories, either measured or estimated from body size. 1 MET is approximately 1 kcal · kg^{-1} · h^{-1} on average.

meta-analysis—Quantitative procedure for summarizing the effects of a number of research studies on a common topic.

metabolic syndrome X—Co-occurrence of obesity (especially visceral adiposity) with diabetes, hypertension, and hyperlipidemia, a constellation of risk factors of coronary heart disease.

metastasize—To spread by metastasis, the process whereby tumors spread to parts of the body other than the originating part.

Mill's canons—Key criteria (strength of association, temporal sequence, dose response, consistency, and biological plausibility) that, if satisfied, indicate the likelihood that a statistical association between a risk factor and a disease outcome is causal.

mineralocorticosteroids—A group of hormones (the most important being aldosterone) that regulate the balance of water and electrolytes (ions such as sodium and potassium) in the body. The hormones act on the kidneys, specifically, on the kidney tubules.

moderator—A variable that influences the relationship between two other variables or influences how an intervention or mediator affects the outcome.

monocyte—A large white blood cell (i.e., leukocyte) differentiated from stem cells in bone marrow that has a single nucleus. Monocytes constitute about 5% of the leukocytes circulating in the blood.

mood—An affective state that is accompanied by anticipation, even unconscious, of pleasure or pain; moods can last less than a minute or as long as days, even weeks or months when disordered.

morbidity—The state of being diseased.

muscle dysmorphia—Pathological preoccupation with muscularity that can occur in both men and women.

muscular endurance—The capacity to exert force repeatedly.

muscular strength—The capacity to exert force against resistance.

myocardial infarction—Irreversible injury or death of heart muscle cells resulting from sudden insufficiency of blood flow; commonly called a heart attack.

natural history—Observed fluctuation in people's attributes, behavior, or health that is not the result of controlled experimental manipulation.

natural killer (NK) cell—One of a class of distinct lymphocytes that have innate immune properties and are key cells in natural surveillance and destruction of viruses, tumor cells, bacteria, protozoa, and other foreign microorganisms.

neuroimaging—Methods to measure brain activity using techniques such as functional magnetic resonance imaging.

neuropeptide Y—Amino acid peptide that inhibits the locus coeruleus from firing in vitro, providing feedback inhibition to locus coeruleus neurons.

neurotransmitter—Any specific chemical agent that is released by a presynaptic nerve cell upon excitation and that crosses the synapse to stimulate, inhibit, or modify the postsynaptic cell, serving as the basis of communication between neurons.

neutrophil—The most-active phagocytic granulocyte. Neutrophils constitute about 80% of granulocytes and 50% to 65% of all leukocytes in the blood.

noradrenaline—See *norepinephrine*.

noradrenergic—Relating to cells or fibers of the autonomic or central nervous system that use norepinephrine as their neurotransmitter.

norepinephrine—The main neurotransmitter of peripheral sympathetic nerves and a key neuromodulator in the brain. Also acts as a hormone released by the adrenal medulla; its principal effects are excitatory. Also known as *noradrenaline*.

nucleus accumbens—A collection of neural cell bodies located in the basal forebrain near the ventral striatum. Helps regulate reward-motivated behavior.

nulliparity—Condition of not having given birth.

obesity—An excessively high amount of body fat or adipose tissue in relation to lean body mass. The amount of body fat includes both the distribution of fat throughout the body and the size of the adipose tissue deposits. Body fat distribution can be estimated by skinfold measurements, waist-to-hip ratio, ultrasound, dual X-ray absorptiometry, computed tomography, or magnetic resonance imaging.

obsessive-compulsive disorder (OCD)—A disorder characterized by a recurrent, persistent, and unwanted idea, thought, or impulse to carry out an unwanted act that the individual cannot voluntarily suppress, typified by repetitive acts or rituals to relieve anxiety.

odds ratio (OR)—The ratio of the odds of exposure to a risk factor (i.e., chance of having versus not having the risk factor) in the diseased group, *a/b*, to the odds of exposure to the risk factor in the nondiseased group, *c/d*. Used in cross-sectional or case–control studies where exposure to risk cannot be observed.

oncogenes—Genes that promote abnormal cell division, usually by transforming the DNA of a host cell.

opsonization—Coating by antibodies or complement of the cell walls of bacteria or viruses, making it easier for immune cells to inject cytotoxic enzymes into foreign cells.

osteoblasts—Cells that arise from fibroblasts and, as they mature, are associated with the production of bone.

osteoclasts—Large, multinucleate cells formed from differentiated macrophages, responsible for the breakdown of bone.

osteocytes—Osteoblasts that have become embedded within the bone matrix, occupying a flat oval cavity and sending slender cytoplasmic processes through the canaliculi (tiny channels), which make contact with other osteocytes.

osteoid matrix—A framework composed of newly formed osteocytes prior to calcification that provides the infrastructure for the mineralization of bone (e.g., by calcium and phosphorus) and, along with trabecular bone, gives bone its mechanical, elastic, and tensile strength.

osteopenia—Reduced bone mass due to inadequate osteoid synthesis. May lead to osteoporosis.

osteoporosis—A disease characterized by abnormally low bone mass and microstructural deterioration of bone tissue that leads to brittle bones and increased risk of fractures after minimal trauma. Osteoporosis is commonly defined as a bone mineral density more than 2.5 standard deviations below the average in young adults.

osteosarcoma—Cancer of bone.

outcome-expectancy value—The value or valence placed on an outcome expectation.

overweight—Excessive body weight. Usually expressed in relation to height compared with some standard of acceptable or desirable weights.

oxidation—A chemical reaction whereby the atoms in a compound lose electrons during combination with oxygen.

pandemic—An epidemic that spreads widely across a region or the world.

parasympathetic nervous system—One of three divisions of the autonomic nervous system. The parasympathetic nervous system arises from the cranial nerves and the sacral portions of the spinal cord and is involved primarily in energy conservation.

parathyroid hormone—A peptide hormone that stimulates osteoclasts to increase blood calcium, the opposite effect to that of calcitonin.

parity—Condition of having given birth.

pathogen—That which causes a disease.

perceived behavioral control—The degree to which an individual believes that he or she is able to have an effect on a specific outcome, which ranges along a continuum from no control to total control.

perceived exertion—The subjective judgment of strain or effort during physical activity, involving quantity rather than quality of sensations.

performance-related fitness—The ability to perform physical tasks. Components of performance-related fitness include psychomotor skills, maximal and submaximal cardiorespiratory power, muscular strength, power and endurance in the limbs and trunk for propulsion, body size, and body composition.

periaqueductal gray area—Gray matter that surrounds the duct between the third and fourth ventricles of the brain; processes neural signals associated with pain and aversive behavior.

person with a disability—A person identified as having an activity limitation or who uses assistance or who perceives him- or herself as having a disability.

person-year—A commonly used denominator in the computation of rates that equalizes risk exposure among groups. One person observed for one year equals one person-year.

Peyer's patches—Glandular, mucosal masses of lymphatic tissue located in the small intestine and tonsils.

phagocytic cell—A cell that can ingest and digest other cells. Neutrophils ingest mainly bacteria. Macrophages and monocytes scavenge mainly degenerated cells and dead tissue.

phagocytosis—The process of ingestion and digestion by cells of other cells, bacteria, dead tissue, and other organic and inorganic matter.

phobia—An obsessive, persistent, and unrealistic fear of an external situation or object that is out of proportion to the actual threat or danger.

phospholipase—Enzyme that catalyzes the hydrolysis of phosphate from a phospholipid.

phospholipid—A lipid compound, such as lecithin, that contains phosphorus and is found in lipoproteins.

physical activity—Bodily movement produced by skeletal muscle contraction that requires energy expenditure. Characterized by features including frequency, intensity, timing, and type.

physical activity survey—A self-report questionnaire used to assess physical activity, usually administered by mail, telephone, fax, or Internet.

physical fitness—The capacity to meet the present and potential physical challenges of life successfully; a set of personal attributes, such as muscular strength, cardiorespiratory capacity, and agility, that relate to the ability to perform physical activity.

plasmin—A proteolytic enzyme that hydrolyzes (i.e., dissolves) fibrin. Formed in the blood from plasminogen by tissue-type plasminogen activator (t-PA) and trypsin or by drugs such as streptokinase.

plasminogen—The biologically inactive precursor of plasmin.

polyp—A mass (a tumor, inflammation, lesion, or malformation) that projects outward from a tissue surface.

polysomnography—Simultaneous measurement of multiple physiological indicators of sleep stages, such as brain waves, respiration, and muscle and chin movements to detect rapid eye movement.

population attributable risk—Theoretical percentage reduction in morbidity or mortality rate that might occur if all individuals with a specific risk factor eliminated that factor.

positron emission tomography (PET)—Method of measuring the dynamic activity of a living brain by detecting positrons emitted by radioactive glucose, or analog chemicals, administered orally or by injection.

post–traumatic stress disorder—Anxiety and behavioral disturbances that develop within the first month after exposure to an extreme trauma.

preferred exertion—The level of exertion that someone finds comfortable and is motivated to endure.

prefrontal cortex—The inferior part of the frontal cerebral cortex; believed to store memories of the consequences of behaviors or experiences that were aversive or pleasurable, permitting an emotion to be sustained long enough to direct behavior toward the goal that is appropriate for that emotion.

prevalent cases—The number of persons in a population who have a particular disease or condition at some specific point in time.

primary osteoporosis—Age-related (type I or senile) bone loss and postmenopausal (type II) bone loss.

primary prevention—Preventing the development of disease in a susceptible population.

processes of change—One of the three components of the transtheoretical model of stages of change; 10 covert and overt activities that are used to change thinking or affect behavior or relationships.

prodromal symptom—An early or premonitory symptom of a disease.

prospective cohort study—A research design in which baseline information on potential risk factors is collected from members of a large group of people having a common characteristic (i.e., a cohort) and the people are followed over time to track the incidence of disease.

prostaglandins—A class of hormonelike amino acid derivatives that regulate the dilation and constriction of smooth muscle and play a key role in inflammation. Prostaglandins are found in blood vessels, the intestines, the lungs, and the uterus and in hormones that have an antagonistic influence on lipid metabolism.

prostate-specific antigen (PSA)—A protein made by prostate cells. High levels may predict prostate cancer.

protease—An enzyme that catalyses the splitting of the interior peptide bonds in a protein.

punishment—Consequences of a specific behavior that decrease the frequency of the behavior.

randomized controlled trial—A research design in which participants are selected for study and are randomly assigned to receive an experimental manipulation or a control condition. Measurements are made before and after the intervention period in both groups to assess the degree of change in the outcomes of interest between the intervention and control conditions.

raphe nucleus—One of the major nuclei for the production of serotonin, located in the center line of the brain stem.

reasonable weight—A realistically attainable body weight that is influenced by the impact of weight gain on a person, his or her individual history, and the circumstances that contribute to his or her "settling point" and likelihood of successfully maintaining weight loss.

receptor—A structural protein molecule, usually on the cell surface or within the cytoplasm, that combines with a specific factor, such as a hormone or neurotransmitter; the interaction of the factor and the receptor results in a change in cell function.

reciprocal determinism—The central concept of causation for social cognitive theory, which describes the bidirectional, interacting influence of determinants of behavior; a mutually influencing relationship among two or more variables.

reinforcement—Consequences of a target behavior that increase the frequency of the behavior.

reinforcement control—Behavior change strategy that manipulates the consequences of the target behavior to increase the frequency of the behavior.

relapse prevention—Set of strategies designed to help keep people from returning to undesired behavior after successful behavior modification.

relative intensity—Work rate expressed in relation to maximal intensity, maximal aerobic capacity, or maximal workload.

relative risk (RR)—The ratio of the risk of disease in an exposed group, $a/(a + b)$, to the risk in an unexposed group, $c/(c + d)$, where a and c are incident cases and b and d are nonincident cases. Used in prospective studies where exposure to risk can be observed. Also known as the *risk ratio*.

reliability—Characteristic of a measure that includes precision, accuracy, and stability over time; freedom from measurement error or random error.

research design—Manner in which study participants are grouped or classified according to levels of the independent variable, modifiers, and confounders to determine influences on the dependent variable.

reverse cholesterol transport—Return of excess cholesterol from extrahepatic tissue to the liver for metabolism. Reverse cholesterol transport involves esterification and storage of cholesterol in the core of the HDL molecule by the enzyme lecithin:cholesterol acyltransferase, which is regulated by apolipoprotein A-1.

risk difference—An estimate of the amount of risk attributed to a risk factor, calculated as the risk (i.e., incidence rate) of disease in the group exposed to the risk factor minus the risk of disease in the unexposed group. Also called the *attributable risk*.

risk factor—A clearly defined characteristic that has been associated with the increased rate of a subsequently occurring disease.

risk ratio (RR)—See *relative risk*.

sarcoma—A tumor of connective tissue cells, usually malignant.

saturated fat—A fatty acid with all potential hydrogen-binding sites filled (totally hydrogenated), which is associated with high risk of atherosclerosis.

secondary osteoporosis—Osteoporosis that is caused by another disease but may not be independent of age or menopause.

secondary prevention—Early diagnosis and prompt treatment to shorten the duration of an illness, reduce its severity, and limit sequelae (subsequent effects).

secular trend—A naturally occurring change in the population.

selectin molecules—A type of adhesion molecule expressed by the endothelium of venules, which bind with leukocytes and cause them to roll along a "sticky" endothelial surface of the blood vessel; mediate the first step of extravasation.

self-concept—Organized configuration of perceptions about one's attributes and qualities that are within conscious awareness.

self-efficacy—Perception of one's capability to carry out a behavior with a known outcome; expectations of personal mastery regarding initiation and persistence of a behavior.

self-esteem—A person's evaluation of his or her self-concept and feelings associated with that evaluation.

self-monitoring—An individual's assessment of the antecedents, consequences, and characteristics of attempts to engage in or avoid a target behavior.

self-motivation—Internal factor that arouses, directs, and integrates a person's behavior; sustains a person to evaluate his or her own performance and then to seek to meet personal standards of achievement in the absence of external reinforcement.

self-regulation—Ways in which a person modifies his or her own behavior based on the assumption that behavior is under the person's direct control and is guided by internalized standards whose achievement will elicit positive self-evaluation.

serotonergic—Denoting or relating to activity of neurons that produce or respond to serotonin.

serotonin—A synaptic transmitter produced and secreted by the raphe nuclei; general suppressor of neural gain. Also known as 5-hydroxytryptamine (5-HT).

set point theory—The idea that the body has an internal control mechanism—that is, a set point—located in the lateral hypothalamus of the brain that regulates metabolism to maintain a certain level of body fat.

settling point theory—The idea that weight loss and gain in most humans are determined mainly by the patterns of diet and physical activity that they "settle" into as habits based on the interaction of their genetic dispositions, learning, and environmental cues to behavior.

sinoatrial node—A small mass of specialized cardiac muscle cells located in the right atrium of the heart that emits the electrical signal that determines the intrinsic rate of the heartbeat.

social cognitive theory—A theory of human behavior, which evolved from social learning theory, that views behavior as a function of social cognitions; its key concept is that the characteristics of a person, environment, and behavior mutually influence one another.

social ecology—The study of human and natural ecosystems, the interrelations of culture and nature, and especially how people function in natural systems during change. Applied to physical activity, it suggests that interventions should blend personal and environmental resources to focus on developing social support networks and community partnerships to promote physical activity.

state anxiety—The immediate response to a conscious or unconscious threat that has somatic and cognitive symptoms, including elevated heart rate, muscle tension, visceral motility, transient feelings of lack of control, low confidence, and uncertainty.

statin—One of a family of drugs (e.g., lovastatin, pravastatin, and simvastatin) that lower LDL levels by inhibiting the enzyme HMG CoA reductase.

stenosis—Narrowing or stricture of a duct (e.g., a blood vessel) or a canal.

stimulus control—Strategies to change the frequency of a target behavior by modifying the antecedents of the behavior.

strength of association—One of Mill's canons, which states that there must be a large and clinically meaningful difference in disease risk between those exposed and those not exposed to a risk factor in order to establish causality.

stressor—A force that acts on a biological system to cause stress; an imbalance or disruption in homeostasis.

stroke—The loss or impairment of bodily function resulting from injury or death of brain cells after insufficient blood supply.

surveillance—The tracking of population trends in a behavior, such as physical activity, over time.

sympathetic nervous system (SNS)—One of three divisions of the autonomic nervous system. The sympathetic nervous system arises from the thoracic and lumbar portions of the spinal cord and is involved primarily in activities that require energy expenditure.

telomerase—An enzyme that blocks the shrinking of telomeres, thus resulting in uncontrolled division of a cell into a tumor.

telomeres—Structures located at the end of chromosomes that shrink each time a cell divides until they reach a critical length, usually at maturation, that inhibits the cell from dividing further, after which the cell dies.

temperament—Mainly stable, core component of personality that affects an individual's emotional responsiveness and predisposition to changing moods.

temporal sequence—One of Mill's canons, which states that exposure to a risk factor must precede development of the disease in order to establish causality.

thalamus—A brain region in the diencephalon composed of sensory relay nuclei with bidirectional connections to many areas in the cerebral cortex.

theory—Formulation of underlying principles of certain observed phenomena that have been verified to some degree and are used to explain and predict;

a symbolic model used to guide the design, execution, and interpretation of research.

3-methoxy-4-hydroxyphenylglycol (MHPG)—The major metabolite of norepinephrine, secreted in the urine.

thrombin—A proteolytic enzyme in blood that converts fibrinogen to fibrin by hydrolysis.

thrombosis—Formation, development, or presence of a blood clot within a vessel.

tissue-type plasminogen activator (tPA)—Activates conversion of plasminogen from plasmin in the blood. Released from endothelial cells in blood vessels.

T lymphocyte—A long-lived (months to years) lymphocyte derived in the thymus gland. A key cell of cell-mediated, adaptive immunity possessing cytotoxic or memory abilities.

total peripheral resistance (TPR)—The total resistance to blood flow in the systemic circulation; the quotient produced by dividing the mean arterial pressure by the cardiac output.

trabecular bone—Adult bone consisting of mineralized, regularly ordered parallel collagen fibers that are more loosely organized than those of cortical bone; found in adult flat bones, vertebrae, and ends of long bones.

trait—The tendency to respond to an internal or external event in a particular manner. Traits are relatively consistent over time, but changes in traits are also possible.

trait anxiety—Chronic generalized anxiety that predisposes a person to appraise events as threatening.

transforming growth factor-beta (TGF-β)—A cytokine secreted by platelets, macrophages, and lymphocytes that increases IL-1 production by macrophages, increases IgA formation, attracts monocytes and macrophages, and aids wound healing by inhibiting inflammation after cell injury.

transient ischemic attack (TIA)—A temporary paralysis, numbness, speech difficulty, or other neurological symptoms that start suddenly but disappear within 24 hours (typically within several hours).

transtheoretical model (TTM) of stages of change—A dynamic model of intentional behavior change that is based on the stages and processes individuals go through to bring about long-term behavior change.

triglyceride—The main constituent of fats and oils; an ester composed of three fatty acid molecules and one glycerol molecule.

trypsin—Proteolytic enzyme formed in the small intestine that activates conversion of plasmin to plasminogen in the blood.

tumor necrosis factor-alpha (TNF-α)—A cytokine produced primarily by monocytes and lymphocytes that activates the killing of tumor cells by macrophages, plays a role in antiviral activity, and is a major mediator of the inflammatory acute-phase response. High levels of TNF-α have harmful effects, including inflammation and muscle wasting.

tumor necrosis factor-beta (TNF-β)—A cytokine secreted by T lymphocytes that activates tumor lysis, enhances phagocytosis by macrophages, and mediates inflammation.

tumor suppressor gene—A gene that slows down or terminates cell division before progression to a tumor.

type 1 diabetes—A form of diabetes that develops when the body's immune system destroys pancreatic beta cells, the only cells in the body that make the hormone insulin, which regulates blood glucose. This form of diabetes usually strikes children and young adults, who need supplemental insulin daily to survive. Also called *insulin-dependent diabetes mellitus (IDDM)* or *juvenile-onset diabetes*.

type 2 diabetes—A form of diabetes that usually begins as insulin resistance, a disorder in which the cells do not use insulin properly. As the need for insulin rises, the pancreas gradually loses its ability to produce insulin. Type 2 diabetes is increasingly being diagnosed in children and adolescents. Also called *non-insulin-dependent diabetes mellitus (NIDDM)* or *adult-onset diabetes*.

unintentional injury—An injury that is judged to have occurred without anyone intending that harm be done.

up-regulation—Increased sensitivity developed after repeated administration of a pharmacologically or physiologically active substance or in response to abnormally low levels of a substance, which is often characterized by an initial increase in the affinity of receptors for the substance or an increase in the number of receptors.

vagal tone—Basal level of parasympathetic activation of the vagus nerve.

value (of an outcome)—The reinforcement or incentive value of an expected outcome, which can be something an individual wants to obtain or to avoid.

ventral striatum—Area of the brain around the lateral ventricle that includes the caudate nucleus and putamen; the ventral striatum and the globus pallidus (or pallidum) form the corpus striatum.

ventral tegmental area (VTA)—A group of neural cell bodies in the underside of an area at the top of the brainstem, between the pons and the fourth ventrical of the brain, that contains neurons that secrete dopamine and project to the frontal cortex and the nucleus accumbens; believed to regulate arousal, reinforcement, and pleasure.

very low density lipoprotein cholesterol (VLDL-C)—A subfraction of the total blood cholesterol, composed mainly of triglycerides and cholesterol, that is a precursor to the formation of LDL-C in the blood.

viscosity—A physical property of fluids that determines the internal resistance to shear forces; thickness.

vitamin D—A vitamin produced by the body in response to sunlight exposure that plays an important role in calcium and phosphorous metabolism.

waist circumference—A common measure used to assess abdominal fat content. The presence of excess body fat in the abdomen, disproportionate to total body fat, is considered an independent predictor of ailments associated with obesity.

waist-to-hip ratio—The ratio of waist circumference to hip circumference. For men, a ratio of 0.90 or less is considered safe. For women, a ratio of 0.80 or less is considered safe.

Index

About the Authors

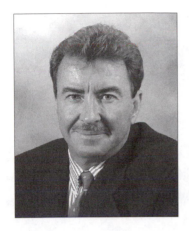

Rod K. Dishman, PhD, is a professor of exercise science and the director of the Exercise Psychology Laboratory at the University of Georgia at Athens and adjunct professor in the School of Public Health at the University of South Carolina at Columbia. He earned his PhD and MS at the University of Wisconsin–Madison. He has served as an exercise consultant to numerous public health agencies in the United States, Canada, and Europe; and he has written or edited six books on physical activity and health.

Dr. Dishman is an American College of Sports Medicine fellow and a member of the jury for selection of the Olympic Prize in Sport Sciences awarded by the International Olympic Committee's Medical Commission. He resides in Athens, Georgia, and enjoys running, resistance exercise and, on occasion, gardening.

Richard A. Washburn, PhD, is a specialist in exercise epidemiology. Dr. Washburn is an associate professor at the University of Kansas at Lawrence. He is a fellow in the American College of Sports Medicine and an author, co-author, and presenter of more than 75 scholarly articles and abstracts on exercise epidemiology and related topics. Dr. Washburn earned his PhD at the University of Wisconsin at Madison and a master's in public health from the University of Pittsburgh. In his free time he enjoys downhill skiing, bicycling, and in-line skating.

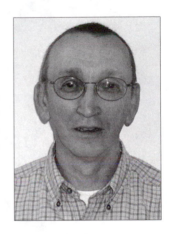

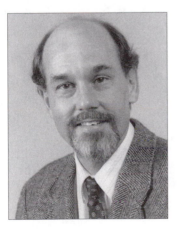

Gregory W. Heath, DHSc, MPH, has been contributing to the field of exercise science and health promotion for 25 years. Dr. Heath is at the Centers for Disease Control and Prevention in Atlanta and is lead health scientist in the Physical Activity and Health Branch. He is also adjunct associate professor of exercise science at the University of Georgia at Athens. He has extensive experience in conducting studies and data analyses in the areas of physical activity epidemiology and public health practice.

Dr. Heath is a fellow in the Council on Epidemiology and Prevention, the American Heart Association, and the American College of Sports Medicine. He earned his doctor of health science degree in applied physiology and nutrition and his master's of public health in epidemiology from Loma Linda University.

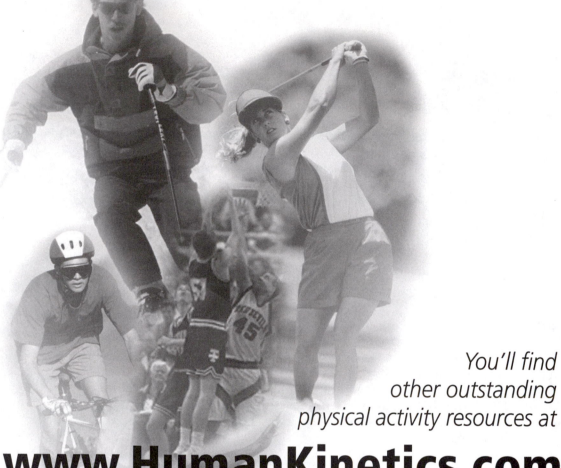